Quality of Life in Asia

Volume 16

This series, the first of its kind, examines both the objective and subjective dimensions of life quality in Asia, especially East Asia. It unravels and compares the contours, dynamics and patterns of building nations by offering innovative works that discuss basic and applied research and emphasizing inter- and multi-disciplinary approaches to the various domains of life quality. The series appeals to a variety of fields in humanities, social sciences and other professional disciplines. Asia is the largest, most populous continent on Earth, and it is home to the world's most dynamic region, East Asia. In the past three decades, East Asia has been the most successful region in the world in expanding its economies and integrating them into the global economy, offering lessons on how poor countries, even with limited natural resources, can achieve rapid economic development. Yet while scholars and policymakers have focused on why East Asia has prospered, little has been written on how its economic expansion has affected the quality of life of its citizens. This series publish several volumes a year, either single or multiple-authored monographs or collections of essays.

Vincent Tin Sing Law · Ben Yuk Fai Fong
Editors

Ageing with Dignity in Hong Kong and Asia

Holistic and Humanistic Care

Springer

Editors
Vincent Tin Sing Law
Hong Kong Polytechnic University
Hong Kong, China

Ben Yuk Fai Fong
Hong Kong Polytechnic University
Hong Kong, China

ISSN 2211-0550 ISSN 2211-0569 (electronic)
Quality of Life in Asia
ISBN 978-981-19-3063-8 ISBN 978-981-19-3061-4 (eBook)
https://doi.org/10.1007/978-981-19-3061-4

This Springer imprint is published by the registered company Springer Nature Singapore Pte Ltd.
The registered company address is: 152 Beach Road, #21-01/04 Gateway East, Singapore 189721, Singapore

Foreword

I am honoured to write this foreword for the new book on ageing with dignity, particularly in my capacity as the Chairman of the Elderly Commission of the Hong Kong Special Administrative Region Government. My sincere congratulations to the authors and the editors, Dr. Vincent Law and Dr. Ben Fong, who have presented in three main themes, namely policies and development of aged care, holistic and humanistic care for the elderly and capacity building for ageing with dignity. They tally with the objectives of the Elderly Commission in its role in advising the Government on the formulation of a comprehensive policy for the elderly and the associated programmes and services for the older population. The topics cover a wide scope of issues and practical solutions pertaining to the care of the elderly with dignity in a holistic and humanistic manner, together with examples from Asia.

With the increasing ageing population, both locally and in the neighbouring regions, aged care is always on the agenda of the Government, healthcare professionals, academia, service providers, healthcare groups and investors, as well as the elderly themselves, their carers and families. It is a 'mini' industry in its own right because the considerations and approaches are very unique for obvious reasons like degeneration of body and health, changes in family dynamics, retirement and potential financial difficulties, social disconnection, long-term care, end-of-life matters, etc. The editors have engaged academics and experts in the production of this special and timely publication to allow for discussion and implementation of the initiatives to aged care and related policy and projects. It is a useful reference and practical resource for policymakers, academics, students, healthcare practitioners, operators and community social workers in better understanding of the needs of the elderly, particularly in attention to dignity, as well as the holistic and humanistic consideration in service delivery.

Dr. Lam Ching-choi, SBS, JP
Former Chairman, Elderly Commission
Member of Executive Council
The Government of the Hong Kong
Special Administrative Region
Hong Kong, China

Chief Executivc Officer, Haven
of Hope Christian Service
Hong Kong, China

Preface

Development of this book was provoked by the worldwide challenges faced by ageing population and opportunities to deal with the related health needs in long-term care, community health and social services. People age naturally but not all of them age with dignity, which is constructed with respect, love, identity, integrity, status, autonomy, protection and human right. Dignity is important to the elderly, family, relatives and friends in the social and cultural contexts. Elderly people should feel being valued by the family and the community for recognition of their contribution to the society. They are traditionally considered 'gems in the family' in the Chinese culture. The elderly should be supported to live a healthy life with quality and with thoughts, preferably independently, and be encouraged to serve the community in different roles and capacities.

In healthcare, dignity entails more than professionalism. There must be empathy, compassion and safety in the care of the older adults when they are frail with deterioration in physical and psychosocial well-being and suboptimal intrinsic capacity from ageing. The older adults must be respected and protected when they are sick.

To achieve the goal of ageing with dignity, it is imperative to proactively engage various stakeholders to conceive and apply holistic and humanistic approaches in elderly care and services. Against such background, this book aims to serve as a useful reference and practical resource for stakeholders of elderly care which include policymakers, healthcare practitioners, the health sector, academics, community health workers, as well as carers of the elderly.

This book is structured into three main parts: (I) Policies and Development of Aged Care, (II) Holistic and Humanistic Care for Elderly and (III) Capacity Building for Ageing with Dignity.

Part I focuses on public policies and development of care for the elderly in relation to ageing with dignity. Integrated care models, community care policy, social construct of "dirty work", palliative care, elderly healthcare voucher scheme, dignity issues of electronic health records, as well as age-friendly city are covered.

In Chap. 1, Martin C. S. Wong provides an overview of the ageing issues of the Asian countries or regions. Important issue of increasing prevalence of citizens suffering from comorbid conditions was discussed. The chapter ends by exploring the impacts of ageing on healthcare and social issues.

Chapter 2 by Cheryl C. W. Ho, Ben Yuk Fai Fong and Ellen Ku provides insights on the application of integrated care to tackle the ever-increasing demand for aged care. The use of Complementary and Alternative Medicine (CAM) and Integrative Medicine (IM) as essential elements of integrated care are illustrated with Asian examples.

Chapter 3 by Ray Choy outlines the policies, mechanisms and social welfare services for the older adults in Hong Kong. The concept of community care was revisited while the concept of ageing in place in Hong Kong was discussed. The chapter ends by discussing the implementation issues of primary care in Hong Kong.

In Chap. 4, Tommy K. C. Ng and Ben Yuk Fai Fong review the needs of care and service gaps in primary care for the elderly. Started with background on primary care services, the authors assess the needs of and service gaps in primary care in Hong Kong. The chapter ends by giving recommendations on meeting needs of care and closing the service gaps for the elderly to age with dignity.

Chapter 5 by Sui Yu Yau, Yin King Lee, Siu Yin Li, Sze Ki Lai, Sin Ping Law and Shixin Huang call for the pressing needs of understanding how "dirty work" is being socially constructed. The authors view "dirty work" as a critical factor of the "residential care homes for the elderly" (RCHE) workforce crisis in Hong Kong. The chapter concludes by discussing the development of public policy initiatives to tackle the "dirty work" workforce crisis.

In Chap. 6, Hilary H. L. Yee and Vincent Tin Sing Law compare the resources on palliative services, Advance Directives (AD) policy, and public awareness on palliative care of Taiwan, Singapore, and Hong Kong. The chapter discusses Government funding and subsidy on palliative care, death taboos, dying at home and technology adoption related to palliative care. Policy recommendations on resource allocation and legal stipulations on palliative care are given.

In Chap. 7, Daniel C. S. Chiu stresses the importance of vaccination as an effective strategy for prevention of infection for the elderly. Vaccination strategies for selected diseases are discussed while that for special groups are illustrated. The chapter ends by depicting the challenging of vaccination for the elderly and provides insights on improving immune response and enhancing coverage rate in the future.

Chapter 8 by Hilary H. L. Yee and Vincent Tin Sing Law gives background on the Elderly Health Care Voucher Scheme (EHCVS) of Hong Kong and discusses its effectiveness from the perspectives of resource utilisation and health promotion. The chapter reviews and analyses factors affecting the use of elderly vouchers and proposes feasible recommendations for the Government.

In Chap. 9, Kar-wai Tong, from a medico-legal perspective, illustrates the use of Electronic Health Records (EHR) as a backbone to support dignified ageing in place. The author discusses dignity in healthcare, dignity of older persons, as well as the roles of and legal risks inherent in EHR. The chapter ends by advising healthcare institutes and professionals to check and take remedy actions regarding possible medico-legal risks in the EHR systems.

In Chap. 10, Fiona C. M. Yuen and Chesney P. Y. Wong depict how an age-friendly city with comprehensive community support and positive attitude towards elderly is pivotal to a discrimination-free city. The chapter analyses the negative labels and potential opportunities for elderly. The chapter also discusses and compares selected Asian and European age-friendly cities and provides insights on future research.

Part II illustrates the perspectives of holistic and humanistic care for the elderly. It covers monitoring of elderly services, social determinants of health, cultural and spiritual needs of the elderly, enhanced and holistic community-based programmes for the elderly, optimal healthy eating, osteosarcopenia, pollution and ageing, as well as pet ownership.

In Chap. 11, Billy S. H. Ho, Kenneth H. H. Chui and Ben Yuk Fai Fong evaluate the gaps in healthcare and social services for the elderly in Hong Kong. With detailed evaluation of barriers to improve healthcare and social services, as well as policies and strategies in Asian countries or regions, the chapter ends by discussing the implications to holistic and humanistic elderly care from the perspective of an ageing-friendly city.

Chapter 12 by Fowie Sze Fung Ng, Roger Watson and Graeme Drummond Smith address the theory and biological and psychological perspectives of longevity, including the physiological aspects of ageing, nutrition and so on. The chapter focuses on the frailty of the older people. Supported by case studies, the chapter ends by providing policy recommendations and implementation to enhance longevity of world citizens.

In Chap. 13, Hongjiang Wu and Katy N. W. Wong introduce the concept of social determinants of health, describe the mechanisms linking social factors and health outcomes with emphasis on social inequities in health among the older adults. The chapter also discusses the key challenges and ways forward in achieving successful ageing from the perspective of social factors.

In Chap. 14, Candy Yuen Yee Tsoi and Yim Fan Chan highlight the importance of cultural and spiritual needs of the elderly. The chapter emphasises the necessity of cultural awareness and integrating concepts of spirituality in aged care. The chapter ends by advising healthcare setting to consider meeting the cultural and spiritual needs of the elderly.

Chapter 15 by Maggie H. Y. Kwong and Carman K. M. Leung reviews community-based programmes for the elderly in Hong Kong from the perspective of holistic home care. To further enhance the dignity of the elderly, the chapter provides community initiative such as town planning, scientific and technological development, healthcare practitioners training, social education, as well as intergeneration connectivity.

In Chap. 16, Carina Y. H. Lam and Fuk Tan Chow introduce the concept for optimal healthy eating for the elderly. Community nutrition intervention, physiological factors related to nutrition, as well as social and psychological issues affecting consumption of nutrients are discussed. The chapter ends by advocating comprehensive practical nutrition policies and programmes which involve policymakers, food manufacturers, community centres and medical professionals.

In Chap. 17, Ben Yuk Fai Fong, Yumi Y. T. Chan, Bryan P. C. Chiu and Karly Oi-wan Chan illustrate the importance of physical activity to promote active ageing for the elderly. Health impacts of physical inactivity of older adults are highlighted while potential benefits of regular exercise are discussed. The chapter analyses factors that shape active and health ageing and concludes by proposed behavioural change interventions from a community perspective.

Chapter 18 by Leon Wai Li, Wing Tung Ho and Sin Yee Lau discusses the importance of treatment of osteoporosis and sarcopenia regarding the prevention of morbidity and mortality in the elderly. The chapter proposed primary prevention, early diagnosis and treatment as important measures in reducing diseases-related falls and subsequence fractures, mortality rate, healthcare costs as well as quality of life of the elderly.

Chapter 19 by Wang-kin Chiu and Ben Yuk Fai Fong analyses the relationship of chemical pollution and health ageing. Various types of pollution such as air, water and food pollution in related to healthy ageing are discussed. The chapter concludes by giving important implications and recommendations on research, policy and education for achieving a cleaner environment which is indispensable for the success of healthy ageing.

In Chap. 20, Andrea Chiu and Ben Yuk Fai Fong discuss loneliness, social isolation and rejection of the elderly. While pet ownership is regarded as helpful in promoting health and increasing the quality of life of older adults, this chapter also review the physical and psychosocial benefits, as well as potential harms of owning pets. The chapter recommends the collaboration of community service animals and community elderly services to improve the dignity of the elderly.

Part III explores the means of building capacity for the elderly to age with dignity. It covers the building of living capacity, lifelong learning, roles of community health practitioners, service-learning, social enterprises in elderly care, social capital enhancement with time banking, doctor-patient relationship, quality assurance in long-term care, medication management, as well as the role of clinical pharmacists in relation to elderly.

In Chap. 21, Catherine K. Y. Kwong and Ben Yuk Fai Fong provide insights on building the living capacity for senior citizens. Based on examples of elderly residence from Singapore, Korea and Australia, the chapter presents opportunities and barriers of providing housing for the elderly to live with comfort and dignity. Accommodations for the elderly in Hong Kong and the barriers of implementation are discussed.

Chapter 22 by Hilary H. L. Yee, Ben Yuk Fai Fong, Tommy K. C. Ng and Vincent Tin Sing Law uses a case study on elderly students to illustrate the health ageing and lifelong learning for the elderly in Hong Kong. The chapter lists the advantages of lifelong education to older adults and analyses the current education policy for older learners in Hong Kong. The chapter concludes by giving new insights and future opportunities on lifelong learning for the elderly.

In Chap. 23, Sean Hon Yin Hui and Ellen Ku discuss the roles and training of Community Health Practitioners (CHPs) and Community Health Coach (CHCs) in elderly care. The importance of training for community workers are emphasised and linked to improving the health statues of elderly in physical, mental, social and spiritual perspectives.

Chapter 24 by Ben Yuk Fai Fong, Tommy K. C. Ng, Hilary H. L. Yee and Bille S. M. Chow relates the experience of service-learning by a group of tertiary students in Hong Kong on contributing to ageing with dignity of the elderly being served. Benefits gained by the elderly being served and the serving students are discussed. The chapter concludes that promotion of healthy lifestyle and self-management of chronic conditions among the elderly help promoting health with dignity.

In Chap. 25, Vincent Tin Sing Law discusses the nature of social enterprises, their roles in elderly care and community services, as well as the impacts of social enterprises on health and well-being of older people. The chapter ends by providing recommendations on further enhancing the roles of social enterprises in elderly care.

In Chap. 26, Tommy K. C. Ng, Ben Yuk Fai Fong and Wilson K. S. Leung explore the enhancement of social capital in the community so as to relieve the burden of increasing elderly services. The chapter analyses the potential of time banking in the community to achieve holistic and humanistic care for the elderly. Analyses on the adoption of time banking in different countries are provided to underpin understanding its operations and effectiveness in enhancing elderly services.

In Chap. 27, Sukhpreet Kaur and Chor Ming Lum view doctor-patient relationship as an essential determinant of quality of healthcare especially in elderly care. Three basic models of doctor-relationship including Active-Passive Model, Guidance-Cooperation Model and Mutual Participation Model are discussed. The chapter concludes by discussing professional ethics in elderly care and ways to achieve highest level of elderly care.

Chapter 28 by Tiffany C. H. Leung and Ray Choy provides an overview of the recent development for quality assurance in long-term and quality indicators community elderly care services in the extant literature. The chapter also discusses the practical implications for healthcare regulators, the private sector and non-profit service providers in long-term and community elderly care service in Hong Kong. Concluding remarks on the current elderly services and identification of possible improvements in the future are given.

In Chap. 29, Sau Chu Chiang, Cheuk Wun Ting, Kei Hong So, Yin Ting Cheung, Chui Ping Lee, Daisy Lee and Gary Chung Hong Chong delineate the practices, significance and challenges in developing a safe medication management service for institutionalised and community-dwelling elderly people. The chapter concludes with practical suggestions for the development of a sustainable ICT-enabled medication management service for the elderly to improve medication adherence, to control chronic diseases and related hospitalisation better, as well as reducing the pressure on caretakers.

In the last chapter, Chap. 30, Wilson W. S. Chiu and Gary Chung Hong Chong analyse the role of clinical pharmacists in the multidisciplinary care of geriatric patients. Based on six case studies, the chapter illustrates the challenges of medication management in older patients and explores the potential for the use of technology in caring for geriatric patients. The chapter concludes that pharmacists with good communication skills can perceive how patients feel to improve their dignity while ageing.

Hong Kong, China

Vincent Tin Sing Law
Ben Yuk Fai Fong

Acknowledgements

The book was partly supported by a grant from the Research Grants Council of the Hong Kong Special Administrative Region, China (Project Reference No.: UGC/IDS24/18), which funded the establishment of the Centre for Ageing and Healthcare Management Research (CAHMR) from 1 November 2018 to 31 May 2022. The editors wish to thank colleagues of CAHMR at the School of Professional Education and Executive Education (SPEED) of The Hong Kong Polytechnic University (PolyU) for the support to the book. A few Team and Associate Members of CAHMR have contributed chapters. The editors also appreciate the involvement of some Fellows of the Hong Kong College of Community Health Practitioners (HKCCHP) for writing up individual chapters. Efforts made by all chapter authors in the preparation and refinement of the manuscripts are acknowledged in the highest honours. Without everyone's heart and time in working for the book since early 2020, we would not be able to complete our committed mission. We are also indebted to Tommy Ng and Hilary Yee for their meticulous review and proof-reading of the manuscript. We also appreciate the encouragement from Dr. Lam Ching-choi, SBS, JP who has kindly written the Foreword for the book. The Editors would like to thank Alexandra Campbell of Springer for her advice and help in the planning and development of the book.

Vincent Tin Sing Law
Ben Yuk Fai Fong

About This Book

The world is facing an increasing ageing population and has to deal with the related health needs in long-term care, community health and social services, particularly for chronic conditions and psychosocial supports. The book advocates the application of the holistic and humanistic approaches in elderly care and services to achieve the goal of ageing with dignity that entails respect, love, identity, integrity, status, autonomy, protection and human right. The book consists of three sections of policy and development of aged care, holistic and humanistic care for older adults, and capacity building for ageing with dignity. Topics include the latest initiatives in aged care, appropriate services and delivery models, lifestyle modification, education, psychosocial and environmental consideration, professional development, technologies and social capital. The chapters review and discuss these issues in a general global coverage, illustrated by local and regional examples, derived from research by the authors. The contents serve as a topical reference to university studies in ageing and related disciplines, but are also useful to policymakers, researchers, community and public health practitioners, health executives and interns in policy, practical and scholarly issues pertinent to care development, delivery model, planning, quality, ethics, health promotion, professional training and monitoring in health services to the older adults. The book is not a clinical practice guide on elderly care. Contributors are academics and practitioners from diversified professional backgrounds of medicine, public health, nursing, pharmacy, Chinese medicine, dietetics, allied health, social sciences, life sciences, health informatics, psychology, sports sciences, business, administration, marketing, hospitality, law, social work, public policy and information technology. A number of the contributors possess international educational background and overseas professional experience.

Contents

Editors and Contributors

About the Editors

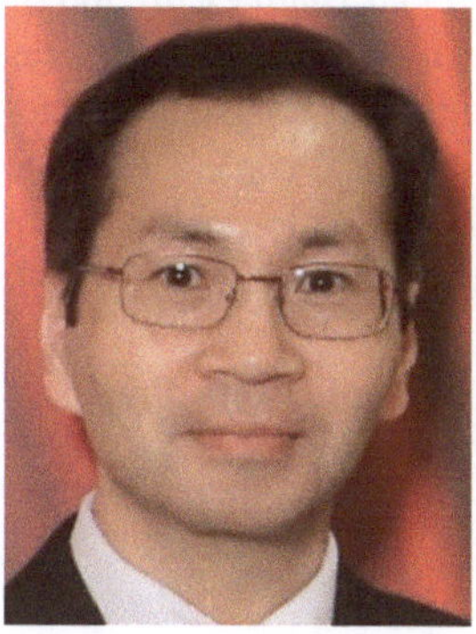

Dr. Vincent Tin Sing Law is Senior Lecturer of School of Professional Education and Executive Development (SPEED) of The Hong Kong Polytechnic University (PolyU). Vincent is also the Founding Member, former Academic Convenor and current Deputy Director of the Centre for Ageing and Healthcare Management Research (CAHMR) of PolyU SPEED. Being an experienced researcher in public policy, Vincent participated in some large-scale consultancy or research projects on public policy and public engagement with the Hong Kong Government in recent years. He authored a few academic journal papers and book chapters on healthcare and sustainability, and published five Chinese books on Chinese wisdom.

https://directory.speed-polyu.edu.hk/staff-directory/en/speed/spd-acadiv-sshd/vincent-law.

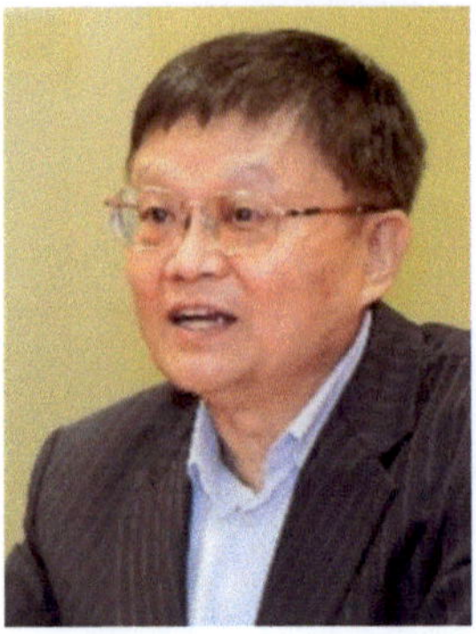

Dr. Ben Yuk Fai Fong is Specialist in Community Medicine, holding Honorary Clinical Associate Professorship at the two local medical schools in Hong Kong, China. He is currently the Professor of Practice (Health Studies) and Associate Division Head of the Division of Science, Engineering and Health Studies of the College of Professional and Continuing Education (CPCE), and Centre Director of the Centre for Ageing and Healthcare Management Research of CPCE of The Hong Kong Polytechnic University (PolyU). He also holds honorary appointments at the Hong Kong Institute of Asia-Pacific Studies and Hong Kong Institute of Integrated Medicine at The Chinese University of Hong Kong. He is President of Hong Kong College of Community Health Practitioners and has contributed to publications, including *The Routledge Handbook of Public Health and the Community* (as lead editor, 2021), *Primary Care Revisited: Interdisciplinary Perspectives for a New Era* (as lead editor, 2020), a training manual for general practitioners in China published by the People's Medical Publishing House in Beijing (as co-editor, published in 2020), over 30 health books in Chinese, and over 40 journal papers.

https://directory.speed-polyu.edu.hk/staff-directory/en/speed/spd-acadiv-aacadiv/ben-fong.

Contributors

Chan Karly Oi-wan College of Professional and Continuing Education, The Hong Kong Polytechnic University, Hong Kong, China

Chan Yim Fan Hong Kong College of Paediatric Nursing, Hong Kong, China

Chan Yumi Y. T. Hong Kong College of Community Health Practitioners, Hong Kong, China

Cheung Yin Ting School of Pharmacy, Faculty of Medicine, The Chinese University of Hong Kong, Hong Kong, China

Chiang Sau Chu Hong Kong Pharmaceutical Care Foundation, Hong Kong, China

Chiu Bryan P. C. Hong Kong College of Community Health Practitioners, Hong Kong, China

Chiu Daniel C. S. Faculty of Community Health Emergency Management, Hong Kong College of Community Health Practitioners, Hong Kong, China

Chiu Wang-Kin College of Professional and Continuing Education, The Hong Kong Polytechnic University, Hong Kong, China

Chong Gary Chung Hong Hospital Pharmacist, Hong Kong, China

Chow Billie S. M. School of Professional Education and Executive Development, College of Professional and Continuing Education, The Hong Kong Polytechnic University, Kowloon, Hong Kong, China

Chow Fuk Tan Hong Kong College of Community Health Practitioners, Hong Kong, China

Choy Ray Department of Innovative Social Work, City University of Macau, Macau, China

Chu Andrea School of Professional Education and Executive Development, The Hong Kong Polytechnic University, Hong Kong, China

Chu Wilson W. S. Hospital Pharmacist, Hong Kong, China

Chui Kenneth H. H. Hong Kong College of Community Health Practitioners, Hong Kong, China

Fong Ben Yuk Fai School of Professional Education and Executive Development, College of Professional and Continuing Education, The Hong Kong Polytechnic University, Kowloon, Hong Kong, China

Ho Billy S. H. School of Professional Education and Executive Development, The Hong Kong Polytechnic University, Hong Kong, China

Ho Cheryl C. W. Hong Kong College of Community Health Practitioners, Hong Kong, China

Ho Wing Tung Hong Kong College of Community Health Practitioners, Hong Kong, China

Huang Shixin Hong Kong Metropolitan University, Hong Kong, China

Hui Sean Hon Yin Hong Kong College of Community Health Practitioners, Hong Kong, China

Kaur Sukhpreet Hong Kong College of Community Health Practitioners, Hong Kong, China

Ku Ellen Caritas Institute of Higher Education, Hong Kong, China

Kwong Catherine K. Y. Hong Kong College of Community Health Practitioners, Hong Kong, China

Kwong Maggie H. Y. The Hong Kong Polytechnic University, Hong Kong, China

Lai Sze Ki Hong Kong Metropolitan University, Hong Kong, China

Lam Carina Y. H. Hong Kong College of Community Health Practitioners, Hong Kong, China

Lau Sin Yee Hong Kong Children's Hospital, Hospital Authority, Hong Kong, China

Law Sin Ping Hong Kong Metropolitan University, Hong Kong, China

Law Vincent Tin Sing School of Professional Education and Executive Development, College of Professional and Continuing Education, The Hong Kong Polytechnic University, Hong Kong, China

Lee Chui Ping School of Pharmacy, Faculty of Medicine, The Chinese University of Hong Kong, Hong Kong, China

Lee Daisy School of Professional Education and Executive Development, The Hong Kong Polytechnic University, Hong Kong, China

Lee Yin King Hong Kong Metropolitan University, Hong Kong, China

Leung Carman K. M. The Hong Kong Polytechnic University, Hong Kong, China

Leung Tiffany C. H. Faculty of Business, City University of Macau, Macau, China

Leung Wilson K. S. School of Professional Education and Executive Development, College of Professional and Continuing Education, The Hong Kong Polytechnic University, Kowloon, Hong Kong, China

Li Leon Wai Hong Kong College of Community Health Practitioners, Hong Kong, China

Li Siu Yin Hong Kong Metropolitan University, Hong Kong, China

Lum Chor Ming The Chinese University of Hong Kong, Hong Kong, China

Ng Fowie Sze Fung Tung Wah College, Hong Kong, China

Ng Tommy K. C. School of Professional Education and Executive Development, College of Professional and Continuing Education, The Hong Kong Polytechnic University, Kowloon, Hong Kong, China

Smith Graeme Drummond Caritas Institute of Higher Education, Hong Kong, China

So Kei Hong Hong Kong Pharmaceutical Care Foundation, Hong Kong, China

Ting Cheuk Wun School of Pharmacy, Faculty of Medicine, The Chinese University of Hong Kong, Hong Kong, China

Tong Kar-wai City University of Hong Kong, Hong Kong, China

Tsoi Candy Yuen Yee Hong Kong College of Education & Research in Nursing, Hong Kong, China

Watson Roger Southwest Medical University, Luxhou, China

Wong Chesney P. Y. Department of Surgery, Queen Mary Hospital, Hospital Authority, Hong Kong, China

Wong Katy N. W. Hong Kong College of Community Health Practitioners, Hong Kong, China

Wong Martin C. S. JC School of Public Health and Primary Care, Faculty of Medicine, The Chinese University of Hong Kong, Hong Kong, China

Wu Hongjiang The Chinese University of Hong Kong, Hong Kong, China

Yau Sui Yu Hong Kong Metropolitan University, Hong Kong, China

Yee Hilary H. L. Department of Rehabilitation Sciences, The Hong Kong Polytechnic University, Kowloon, Hong Kong, China

Yuen Fiona C. M. Department of Oncology, Princess Margaret Hospital, Hospital Authority, Hong Kong, China

List of Figures

List of Tables

Part I
Policies and Development of Aged Care

Chapter 1
Ageing and Its Impacts on Healthcare and Social Issues

Martin C. S. Wong

Abstract The Asian population is ageing rapidly with a profound demographic shift. It has been estimated that by the year 2050, there will be 1.3 billion (~25%) of Asian at the age of 60 or above. This will be more than twice the number in 2016. The most severely affected regions include the East and North-East Asia (36.8%), followed by the North and Central Asia (24.5%). Among the Asian countries and regions, the longest life expectancy was reported in Hong Kong (85.3 years), Japan (85.0 years), Macau (84.7 years), Singapore (84.1 years) and South Korea (83.5 years). There exists a linear relationship between country-specific Gross-Domestic Product (GDP) and the level of population ageing. The older population in the less developed countries are experiencing quicker increase than the more developed countries. Such change is translated to having 80% of the elderly worldwide living in the less developed nations. The chapter explores the impacts of ageing on healthcare and social issues.

Keywords Ageing · Impacts · Multimorbidity · Social protection · Elder abuse

The Asian population is ageing rapidly with a profound demographic shift (Research Institute for ASEAN & East Asia, 2021). It has been estimated that by the year 2050, there will be 1.3 billion (~25%) of Asian at the age of 60 or above and this is more than twice the number in 2016 (United Nations ESCAP, 2016). The most severely affected regions include the East and North-East Asia (36.8%), followed by the North and Central Asia (24.5%). Among the Asian countries and regions, the longest life expectancy was reported in Hong Kong (85.3 years), Japan (85.0 years), Macau (84.7 years), Singapore (84.1 years) and South Korea (83.5 years) (Worldmeters, 2021). There exists a linear relationship between country-specific Gross-Domestic Product (GDP) and the level of population ageing (United Nations ESCAP, 2016). The older population in less developed countries are experiencing quicker increase than the more developed countries. Such change is translated to having 80% of the

M. C. S. Wong (✉)
JC School of Public Health and Primary Care, Faculty of Medicine, The Chinese University of Hong Kong, Hong Kong, China
e-mail: wong_martin@cuhk.edu.hk

V. T. S. Law and B. Y. F. Fong (eds.), *Ageing with Dignity in Hong Kong and Asia*, Quality of Life in Asia 16, https://doi.org/10.1007/978-981-19-3061-4_1

elderly worldwide are living in these less developed nations (United Nations, 2015). For instance, whilst Vietnam may take 19 years to move from an ageing to an aged country, France took 115 years (Kinsella & Gist, 1995; UN Census Bureau, 2005; Viet Nam GSO, 2010 as cited in United Nations ESCAP, 2016). This disparity is particularly noticeable in Asia, as the region comprises of countries from both ends of the GDP distribution (United Nations ESCAP, 2016).

The underlying causes of the ageing population in Asia include two major drivers, namely a drastic decline in fertility and a steady rise in life expectancy. The South and South-West regions as well as the South-East Asia sub-regions are examples where within the 40 years of time, the fertility rate of both regions has dropped by around 50% (United Nations ESCAP, 2016). In addition, Asian countries have improved living standards, nutritional levels, technological advancement in medicine and better access to healthcare, which have accounted for its increased life expectancy. Whilst longevity should be celebrated, its associated issues brought to the society need to be addressed.

1.1 Multimorbidity

The first and probably the most important issue is an increasing number of citizens who suffer from comorbid conditions. Multimorbidity, defined as the coexistence of two or more chronic conditions, is prevalent among the elderly populations (Marengoni et al., 2011). A systematic review reported that multimorbidity is affecting the majority (around 76.5%) of Chinese elderlies (Hu et al., 2015), and its burden is growing in ageing communities (Kim et al., 2012). It is associated with a variety of adverse health outcomes, including disability, suboptimal self-care, poor health-related quality of life (HRQL), hospital admissions, complicated individual management and premature mortality (Marengoni et al., 2011). Asian countries and regions, including mainland China, Hong Kong, Japan and Singapore, are no exception to the impact. According to estimations, the long-term care expenditure for elderly in Hong Kong is projected to increase from 1.4% of Hong Kong's GDP in 2004 to 4.9% by 2036 (Chung et al., 2009, 2016). In addition, ageing is associated with frailty, which is known as an age-related clinical condition presented with a deterioration in physiological capacity across several organ systems, leading to an increased susceptibility to stressors (Dent et al., 2019).

1.2 Impacts on Healthcare

Second, the issue is the burden on healthcare and the healthcare system. Non-communicable diseases (NCDs) are commonly found in the ageing population. For instance, the number of women with moderate or severe hypertension is increasing starting from the age of 50 (National Institutes of Health, 2011). In addition, elderly with NCDs can be more vulnerable to other diseases. For instance, hypertension, diabetes and lipid disorders are clustered with cerebrovascular and cardiovascular diseases. As a result, an ageing population may create a high demand in our healthcare system and induce a substantial economic and healthcare burden (National Institutes of Health, 2011). Even after hospital discharge, burdens on healthcare can be observed in hospital re-admissions due to the limited capacity of the outpatient services, and inadequate staff and training in elderly care.

When the resources for outpatient service are insufficient, it will create a burden on inpatient services. For example, the government of Singapore offers heavy subsidies to inpatient services (Nurjono et al., 2018). Elderly people may, therefore, prefer hospital treatment to long-term care in healthcare centres. It may lead to underdevelopment of different healthcare centres, rendering them inadequate to cope with the burden induced by hospital discharges (Lim et al., 2017). Therefore, their diseases (especially for NCDs) may be sub-optimally managed, resulting in avoidable hospital admissions which are undesirable for the healthcare system. The situation in Hong Kong is similar (Ng et al., 2019). Although elderly patients are often provided with discharge plans, there is no guarantee that they can receive suitable care in community care centres (Lau et al., 2018). The coordination in services between hospitals and the community is inconsistent in terms of their communication but also the resources required to achieve connectedness.

Moreover, there are many elderly patients with multiple morbidities. In Hong Kong, participation in preventive care is still not commonly observed (Lam, 2017) as it usually requires out-of-pocket payments, and this lowers their incentive to receive regular medical assessments. Thus, different health issues (often complications) might be identified at a later stage, making treatment more demanding and challenging. As they suffer from multiple chronic diseases, they require more attention and care than other patients do. However, primary care professionals find it difficult to handle (Woo et al., 2013), especially when an elderly patient presents with multiple medical conditions also demands physical, psychological and social care in an integrated manner. These responsibilities may be overwhelming at the expense of reducing health service quality. Despite Hong Kong has a low mortality rate, there is still potential to minimise the number of avoidable deaths if it can provide a better primary care for elderly patients (Chau et al., 2011).

Furthermore, the development of primary care in many Asian countries remains slow. Generally, there is inadequate manpower in the healthcare system in many countries or regions, including Malaysia, Hong Kong and Singapore (Akil et al., 2014; Ng et al., 2011; Schoeb, 2016). This has resulted in huge pressure on the healthcare system, especially when more trained staff is needed to provide adequate elderly services. Healthcare providers might not be, however, familiar with holistic patient management in the community (Woo et al., 2013).

Other than the manpower issue, financial resource is also a significant concern. Healthcare expenditure in the elderly populations is high in Asia regions, including Singapore, Japan, China and Hong Kong, and the trend is expected to continue in the next decade (Food & Health Bureau, 2018; Hedrich et al., 2016; Legislative Council Secretariat, 2019). However, the aforementioned trend prediction only includes different medical costs such as long-term treatment, but not expenses in community care. It is well known that community care could provide elderly people with holistic care and relieve the overwhelmed workload of hospitals (He & Tang, 2021). With the growing demand of elderly healthcare, there is no doubt that it could exert a huge impact on stakeholders in the society.

To relieve the burden of the healthcare system, it requires the support and cooperation from both the public and private sectors to provide comprehensive care to the older adults (Yip, 2019). The World Bank proposed a mechanism which combines insurance, tax, savings and different forms of out-of-pocket payment to improve the healthcare financing in the long run (Gottret & Schieber, 2006). However, the mechanisms will work differently according to the socioeconomic situations in different countries.

1.3 Social Issues

The continuing trend of ageing population is expected to bring adverse effects on the society such as increasing cases of elder abuse and burden of social protection. The ageing population accompanied with the decline in fertility rate is projected to cause a significant decrease of the working-age population (from 70% of the population at working-age to 50% by the end of 2100) and increase in government financial pressure (Chomik & Piggott, 2015; United Nations ESCAP, 2016).

Social issues surrounding an ageing population should not be overlooked. Elder abuse, defined as "single or repeated act, or lack of appropriate action, occurring within any relationship where there is an expectation of trust, which causes harm or distress to an older person", can lead to physical injury, emotional distress, financial loss and even premature death among older adults (World Health Organization, 2021). Studies have reported that across Asian countries, the prevalence rate of elder abuse varies greatly, ranging from 0.02% to 62%, depending on the geographical region and event setting (Yan et al., 2015). Among different forms of elder abuse, emotional or verbal abuse is the most common form with an average prevalence of 8.8%, followed by financial exploitation (4.7%), negligence (3.1%), and physical abuse (2.8%) (Pillemer et al., 2016). Such figures show that elder abuse could be a widespread phenomenon that endangers the quality of life of the elderly populations, as well as their physical and mental health. When considering the health outcomes, systematic reviews have reported that elder abuse could strongly be associated with clinical depression and anxiety among the elderly individuals (Dong et al., 2013). The number of abuse cases is likely be increasing with the ageing population as the increase in old-age dependency ratio could be translated into higher stress among caregivers, and thus potentially lead to even more cases of elder abuse (Schiamberg et al., 2011). Specifically, as Asian cultures often emphasise on family harmony and filial piety, the relatives of the elderly people are expected to be their caregivers. However, the expectations and interpretations of "taking care" can vary greatly between the caregiver and the elder people, and once the divergence is large, it could result in conflicts and abusive behaviours with the elderly populations becoming the victims (Yan et al., 2015).

In addition, the ageing population also impose challenges on the social protection system with increasing financial pressure. Social protection for elderly people can be divided into two main categories: the healthcare and pension systems (Chomik & Piggott, 2015; International Labour Organization, 2017). Regarding the healthcare system, the ageing population is estimated to bring financial pressure to the government with the increasing demand from old-age individuals for medical services, along with the need for better medical equipment and human resources to meet such demand. Previous research has projected that the ageing population would have directly caused the public health expenditure to increase 50% of its share of GDP among Asian countries by 2030, and the proportion of healthcare expenditure on GDP is expected to rise in a drastic manner (Soto et al., 2012). Older individuals also face greater financial risk. For most Asian countries, public health insurance and medical scheme only cover around 50% of the total cost and it still requires a high level of out-of-pocket medical expenses (Chomik & Piggott, 2015).

In the light of the pension system, many Asian countries do not have enough protection to secure the income of the elderly people after retirement. The declining fertility hampers an important source of income for older individuals, as the Asian cultures tend to rely on family support and household transfer as the main source of post-retirement income (Ladusingh & Maharana, 2018). It has been reported that less than 30% of the current working population in Asia has access to the contributory pension system (United Nations ESCAP, 2016), and the relative poverty rates of elderly people are also high among Asian countries. For instance, Korea has around 40% of individuals older than 60 years in poverty, and this proportion is similarly high in China (39%), India (22.9%), and Japan (19.6%) (Organisation for Economic Co-operation and Development, 2019). These figures show that many Asian countries are still not fully prepared for the rapid ageing of their populations, and without proper policy interventions, old-age poverty would become a widespread and persistent problem in Asia.

1.4 Age-Related Policies

In this context, the United Nations Population Fund (UNFPA) has offered some recommendations for the governments in Asia and the Pacific (UNFPA & HelpAge International, 2011; United Nations ESCAP, 2016). Some major proposals include the development and implementation of well-rounded policies to cope the ageing issues, provision of the necessary resources, both financial and human, for such policies, and enhancing the technical capability of the responsible parties. Sectoral policies on ageing should be based on research data at the national and regional levels, thus enabling the delivery of well-rounded medical care tailored to the needs of the older adults via reorientation of the health systems.

1.5 Conclusion

In summary, many nations in the world encountered population ageing as one of the top challenges. Its impact is expected to rise in a drastic manner, especially in developing countries. The impact of ageing on healthcare and social issues is substantial. Public health policymakers should plan and formulate strategies that could reduce its impact by targeted measures that are tailored to the general population. More resources should be dedicated to address these ageing-related problems, including the adoption of a multi-sectoral approach and engagement of relevant stakeholders. In addition, more research should examine the various health-related interventions to mitigate its influence on the individuals and the community.

Acknowledgements The author wishes to acknowledge Mr Peter Tin, Research Assistant of the JC School of Public Health and Primary Care of The Chinese University of Hong Kong, for his assistance in the literature review.

References

Akil, S. M. S., Abdullah, S., & Sipon, S. (2014). Challenges in managing elderly care centres in Malaysia. *International Journal of Arts & Sciences, 7*(3), 129.

Chau, P. H., Woo, J., Chan, K. C., Weisz, D., & Gusmano, M. K. (2011). Avoidable mortality pattern in a Chinese population—Hong Kong, China. *European Journal of Public Health, 21*(2), 215–220. https://doi.org/10.1093/eurpub/ckq020

Chomik, R., & Piggott, J. (2015). Population ageing and social security in Asia. *Asian Economic Policy Review, 10*, 199–222. https://doi.org/10.1111/aepr.12098

Chung, R. Y., Mercer, S. W., Yip, B. H., Chan, S. W., Lai, F. T., Wang, H. H., Wong, M. C., Wong, C. K., Sit, R. W., Yeoh, E. K., & Wong, S. Y. (2016). The association between types of regular primary care and hospitalization among people with and without multimorbidity: A household survey on 25,780 Chinese. *Scientific Reports, 6*(1), 1–9. https://doi.org/10.1038/srep29758

Chung, R. Y., Tin, K. Y., Cowling, B. J., Chan, K. P., Chan, W. M., Lo, S. V., & Leung, G. M. (2009). Long-term care cost drivers and expenditure projection to 2036 in Hong Kong. *BMC Health Services Research, 9*(1), 1–14. https://doi.org/10.1186/1472-6963-9-172

Dent, E., Martin, F. C., Bergman, H., Woo, J., Romero-Ortuno, R., & Walston, J. D. (2019). Management of frailty: Opportunities, challenges, and future directions. *The Lancet, 394*(10206), 1376–1386. https://doi.org/10.1016/S0140-6736(19)31785-4

Dong, X. Q., Chen, R. J., Chang, E. S., & Simon, M. (2013). Elder abuse and psychological well-being: A systematic review and implications for research and policy—A mini review. *Gerontology, 59*, 132–142. https://doi.org/10.1159/000341652

Food and Health Bureau. (2018). *Statistics*. https://www.fhb.gov.hk/statistics/en/dha/dha_summary_report.htm

Gottret, P. E., & Schieber, G. (2006). *Health financing revisited: A practitioner's guide*. World Bank Publications.

He, A. J., & Tang, V. F. (2021). Integration of health services for the elderly in Asia: A scoping review of Hong Kong, Singapore, Malaysia, Indonesia. *Health Policy, 125*(3), 351–362. https://doi.org/10.1016/j.healthpol.2020.12.020

Hedrich, W., Tan, J., Chalmers, B., & Yeo, J. (2016). *Advancing into the golden years-cost of healthcare for Asia Pacific's elderly*. Marsh & McLennan Companies. https://www.mmc.com/content/dam/mmc-web/insights/publications/2018/dec/healthy-societies/Advancing-into-the-Golden-Years/APRC%20Ageing%20report.pdf

Hu, X., Huang, J., Lv, Y., Li, G., & Peng, X. (2015). Status of prevalence study on multimorbidity of chronic disease in China: Systematic review. *Geriatrics & Gerontology International, 15*(1), 1–10. https://doi.org/10.1111/ggi.12340

International Labour Organization. (2017). *Ageing and social protection in Asia and the Pacific*. https://www.ilo.org/wcmsp5/groups/public/---asia/---ro-bangkok/documents/briefingnote/wcms_614170.pdf

Kim, K. I., Lee, J. H., & Kim, C. H. (2012). Impaired health-related quality of life in elderly women is associated with multimorbidity: Results from the Korean National Health and Nutrition Examination Survey. *Gender Medicine, 9*(5), 309–318. https://doi.org/10.1016/j.genm.2012.08.001

Ladusingh, L., & Maharana, B. (2018). How sustainable is the familial support of elderly in Asia? *Population Ageing, 11*, 349–366. https://doi.org/10.1007/s12062-017-9192-4

Lam, A. H. Y. (2017). Strategies of Hong Kong's healthcare system in ageing population. In *Official Conference Proceedings of the Asian Conference on Ageing & Gerontology*. The University of Hong Kong.

Lau, J. Y. C., Wong, E. L. Y., Chung, R. Y., Law, S. C., Threapleton, D., Kiang, N., Chau, P., Wong, S. Y. S., Woo, J., & Yeoh, E. K. (2018). Collaborate across silos: Perceived barriers to integration of care for the elderly from the perspectives of service providers. *The International Journal of Health Planning and Management, 33*(3), e768–e780. https://doi.org/10.1002/hpm.2534

Legislative Council Secretariat. (2019). *Government expenditure on the elderly* (RT02/19-20). https://www.legco.gov.hk/research-publications/english/1920rt02-government-expenditure-on-the-elderly-20191213-e.pdf

Lim, W. S., Wong, S. F., Leong, I., Choo, P., & Pang, W. S. (2017). Forging a frailty-ready healthcare system to meet population ageing. *International Journal of Environmental Research and Public Health, 14*(12), 1448. https://doi.org/10.3390/ijerph14121448

Marengoni, A., Angleman, S., Melis, R., Mangialasche, F., Karp, A., Garmen, A., Meinow, B., & Fratiglioni, L. (2011). Ageing with multimorbidity: A systematic review of the literature. *Ageing Research Reviews, 10*(4), 430–439. https://doi.org/10.1016/j.arr.2011.03.003

National Institutes of Health. (2011). *Global health and ageing*. https://www.who.int/ageing/publications/global_health.pdf

Ng, A. T. S., Sy, C., & Li, J. (2011). A system dynamics model of Singapore healthcare affordability. In *Proceedings of the 2011 Winter Simulation Conference (WSC)* (pp. 1–13). IEEE. https://doi.org/10.1109/WSC.2011.6147853

Ng, T. K. C., Fong, B. Y. F., & Kwong, C. K. Y. (2019). Transition of hospital acute-centric to long term care in an ageing population in Hong Kong—Is it an issue of service gap? *Asia-Pacific Journal of Health Management, 14*(1), 11–15. https://doi.org/10.24083/apjhm.v14i1.207

Nurjono, M., Yoong, J., Yap, P., Wee, S. L., & Vrijhoef, H. J. M. (2018). Implementation of integrated care in Singapore: a complex adaptive system perspective. *International Journal of Integrated Care, 18*(4). https://doi.org/10.5334/ijic.4174

Organisation for Economic Co-operation and Development. (2019). Old-age income poverty. In *Pension at a glance 2019: OECD and G20 Indicators*. https://doi.org/10.1787/b6d3dcfc-en

Pillemer, K., Burnes, D., Riffin, C., & Lachs, M. S. (2016). Elder abuse: Global situation, risk factors, and prevention strategies. *The Gerontologist, 56*(Suppl 2), S194–S205. https://doi.org/10.1093/geront/gnw004

Research Institute for ASEAN and East Asia. (2021). *Ageing in Asia*. https://www.eria.org/database-and-programmes/topic/ageing-in-asia

Schiamberg, L. B., Barboza, G. G., Oehmke, J., Zhang, Z., Griffore, R. J., Weatherill, R. P., von Heydrich, L., & Post, L. A. (2011). Elder abuse in nursing homes: An ecological perspective.

Journal of Elder Abuse and Neglect, 23(2), 190–211. https://doi.org/10.1080/08946566.2011.558798

Schoeb, V. (2016). Healthcare service in Hong Kong and its challenges: The role of health professionals within a social model of health. *China Perspectives, 2016*(2016/4), 51–58. https://doi.org/10.4000/chinaperspectives.7118

Soto, M., Shang, B., & Coady, D. (2012). New projections of public health spending, 2010–2050. In B. Clements, D. Coady, & S. Gupta (Eds.), *The economics of public health care reform in advanced and emerging countries* (pp. 37–54). International Monetary Fund. https://doi.org/10.5089/9781616352448.071

UNFPA & HelpAge International. (2011). *Overview of available policies and legislation, data and research, and institutional arrangements relating to older persons—Progress since Madrid.* https://www.unfpa.org/sites/default/files/pub-pdf/Older_Persons_Report.pdf

United Nations ESCAP. (2016) *Ageing in Asia and the Pacific: Overview.* https://mipaa.unescapsdd.org/files/documents/SDD%20Ageing%20Fact%20Sheet%20Overview.pdf

United Nations, Department of Economic and Social Affairs, Population Division. (2015). *World Population Ageing 2015* (ST/ESA/SER.A/390). https://www.un.org/en/development/desa/population/publications/pdf/ageing/WPA2015_Report.pdf

Woo, J., Mak, B., & Yeung, F. (2013). Age-friendly primary health care: An assessment of current service provision for older adults in Hong Kong. *Health Services Insights, 6*, HSI-S12434. https://doi.org/10.4137/HSI.S12434

World Health Organization. (2021). *Elder abuse: Fact sheet.* https://www.who.int/news-room/fact-sheets/detail/elder-abuse

Worldmeters. (2021). *Life expectancy of the world population.* https://www.worldometers.info/demographics/life-expectancy/

Yan, E., Chan, K. L., & Tiwari, A. (2015). A systematic review of prevalence and risk factors for elder abuse in Asia. *Trauma, Violence, & Abuse, 16*(2), 199–219. https://doi.org/10.1177/1524838014555033

Yip, W. (2019). Healthcare system challenges in Asia. *Oxford Research Encyclopedia of Economics and Finance.* https://doi.org/10.1093/acrefore/9780190625979.013.245

Chapter 2
Moving Towards Integrated Models of Aged Care Across Boundaries in Asia

Cheryl C. W. Ho, Ben Yuk Fai Fong, and Ellen Ku

Abstract The demand for aged care has been increasing continuously. Integrated care covers comprehensive areas of medical and health services and is essential in improving the fragmented primary services, aiming to achieve high quality of care to the older adults and their families. Holistic care philosophy, acknowledging the existence of a very close relationship between body, mind and soul (spirit) and focusing on individualism, emphasises that every dimension of human is distinctive and unique as well as being connected to each other. Medicine in particular appears to have become distracted from its duty to care, comfort and console, while focusing preferentially on its duty to ameliorate, attenuate and cure. Such a 'decoupling' of medicine in its humanistic character from the scientific knowledge is exerting negative effects on the patient's experience of illness. While conventional Western medicine has established its solid foundation based on state-of-the-art technology, objective clinical evidence, well-defined therapeutic mechanisms, standardisation of treatment and rigorous research methodology, it is limited by the lack of holistic and humanistic approach, individualised treatment and awareness of the interrelationship between the environment, psychosocial factors and the physical illness. In contrast, the time-honoured complementary and alternative medicine (CAM) has founded a distinct system to strive for the balance and harmony between the environment, spiritual, mental and physical well-being with a holistic approach, that emphasises patient-practitioner therapeutic relationship and tailor-made management. It is generally perceived as a more natural treatment modality and the use of CAM has been increasingly accepted in developed countries. To reconcile the two completely different systems of medical practice, the concept of 'Integrative Medicine' has emerged in recent years. Integrative Medicine combines conventional

C. C. W. Ho
Hong Kong College of Community Health Practitioners, Hong Kong, China

B. Y. F. Fong (✉)
College of Professional and Continuing Education, The Hong Kong Polytechnic University, Hong Kong, China
e-mail: byffong@gmail.com

E. Ku
Caritas Institute of Higher Education, Hong Kong, China

V. T. S. Law and B. Y. F. Fong (eds.), *Ageing with Dignity in Hong Kong and Asia*, Quality of Life in Asia 16, https://doi.org/10.1007/978-981-19-3061-4_2

Western medicine and CAM in the disease management. It aims to synergise the strengths and compensate the shortcomings of conventional Western medicine and CAM so as to provide the best patient care: delivery of medical care based on robust evidence and theoretical basis through a holistic, individualised approach of healing the mind, body and spirit.

Keywords Integrated care · Complimentary and alternative medicine · Integrative medicine · Traditional Chinese medicine

2.1 Introduction

The demand for aged care has been increasing continuously. Integrated care covers comprehensive areas of medical and health services, which are essential in improving the fragmented primary services, aiming to achieve high quality of care to the older adults and their families. There are concerns about medical care without humane care (Ferry-Danini, 2018). Marcum (2008, p. 393) has suggested that patients should receive humane care, not only technical care. The humanistic approach is to focus on the entire person and not only on curing the disease (Solomon, 2015, p. 11).

Holistic care philosophy, while acknowledging the existence of a very close relationship between body, mind and soul (spirit) and focusing on individualism, emphasises every dimension of human being distinctive and unique as well as being connected to each other. Medicine in particular appears to have become distracted from its duty to care, comfort and console, with focusing preferentially on its duty to ameliorate, attenuate and cure bodily conditions. Such a 'de-coupling' of medicine from its humanistic character to the scientific knowledge is exerting negative effects on the patient's experience of illness. Therefore, integrity is also one of the major concerns of the current aged care system, which emphasises that holistic treatment/health care should be concerned about spiritual gains a person has experienced in fixing the physical disorders (Demirsoy, 2017).

2.2 Major Diseases in Elderly in Asia

Gu et al. (2013) have done a research on mortality of age 65 for five eastern and eastern Asia areas i.e. China, Hong Kong, Japan, Republic of Korea and Singapore. It was found that around 30 to 40% of females and 20% to 40% males died from stroke and heart diseases, while the mortality of stroke in the studied places except China had dropped over 50% from 1980–1985 to 2005–2010. The mortality of heart diseases in all five places had decreased as well. Cancer was the cause of around 20% of mortality over the period. The mortality rate remained stable from 1980–1985 to 2005–2010. For older elderly, the rate of dying from cancer in all five places had risen over the period. Cancer was one of the most dominant causes of death (Ghaljeh et al., 2019). Each year, nearly 8 million people died from cancer (Jemal et al., 2011). Current treatment of cancer still causes anxiety and physical discomfort to patients (Cornelis et al., 2020). Therefore, the demand of integrated medicine has increased as it is believed that the application of complementary and alternative medicine (CAM) may reduce the drawbacks of western medicine (WM) in curing cancer.

As current WM treatment by interventional radiologist (IR) may cause anxiety and pain, medication for pain relief and calming down would be given. Many factors can cause stress to patients such as their fear towards the result of the treatment, staying in an unfamiliar environment, etc. Using IM with the help of lowest invasive image-guided procedures may reduce stress in patients than only using IR (Cornelis et al., 2020).

2.3 Western Medicine and Complementary and Alternative Medicine

Conventional western medicine has established its solid foundation based on state-of-the-art technology, objective clinical evidence, well-defined therapeutic mechanisms, standardisation of treatment, and rigorous research methodology. WM is limited by the lack of focuses on holistic and humanistic approach, individualised treatment and awareness of the inter-relationship among the environment, psychosocial factors and the physical illnesses.

In contrast, the time-honoured complementary and alternative medicine has founded a distinct system to strive for the balance and harmony among the environment, spiritual, mental and physical well-being with a holistic approach that emphasises patient-practitioner therapeutic relationship and tailor-made management. It is generally perceived as a more natural treatment modality and the use of CAM has been increasingly accepted in many countries.

2.3.1 Integrative Medicine

To reconcile the two completely different systems of medical practice, the concept of 'Integrated Medicine' (IM) has emerged in recent years. Integrative medicine combines conventional western medicine and CAM in disease management. It aims to synergise the strengths and compensate the shortcomings of conventional western medicine and CAM so as to provide the best patient care in the delivery of medical care based on robust evidence and theoretical basis through a holistic, individualised approach of healing the mind, body and spirit. In 1978, Angelica Thieriot firstly suggested the Planetree model to use IM as a method to achieve patient-centred care (George, 2015).

Table 2.1 Five common types of CAM methods

Types of CAM	Example
Alternative medical systems	Traditional Chinese medicine, Ayurveda, homeopathic medicine, chiropractic, naturopathic medicine, etc
Mind–body interventions	Meditation, prayer, mental healing, art, dance, music therapy, etc
Biologically based therapies	Foods, herbs, vitamins, dietary supplements, aromatherapy, etc
Manipulative and body-based methods	Chiropractic or osteopathic manipulation, and massage, etc
Energy therapies Biofield therapies	Qi gong, therapeutic touch Bioelectromagnetic-based therapies

IM focuses on each patients' own health needs. It allows the care providers to find out the most ideal treatment/care plans through knowing each patients' value (Maizes, 1999). It also focuses on prevention, which consists of five areas: physical activity, nutrition, screening, stress management and spirituality. The definition of IM can be very broad that folk medicines like praying or the application of herbal teas are also included (George, 2015).

There are five common types of CAM methods, (1) alternative medical systems, (2) mind–body interventions, (3) biologically based therapies, (4) manipulative and body-based methods and (5) energy therapies biofield therapies (Suzuki, 2004) (Table 2.1). Each type of these CAMs can be adopted to heal patients as IM methods.

2.4 Development of IM in Asia

Some of the CAM methods are found in Asia, like Korean Medicine (KM) and Korea herb, Kampo medicines (traditional Japanese herbal medicines), and Qi Gong, Tai Chi Chuan in China. The collaboration of WM and CAM has been developing well in Asian countries. Rather than adopting their local CAM, CAM methods originated from other countries are also used as IM therapy in these countries.

2.4.1 Development of IM in China

China has paid a lot of effort in combining the use of WM and traditional Chinese medicine (TCM). According to Wang and Xiong (2012), China tried to use IM in different diseases like multiple organ dysfunction syndrome (MODS), hepatic fibrosis, acute respiratory distress syndrome (ARDS) and severe acute respiratory syndrome (SARS), etc. Through the use of IM, a new theory, 'bacteria and bacterial toxin treated simultaneously' was developed to enhance the diagnosis procedure of

MODS. The mortality rate of MODS has been decreased by reducing the course of the disease (Wang & Xue, 1998). Liver fibrosis, a common end stage of many chronic liver diseases, was found to be reversible through combining TCM and WM. The new drug 'Fu Zheng Hua Yu Capsules' was invented by using TCM theory to find out the pathogenesis of the disease and using drug manufacturing method in WM to treat the disease (Liu, 1998). Another example of IM in China is treating ARDS with standard WM treatment and purgation by taking laxatives. Purgation was applied because TCM believed that 'lung and large intestine are related'. It is known that 65% of death cases of acute haemorrhagic necrotising pancreatitis was directly related to ARDS, where the average cure rate has boosted from 80 to 97% after using IM (Wen et al., 2004). In addition, an experiment of comparing the application of IM with that of WM alone, the control group, to SARS patients has been done. It was found that the duration of weakness was reduced by 36 hours on average, short breath, dyspnea and muscle aching pain were reduced by 48 hours, 24 hours, and 48 hours than the control group (WM treatment group) respectively on average (Wang et al., 2003). China has actively applied IM and done a lot of related researches.

2.4.2 Development of IM in Japan

Kampo medicine is a CAM that Japanese doctors are proud of. According to the research by Imanishi et al. (1999), over 70% of respondents were practising with CAM with WM where 96% of them were adopting Kampo medicine. Beside Kampo medicine, the Japanese doctors also adopt other CAM as IM therapy. In 1999, 8% of respondents reported that they adopted other CAM methods (Imanish et al., 1999). Japan has a positive attitude on IM, Japan Society for Integrative Medicine (JIM) was founded in 2001 to keep on developing the IM in Japan (Suzuki, 2004). In 2018, Motoo et al. (2018) conducted a survey on using CAM and found that over half of the respondents received CAM from physicians and around 90% of those who used CAM received different treatment methods other than Kampo medicine.

2.4.3 Development of IM in Korea

IM was introduced in the nineteenth century which is currently included in the national health insurance (Han et al., 2016). IM has also been used widely with WM in Korea. Park et al. (2018) did a research on the result of using IM to cure acute stroke with WM and found that IM was associated with reducing the mortality rate at 3 and 12 months. However, the development of IM is not as good as the development in China. As IM and WM are two separate systems in Korea, most of the hospitals only adopt one type of medicine (Park et al., 2018). This has led to a lower chance of combining IM and WM in Korea. In order to encourage the collaboration between

IM and WM, the Korean government amended the medical law in 2010. Since then, the medical employers are granted to employ WM doctors, IM doctors and dentists in the same clinic (Jo et al., 2016). Yet, the surveys have found that the collaborative treatment of IM and WM is still refused by conventional hospitals. According to Leem et al. (2020), many IM hospitals and only a few conventional hospitals conducted KM and WM collaborative treatments in 2010. After 10 years, WM doctors are still not interested in treating patients by combining WM with IM. They also showed lower understanding in IM than IM doctors' understanding in WM (Leem et al., 2020).

The IM development in Korea is not only being measured by the collaboration between WM and KM but also the collaboration of other alternative medicine with WM. Jeong et al. (2010) conducted research on using Chinese herbal medicine as IM treatment to heal cancers. In addition, the research of Kim et al. (2004) found that nearly 80% of experimental subjects had been treated with at least one type of CAM with WM. The major reasons for application in the research were found to be nutritional support and physical strengthening. The development of IM in Korea is slow when compared to Japan and China. The integrative use of WM and IM can be strengthened.

2.4.4 Development of IM in India

The Indian traditional CAM is called Ayurveda, which has been developed systematically for more than 3000 years (Kumar & Gulia, 2016). Ayurveda can treat sleep disorders by focusing on the physical, mental and spiritual aspects of a person (Kumar & Gulia, 2016; Patwardhan, 2010). Although Ayurveda is common in India, it is not famous in the world due to lack of scientific evidence (Rao & Gandhi, 2014). Other than Ayurveda, Unani, Siddha and Homoeopathy are CAM systems that are also widely accepted in India. Since these traditional Indian therapies usually use Indian resources, these treatments are more affordable than WM (Joseph et al., 2019).

In order to deal with the medical care needs in India, the National AYUSH Mission (NAM) has introduced in their five-year plan (2012–2017) to advocate Ayurveda, Unani, Siddha and Homoeopathy (AYUSH) in India including rural areas (Joseph et al., 2019). Under NAM, the government would provide funding to help the setup of AYUSH wings in various places across India (Joseph et al., 2019). AYUSH, IPC Heart Care Center, Mumbai, Institute of Preventive Medicine (IPM) and International Society for Prevention of Atherosclerosis and Thrombosis (IPSAT) co-operate to facilitate the development of IM in India and create the Global Alliance of Traditional Health Systems (GATHS), a platform to group different CAM providers together (Rao & Gandhi, 2014). The platform has set standards and to make holistic care easier (Rao & Gandhi, 2014). In addition, Mind–Body Spirit Society of India has also been created to support IM in India (Rao & Gandhi, 2014). In 2010, the idea of IM was introduced in the World Ayurveda Conference (Rao & Gandhi, 2014).

WM in India have started to adopt different CAM methods in IM treatments. For instance, a Robotic Surgeon in Medanta-Hospital used yoga before and after surgery

(Rao & Gandhi, 2014). Joseph et al. (2019) have also done a study about the usage of CAM by WM doctors in Mangalore, an urban area in India. The study revealed that around 75% of respondents suggested IM to patients. Most of them suggested yoga to their patients (Joseph et al., 2019). Other CAMs like Ayurveda, Chiropractic and Acupuncture, etc. are also suggested. Although some CAM methods may not be popular in India, there are CAM methods that are widely accepted by Indian WM doctors.

2.4.5 Development of IM in Malaysia

CAM is defined in the Laws of Malaysia as medicine which targets to maintain both physical and mental health of a person through prevention and treatment (Kaur et al., 2019). Herbal medicine is one of the Malaysian traditional medicines which has taken advantage of the abundant plants in Malaysian rainforest by using herbs to cure patients (Tan et al., 2020). There are around 12,500 species of seed plants in the Malaysian rainforest. Around 10% of those seed plants have proved to be useful in the medical aspect (Tan et al., 2020).

Siti et al. (2009) found that almost 70% of respondents had used CAM in both urban and rural areas of Malaysia. Moreover, biologically based therapies are the most popular CAM method that nearly 90% of them use these therapies for both health problems and maintaining health. Other types of CAM are far less common in Malaysia. The usage of mind–body medicine, manipulative and body-based therapies as well as whole medical system used for health problems are 11.1%, 27% and 1.9%, respectively, while the usage of these CAMs for maintaining health are 41%, 26.4% and 1.5% respectively (Siti et al., 2009). In the research by Silcanathan & Low (2015), it was found that over 70% of the respondents used CAM in the year prior to the research.

The government launched a national policy to promote IM to provide a more holistic care to patients in 2001 (Kaur et al., 2019). Originally, traditional and complementary medicine (T&CM) in Malaysia was operating in a self-regulation mode that around 16,050 CAM providers had registered with the government (Kaur et al., 2019). In 2016, the traditional and complementary medicine Act [Act 775] was launched and the mode of regulating T&CM was changed (Kaur et al., 2019). Later, the T&CM Council was set up to govern T&CM.

2.4.6 Development of IM in Thailand

Thai traditional medicine (TTM) is a holistic medicine which could be applied to different health conditions. It uses herbs and massage for treatment as well (Nootim et al., 2020). In order to promote TTM for enhancing the people's health, the Ministry of Public Health in Thailand added TTM to the national healthcare system in 2011

(Senachai, 2020, p. 3319). Yet, there is a lack of study to find out the effectiveness of combining TTM and WM as IM (Nootim et al., 2020). After that, Nootim et al. (2020) conducted a research and found that both cancer patients and health providers felt satisfactory in using TTM as IM. But still, more research has to be done in investigating the combined use of TTM and WM.

2.5 Alternative Medicine in Integrated Model

2.5.1 Traditional Chinese Medicine

The use of WM with Chinese herbal medicine is beneficial to the cancer patients. According to Li and Lin (2011), TCM can be used to improve the patient's body to fight cancers by strengthening their internal energy and improve their physique, enhancing qi and nourishing yin, and clearing away heat and resolving toxicity inside the body. It is also found that the toxicity is greatly reduced while the effectiveness of radiotherapy and chemotherapy is raised by TCM. Moreover, there are around three hundred Chinese herbal combinations out of three thousand different species of samples containing constituents that can kill cancer cells directly (Wang & Xiong, 2012). In addition, some Chinese herbs can strengthen immunity which can assist the patients to fight cancers. As TCM is effective in curing cancer, a new model 'China Model for Cancer Treatment' which integrates TCM and modern treatment was created (Li & Lin, 2011).

2.5.2 Naturopathic Medicine

According to Maizes (1999), healing by the bodies of patients themselves but not intervention from physicians is one of the main definitions of IM. Naturopathic medicine (NM) emphasises the natural healing ability of the bodies rather than other means of intervention (Armstrong et al., 2018). To assist the self-healing of the patients, NM advocates nutritional improvement, herbal medicine, homoeopathy, lifestyle improving and mind–body medicine (Armstrong et al., 2018). Some preclinical and clinical researches have proved that increasing the intake of specific kinds of nutrients can encourage the immunity to produce anti-tumour response (Takaki et al., 2017). Yet, some CAM treatment may interact with WM treatment. Therefore, patients should inform their practitioners all treatments they are undertaking (Cornelis et al., 2020).

2.5.3 Mind–Body Interventions

The healing of cancers or chronic conditions takes more time with the presence of psychological stress (Guo & DiPietro, 2010). They will also be under greater stress due to different reasons such as pain and financial burden. Therefore, mind care should also be focused under IM. Currently most settings of medical facilities are designed functionally for sophisticated equipment to be used (Cornelis et al., 2020). People may feel pressured and anxious in this kind of 'strange' setting. Concerning the feelings of patients, some facilities are designed by using a human-centred approach at an affordable price. For instance, avoiding noise and providing enough spaces for daily needs by making good use of advanced technologies like VR to minimise additional stress (Schuster & Weber, 2003). Hospitals should be aware of their settings to avoid causing unnecessary stress to patients (Frasca-Beaulieu, 1999).

Communication between patients and medical staff is related to patient's stress (Cornelis et al., 2020). Communicating in a neutral or positive way instead of a negative way may help patients to relax and to build their self-confidence (Lang & Hamilton, 1994). Maizes (1999) suggested that helping patients to have a better understanding of the illness they are facing is a useful way to help the patient to heal.

2.5.4 Music Therapy

Listening to music can lighten stress and pain (Lunde et al., 2019). Not only for anxiety and pain, music therapy has been proved to reduce various symptoms (Lopez et al., 2019). It is effective in both active and passive ways (Cornelis et al., 2020). This means that negative feelings and pain can be relieved by either the patients playing music or listening to music. With the application of music therapy, the use of medication like analgesia and sedation can be reduced (Koch et al., 1998).

2.5.5 Meditation

Prevention is one of the vital topics in IM. Practising meditation can achieve prevention through enhancing well-being in spiritual and stress management aspects (Maizes, 1999). During meditation, people have to concentrate and control themselves to be calm (Walsh & Shapiro, 2006). People learn how to be relaxed (Maizes, 1999). Yoga, qi gong and tai chi chuan are examples of meditation (Cornelis et al., 2020). Moreover, people can practise more than one meditation treatments at a time. Oh et al. (2012) used qi gong and mindfulness together to treat cancer patients.

2.5.6 Stress Management Techniques

Stress management techniques are not high-risk interventions. All patients except those who have psychotic problems can receive these techniques (Deng, 2019). There are many types of techniques to manage stress like deep breathing, progressive muscle relaxation and guided imagery. They have been proved to be effective in reducing anxiety and pressure (Trijsburg et al., 1992). Through the advancement of technologies, like virtual reality (VR), digital sedation (DS) has been added to be the distraction of pain and attention during treatments (Cornelis et al., 2019; Li et al., 2011). Research has proved that VR can distract patients from real environments like hurt, burns and punctures (Chan et al., 2018). VR can draw patients' attention from pain by visual attraction while DS draws patients' all attention as it gives visual and auditory attraction as well as requires verbal response (Hoffman et al., 2004). DS has already been developed to be more effective in distracting patients than normal video games (Hoffman et al., 2006).

2.5.7 Biologically Based Therapies and Food, Herbs and Supplements

According to Lin et al. (2019) who analysed 10 randomly selected clinical trials which all related to nutrition or herbal treatments and cancer patients, herbs and supplements can aid cancer treatment. Marx et al. (2017) also did a research on applying ginger capsules as supplements to cancer patients and found to be successful in helping them.

2.6 Conclusion

When people become older, the risk of suffering from chronic diseases increases. Current WM only emphasises on eliminating the disease but ignoring the damage to the patients' bodies and patients' stress. By combining the treatments of WM and CAM, the effectiveness of treatment and maintaining the quality of life can be improved, for example, reducing the negative feelings of patients, relieving pain during treatment etc. Yet, the use of CAM under IM must be under the advice of health professionals to avoid negative effects from mixing treatments. It is known that Asian countries have their own CAM and IM system at different stages of development. The development of IM in China, Japan, India and Malaysia are relatively more mature than that in Korea and Thailand. If the use of IM increases, aged care will become more holistic and humanistic. Then, elderly can enjoy better healthcare and quality of life.

References

Armstrong, K., Lanni, T., Anderson, M. M., & Patricolo, G. E. (2018). Integrative medicine and the oncology patient: Options and benefits. *Supportive Care in Cancer, 26*,. https://doi.org/10.1007/s00520-017-4007-y

Chan, E., Foster, S., Sambell, R., & Leong, P. (2018). Clinical efficacy of virtual reality for acute procedural pain management: A systematic review and meta-analysis. *PLoS ONE, 13*(7), e0200987. https://doi.org/10.1371/journal.pone.0200987

Cornelis, F. H., Monard, E., Moulin, M. A., Vignaud, E., Laveissiere, F., Ammar, M. B., Nouri-Neuville, M., Barral., M., & Lombart, B. (2019). Sedation and analgesia in interventional radiology: Where do we stand, where are we heading and why does it matter?. *Diagnostic and Interventional Imaging, 100*(12), 753–762. https://doi.org/10.1016/j.diii.2019.10.002

Cornelis, F. H., Najdawi, M., Ammar, M. B., Nouri-Neuville, M., Lombart, B., Lotz, J-P., Cadranel, J., & Barral, M. (2020). Integrative medicine in interventional oncology: A virtuous alliance. *Medicina, 56* (35). https://doi.org/10.3390/medicina56010035

Demirsoy, N. (2017). Holistic care philosophy for patient-centered approaches and spirituality. *INTECH, 6*,. https://doi.org/10.5772/66165

Deng, G. (2019). Integrative medicine therapies for pain management in cancer patients. *The Cancer Journal, 25*(5), 343–348. https://doi.org/10.1097/PPO.0000000000000399

Ferry-Danini, J. (2018). A new path for humanistic medicine. *Theoretical Medicine and Bioethics, 39*, 57–77. https://doi.org/10.1007/s11017-018-9433-4

Frasca-Beaulieu, K. (1999). Interior design for ambulatory care facilities: How to reduce stress and anxiety in patients and families. *Journal of Ambulatory Care Management, 22*(1), 67–73. https://doi.org/10.1097/00004479-199901000-00011

George, M. (2015). Integrative medicine is integral to providing patient-centered care. *Annals of Allergy, Asthma & Immunology, 114*(4), 261–264. https://doi.org/10.1016/j.anai.2015.01.001

Ghaljeh, M., Rezaee, N., Imanigoghari, Z., & Rafati, F. (2019). End of life holistic care for cancer patients: A qualitative study. *Journal of Clinical and Diagnostic Research, 13*(8), LC06-LC09. https://doi.org/10.7860/JCDR/2019/39814.13075

Gu, D., Li, N., Gerland, P., Spoorenberg, T., Andreev, K., & Heilig, G. (2013). Old age mortality in Eastern and South-Eastern Asia. *Demographic Research, 29*(38), 999–1038. https://doi.org/10.4054/DemRes.2013.29.38

Guo, S., & DiPietro, L. A. (2010). Factors affecting wound healing. *Journal of Dental Research, 89*(3). https://doi.org/10.1177/0022034509359125

Han, S. Y., Kim, H. Y., Lim, J. H., Cheon, J., Kwon, Y. K., Kim, H., Yang, Y., & Chae, H. (2016). The past, present, and future of traditional medicine education in Korea. *Integrative Medicine Research, 5*(2), 73–82. https://doi.org/10.1016/j.imr.2016.03.003

Hoffman, H. G., Seibel, E. J., Richards, T. L., Furness, T. A., Patterson, D. R., & Sharar, S. R. (2006). Virtual reality helmet display quality influences the magnitude of virtual reality analgesia. *The Journal of Pain, 7*(11), 843–850. https://doi.org/10.1016/j.jpain.2006.04.006

Hoffman, H. G., Sharar, S. R., Coda, B., Everett, J. J., Ciol, M., Richards, T., & Patterson, D. R. (2004). Manipulating presence influences the magnitude of virtual reality analgesia. *Pain, 111*(1–2), 162–168. https://doi.org/10.1016/j.pain.2004.06.013

Imanishi, J., Watanabe, S., Satoh, M., & Ozasa, K. (1999). Japanese doctors' attitudes to complementary medicine. *The Lancet, 354*(9191), 1735–1736. https://doi.org/10.1016/S0140-6736(05)76729-5

Jemal, A., Bray, F., Center, M., Ferlay, J., Ward, E., & Forman, D. (2011). Global cancer statistics. *CA: A Cancer Journal for Clinicians, 61*(2), 69–90. https://doi.org/10.3322/caac.20107

Jeong, J. S., Ryu, B. H., Kim, J. S., Park, J. W., Choi, W. C., & Yoon, S. W. (2010). Bojungikki-tang for cancer-related fatigue: A pilot randomized clinical trial. *Integrative Cancer Therapies, 9*(4), 331–338. https://doi.org/10.1177/1534735410383170

Jo, H. J., Kwon, M. S., Kim, J. H., Jo Choi, D. H., Han, J. S., Lee, S. H., Kim, Y. S., & Nam, S. S. (2016). An retrospective analysis of 1549 patients under the cooperative medical care consulted to the Department of Acupuncture and Moxibustion in a Korean medical hospital. *Journal of Acupuncture Research, 33*(4), 109–119. https://doi.org/10.13045/acupunct.2016059

Joseph, N., Talwar, C., Sikdar, I., Sengupta, M., Sayed, D. A., & Mahajan, I. (2019). Experiences and perceptions toward integrative, complementary, and alternative medicine among conventional medicine practitioners of Mangalore, India. *Journal of Manipulative and Physiological Therapeutics, 42*(7), 492–502. https://doi.org/10.1016/j.jmpt.2018.12.009

Kaur, J., Hamajima, N., Yamamoto, E., Saw, Y. M., Kariya, T., Soon, G. C., Amin, A., Halim, A. N., Aziz, F. A., & Sharon, S. H. (2019). Patient satisfaction on the utilization of traditional and complementary medicine services at public hospitals in Malaysia. *Complementary Therapies in Medicine, 42*, 422–428. https://doi.org/10.1016/j.ctim.2018.12.013

Kim, M. J., Lee, S. D., Kim, D. R., Kong, Y. H., Sohn, W. S., Ki, S. S., Kim, J., Kim, Y. C., Han, C. J., Lee, J. O., Nam, H. S., Park, Y. H., Kim, C. H., Yi, K. H., Lee, Y. Y., & Jeong, S. H. (2004). Use of complementary and alternative medicine among Korean cancer patients. *The Korean Journal of Internal Medicine, 19*(4), 250–256. https://doi.org/10.3904/kjim.2004.19.4.250

Koch, M. E., Kain, Z. N., Ayoub, C., & Rosenbaum, S. H. (1998). The sedative and analgesic sparing effect of music. *Anesthesiology, 89*, 300–306. https://doi.org/10.1097/00000542-199808000-00005

Kumar, V. M., & Gulia, K. K. (2016). Sleep medicine in ayurveda. *Sleep Medicine Reviews, 25*, 131. https://doi.org/10.1016/j.smrv.2015.02.006

Lang, E. V., & Hamilton, D. (1994). Anodyne imagery: An alternative to i.v. sedation in interventional radiology. *American Journal of Roentgenology, 162*, 1221–1226. https://doi.org/10.2214/ajr.162.5.8166014

Leem, J., Kim, K. I., Seo, J. H., Cheong, M. J., & Youn, I. (2020). Korean medicine doctors' views on Western medicine and Korean medicine collaborative treatment in Korea: Study protocol for a qualitative study. *European Journal of Integrative Medicine, 37*, 101141. https://doi.org/10.1016/j.eujim.2020.101141

Li, A., Montano, Z., Chen, V. J., & Gold, J. I. (2011). Virtual reality and pain management: Current trends and future directions. *Pain Management, 1*(2), 147–157. https://doi.org/10.2217/pmt.10.15

Li, J., & Lin, H. S. (2011). Integrative medicine: A characteristic China model for cancer treatment. *Chinese Journal of Integrative Medicine, 17*(4), 243–245. https://doi.org/10.1007/s11655-011-0712-4

Lin, W. F., Zhong, M. F., Zhou, Q. H., Zhang, Y. R., Wang, H., Zhao, Z. H., Cheng, B. B., & Ling, C. Q. (2019). Efficacy of complementary and integrative medicine on health-related quality of life in cancer patients: A systematic review and meta-analysis. *Cancer Management and Research, 11*, 6663–6680. https://doi.org/10.2147/CMAR.S195935

Liu, P. (1998). Clinic and mechanism study of health-supporting and stasis-resolving decoction on chronic hepatitis B. *Shi Jie Hua Ren Xiao Hua Za Zhi, 6*(7), 60–61.

Lopez, G., Christie, A. J., Powers-James, C., Bae, M. S., Dibaj, S. S., Gomez, T., Williams, J. L., & Bruera, E. (2019). The effects of inpatient music therapy on self-reported symptoms at an academic cancer center: A preliminary report. *Supportive Care in Cancer, 27*, 4207–4212. https://doi.org/10.1007/s00520-019-04713-4

Lunde, S. J., Vuust, P., Garza-Villarreal, E. A., & Vase, L. (2019). Music-induced analgesia: How does music relieve pain? *Pain, 160*(5), 989–993. https://doi.org/10.1097/j.pain.0000000000001452

Maizes, V. (1999). The principles and challenges of integrative medicine. *Western Journal of Medicine, 171*, 148–149.

Marcum, J. A. (2008). Refections on humanizing biomedicine. *Perspectives in Biology and Medicine, 51*(3), 392–405. https://doi.org/10.1353/pbm.0.0023

Marx, W., McCarthy, A. L., Ried, K., McKavanagh, D., Vitetta, L., Sali, A., Lohning, A., & Isenring, E. (2017). The effect of a standardized ginger extract on chemotherapy-induced nausea-related quality of life in patients undergoing moderately or highly emetogenic chemotherapy: A double blind, randomized, placebo controlled trial. *Nutrients, 9*(8), 867. https://doi.org/10.3390/nu9080867

Motoo, Y., Yukawa, K., Arai, I., Hisamura, K., & Tsutani, K. (2018). Use of complementary and alternative medicine in Japan: A cross-sectional internet survey using the Japanese version of the international complementary and alternative medicine questionnaire. *JMA Journal, 2*(1), 35–46. https://doi.org/10.31662/jmaj.2018-0044

Nootim, P., Kapol, N., Bunchuailua, W., Poomprauek, P., & Tungsukruthai, P. (2020). Current state of cancer patient care incorporating Thai traditional medicine in Thailand: A qualitative study. *Journal of Integrative Medicine, 18*, 41–45. https://doi.org/10.1016/j.joim.2019.12.004

Oh, B., Butow, P. N., Mullan, B. A., Clarke, S. J., Beale, P. J., Pavlakis, N., Lee, M. S., Rosenthal, D. S., Larkey, L., & Vardy, J. (2012). Effect of medical qigong on cognitive function, quality of life, and a biomarker of inflammation in cancer patients: A randomized controlled trial. *Supportive Care Cancer, 20*, 1235–1242. https://doi.org/10.1007/s00520-011-1209-6

Park, M., Hunter, J., & Kwon, S. (2018). Evaluating integrative medicine acute stroke inpatient care in South Korea. *Health Policy, 122*(4), 373–379. https://doi.org/10.1016/j.healthpol.2018.02.004

Patwardhan, B. (2010). Ayurveda and integrative medicine: Riding a tiger. *Journal of Ayurveda and Integrative Medicine, 1* (1), 13–15. https://doi.org/ https://doi.org/10.4103/0975-9476.59820

Rao, G. H. R., & Gandhi, P. G. (2014). Integrative medicine: Global perspective. *Journal of Homeopathy & Ayurvedic Medicine, 3*(2), 150. https://doi.org/10.4172/2167-1206.1000150

Schuster, R. J., & Weber, M. L. (2003). Noise in the ambulatory health care setting. *Journal of Ambulatory Care Management, 26*(3), 243–249. https://doi.org/10.1097/00004479-200307000-00007

Senachai, P. (2020). The problems associated with the integration of Traditional Thai Medicine (TTM) in public health policy. *Opción, 36*(26), 3319–3352.

Siti, Z. M., Tahir, A., Ida Farah, A., Ami, F., & S. M., Sondi, S., Azman, A. H., Maimunah, A. H., Haniza, M. A., Siti Haslinda, M. D., Zulkarnain, A. K., Zakiah, I., & WanZaleha, W. C. (2009). Use of traditional and complementary medicine in Malaysia: A baseline study. *Complementary Therapies in Medicine, 17*(5–6), 292–299. https://doi.org/10.1016/j.ctim.2009.04.002

Solomon, M. (2015). *Making medical knowledge*. Oxford University Press.

Suzuki, N. (2004). Complementary and alternative medicine: A Japanese perspective. *Hindawi, 1*(2), 113–119. https://doi.org/10.1093/ecam/neh029

Takaki, H., Cornelis, F. H., Kako, Y., Kobayashi, K., Kamikonya, N., & Yamakado, K. (2017). Thermal ablation and immunomodulation: From preclinical experiments to clinical trials. *Diagn. Intero. Imaging, 98*(9), 651–659. https://doi.org/10.1016/j.diii.2017.04.008

Tan, T. Y. C., Lee, J. G., Yusof, N. A. M., Teh, B. P., & Mohamed, A. F. S. (2020). Malaysian herbal monograph development and challenges. *Journal of Herbal Medicine, 23*,. https://doi.org/10.1016/j.hermed.2020.100380

Trijsburg, R. W., van Knippenberg, F. C., & Rijpma, S. E. (1992). Effects of psychological treatment on cancer patients: A critical review. *Psychosomatic Medicine, 54*(4), 489–517. https://doi.org/10.1097/00006842-199207000-00011

Walsh, R., & Shapiro, S. L. (2006). The meeting of meditative disciplines and western psychology: A mutually enriching dialogue. *American Psychologist, 61*(3), 227–239. https://doi.org/10.1037/0003-066x.61.3.227

Wang, J., & Xiong, X. (2012). Current situation and perspectives of clinical study in integrative medicine in China. *Evidence-Based Complementary and Alternative Medicine, 2012*, 268542. https://doi.org/10.1155/2012/268542

Wang, J. D., & Xue, L. (1998). Bacteria, bacterial toxin and inflammatory mediator treated simultaneously is a new strategy for the treatment of severe sepsis. *Zhongguo Wei Zhong Bing Ji Jiu Yi Xue, 10*(6), 323–325.

Wang, R. B., Liu, J. M., Jiang, Y. Y., Wu, Y. Z., Wang, X. J., Chi, P. P., & Sun, F. X. (2003). Preliminary study on clinical efficacy of integrative Chinese and western medicine in treating severe acute respiratory syndrome. *Chinese Journal of Integrative Medicine, 9*, 209. https://doi.org/10.1007/BF02838035

Wen, Q. P., Chen, H. L., & Guan, F. L. (2004). Effect of Qingyitang on acute lung injury induced by severe acute pancreatitis in rats. *World Chinese Journal of Digestology, 12*(6), 1341–1345.

Chapter 3
Implementation of Community Care Policy for Older Adults in Hong Kong

Ray Choy

Abstract Compared to other economies including the Organisation for Economic Co-operation and Development countries and mainland China, the trend of ageing in Hong Kong Special Administrative Region will be one of the fastest. Hong Kong is already an aged society taken into account of an annual 3% increase of the population of older adults from 2014 to 2019. The government of Hong Kong has formulated policies, provided a number of social welfare services for the senior citizens, established the Elderly Commission and made 'Care for the Elderly' as a policy objective. In 2014, the Elderly Services Programme Plan was introduced. Concerning social welfare services, Hong Kong puts emphasis on community care and ageing in place. Due to the voluminous demand of residential services in Hong Kong, the waiting list for quality homes for older adults is long. The needs of such services are clearly expressed as the existing residential homes cannot accommodate the demand. Community care is therefore extensively introduced to support the older adults residing in the community as far as possible. In addition to social welfare, medical and health services are highly needed for those who stay in the community. Primary healthcare is one of the policy directives in Hong Kong in this regard. The chapter will first outline the policies, mechanisms and social welfare services for older adults in Hong Kong. Emphasis will be put on community care. The concepts will be reviewed and revisited. As a community-based health service for older adults, primary healthcare will also be discussed.

Keywords Community care policy · Social welfare services · Primary healthcare · Older adults · Hong Kong

---

R. Choy (✉)
Department of Innovative Social Work, City University of Macau, Macau, China
e-mail: raychoy@cityu.mo

V. T. S. Law and B. Y. F. Fong (eds.), *Ageing with Dignity in Hong Kong and Asia*, Quality of Life in Asia 16, https://doi.org/10.1007/978-981-19-3061-4_3

Table 3.1 Countries or areas with the largest percentage point increase in the share of older persons aged 65 years or over between 2019 and 2050

Number	Countries or areas	Percentage
1	Republic of Korea	23
2	Singapore	20.9
3	Taiwan	19.9
4	Macao	17.7
5	Maldives	17.2
6	Thailand	17.2
7	Hong Kong	17.2

Source of information United Nations, 2019, p. 8

3.1 Ageing Population in Hong Kong

In 2020, the population in Hong Kong Special Administrative Region (HKSAR) was 7,481,800, 18.3% of which were 65 years of age and over. The ageing rate has risen rapidly in the last five years with an annual 3% increase from 2015 (Census and Statistics Department, 2021, p. 4). It is anticipated that with such a steady increase, the cohort of senior citizens at the age of 65 and above will reach 31% in 2039—22% in 2024, 26% in 2029 and 29% in 2034, respectively (Census & Statistics Department, 2020b, p. 7). In 2039, almost one in three Hong Kong citizens will be older adults. The population-mix is partly due to the decrease of the fertility rate—from 8.2 (per 1,000 population) in 2015 to 5.8 in 2020 (Census and Statistics Department, 2021, p. 5). Due to the low fertility rate, the population of children and youth aged under 15 has been decreasing gradually. As a result of the changing age structure of the Hong Kong population on two fronts, the older adults' dependency ratio has been increased steadily—from 124 in 1991 to 168 in 2006 and to 441 in 2019 (Census & Statistics Department, 2020b, p. 6; Chui, 2008, p. 170).

Like other affluent and established cities, the advances in science, and medical and health technology, the rising living standards, and the provision of affordable medical and social services in Hong Kong have made the life expectancy of the citizens one of the longest in the world—82 years and 88 years for males and females in 2019, respectively (Census & Statistics Department, 2020a, p. 7). Following Japan, Hong Kong is ranked the second highest as far as ageing population in Asia is concerned, exceeding all the Organisation for Economic Co-operation and Development countries and mainland China (Elderly Commission, 2017, p. 8).

It is worth mentioning that according to the United Nations' figures, Hong Kong is the 7th rank in the countries or areas with the largest growth rate in the age group of 65 years or over between 2019 and 2050. The ageing rate in Asia should be particularly noted as the first to seven ranks are occupied by Asian countries or areas (United Nations, 2019, p. 8) (Table 3.1).

3.2 Community Care Policy—Formulation and Initiatives

In view of the changing landscape of its population, in 1997 the government of Hong Kong made 'Care for the Elderly' as the policy objective. The objective of this policy is 'to improve the quality of life of the elderly population and to provide them with a sense of security, a sense of belonging and a feeling of health and worthiness' (Elderly Commission, 2021). The Elderly Commission (EC), established in the same year, is tasked with providing advice and making recommendations for the HKSAR government in the policy for caring the older adults. Programmes and services have to be planned and developed to ensure that the policy objectives are met (Elderly Commission, 2021).

With the advice of the EC, the Labour and Welfare Bureau (a policy bureau) of the Hong Kong government is responsible for the formulation and implementation of a policy for the older adults in Hong Kong. Undoubtedly, the welfare of the senior citizens is related to a spectrum of services including retirement protection, medical and health services, social care, employment (work re-skilling and re-employment), housing, transport and recreational facilities, and a number of other policy bureaux and departments are involved in policy formulation and service provision. To have a blueprint for future development, the EC was asked in 2014 to formulate the Elderly Services Programme Plan (ESPP) to outline a work plan of serving older adults in Hong Kong in the long term.

The vision and mission of the ESPP are 'to uphold the spirit of respecting, loving and caring for the elderly' (Elderly Commission, 2017, p. 13). An overarching aim of the ESPP is to uphold the Hong Kong government's policy directive of ageing in place, i.e., to reduce institutionalisation through providing community care extensively (Elderly Commission, 2017, p. 14). The ESPP proposes an Elderly Care Service Model (ECSM) which is made up by five components, namely, Active Ageing, Community Support, Community Care, Residential Care and End-Of-Life Care (Elderly Commission, 2017, p. 16). As a continuum of care, such a model is set up based on the increasing frailty and care needs, i.e., from the first service model—Active Ageing (for those who are relatively young, healthy and independent) to the last stage of End-of-Life Care (when the individuals become frail and less independent, they need more care and professional services gradually). Details of the service models can be found in Table 3.2.

3.2.1 Elderly Care Service Delivery Models in Hong Kong

Taking the first two service components of the ECSM—Active Ageing and Community Support into consideration, active ageing is aimed at facilitating the older adults in having an engaged and productive life, which is beneficial to their well-being and

Table 3.2 Elderly Care Service Delivery Model in Hong Kong

Increasing frailty and care needs →

Active Ageing	Community Support	Community Care	Residential Care	End-of-life Care
•Healthy lifestyle •Active social participation	•Health maintenance •Reduction in health risks •Illness prevention	•Carer support •Center-based service •Home-based service •Resipite	•24-hour assistance in daily living	•Quality of life and dignity at last stage of life

Source of information Adapted from Elderly Commission, 2017, p. 16

is conducive to getting old in their home environment (Elderly Commission, 2017, p. 17). Kwok (2013) states that 'ageing is not a barrier to an active social life' (Kwok, 2013, p. 675). With reference to the World Health Organization's (2002) 'Active Aging: A Policy Framework', the EC has worked out an implementation plan in this respect. The framework includes three major components, namely security, health maintenance and participation (Chan & Liang, 2013, p. 31).

The first-tier service model of the ECSM outlines healthy lifestyle and active social participation, the individuals concerned like retirees, the 'young-old' and those who are fit, healthy and independent can fulfil their needs by themselves, and by using personal and social networks, family resources and generic services. They may not need professional help at this stage. Specifically, both Chui (2012) and Tam (2011) identify that learning or lifelong learning is crucial for active ageing. In Hong Kong, the EC launched in 2007 a school-based Elder Academy (EA) Scheme which is attached to primary, secondary and post-secondary institutions. The objectives of the EA include promoting lifelong learning, maintaining physical and mental well-being, widening social networks and fostering sense of worthiness of the senior students. It should be noted that intergenerational communication and learning between the senior and younger students is encouraged (Elder Academy, 2020).

Community Support, the second-tier service model, highlights reducing health risks, prevention of serious illness and maintaining current health status; such tasks can be carried out by the individuals with relevant health advice and support. Community-wide health promotion is therefore of vital importance for the ageing adults. As discussed in the last part of this chapter, primary healthcare plays a significant role in such services. To provide community support, the ESPP emphasises the importance of creating an age-friendly environment and, affordable and comprehensive programmes which can meet the physiological, psychological and social needs of the older adults. Examples may include accessible recreational and sports facilities, and affordable transportation fare to enhance mobility. Wong et al. (2015) put forward eight domains in assessing the age-friendliness of districts in Hong Kong, namely outdoor spaces and buildings, transportation, social participation, respect and social inclusion, civic participation and employment, communication and information (Wong et al., 2015). Comparing the neighbourhood environment related to the health of senior citizens living in Hong Kong, Singapore and Tokyo, Loo et al. (2017) recommend that simply creating a walkable urban environment and fostering peer support groups can already promote a more active lifestyle, support ageing in place and enhance the health of the seniors (Loo et al., 2017). In addition to age-friendly facilities, environmental safety, information and communication, Han et al. (2021) propose that public transportation and accessibility, societal attitude of the general public such as respect and discrimination prevention are also policy factors to enhance the well-being of older adults (Han et al., 2021). Wen et al. (2021) have similar findings in examining productive engagement of senior citizens in Hong Kong—social atmosphere as well as the built environment and social service provision are the key determinants (Wen et al., 2021).

The ESPP points out that a range of services has been provided by the public and private sectors, and other the civil groups (Elderly Commission, 2017, p. 17). Such multi-sectoral approach can alleviate the burden of provision of services on the government. As the ECSM describes, the last two tiers service models, i.e., Residential Care involves 24-hour residential care and assistance while End-of-life Care would very often involve hospital admissions and institutionalisation, this paper will focus on the Community Care mode which will be discussed in detail in the succeeding section.

3.3 The Concept of Community Care Re-Visited

3.3.1 Community Care

The concept of community care has been extensively studied and adopted in Hong Kong, a British colony until 1997 when the sovereignty was returned to China. Community care has once dominated the studies and research of social policy, and community services in the United Kingdom (UK) and her colonies, and the Commonwealth nations in 1980s. Though the notion of community care varies, it emphasises that care is provided for those in need, for example, older adults (Chen, 2012). Central to the concept of community care, supporting those who are in need to continue to reside in their own home and stay in the community is one of the core ideologies. Community care or '*care in the community*' is considered as an alternative or a better option than hospitalisation and institutionalisation. The emergence of community care was against the institutional care, largely due to the stigmatisation of being institutionalised, and the scandals of poor care and abuse taken place in large institutions in the UK and Australia in the latter part of the last century (Chen, 2012).

Apart from the historical and ideological perspectives, the economic and financial factors in the UK in the 1980s also made a policy shift of moving away from institutional service to community care. Johnson (1987) points out that '…recent events have…strengthened the commitment of governments to community care since it appears to offer the opportunity to cut public expenditure and reduce the role of the state…defining community care as *care by the community* (italics added) is more in line with the ideas of welfare pluralism' (Johnson, 1987, p. 67). Welfare pluralism or 'mixed economy of care' suggests that health and social care can be provided by various sectors—the informal, non-governmental, private and statutory (Chen, 2012; Johnson, 1987). Such financial considerations are still considered in policy formulation for senior citizens in Hong Kong due to, among other factors, the rising demand for healthcare services and escalating medical costs (Yip & Hsiao, 2006).

Concerning the first and second components of ECSM, older adults in Hong Kong can meet their care needs by utilising the resources from the informal sector (family, friends and social networks), voluntary organisations (non-governmental organisations (NGO), neighbourhood centres, ethnic and religious groups) and the commercial sector (family doctors and private companies). From an ecological perspective, families—the basic units of any societies provide immediate care and attention for their members (Chan & Philips, 2002). However, when family care can no longer support the frail or sick members, services have to be brought in (or bought) one way or the other. It is particularly the case in highly urbanised cities such as Hong Kong when young couples are engaged in full-time employment, leaving their parents or those who are in need alone or in the hands of foreign domestic helpers. As early as the 1980s, Payne suggests that care by the community is a service model involving outsiders in providing care in various way (cited in Chen, 2012). While the home environment is the location of care, community care was originally referred to domiciliary services offered by different kinds of staff. Domiciled care was advocated by the UK government under the rule of Margaret Thatcher (Chen, 2012). The current home-based services in Hong Kong including the traditional home help service and other expanded ones are models of such domiciliary services.

There is no doubt that families play a primary role in taking care of their members, the question is whether they have the resources and technical know-how to provide such support like round-the-clock care, the skills and knowledge to look after, for example, parents with cognitive impairments and other kinds of disorders. Walker (1982), one of the prominent figures in discussing community care policy in the UK, has already advocated in 1980s that *care for the community* should be provided by the government to support the caregivers (Walker, 1982).

3.3.2 Ageing in Place

The concept of community care has been discussed in the UK and British affiliates for several decades. In Australia, community health centres and geriatric centres were set up in 1970s to carry out a community health programme. The programme considers primary care as the appropriate point of entry to a comprehensive health system.

Chen (2012), however, contends that the concept of community care is not so prominent in the United States (US). Instead, key locality terms such as home-based and community-based have been adopted in social policy studies and provision of community services in the US. Other terms like long-term care (LTC) which is programme-oriented have been used. A wider concept of social support or social support network is extensively examined in the American studies in general and is applied to ageing studies in particular (Chen, 2012). The American terms which are locality-based help to clearly distinguish the place—location of care, be it a home or a community. Nevertheless, even for the term 'community-based', we need to specify what kinds of services are included. As we can see in the discussion about Hong Kong scene in the following section of this chapter, it is commonly agreed that when concept is translated to practice, community care includes home-based, centre-based and community-based services.

Though the notion of ageing in place did not gain much attention in the sector for senior citizens, its history can be traced back to the Franklin Roosevelt era in the US—the principles of ageing in place were already applied in adopting a place for older adults (Chen, 2012). The principles have been further developed in the past few decades by addressing the need to help older adults stay in the community in which they have been living. The sense of belonging and security of the older adults would not be lost due to the change of a familiar physical and social neighbourhood.

The concept of ageing in place is defined by Davey et al. (2004) as 'remaining living in the community with some level of independence, rather than in residential care' (Davey et al., 2004, p. 133). It has played a prominent role in the formulation of social policies for senior citizens in ageing societies in recent decades. He and Chou (2019) have outlined a number of studies showing the merits of this notion. Firstly, most of the of older adults tend to stay in their homes as far as possible (Frank, 2002; Gitlin, 2003). Secondly, home-dwelling older adults can have a sense of independence, autonomy and dignity, and the established social support networks and thereby their psychological and physical well-being can be improved (Keeling, 1999; Lawler, 2001). Thirdly, as discussed earlier, the cost of community living is lower than that of institutional and nursing care, and hospital services (Tinker, 1997; World Health Organization, 2007). The financial consideration is one of the key factors not only for the government but for many older community dwellers as well. In a scope review of 34 articles, Pani-Harreman et al. (2021) found that ageing in place is related to personal characteristics, place, social networks, support and technology (Pani-Harreman et al., 2021). Concerning Hong Kong, Chan and Pang (2007) have examined a range of LTC facilities and identified that ageing in place and family care were the best approach (Chan & Pang, 2007). The investigation conducted by Hui and Yu (2009) shows similar findings—senior citizens either born in Hong Kong or in the mainland tend to be more satisfied with their current residence than those with other origins (Hui & Yu, 2009).

3.3.3 The 'Place' and the Hong Kong Situation

Ageing in place, however, is by no means a homogeneous concept. One can comfortably presume that ageing in place means the older adults living in their own home at their advanced stage of life. Yet, the emergence of retirement villages and senior housing, especially promoted by the commercial sector, has made the boundary of 'the place' blurred. The situation is complex as the levels of care and attention can be varied depending on the needs and health status of the residents living in those life-care communities or continuing care (retirement) communities (CCRC) (Chen, 2012). Many older citizens choose to move to a retirement village or senior housing to prepare for their advanced age or at a time when they can manage the task of moving away from their own home and settling in the new residential setting. In the new home (purchased or rented), a range of social services, and medical and health support is available upon request, subject to the physical conditions and the needs of the residents. The new settlers can live on their own without seeking any help from the helping personnel if their health conditions allow. The purposefully built accommodation units for senior citizens can be easily converted to assisted living residences if needs arise. Alternatively, when the residents face more frailty and inability to care for themselves, they may move to another unit or wing of the campus to receive a higher level of care. There is no difference between the latter part of accommodation mode and traditional nursing homes. The only difference is the timing of moving—for those who opt for retirement villages and senior housing, they have to move in first to help settle in a new environment earlier.

The American Association of Homes for the Aging (AAHA) covers a spectrum of accommodation options for senior citizens. The AAHA is committed to support people to stay in such residence as they age. Ageing in place is sometimes called 'ageing in place through home modifications' (Chen, 2012). The ageing in place as such is based on the belief of 'naturally occurring retirement communities' which helps the individuals grow old without having to move at an advanced age or in a sick or frail condition to avoid relocation stress or transfer trauma (Chen, 2012).

Retirement villages and senior housing have been operated by NGOs and the private sector in countries like Australia and Canada for a certain period of time. Such mode of accommodation is relatively novel in Hong Kong. With reference to the concept of ageing in place, the Hong Kong Housing Society has developed the Senior Citizen Residence Scheme projects in 2003 and 2004 which provide a friendly housing option for those who are aged 60 or above. Under a 'long-lease' arrangement, the residence integrates housing, recreation and medical and care services for the residents (Hong Kong Housing Society, 2019). Though the projects are small in scale and are designed for the middle-income groups, they have offered one more ageing in place option for Hong Kong citizens. Such residences can also meet the housing needs of those who can afford, bearing in mind that the highest residential satisfaction of older dwellers in Hong Kong is related to the structural domain including interior and exterior housing characteristics, and security (Phillips et al., 2004). The research findings came as no surprise in view of the living conditions of Hong Kong citizens in a densely populated city.

The nearby city Macau also follows suit. The 2021 Policy Address of Macau SAR government has announced the construction of housing for senior citizens which is a new housing product in this city (The Government of the Macao Special Administrative Region, 2021).

3.4 Implementation of Community Care Policy in Hong Kong—Community Care and Support Services

In the third service mode of the ECSM, i.e., community care, community care services should be provided at different levels. The first level is carer support—to facilitate the Hong Kong older adults to continue to live in their own home and in the community as long as they can. The services should be provided for the senior family members and their caregivers. Hong Kong is a Chinese society by nature but the number of parents having adult children living with them is on the decreasing trend as a result of the change of cultural and traditional factors. The percentage of older adults having co-residence with their adult children dropped significantly (Census & Statistics Department, 2010; Chui, 2008). It implies that the older adults either live with their spouses or on their own, which have implications for social and health service providers.

Co-living with older parents appears to show filial piety of the children, especially the grown-up ones. Nevertheless, filial piety—a traditional and well-respected cultural belief or social value influencing parental care and parent–child relationships in Chinese societies—has to be updated or interpreted with caution. According to Chong and Liu (2016), satisfaction derived from filial piety can be conducive to well-being. Older parents enjoy the company of their children and grandchildren. At the same time, a more realistic and contemporary reciprocal notion of filial piety is identified—older parents or grandparents are prepared to give more to their children and other offspring, rather than only to receive, for example, taking care of the younger generations. Positive ageing can be achieved by such caring engagement (Chong & Liu, 2016). A report of the Hong Kong government indicates that nearly 40% of families are having grandparents as caregivers in addition to parents for their children (Family Health Service, Department of Health, 2018). The magnitude of grandparenting can easily be underestimated due to the structural change of households mentioned before. The positive ageing effects, however, are not conclusive. Such intergenerational care or skipped-generational care does not necessarily enhance the well-being of grandparent carers. They face more health, psychosocial and economic problems in the provision of care, compared with those who occasionally or seldom provide care (Chan et al., 2019).

3.4.1 Community Care Services

Hong Kong has provided family and community care since the 1970s to support older people to live in the own home independently (Chui, 2008). According to the Social Welfare Department (SWD) of the Hong Kong government, the services aimed at promoting the welfare of senior citizens provide a spectrum of services to help them live in the community as long as they wish (Social Welfare Department, 2021). In addition to the Home Help Service mentioned above, Integrated Home Care Services (IHCS) and Enhanced Home and Community Care Services (EHCCS) were introduced in 2000 and 2003 respectively. Such home-based community support are the services delivered to the homes of the older service users to support them to stay in their home and community environment or to prolong their domestic way of living as far as possible. The services which have been expanded both in scope and in professionalism including personal care, meal service, rehabilitation exercise, respite, escort service and home modifications offered by social workers and community nurses, depending on the needs and frailty of the service users. The aims of such services are to support the older service recipients to live in the home and community environment when such care cannot be rendered by their families during the day (Social Welfare Department, 2021).

In a review of scholarly work in ageing in place from 2000 to 2010, Vasunilashorn et al. (2012) found that the topics were initially related to the environment and services. With the rapid development of information and communication technology, more scholarly work touched on technology, and health and functioning of the individuals (Vasunilashorn et al., 2012). How to make use of technology and to modify the homes of the older adults to meet their changing needs is certainly on the agenda of enhancing community care services in Hong Kong.

Lai et al. (2009) particularly evaluated the effectiveness of community occupational therapy in IHCS and EHCCS. They found that the community-based therapy had contributed to functional training, modifying the home living environment, providing advice in the use of assistive devices and education for senior adults and their carers. The activities of daily living of the older adults were expanded and quality of life improved. Home visits arranged by occupational therapists were also found effective to reduce the risk of falls (Lai et al, 2009). Overall, the majority of both EHCCS services users and their caregivers agreed that the services could enhance home safety, reduce admission to hospitals, enable the older service users to stay in their home environment continuously, and lower the demand for residential care homes (Social Welfare Department, 2008, pp. 27–32).

3.4.2 *Community Support Services*

In addition to home-based services, centre-based services are run by a number of centres including Social Centres, Neighbourhood Centres and District Community Centres. The centre services are aimed at providing community support for older service users and their carers in the local communities, and at neighbourhood and district levels. Counselling service, educational and developmental activities are organised in these centres (Social Welfare Department, 2021).

The spirit of community care or ageing in place is to provide a range of services for older individuals and their caregivers so that older adults can live in a physical and social environment which they are familiar and prefer. However, family support, home-based or community-based care may come to a point that the services can no longer cater for the deteriorating health needs of the older individuals or the needed support has already gone beyond the means of the carers. Residential care is then required. In Hong Kong, however, there is a long waiting list for the subsidised nursing homes, and care and attention homes (Chan & Philips, 2002; The Government of the Hong Kong Special Administrative Region, 2021). For those who are in need and cannot afford to wait, they can go to the non-subsidised sector which often offers more costly but poorer quality of residential care. Under such circumstances, the community care or ageing in place services in fact play a prominent role in supporting and sustaining a quality community living for older adults in Hong Kong before they no longer benefit from it. Critics in Hong Kong therefore argue that community care or ageing in place is a solution for Hong Kong older adults due to the shortage of residential care in this city (Chan & Philips, 2002). Furthermore, a number of gerontologists criticise that family self-reliance has dominated policy formulation in Hong Kong as the government tends to maintain its role in providing a basic safety net to the neediest individuals only. Promoting community care and ageing in place cannot address the imbalance in LTC and help those with dependency. They advocate for social structural changes so that older adults can have more productive participation and remain independent for as long as possible (Cheng et al., 2013).

3.5 Implementation of Primary Healthcare in Hong Kong

Community care is aimed at supporting older adults to live in the community as far as possible. Apart from social welfare services, medical and healthcare provided by the private and public sectors are an integral part in such community-based services. The private general practitioners, Chinese medicine practitioners, family doctors and other professionals located in the geographical community of the older adults provide the first level of care when assistance is needed. Following the release of the 'Primary Care Development in Hong Kong: Strategy Document' in 2010, one of the significant healthcare movements in Hong Kong in the last decade is to promote primary care in the communities with a view of reforming the healthcare system, i.e., reducing the utilisation of hospital services (Food & Health Bureau, 2010).

In primary healthcare, cross-sectoral and inter-organisational coordination should be enhanced. More collaboration and better integration of social welfare and health services is particularly needed, bearing in mind a number of healthcare professionals including nurses and therapists are employed by social welfare agencies. Through the provision of comprehensive, holistic, preventive and continuing healthcare services in the communities, the awareness in disease prevention and self-health management of older adults will be strengthened. Greater support for individuals with chronic diseases will be provided to prevent unnecessary and immature hospitalisation and institutionalisation.

It is planned that community-based district health centres (DHC)—the first point of contact in a healthcare process, will be set up in all districts in Hong Kong. The Chief Executive of the Hong Kong government announced in 2017 that the government is determined to step up efforts to promote individual and community involvement, enhance coordination among various medical and social sectors and strengthen district-level primary healthcare services. Through these measures, the government aims to encourage the public to take precautionary measures against diseases, enhance their capability in self-care, change the current focus of healthcare services from treatment to prevention and reduce the demand for hospitalisation (The Hong Kong Special Administrative Region of the People's Republic of China, 2017). Operating through district-based medical-social collaboration and public–private partnership, the DHCs will provide services in health promotion, health assessment, chronic disease management and community rehabilitation (The Hong Kong Special Administrative Region of the People's Republic of China, 2018). Though the primary healthcare is not solely for the senior citizens, older adults who very often have more medical and health needs will benefit from such community initiatives.

On the other hand, the Department of Health (DH) of the Hong Kong government adopts a healthy life course approach according to the developmental needs of Hong Kong citizens. Concerning the senior target group, the DH provides a range of services such as health assessment, counselling, health education and promotion, disease prevention and curative treatment to cater to the needs of this particular age group. The aim of these services is to address the multiple health needs of the citizens by providing integrated primary healthcare services to them. Preventive, promotive and curative services are rendered from a family medicine perspective using a multi-disciplinary team approach (Department of Health, 2019).

3.6 Conclusion

Like all other developed cities, Hong Kong faces the issue of ageing. What made the demographic, health and social issue particularly challenging is the lack of land resources. Building and establishing massive homes of senior citizens is not a simple task. Even if such residential homes are available, whether placing older adults in such a care setting is subject to discussion. The benefits of supporting older adults to live in their own home and a community they are familiar with is well-evidenced. To provide an option for residential care and to solve the shortage of such services, the Hong Kong government has adopted a community care policy for caring the individuals in their advanced stages of life. The latest development is that more healthcare services have been incorporated in such community care and support services to meet the more frailty and health needs. It also goes hand in hand with the Hong Kong government's recent endeavours in introducing primary healthcare, and integrating the medical-social welfare services for senior citizens.

References

Census and Statistics Department. (2010). *Thematic household survey report no. 44—Relationships among family members.* https://www.statistics.gov.hk/pub/B11302442010XXXXB0100.pdf

Census and Statistics Department. (2020a). *Hong Kong life tables 2014–2069.* https://www.censtatd.gov.hk/en/data/stat_report/product/B1120016/att/B11200162020aXXXXB0100.pdf

Census and Statistics Department. (2020b). *Hong Kong population projections 2020b–2069.* https://www.statistics.gov.hk/pub/B1120015082020bXXXXB0100.pdf

Census and Statistics Department. (2021). *Hong Kong in figures 2021 edition.* https://www.censtatd.gov.hk/en/data/stat_report/product/B1010006/att/B10100062021AN21B0100.pdf

Chan, C. M. A., & Liang, S. E. (2013). Active aging: Policy framework and applications to promote older adult participation in Hong Kong. *Ageing International, 38*, 28–42. https://doi.org/10.1007/s12126-012-9166-z

Chan, C. M. A., & Philips, D. R. (2002). Policy on ageing and long-term care in Hong Kong. In D. R. Phillips, & A. C. M. Chan (Eds.), *Ageing and long-term care: National policies in the Asia-Pacific* (pp. 23–67). Institute of Southeast Asian Studies. https://doi.org/10.1355/9789812307163-006

Chan, H. M., & Pang, S. (2007). Long-term care: Dignity, autonomy, family integrity, and social sustainability: The Hong Kong experience. *Journal of Medicine and Philosophy, 32*(5), 401–424. https://doi.org/10.1080/03605310701631661

Chan, K. L., Chen, M., Lo, K. M. C., Chen, Q., Kelley, S. J., & Ip, P. (2019). The effectiveness of interventions for grandparents raising grandchildren: A meta-analysis. *Research on Social Work Practice, 29*(6), 607–617. https://doi.org/10.1177/1049731518798470

Chen, S. (2012). Historical and global perspectives on social policy and "aging in community." *Ageing International, 37*, 1–15. https://doi.org/10.1007/s12126-011-9136-x

Cheng, S. T., Lum, T., Lam, L. C. W., & Fung, H. H. (2013). Hong Kong: Embracing a fast aging society with limited welfare. *The Gerontologist, 53*(4), 527–553. https://doi.org/10.1093/geront/gnt017

Chong, A. M. L., & Liu, S. (2016). Receive or give? Contemporary views among middle-aged and older Chinese adults on filial piety and well-being in Hong Kong. *Asia Pacific Journal of Social Work and Development, 26*(1), 2–14. https://doi.org/10.1080/02185385.2015.1131619

Chui, E. (2008). Ageing in place in Hong Kong—Challenges and opportunities in a capitalist Chinese city. *Ageing International, 32*, 167–182. https://doi.org/10.1007/s12126-008-9015-2

Chui, E. (2012). *Elderly learning in Chinese communities: China, Hong Kong, Taiwan and Singapore.* In G. M. Boulton-Lewis, & M. Tam (Eds.), *Active Ageing, Active Learning. Education in the Asia-Pacific Region: Issues, Concerns and Prospects* (pp. 141–161). Springer. https://doi.org/10.1007/978-94-007-2111-1_9

Davey, J., de Joux, V., Nana, G. & Arcus, J. (2004). *Accommodation options for older people in New Zealand*. New Zealand Institute for Research on Ageing. https://thehub.swa.govt.nz/resources/accommodation-options-for-older-people-in-aotearoanew-zealand/

Department of Health. (2019). *Elderly health service*. https://www.dh.gov.hk/english/main/main_ehs/main_ehs.html

Elder Academy. (2020). *About elder academy*. https://www.elderacademy.org.hk/en/aboutea/index.html

Elderly Commission. (2017). *Elderly services programme plan*. https://www.elderlycommission.gov.hk/en/download/library/ESPP_Final_Report_Eng.pdf

Elderly Commission. (2021). *Introduction*. https://www.elderlycommission.gov.hk/en/About_Us/Introduction.html

Family Health Service, Department of Health. (2018). *The parenting practices in Hong Kong: A community survey on parents of 4-year-old children*. https://www.fhs.gov.hk/english/archive/files/reports/report-pp-2014_full.pdf

Food and Health Bureau. (2010). *Primary care development in Hong Kong: Strategy document*. https://www.fhb.gov.hk/download/press_and_publications/otherinfo/101231_primary_care/e_strategy_doc.pdf

Frank, J. B. (2002). *The paradox of ageing in place in assisted living*. Praeger; Illustrated edition.

Gitlin, L. (2003). Conducting research on home environments: Lessons learned and new directions. *The Gerontologist, 43*(5), 628–637. https://doi.org/10.1093/geront/43.5.628

Han, J., Chan, E. H. W., Qian, Q. K., & Yung, E. H. K. (2021). Achieving sustainable urban development with an ageing population: An "age- friendly city and community" approach. *Sustainability, 13*(15), 8614. https://doi.org/10.3390/su13158614

He, A. J., & Chou, K. L. (2019). Long-term care service needs and planning for the future: A study of middle-aged and older adults in Hong Kong. *Ageing & Society, 39*(2), 221–253. https://doi.org/10.1017/S0144686X17000824

Hong Kong Housing Society. (2019). *Senior citizen residences scheme*. https://www.hkhs.com/en/our-business/elderly-housing/senior-citizen

Hui, E. C. M., & Yu, K. H. (2009). Residential mobility and aging population in Hong Kong. *Habitat International, 33*(1), 10–14. https://doi.org/10.1016/j.habitatint.2008.02.001

Johnson, N. (1987). *The welfare state in transition: The theory and practice of welfare pluralism*. Wheatsheaf Books Ltd.

Keeling, S. (1999). Ageing in (a New Zealand) place: Ethnography, policy and practice. *Social Policy Journal of New Zealand,* 13, 95–114. https://www.msd.govt.nz/about-msd-and-our-work/publications-resources/journals-and-magazines/social-policy-journal/spj13/ageing-in-place-ethnography-policy-practice.html

Kwok, Y. C. J. (2013). Projecting sustainable living environment for an ageing society: The case of Hong Kong. *Procedia Environmental Sciences, 17*, 675–684. https://doi.org/10.1016/j.proenv.2013.02.084

Lai, W. L., Chan, J. P. Y., Choi, P. K. K., Ngai, L. C. T., Mar, C. S. F., Chan, E. Y. L., Lam, P. Y. P., & Lam, F. N. Y. (2009). Occupational therapy in the integrated elderly and community support services for the elderly in Hong Kong. *Hong Kong Journal of Occupational Therapy, 19*(1), 27–30. https://doi.org/10.1016/S1569-1861(09)70041-5

Lawler, K. (2001). *Ageing in place: Coordinating housing and health care provision for America's growing elderly population*. Joint Center for Housing Studies of Harvard University and Neighbourhood Reinvestment Corporation. https://www.jchs.harvard.edu/sites/default/files/media/imp/lawler_w01-13.pdf

Loo, B. P. Y., Lam, W. W. Y., Mahendran, R., & Katagiri, K. (2017). How is the neighborhood environment related to the health of seniors living in Hong Kong, Singapore, and Tokyo? Some insights for promoting aging in place. *Annals of the American Association of Geographers, 107*(4), 812–828. https://doi.org/10.1080/24694452.2016.1271306

Pani-Harreman, K. E., Bours, G. J. J. W., Zander, I., Kempen, G. I. J. M., & van Duren, J. M. A. (2021). Definitions, key themes and aspects of 'ageing in place': A scoping review. *Ageing and Society, 41*(9), 2026–2059. https://doi.org/10.1017/S0144686X20000094

Phillips, D. R., Siu, O. L., Yeh, A. G. O., & Cheng, K. H. C. (2004). Factors influencing older persons' residential satisfaction in big and densely populated cities in Asia: A case study in Hong Kong. *Ageing International, 29*, 46–70. https://doi.org/10.1007/s12126-004-1009-0

Social Welfare Department. (2008). *Social Welfare Department review (2005–2006 and 2006–2007).* https://www.swd.gov.hk/doc/annreport/SWD_e-review_en_w.pdf

Social Welfare Department. (2021). *Community support services for the elderly.* https://www.swd.gov.hk/en/index/site_pubsvc/page_elderly/sub_csselderly/id_introduction/

Tam, M. (2011). Active ageing, active learning: Elder learning in Hong Kong. In G. M. Boulton-Lewis, & M. Tam (Eds.), *Active Ageing, Active Learning. Education in the Asia-Pacific Region: Issues, Concerns and Prospects* (pp. 161–174). Springer. https://doi.org/10.1007/978-94-007-2111-1_10

The Government of the Hong Kong Special Administrative Region. (2021). *LCQ20: Residential care homes for elderly.* https://www.info.gov.hk/gia/general/202103/17/P2021031700222.htm

The Government of the Macao Special Administrative Region. (2021). *Highlights of policy address of fiscal year of 2021 of the Macao Special Administrative Region (MSAR).* https://www.policyaddress.gov.mo/data/policyAddress/2021/en/2021_summary_e.pdf

The Hong Kong Special Administrative Region of the People's Republic of China. (2017). *The Chief Executive's 2017 Policy Address.* https://www.policyaddress.gov.hk/2017/eng/index.html

The Hong Kong Special Administrative Region of the People's Republic of China. (2018). *The Chief Executive's 2018 Policy Address.* https://www.policyaddress.gov.hk/2018/eng/

Tinker, A. (1997). Housing for elderly people. *Reviews in Clinical Gerontology, 7*(2), 171–176. https://doi.org/10.1017/S095925989700018X

United Nations. (2019). *World population ageing 2019 highlights.* https://www.un.org/en/development/desa/population/publications/pdf/ageing/WorldPopulationAgeing2019-Highlights.pdf

Vasunilashorn, S., Steinman, B. A., Liebig, P. S., & Pynoos, J. (2012). Aging in place: Evolution of a research topic whose time has come. *Journal of Aging Research, 2012*, 1–6. https://doi.org/10.1155/2012/120952

Walker, A. (Ed.). (1982). *Community care: The family, the state and social policy.* Blackwell Martin Robertson.

Wen, Z., Mok, K. H., & Amoah, P. A. (2021). Productive engagement and ageing in productivist welfare regimes: Questing for an age-friendly city in Hong Kong. *Ageing and Society, 1–23.* https://doi.org/10.1017/S0144686X21000167

Wong, M., Chau, P. H., Cheung, F., Phillips, D. R., & Woo, J. (2015). Comparing the age-friendliness of different neighbourhoods using district surveys: An example from Hong Kong. *PLoS ONE, 10*(7), e0131526. https://doi.org/10.1371/journal.pone.0131526

World Health Organization. (2002). *Active aging: A policy framework.* https://apps.who.int/iris/handle/10665/67215

World Health Organization. (2007). *Global age-friendly cities: A guide.* https://apps.who.int/iris/handle/10665/43755

Yip, W., & Hsiao, W. (2006). A systematic approach to reforming Hong Kong's health financing: The Harvard proposal. In G. M. Leung & J. Bacon-Shone (Eds.), *Hong Kong's health system—Reflections, perspectives and visions* (pp. 447–459). Hong Kong University Press.

Chapter 4
Needs of Care and Service Gaps in Primary Care for Older Adults in Hong Kong

Tommy K. C. Ng, Ben Yuk Fai Fong, and Hilary H. L. Yee

Abstract Long waiting time of inpatient and outpatient services as well as shortage of healthcare manpower and hospital beds are noticeable issues affecting the whole quality of care. Over-reliance on secondary care can lead to a heavy burden on the healthcare system. Older adults are more likely to use acute-centric care because of their financial affordability. In Hong Kong, the charges of accident and emergency service in public hospitals is only HK$180 for residents, and so the patients, particularly the older adults of lower socioeconomic status, would like to utilise this service for all their health problems. To relieve over-reliance of secondary care services, meeting the needs of care for older adults is an essential pathway that identifies the service gaps to facilitate improvement of care delivery. The Hong Kong government is working towards a well-developed primary care to optimise the overall delivery of healthcare service because sufficient preventive service, such as health screening and immunisation, can result in reduced utilisation of secondary care. Thus, a strong primary care is more likely to achieve better population health despite the spending on health needs would increase. Likewise, understanding the healthcare needs and service gap of the older adults can make good use of the healthcare spending to obtain effective and practical overcomes. Furthermore, it is important to ensure healthcare needs of the older adults can be met so as to reach health equity. Besides, affordable and accessible primary care service for older adults is utterly vital for the development of a promising healthcare system in Hong Kong.

Keywords Primary care · Needs of care · Older adults · Delivery of healthcare service

T. K. C. Ng (✉) · B. Y. F. Fong
School of Professional Education and Executive Development, College of Professional and Continuing Education, The Hong Kong Polytechnic University, Kowloon, Hong Kong, China
e-mail: tommy.ng@cpce-polyu.edu.hk

H. H. L. Yee
The Hong Kong Polytechnic University, Kowloon, Hong Kong, China
e-mail: hiulam.yee@polyu.edu.hk

V. T. S. Law and B. Y. F. Fong (eds.), *Ageing with Dignity in Hong Kong and Asia*, Quality of Life in Asia 16, https://doi.org/10.1007/978-981-19-3061-4_4

4.1 Introduction

Ageing population is one of the major global challenges and issues, and will aggravate the demand on social and health services. It is estimated that the older adults population would be accounting for about 15.7% of the total population by 2021. According to the Census and Statistics Department (2017), the projected life expectancies from 2016 to 2066 for male and female would be raised from 81.3 to 87.1 and 87.3 to 93.1, respectively. The percentage of aged 65 years and above would be doubled from 16 to 34% in this period. However, total fertility rate is projected to decrease from nearly 1200 live births per thousand women in 2016 to less than 1170 in 2066. Older adults population has greater needs for healthcare as 75% of older adults aged 65 years old or above are suffering from at least one chronic disease such as diabetes, heart disease or chronic bronchitis (Elderly Commission, 2021). Moreover, increased longevity would be accompanied by a decline in functional capacity and an increase in care needs (Yu et al., 2019). The older age group occupies more than 46% of inpatient hospital beds, and spends six times more bed-days than the younger group (Elderly Commission, 2021; Food & Health Bureau, 2010). It reflects that ageing issues would become severe in Hong Kong, and the ageing population induces rapid increase in demand for inpatient service, causing a heavy burden to the healthcare system (Kwok et al., 2017). Although ageing population only moderately contributes to the growth of healthcare expenditure on acute care, it strongly increases the long-term care expenditures (de Meijer et al., 2013).

The healthcare system in Hong Kong encompasses the dual track of public and private sectors that operate independently. The public sector serves as a safety net for the entire community by providing affordable services while the private sector provides an alternative for civilians. Both public and private sectors shared nearly equal total health expenditure from 2006 to 2017, with Gross Domestic Product 3.2% and 3.0%, respectively (Hong Kong's Domestic Health Accounts, 2019). In public expenditure, inpatient accounted for 32% while outpatient curative care accounted for 26% in 2018/19 (Food & Health Bureau, 2020). Public health expenditure has increased by more than doubled, 38 to 85 billion dollars, from 2006 to 2017. For private health expenditure, outpatient care, inpatient care and medical goods accounted for 38%, 24% and 19%, respectively. Although health expenditure has continuously increased since 1989, such growth has not reflected that the needs of an ageing population have been effectively and adequately addressed. Nevertheless, the majority of the expenditure has gone to public hospitals but very little on primary care, such as long-term care and preventive care. Since the public sector is heavily subsidised while private practitioners in the community are expensive, the general public, especially the older adults, rely on the services of public sector causing over-reliance. Although the healthcare system is shared equally by the public and private sectors, inequality in primary care exists which caused over-reliance on public health services.

The demand for healthcare service exceeds the supply as reflected by the longer waiting time for hospital services and shortage of healthcare professionals. It is noted that public hospitals provide care to more than 90% of inpatients by only 40% of doctors in Hong Kong (Our Hong Kong Foundation, 2018). The waiting time for semi-urgent and non-urgent patients in accident and emergency services and specialist outpatient services in public hospitals increased by 20 to 40 minutes and 25 weeks in average respectively (Legislative Council Secretariat, 2018). It is noted that the longest waiting time of new cases of otorhinolaryngology and optometry are 148 and 134 weeks respectively (Hospital Authority, 2021). Together with the estimated shortfall of more than 1000 doctors and 1600 nurses by 2030, massive pressure would be added to meeting public healthcare needs (The Government of the Hong Kong Special Administrative Region, 2017).

In addition, focusing on hospital acute-centric care leads to various issues, including long waiting time for non-urgent patients at not only accident and emergency department but also at specialist outpatient clinics. Therefore, the traditional model of financing and delivery of care has created huge problems in terms of accessibility, equity, sustainability and patients' best interests, while a powerful primary healthcare will lead to better health of the population at lower cost, relieve the over-reliance of the service of public sector and result in greater user satisfaction (Atun, 2004; Fong et al., 2020). To ease the burden of public health sector from an increasing ageing population, strengthening the provision of primary care is the most cost-effective way (Atun, 2004; Fong et al., 2020). Evidence has shown that primary care could bring positive health outcomes with lower cost as it emphasises more on prevention and continuous management of chronic conditions at the first level. Moreover, the convenient primary care services can significantly lead to a decline of visits to emergency department (Pinchbeck, 2019). Hence, emphasis on primary care can alleviate the financial burden of the healthcare system. Therefore, it is imperative to evaluate the needs of care and service gaps for older adults in Hong Kong.

4.2 Primary Care Services in Hong Kong

In an effective healthcare system, primary care is indispensable and essential. High quality primary care is associated with several positive outcomes, including improved health outcomes, reduced mortality and hospitalisation, improved preventive care and equitable distribution of health (Chung et al., 2019). Private healthcare service providers provide higher quality of healthcare, but more expensive services compared to public ones. Therefore, residents are used to using a combination of services from both public and private sectors to meet a wide range of healthcare needs (Chung et al., 2019).

To enhance primary healthcare for the older adults and their self-care ability, the Elderly Health Service, including elderly health centres and visiting health teams, was established in 1998. There are 18 elderly health centres operating in all 18 administrative districts of Hong Kong. Elderly health centres provide primary care service, such as health assessment, physical examination, curative treatment, health education and promotion services, to the members of the centres. Older adults who are aged

65 and above can apply for membership of the elderly health centres (Department of Health, 2019). The elderly health centres provide more opportunities for older adults to utilise primary care services. Nevertheless, the waiting time for membership at these centres ranges from 9 to 42 months, and so the older adults cannot readily receive updated health information or health assessment at all times (Elderly Health Service, 2021).

To provide accessible public primary care services for the older adults and the financially vulnerable, the Hospital Authority (HA) of Hong Kong manages more than 70 general outpatient clinics covering different districts. For patients with stable conditions, the clinics will arrange the next appointment and the patients only need to return to the clinic for follow-up consultation next time. For patients with episodic disease, they are required to reserve consultation timeslots through the telephone appointment system or mobile application. According to the Hospital Authority (2020), there were more than 6,000,000 primary care attendances, including general outpatient clinics and family medicine specialist clinics under HA in 2019 to 2020. It means the number of daily primary care attendance in the public sector is increased by 16,000 from 2019 to 2020. However, about one-third of the doctors working in the general outpatient clinics do not have formal training in family medicine (Wong et al., 2010). Apart from public general outpatient clinics, patients can receive primary care by choosing private service and pay either on their own pocket or by private insurance. The major supplier of primary care in Hong Kong is the private sector, which provides about 70% of outpatient consultations (Wong et al., 2010).

The Hong Kong Government has strived to reform the healthcare system by enhancing primary care development since 2008, from introducing 'Primary Care Development in Hong Kong: Strategy Document' in 2010, initiating Elderly Health Care Voucher Pilot Scheme and Elderly Vaccination Subsidy Scheme, to establishing District Health Centres (DHCs) across Hong Kong in 2019. To facilitate the use of primary care in the private sector, the Government has changed the Elderly Health Care Voucher Scheme to a recurrent programme since 2014. Each eligible older adult receives an annual voucher amount of HK$2,000 to seek medical consultations with private doctors. The older adults can accumulate a maximum amount of HK$8,000 of vouchers. In 2019, eligible older adults had additional voucher amount HK$2,000 on optometry services in order to encourage the use on other primary care services.

To enhance and strengthen the use of district primary care services in Hong Kong, the first DHC in Hong Kong was established in Kwai Tsing in September 2019. The centre provides services in health promotion, health assessment, chronic disease management, rehabilitation and other preventive services for citizens living in the Kwai Tsing district, which covers 6.7% of the total population of Hong Kong. Most of the charges of service for chronic disease management programme are HK$150 except medical consultation, which is the basic medical consultation fee minus HK$250. Health promotion activities and nurse counselling and education are free of charge. The reasonable price of various primary care services may attract more citizens to utilise the primary care services. Two more district health centres at Sham Shui Po and Wong Tai Sin would be operated before the end of June 2021 and the end of June 2022, respectively.

4.3 Assessing the Needs of Primary Care in Hong Kong

Undoubtedly, ageing population is one of the major concerns in Hong Kong. The elderly dependency ratio, meaning the number of aged 65 and above supported by 1000 persons aged between 15 and 64, was increased from 172 in 2009 to 249 in 2019 and it is showing an increasing trend (Census & Statistics Department, 2020). It reflects the decrease in labour force while the economic and social burdens to the government are monstrous. On the other hand, older adults who experience various chronic health conditions may require long-term care because of the chronic diseases, such as diabetes, hypertension and dementia. According to Centre for Health Protection (2017), the prevalence of hypertension and diabetes among those aged 65 to 84 was 64.8% and 25.4%. From a study examining the health profiles of patients aged 60 or above in primary care of Hong Kong, the patients had 4.1 chronic conditions and 2.5 medications on average (Zhang et al., 2020). 75% and 46% of the patients have hypertension and dyslipidaemia (Zhang et al., 2020). The complications of hypertension and diabetes can lead to other chronic diseases. Early prevention, diagnosis and treatment can reduce the risk of long-term complications. Therefore, primary care services for older people should focus on health education about the awareness, prevention and management of the chronic diseases. Moreover, more than half of the persons aged 60 or above anticipated the needs for long-term care services (He & Chou, 2019).

To understand the needs of primary care, the experience of primary care services have to be assessed. Primary Care Needs Assessment Tool (PCAT), developed by John Hopkins Primary Care Centre, is designed for assessing the patients' experience of primary care. It measures attributes of primary care relating to organisation and service delivery at the population level. There are four core dimensions: (1) *first contact* is the accessibility to and use of primary care services in first place, (2) *continuity* means the longitudinal use of a regular source of primary care over time, (3) *coordination* is the interpersonal linkage of care between providers for their health problems, (4) *comprehensiveness* refers to the availability of the ranges of preventative services. There are also three derivate dimensions: (1) *family centredness* means the inclusion of family members during assessment and treatment planning, (2) *community orientation* refers to service provider's knowledge of the community's characteristics and health needs, (3) *cultural competence* refers to patient's willingness to recommend primary care providers to others (Wei et al., 2015; Yang et al., 2013). Adopted in different healthcare systems across countries, PCAT has been translated into different languages and validated into different versions.

A comparison study adopting PACT was conducted to compare the quality of public primary care between Hong Kong and Shanghai (Wei et al., 2015). 1994 and 811 respondents from Hong Kong and Shanghai were recruited respectively to assess their perceived quality of primary care with respect to socioeconomic characteristics and health status. It was found that Hong Kong respondents were less likely to see a doctor on the same day when getting sick and less likely to consult the same doctors over time as the appointment system in government outpatient clinics does not have such function (Wei et al., 2015). In addition, government outpatient clinics in Hong Kong were reported to provide rather limited preventive services such as vaccination and follow-up care for people with hypertension and diabetes, compared to wider ranges of services in Shanghai such as mental healthcare and communicable disease prevention. These resulted in lower score in first contact accessibility, continuity and comprehensiveness domains in PACT. Regarding community orientation and cultural competence, traditional Chinese medicine (TCM) in Hong Kong has limited integration with government outpatient clinics and public TCM clinics. However, referral to specialists and service coordination scored higher in Hong Kong than Shanghai, mainly due to the management of the HA.

Although there are some elderly health centres and general outpatient clinics established across 18 districts in Hong Kong, the accessibility of primary care services can still be further improved. Transportation is one of the determinants of accessibility of primary care services. Older adults are most likely to take public transports, such as a bus and minibus, to the primary care service centres but the safety of the public transport is the concern for the older adults (Woo et al., 2013). The affordability of public transport is acceptable for older adults because they only need to pay HK$2 for any trip of public transport. Nevertheless, older adults may not afford the self-financing barrier-free transport, including Rehabuses and barrier-free taxis, which they need for reasons of mobility impairment (Woo et al., 2013). Likewise, some older adults who pay by themselves consider the total consultation charges in public health sector as 'expensive' (consultation fee, drug costs and travelling costs). The median out-of-pocket health cost among the patients aged 60 or above utilising public primary care clinics is HK$1,000 (Zhang et al., 2020). Therefore, accessibility of primary care services and affordability of expenses derived by the services among older adults needs to be addressed.

4.4 Service Gaps in Primary Care in Hong Kong

There is inequality in receiving primary care under the mixed public–private healthcare system, reflected from studies conducted in Hong Kong with the use of PACT. People with higher income experienced significantly better overall primary care quality compared to people with the lowest income, indicating that low-income citizens cannot obtain equal primary care (Owolabi et al., 2013). Consistent with studies that showed people with higher incomes had better utilisation of primary care, higher income was associated with higher first contact utilisation and comprehensiveness PACT scores (Owolabi et al., 2013). Wong et al. (2010) evaluated the performance of primary care in general outpatient clinics and private providers by adopting PACT Adult Edition in Hong Kong to find out the experience of primary care. It was found that those who received primary care in private general practices (GPs) had better experience than in general outpatient clinics (GOPCs), particularly in the domains' first contact and continuity of care.

In addition, the younger, richer, less chronically ill and more educated residents utilised services in private GPs more often (Wong et al., 2010). Similarly, 68.6% of respondents had regular utilisation of primary care in the private sector, while those who were older, more income-poor, more deprived and more multimorbid visited the public sector for primary care (Chung et al., 2019). Although private care is more convenient, timely and of better quality, affordability is the main concern and becomes a barrier for the older adults who normally opt for public services (Liu et al., 2012). People with long-term chronic diseases tend to receive care in the public sector as repeated visits in the private will cause heavy financial burdens in the long run. Private insurance also plays a role in affecting first contact utilisation and comprehensiveness of care compared to people who only pay out of pocket. The choice of primary care service provider becomes dependent on the ability to pay and resulted in utilisation biased towards the higher income group. Older adult is the vulnerable group with comorbidity of chronic diseases but also financially unaffordable to rely on private primary care sources.

Although the public healthcare system in Hong Kong brings excellent health outcomes, the mixed public–private financing and service delivery in terms of access, coordination and affordability bear criticisms and build service gaps (Wong et al., 2017). Hong Kong people are more likely to have access to same-day or next-day medical care, but due to the 'doctor-shopping' culture and the overemphasis on acute episodic care, only 60% of the population consult a regular healthcare service (Ho, 2020). The Hong Kong Government has enhanced the delivery of primary care services by introducing different health programmes and subsidy schemes, but Hong Kong remains the lowest rate of regular source of care, including regular doctor or clinic, and the highest rate of cost-related accessibility problems, compared to other developed countries (Wong et al., 2017). Many Hong Kong people are yet to be familiar with the principles of family medicine or the importance of primary care. Therefore, the existing health programmes seem ineffective in improving the utilisation of primary care, for which much more work needs to be done as it is a much less costly, holistic and humanistic care to all people in the population. It enhances the wish of ageing with dignity among the older adults as community empowerment is a core objective.

The launching of a recurrent programme called Elderly Health Care Voucher Scheme in 2014 aims to provide partial subsidy and encourage the use of private primary care service. But the effectiveness of supplementing existing public healthcare services remains relatively low. Although the voucher scheme provides financial incentives for older people to choose primary care services in the private sector, the scheme was not found to be significantly associated with a reduction in the utilisation of general outpatient clinics, hospitalisation and accident and emergency in the public sector (Cheung et al., 2020; Yeoh et al., 2020). It indicates that the older adults still opt for public health services even they have used the elderly healthcare vouchers. Thus, the voucher scheme may not have great impact to alleviate the burden of the public health sector. In addition, the older adults perceived the scheme as a social welfare but not an initiative to choose private healthcare services such as prevention or disease management on top of the public primary healthcare (Lai et al., 2018). Instead, they use the vouchers on other purposes such as spending on spectacles when visiting optometrists (Lai et al., 2018). Some of them use the vouchers for one-off purpose like expensive magnetic resonance imaging scan. The lack of planning on health precaution by a proper utilisation of the vouchers may explain why there were 182,000 older adults who had forfeited their voucher amounts due to exceeded accumulation limit (The Government of the Hong Kong Special Administrative Region, 2020). Therefore, the scheme has a huge gap to effectively promote the utilisation of primary care among the older adults, particularly in the private sector. Moreover, the government offers Vaccination Subsidy Scheme, which provides subsidised seasonal influenza and pneumococcal vaccination to eligible residents aged 50 years and above, but the participation rate could not reach even 50% (Centre for Health Protection, 2021). All these schemes and programmes have indicated that primary care services in Hong Kong are neither satisfactory nor effective, particularly among the older population. A systems approach in reviewing the healthcare system is urgent to seriously consider if the existing structure of having a health department and a hospital authority under the bureau still works in the local settings because the last restructuring took place 30 years ago with the hope to better manage public hospitals under one organisation. Experience of both the public and health professionals is not positive. Simple performance indicators are not favourable and there has been voices suggesting to reform the structure with a primary care-led system.

4.5 Concluding Remarks

Hong Kong, a developed and busy metropolitan city, is facing a challenge of improving the fragmented and inefficient primary care system. The Hong Kong government has implemented various programmes and schemes to promote primary care service, with a hope to shift the demand and pressure of the public healthcare system to the private sector and to upgrade the quality of care and life among older adults with dignity. Nevertheless, the implemented programmes and schemes have not effectively addressed the needs of the older adults in Hong Kong. There are many elderly health centres, clinics and district health centres in Hong Kong, but they have not fulfilled the needs of the older adults. For health promotion, education and prevention, it is insufficient and rarely found in the public primary care services, because the public sector focuses more on secondary care and disease treatment. The establishment of district health centres may facilitate and encourage the citizens to attend the health promotion and education services at the district level but there will be only three DHCs by 2022.

Furthermore, the effectiveness of Elderly Health Voucher Scheme is doubtful. The scheme is intended to encourage older adults to use private primary care services. However, the attendance of accident and emergency services among older adults aged

65 or above was increased by 18% from 2008 to 2017 (Legislative Council Secretariat, 2019). The semi-urgent and non-urgent attendance to accident and emergency department remained more than 60% in 2017–2018. It also shows that the older adults will still prefer public health services if they need to seek medical consultation. Therefore, it may not be enough to promote primary care in the private sector with financial incentives only (Liu et al., 2012). Public education of the importance of primary care and health prevention is utterly essential and indispensable in addressing the over-reliance on secondary care, particularly among the older adults in Hong Kong.

The health expenditure in Hong Kong was increased over the past decade but the long waiting time and overcrowding of accident and emergency department have not been solved. The preventable or avoidable hospital admissions could not be found with the greater investment in primary care (van Gool et al., 2021). To achieve a better primary care performance, understanding and meeting the needs of the population is fundamental to narrow the service gap of primary care. In summary, service gaps include the affordability to access primary care service, insufficient intention to use a regular source of primary care and the availability of the ranges of preventative services. To encourage older adults to use a regular source of primary care, the government should pay more attention and efforts to educate and promote the importance of primary care, otherwise the investment to primary care will be worthless.

Acknowledgements The work described in this paper was partially supported by a grant from the Research Grants Council of the Hong Kong Special Administrative Region, China (Project Reference No.: UGC/IDS24/18).

References

Atun, R. (2004). *What are the advantages and disadvantages of restructuring a health care system to be more focused on primary care services?* Copenhagen, WHO Regional Office for Europe, Health Evidence Network report. http://www.euro.who.int/document/e82997.pdf

Census and Statistics Department. (2017). *Hong Kong population projections 2017–2066. Hong Kong: Hong Kong Special Administrative Region Government*. https://www.statistics.gov.hk/pub/B1120015072017XXXXB0100.pdf

Census and Statistics Department. (2020). *Hong Kong annual digest of statistics*. https://www.statistics.gov.hk/pub/B10100032020AN20B0100.pdf

Centre for Health Protection. (2017). *Report of population health survey 2014/2015*. https://www.chp.gov.hk/files/pdf/dh_phs_2014_15_full_report_eng.pdf

Centre for Health Protection. (2021). *Statistics on vaccination programmes in the past 3 years*. https://www.chp.gov.hk/en/features/102226.html

Cheung, J. T., Wong, S. Y., Chan, D. C., Zhang, D., Luk, L. H., Chau, P. Y., Yip, B. H., Lee, E. K., Wong, E. L., & Yeoh, E. K. (2020). Can voucher scheme enhance primary care provision for older adults: Cross-sectional study in Hong Kong. *BMC Geriatrics, 20*(1), 1–8. https://doi.org/10.1186/s12877-020-01851-x

Chung, R. Y. N., Chan, D., Chau, N. N. S., Huang, S., Wong, H., & Wong, S. Y. S. (2019). Poverty affects access to regular source of primary care among the general population in Hong Kong. *Social Policy & Administration, 53*(6), 854–871. https://doi.org/10.1111/spol.12538

de Meijer, C., Wouterse, B., Polder, J., & Koopmanschap, M. (2013). The effect of population aging on health expenditure growth: A critical review. *European Journal of Ageing, 10*(4), 353–361. https://doi.org/10.1007/s10433-013-0280-x

Department of Health. (2019). *Elderly health service.* https://www.dh.gov.hk/english/main/main_ehs/main_ehs.html

Elderly Commission. (2021). *Report on healthy ageing executive summary.* https://www.elderlycommission.gov.hk/en/library/Ex-sum.htm#2

Elderly Health Service. (2021). *Waiting time of enrolment for elderly health centres.* https://www.elderly.gov.hk/english/about_us/waiting_time.html

Food and Health Bureau. (2010). *Primary care development in Hong Kong: Strategy document.* https://www.fhb.gov.hk/download/press_and_publications/otherinfo/101231_primary_care/e_strategy_doc.pdf

Food and Health Bureau. (2020). *Hong Kong's domestic health accounts (DHA).* https://www.fhb.gov.hk/statistics/download/dha/en/a_estimate_1819.pdf

Fong, B. Y. F., Law, V. T. S., & Lee, A. (2020). Primary care revisited: Interdisciplinary perspectives for a new era. *Springer, Singapore.* https://doi.org/10.1007/978-981-15-2521-6

He, A. J., & Chou, K. K. (2019). Long-term care service needs and planning for the future: A study of middle-aged and older adults in Hong Kong. *Ageing and Society, 39*(2), 221–253. https://doi.org/10.1017/S0144686X17000824

Ho, M. K. (2020). Strengthening primary care in Hong Kong: Fostering continuity of care from a health system perspective. *Hong Kong Medical Journal*, *26*(6), 543–545. https://doi.org/10.12809/hkmj198368

Hong Kong's Domestic Health Accounts. (2019). *Estimates of health expenditure, 1989/90–2017/18 (SHA 2011).* https://www.fhb.gov.hk/statistics/download/dha/en/dha_summary_report_1718.pdf

Hospital Authority. (2020). *Hospital Authority statistical report 2019–2020.* https://www3.ha.org.hk/data/HAStatistics/DownloadReport/13?isPreview=False

Hospital Authority. (2021). *Waiting time for stable new case booking at specialist out-patient clinics.* https://www.ha.org.hk/haho/ho/sopc/dw_wait_ls_eng.pdf

Kwok, C. L., Lee, C. K., Lo, W. T., & Yip, P. S. (2017). The contribution of ageing to hospitalization days in Hong Kong: A decomposition analysis. *International Journal of Health Policy and Management*, *6*(3), 155. https://doi.org/10.15171/ijhpm.2016.108

Lai, A. H. Y., Kuang, Z., Yam, C. H. K., Ayub, S., & Yeoh, E. K. (2018). Vouchers for primary healthcare services in an ageing world? The perspectives of elderly voucher recipients in Hong Kong. *Health & Social Care in the Community, 26*(3), 374–382. https://doi.org/10.1111/hsc.12523

Legislative Council Secretariat. (2018). *Healthcare workforce.* https://www.legco.gov.hk/research-publications/english/1819issh05-healthcare-workforce-20181102-e.pdf

Legislative Council Secretariat. (2019). *Emergency care services in selected places.* https://www.legco.gov.hk/research-publications/english/1819in05-emergency-care-services-in-selected-places-20190131-e.pdf

Liu, S., Yam, C. H., Huang, O. H., & Griffiths, S. M. (2012). Willingness to pay for private primary care services in Hong Kong: Are elderly ready to move from the public sector? *Health Policy and Planning, 28*(7), 717–729. https://doi.org/10.1093/heapol/czs112

Our Hong Kong Foundation. (2018). *Fit for purpose: A health system for the 21st century research report.* https://www.ourhkfoundation.org.hk/sites/default/files/media/pdf/ohkf_research_report_digital_1201.pdf

Owolabi, O., Zhang, Z., Wei, X., Yang, N., Li, H., Wong, S. Y., Wong, M. C., Yip, W., & Griffiths, S. M. (2013). Patients' socioeconomic status and their evaluations of primary care in Hong Kong. *BMC Health Services Research, 13*(487). https://doi.org/10.1186/1472-6963-13-487

Pinchbeck, E. W. (2019). Convenient primary care and emergency hospital utilisation. *Journal of Health Economics, 68*, 102242. https://doi.org/10.1186/1472-6963-13-487

The Government of the Hong Kong Special Administrative Region. (2017). *LCQ17: Manpower of healthcare professionals.* https://www.info.gov.hk/gia/general/201707/12/P2017071200517.htm

The Government of the Hong Kong Special Administrative Region. (2020). *LCQ18: Elderly health care voucher scheme.* [Press release]. https://www.info.gov.hk/gia/general/202101/13/P2021011300557.htm?fontSize=1

van Gool, K., Mu, C., & Hall, J. (2021). Does more investment in primary care improve health system performance? *Health Policy, 125*(6), 717–724. https://doi.org/10.1016/j.healthpol.2021.03.004

Wei, X., Li, H., Yang, N., Wong, S. Y., Owolabi, O., Xu, J., Shi, L., Tang, L., Li, D., & Griffiths, S. M. (2015). Comparing quality of public primary care between Hong Kong and Shanghai using validated patient assessment tools. *PLoS ONE, 10*(3), e0121269. https://doi.org/10.1371/journal.pone.0121269

Wong, S. Y., Kung, K., Griffiths, S. M., Carthy, T., Wong, M. C., Lo, S. V., Chung, V. C., Goggins, W. B., & Starfield, B. (2010). Comparison of primary care experiences among adults in general outpatient clinics and private general practice clinics in Hong Kong. *BMC Public Health, 10*(1), 397. https://doi.org/10.1186/1471-2458-10-397

Woo, J., Mak, B., & Yeung, F. (2013). Age-friendly primary health care: An assessment of current service provision for older adults in Hong Kong. *Health Services Insights, 6*, HSI–S12434. https://doi.org/10.4137/HSI.S12434

Wong, S. Y. S., Zou, D., Chung, R. Y., Sit, R. W., Zhang, D., Chan, D., Yeoh, E. K., & Woo, J. W. (2017). Regular source of care for the elderly: A cross-national comparative study of Hong Kong with 11 developed countries. *Journal of the American Medical Directors Association, 18*(9), e1–e8. https://doi.org/10.1016/j.jamda.2017.05.009

Yang, H., Shi, L., Lebrun, L. A., Zhou, X., Liu, J., & Wang, H. (2013). Development of the Chinese primary care assessment tool: Data quality and measurement properties. *International Journal for Quality in Health Care, 25*(1), 92–105. https://doi.org/10.1093/intqhc/mzs072

Yeoh, E. K., Yam, C. H., Chong, K. C., Chow, T. Y., Fung, V. L., Wong, E. L., & Griffiths, S. M. (2020). An evaluation of universal vouchers as a demand-side subsidy to change primary care utilization: A retrospective analysis of longitudinal services utilisation and voucher claims data from a survey cohort in Hong Kong. *Health Policy, 124*(2), 189–198. https://doi.org/10.1016/j.healthpol.2019.12.009

Yu, R., Leung, J., Lum, C. M., Auyeung, T. W., Lee, J. S., Lee, R., & Woo, J. (2019). A comparison of health expectancies over 10 years: Implications for elderly service needs in Hong Kong. *International Journal of Public Health, 64*(5), 731–742. https://doi.org/10.1007/s00038-019-01240-1

Zhang, D., Sit, R. W. S., Wong, C., Zou, D., Mercer, S. W., Johnston, M. C., & Wong, S. Y. S. (2020). Cohort profile: The prospective study on Chinese elderly with multimorbidity in primary care in Hong Kong. *British Medical Journal Open, 10*(2), e027279. https://doi.org/10.1136/bmjopen-2018-027279

Chapter 5
The Social Construction of "Dirty Work" for Working in Residential Care Homes for the Elderly

Sui Yu Yau, Yin King Lee, Siu Yin Li, Sze Ki Lai, Sin Ping Law, and Shixin Huang

Abstract The notion of "dirty work" as a socially constructed metaphor of care-giving work in "residential care homes for the elderly" (RCHE) has been one of the most consequential factors contributing to the acute labour shortage in RCHE. It operates within the context of rapid population ageing and increasing social demand for RCHE work. The term "dirty work" is widely used by a variety of stakeholders in social discourses to describe the job nature in RCHE or to explain RCHE staff shortages in Hong Kong. Nevertheless, RCHE workers' insider experiences with the meaning of RCHE work are largely absent from the community and the literature, resulting in the hidden social processes that stigmatise and marginalise these workers. This chapter calls for the pressing needs of understanding how "dirty work" is being socially constructed and how it contributes to a critical factor of the RCHE workforce crisis in Hong Kong. It aims at generating new discussion on the development of public policy to cope with the workforce crisis from a socio-cultural perspective that is largely lacking in the process of making RCHE workforce policy and may facilitate the socio-cultural change in public views on RCHE work.

Keywords Residential care homes for the elderly · Dirty work · Workforce crisis · Health care workforce

S. Y. Yau (✉) · Y. K. Lee · S. Y. Li · S. K. Lai · S. P. Law · S. Huang
Hong Kong Metropolitan University, Hong Kong, China
e-mail: isyyau@hkmu.edu.hk

Y. K. Lee
e-mail: yklee@hkmu.edu.hk

S. Y. Li
e-mail: siyli@hkmu.edu.hk

S. K. Lai
e-mail: sklai@hkmu.edu.hk

S. P. Law
e-mail: ssplaw@hkmu.edu.hk

V. T. S. Law and B. Y. F. Fong (eds.), *Ageing with Dignity in Hong Kong and Asia*, Quality of Life in Asia 16, https://doi.org/10.1007/978-981-19-3061-4_5

5.1 Introduction

The Hong Kong population has been ageing, and there is a huge social demand for residential care services for the elderly. Residential care homes for the elderly (RCHE) provide such services, and they employ personal care workers, health workers (largely equivalent to "certified nursing assistants" in the United States), and nurses to deliver the caregiving work. Yet, while much effort has been dedicated to enhance the provision and retention of these workers, the long-standing concern of acute shortages of the workers persists in the RCHE sector. The notion of "dirty work" as a socially constructed metaphor of caregiving work in RCHE has been a critical factor in RCHE's acute shortages of health care workforce in Hong Kong. It operates within the context of rapid population ageing and increasing social demand for RCHE work. The term "dirty work" is generally used by a variety of stakeholders in social discourses at all levels to describe RCHE work or to explain RCHE staff shortages in Hong Kong. Nevertheless, the RCHE workers' insider experiences with the meaning of RCHE work are largely absent from the community and the literature, in part as a result of hidden social processes in which these workers are often socially stigmatised and marginalised.

The chapter begins by providing the background and the rapid population ageing in the global and Hong Kong context. Then, the increasing demand for RCHE work in relation to the ageing population is discussed and followed by the social construction of "dirty work" and how "dirty work" is regarded as a metaphor of RCHE work and as a critical factor in Hong Kong RCHE's acute staff shortages. This chapter ends by reinforcing the needs to unearth the voice of the RCHE workers through delineating their insider meanings of RCHE work.

5.2 Rapid Population Ageing

The world's population is rapidly ageing. The ageing population plays a pivotal role in the social transformation in the twenty-first century that impacts various sectors of the societies (United Nations, 2021). The number of worldwide older people is more than 1 billion in 2021, which contributes to 13.5% of the global population (World Health Organization [WHO], 2021), and 1 in 6 people will be aged 65 or above by mid-century (Population Division, 2020). According to WHO, the number of individuals aged 60 years or above will be increasing from 900 million to 2 billion from 2015 to 2050 that accounts for 10% (from 12 to 22%) of rising of the total global population. With around 125 million people aged 80 years or above, it is estimated that there will be 434 million people who fall into this age group by 2050 (WHO, 2018b).

When compared to some developed countries or regions, the share of elderly in the population in Hong Kong (17.9%) is similar to that of the United Kingdom

(UK) (18.2%). While Hong Kong ranked fourth in the share of elderly in the population after Japan (28%), Italy (22.4%), and the UK (18.2%) among nine developed countries or regions, it is projected that Hong Kong will rank third in the year 2038 (Wong & Yeung, 2019).

Within Hong Kong, the pace of rapid ageing is faster than in the past due to the low fertility rate and long life expectancy. The population of older persons aged 65 and over had increased from 13.1% in 2010 to 19.1% in 2020 as a percentage of the total population respectively (Census & Statistics Department, 2021b). Yet, the ageing population in Hong Kong is projected at a faster pace in the coming 20 years. The ageing population will be nearly doubled from 1.27 million (17.9%) to 2.44 million (31.9%) between 2018 and 2038. 1 in 3 persons will be elderly by 2038 (Wong & Yeung, 2019). In a United Nations ranking of 201 countries or regions according to the percentage of the population that is aged 60 or above, Hong Kong stood at 35th (21.7%) in 2015, and is projected to move up to sixth place by 2030 (33.6%) and 2050 (40.9%), respectively (Population Division, 2015).

5.3 Hong Kong Context: Increasing Demand for RCHE Work

The increase in ageing population brings challenges to the demand of RCHE work due to the decline of both physical and mental health among ageing population. According to the figures from the Social Welfare Department (2021a), there are various service providers offering residential care services for the elderly including subvented residential care home for the elderly, subvented nursing home, contract homes, self-financing homes participating in nursing home place purchase scheme, and private homes participating in enhanced bought place scheme. All these residential care services support 34,392 places for the elderly (Social Welfare Department, 2021a).

Health care workforce are being trained to respond to the urgent health needs due to chronic illness of the ageing population (WHO, 2016). There is a huge demand for long-term RCHE services, with long waiting lists and times (Social Welfare Department, 2021b). There are about 700 "care and attention homes" serving older adults with moderate levels of impairment, and about 70 "nursing homes" caring for the more severely impaired. These two major types of RCHE provide a mixture of government-subsidised and non-subsidised RCHE services times (Social Welfare Department, 2021b). RCHE employs such care workers as personal care workers (PCWs) to take care of the residents' activities of daily living; as health workers (HWs, largely equivalent to "certified nursing assistants" in the United States) to monitor PCWs' work and are responsible for basic nursing care delivery; and as nurses to provide nursing care and oversee PCWs' and HWs' work.

Due to the increasing demand of RCHE services, there is a lack of manpower in the elderly service sector. According to the Census and Statistics Department (2021a), there are 34,536 people working in residential care services with a vacancy of 2,889 by the end of 2020. For instance, there is 18% vacancy rate (with staff establishment of 7,403.5 and staff strength 6,073.0) for PCWs in 2017 (The Government of the Hong Kong Special Administrative Region [HKSAR], 2017). Moreover, over 90% of RCHE organisations respond that it is challenging to recruit PCWs or other health care workforce in the sector (HKSAR, 2017).

As a response to the increasing demand for RCHE services, the Hong Kong Government has embarked on the identification and allocation of more sites for building RCHEs (Legislative Council Secretariat, 2016). This attempt, however, has been hampered by acute shortages of RCHE workers at various levels, including PCWs, HWs, and nurses. Despite of the effort such as allowing training opportunities to attract new workers, increasing staff salaries for the existing RCHEs and providing resources to recruit more workers (Legislative Council Secretariat, 2013), the problem of acute staff shortages continues (Audit Commission, 2014; Labour and Welfare Bureau and Education Bureau, 2019). Media attention has also focused on the impact of this issue on the availability of care, as when it was questioned "With a lack of carers in Hong Kong, who will look after us as we grow older?" (Zou & Lee, 2016). Even the Social Welfare Department having been providing additional resources for RCHE services, the amount of manpower in the sector is not promising.

5.4 Social Construction of "Dirty Work"

According to Hughes (1951), dirty work refers to any tasks or jobs that are regarded as disgusting and degrading. The nature of dirty work "may be a symbol of degradation, something that wounds one's dignity... it may be dirty work in that it in some way goes counter to the more heroic of our moral conceptions" (Hughes, 1951, p. 319). The concept of "dirty work" has been applied to various occupations such as public police officers, private security industry, vacant property employees, domestic labour, and health care workers (Anderson, 2000; Clarke & Ravenswood, 2019; Deery et al., 2019; Dick, 2005; Fisher & Kang, 2013; Lofstrand et al., 2016; Olwig, 2018; Ostaszkiewicz et al., 2016).

A society delegates dirty work to groups who are then being stigmatised and become "dirty workers" (Hughes, 1951, 1962). Although research suggests that individuals performing dirty works usually possess high job-related esteem, it is challenging for dirty workers to construct a positive sense of self and an esteem-enhancing social identity (Ashforth & Kreiner, 1999). The characteristic of stigmatisation of dirty work leads to negative stereotypes of the job individuals do and who they are (Amrith, 2017; Deery et al., 2019).

Dirty work is physically, socially, and morally tainted tasks (Hughes, 1958). Ashforth and Kreiner (1999) further enhance the conceptual rigour of Hughes's (1958) work on the three tainted tasks. Physical taint is associated with jobs that are directly related to garbage, death, effluent, or jobs to be in noxious or dangerous nature. Social taint refers to jobs requiring direct contact with stigmatised individuals or jobs with subservient roles (Ashforth & Kreiner, 1999). While moral taint happens where jobs carry "sinful or of dubious virtue" or are "deceptive, intrusive, confrontational, or that otherwise defy morns of civility" (Ashforth & Kreiner, 1999, p. 415). Due to the taint attached to different forms of work, some works are seen to be dirtier than others (Mendonca & D'Cruz, 2021; Sanders, 2010). The low occupational prestige attached to physical taint and the low status and skill associated with physical dirt are often socially constructed as inferior and socially invaluable (Deery et al., 2019; Dick, 2005).

The "dirtiness" of a work is a social construction that is imputed by individuals' subjective perception of "cleanliness" (Ball, 1970). Societies relate "cleanliness" with "goodness", while "dirtiness" is associated with "badness" (Douglas, 1966; Miller, 1997). In order to secure and sustain a positive social identity, dirty workers go through the processes of occupational ideologies (reframing, recalibrating, refocusing) and social weighting (differentiating the outsiders by condemning the condemners and supporting the supporters, and selecting social comparisons) (Ashforth & Kreiner, 1999). Ashforth et al. (2007) further suggested that occupational ideologies, social buffers, confronting clients and the public, and defensive tactics are the tactics for normalising dirty work.

5.5 "Dirty Work" as a Metaphor of RCHE Work and as a Critical Factor in Hong Kong RCHE'S Acute Staff Shortages

Fisher and Kang (2013) specifically defined what dirty work means in relation to care work, nursing, and body-related literature as "physical labor that involves cleaning and caring for the human body, its products, and its environs, particularly where doing so involves handing body parts or products that are intimate, messy, or possibly contaminated" (p. 165). The RCHE work is characterised as "dirty work" due to the immediate contact with human body and dirt, sexualisation with intimate physical contact, and even caring with dying clients (Fisher & Kang, 2013).

Despite being perceived as having great dignity and taking pride in performing the highly responsible, caring and skilful work, RCHE health care workers experienced the "dirty work" nature as "professional ass washer", "cleaning with poop", "physically and emotionally demanding", "satisfying with clients' family members", "verbal and physical abuse by clients and their families", and "dealing with vomit" (Clarke & Ravenswood, 2019; Fisher & Kang, 2013). Amrith (2017) asserts that nurses were shocked once they discovered that they were expected to take care of the mundane needs of clients instead of focusing on the health needs. They view the "dirty work" as taken for granted that is seldom being acknowledged.

In the Hong Kong context, the "work environment" in the RCHE sector is "a socially constructed concept", carrying derogatory connotations that impede RCHE staff recruitment and retention (Choi et al., 2018). Attached to those derogatory connotations are stigmatising labels such as "dirty work", "pee and poop", and "awful smell" that demoralise and devalue the meaning of RCHE work, resulting in discouraging existing staff from staying in the workforce and job seekers from entering the sector (Choi et al., 2018).

The term "dirty work" (also referred to as "obnoxious work", "repulsive work", "taint work", or "stigmatised work") has been most commonly and generally used in social discourses at all levels to describe RCHE work or to explain in part RCHE staff shortages in Hong Kong. In occasions where the issue on RCHE staff shortages is debated, the use of "dirty work" as a metaphor for RCHE work or jobs has been widely adopted by a variety of stakeholders, including interest/pressure groups, labour unions, lawmakers, and even government officials. Due to the nature of dirty work, the RCHE staff may be marginalised in the society. The negative stereotypes on the roles of RCHE workers is impeding the attraction and retention of the workforce (WHO, 2015).

While the term and its synonyms have been fairly defined, the "eTVonline" (an online platform delivering educational services) of Radio Television Hong Kong (the public broadcaster in Hong Kong) has provided a definition for the concept of "repulsive work" at its "liberal studies" area where the term is defined as "a kind of work that is unpopular or that people are unwilling to do" and RCHE work is used as an illustration (Radio Television Hong Kong, 2018). In occasions where the issue on RCHE staff shortages is discussed or deliberated, the use of "dirty work" or its synonym as a metaphor for RCHE work or jobs has been widely adopted by a variety of stakeholders, such as interest/pressure groups (Society for Community Organization & Elderly Rights League (Hong Kong), 2015), labour unions (Radio Television Hong Kong, 2017), advisory bodies of the government on elderly care policy (Radio Television Hong Kong, 2018), government officials (Labour & Welfare Bureau, 2013), and columnists (Lee & Au Yeung, 2013; Wong, 2018).

RCHE manpower policy debates at Legislative Council meetings, to take an instance, have often been inseparable from the use of the stigmatising metaphor to describe RCHE work or jobs, as seen in such descriptions of them as "people are unwilling to take up jobs in elderly homes or other obnoxious jobs" (Legislative Council Secretariat, 2013, p. 2673), "[m]anpower in RCHEs has all along been in short supply due to manpower mismatch, obnoxious job nature…" (Legislative Council Secretariat, 2014, p. 15022), and "no one would be willing to keep on working as a care worker and perform such obnoxious tasks as cleaning the body of elderly people in RCHEs after 10 or 20 years" (Legislative Council Secretariat, 2016, p. 5413). Even health care workers unfolded "meaning through their mastery of work that others shun", how the "less-than-ideal" situation of RCHE work can be empowered remains a question (Fisher & Kang, 2013).

Social discourses or public views about RCHE work could be shaped by the way long-term care (LTC) facilities are portrayed in the media (Miller et al., 2016). An abuse scandal at a local private RCHE in May 2015, for example, had been widely reported and followed up by the media for years (Hong Kong Economic Journal, 2017; Mok & Ngo, 2016; Ngo & Lai, 2015). Such social processes could influence not only RCHE workers' job satisfaction as their "social identification" with the facility they work for affects their job satisfaction (Bjerregaard et al., 2015), but also could undermine the attractiveness of RCHE work and discourage people from entering the sector.

5.6 The Lack of Voice of RCHE Workers on "Dirty Work" in the Literature

While the job satisfaction-turnover literature has identified a wide variety of job/work-related factors in RCHE's staff shortages, such as leadership styles (Chu et al., 2014) and staff autonomy (Culp et al., 2008), the concept of "dirty work" has had little role to play in the analysis. Lying outside this literature, previous studies investigating the conception of RCHE work as "dirty work" are not unheard of, yet they are largely based on a more "top-down" or "analyst-driven" view on RCHE work.

Preceding research could be organised into three main bodies of studies. First, there have been attempts to depict and explain the low social and occupational status of RCHE work as "dirty work" (Amrith, 2017; Ashforth & Kreiner, 1999; Ashforth et al., 2007; Clarke & Ravenswood, 2019; Olwig, 2018). This body of studies tends to acknowledge that RCHE work is "dirty" or suffers from "taint" in one way or another, while believing that something could and should be done about it. Having assumed the existence of the "dirty work", a second body of studies has focused on the negative impacts of the "dirty work" on RCHE staff and staffing outcomes, such as poor self-identify and low personal worth (Ostaszkiewicz et al., 2016); and the lack of new entrants, leaving the jobs to immigrants (Fisher & Kang, 2013; Huang et al., 2012). Third, previous research has also examined how RCHE workers respond to or counteract the negative impact of the "dirty work" on them. Law and Aranda (2010), for instance, have observed attempts to "delegate" "dirty jobs" from more qualified nursing staff to the less qualified ones. Ostaszkiewicz et al. (2016) have noted four types of coping strategies: "accommodating the context", "dissociating oneself", "distancing oneself", and "attempting to elevate one's role status".

Although RCHE work has been socially perceived as a kind of "dirty work", RCHE workers' insider views about the meaning of RCHE work, and their experiences of working with the socially given metaphor and its associated social discourses are largely absent not only in the community but also from the literature. This could be in part a result of the fact that these workers are often socially stigmatised, marginalised and the social process of boundary-making (Ashforth & Kreiner, 1999; Ashforth et al., 2007; Clarke & Ravenswood, 2019). There remains a need to explore insiders' view of RCHE workers about the meanings of RCHE work, their experiences with the "dirty work" metaphor, and their views on how to revitalise their meanings of RCHE work.

A better understanding of the meaning of RCHE work based on the neglected RCHE workers' insider views and experiences will generate new insights into the workforce crisis and important practical implications for policymakers and practitioners as they consider how to deal with the crisis from a socio-cultural perspective that is largely lacking in the public policy arena. Therefore, it urges for the need to unearth the voice of the RCHE workers in order to elicit their meanings and experiences of RCHE work, and the impacts of "dirty work" on them, and to explicate RCHE workers' views on how to revitalise their meanings of RCHE work.

Overall, the emerging RCHE "dirty work" literature has been impeded by a conceptual dominance of a "top-down" approach to understand RCHE work, which is seemingly rooted in researchers' analytical preconceptions of the "dirty work" metaphor, resulting in the voice of RCHE workers on the "dirty work" debate being largely absent from the literature. Do RCHE workers accept the "dirty work" metaphor as socially given to them in the first place? Is it not possible for the "dirty work" metaphor to impact RCHE workers positively? What do RCHE workers have to say about their meanings of RCHE work? Questions such as these deserve further study from a "bottom-up" approach.

5.7 Conclusion

The notion of "dirty work" as a socially constructed metaphor of caregiving work in RCHE in Hong Kong has been a critical factor and workforce crisis in RCHE's acute staff shortages. In the face of rapid population ageing and increasing social demand for RCHE work, a better understanding of the socially stigmatised and marginalised RCHE workers' meanings of RCHE work, their perceptions about the "dirty work" metaphor, the impact of such a "social discourse" on them, and their views on how to revitalise their meanings of RCHE work, will generate new insights into the workforce crisis and important practical implications for policymakers and practitioners as they consider how to deal with the crisis.

The chapter calls for the pressing need to extend our understanding on how "dirty work" is being socially constructed that acts as a critical factor of the RCHE workforce crisis in Hong Kong, and the need of social construction of reframing RCHE work as caring, skilful, and respectful. Yet, assigning meaning and dignity to the RCHE work by unearthing the voice of RCHE workers through exploring their perceptions about the "dirty work" metaphor should be addressed. The health care workers' insider experiences with the impact of such a metaphor, and their meanings of RCHE work, and to examine the workers' views on how their meanings of RCHE work can be revitalised in the face of the "dirty work" hegemony.

The chapter concludes by generating new discussion on the development of public policy initiatives to cope with the workforce crisis from a socio-cultural perspective that is largely lacking in the process of making RCHE workforce policy, and may facilitate the rise of a socio-cultural change in public views on RCHE work.

The results of the discussion will contribute significantly to the "dirty work" debate in the literature and provide important practical implications for policymakers and practitioners in terms of the development of more effective recruitment and retention strategies that counteract the societal hegemony of "dirty work" in the RCHE sector. In addition, the discussion will add significantly to our understanding of the RCHE workforce crisis in Hong Kong from a socio-cultural perspective that is largely absent from the RCHE public "policy cycle" (policy agenda setting, policy formulation, policy implementation, and policy evaluation) (Chui, 2011; Chui et al., 2020; He & Chou, 2019), and contribute to generate new insights from this perspective on the development of policy initiatives to reconstruct the RCHE workforce, resulting in the following intended impacts at various levels in the short, medium, and long term beyond the academia.

In the short term, RCHE public policymakers will benefit from new insights and important practical implications generated from the results of the analysis for the development of policy initiatives to recruit and retain RCHE workers. These initiatives should aim to bring about a "socio-cultural change" in public views on RCHE work away from the socially constructed "dirty work" metaphor towards a positive social identity, in order to improve the attractiveness of the RCHE work environment.

In the medium term, RCHE administrators who have been struggling with developing effective recruitment and retention strategies to tackle the workforce crisis will benefit from the enhanced attractiveness of the RCHE work environment; and RCHE workers who have been struggling with over workload will be benefited from enhanced co-worker support at the facility level.

In the long term, RCHE residents who have been struggling with poorer quality of care as a result of the workforce crisis will be benefited from enhanced quality of care in terms of the indicators such as adequacy of care, responsiveness of care, and so on. After all, all of the stakeholders will grow old and may need residential long-term care in one way or another. They will benefit from a healthy RCHE workforce.

Acknowledgements The work described in this paper was fully supported by a grant from the Research Grants Council of the Hong Kong Special Administrative Region, China (UGC/FDS16/M12/20).

References

Amrith, M. (2017). *Caring for strangers: Filipino medical workers in Asia*. Nordic Institute of Asian Studies (NIAS).

Anderson, B. (2000). *Doing the dirty work?: The global politics of domestic labour*. Zed Books.

Ashforth, B. E., & Kreiner, G. E. (1999). "How can you do it?": Dirty work and the challenge of constructing a positive identity. *Academy of Management Review, 24*(3), 413–434. https://doi.org/10.2307/259134

Ashforth, B. E., Kreiner, G. E., Clark, M. A., & Fugate, M. (2007). Normalizing dirty work: Managerial tactics for countering occupational taint. *Academy of Management Journal, 50*(1), 149–174. https://doi.org/10.2307/20159845

Audit Commission. (2014, October). *Director of audit's report no. 63*. http://www.aud.gov.hk/eng/pubpr_arpt/rpt_63.htm

Ball, D. W. (1970). The problematics of respectability. In J. D. Douglas (Ed.), *Deviance & respectability: The social construction of moral meanings* (pp. 326–371). Basic Books.

Bjerregaard, K., Haslam, S. A., Morton, T., & Ryan, M. K. (2015). Social and relational identification as determinants of care workers' motivation and well-being. *Frontiers in Psychology, 6*, 1460. https://doi.org/10.3389/fpsyg.2015.01460

Census and Statistics Department. (2021a, June). *Hong Kong monthly digest of statistics*. https://www.censtatd.gov.hk/en/data/stat_report/product/B1010002/att/B10100022021aMM06B0100.pdf

Census and Statistics Department. (2021b, February 18). *Population by age and sex group*. https://www.censtatd.gov.hk/en/web_table.html?id=1A

Chui, E. W. T. (2011). Long-term care policy in Hong Kong: Challenges and future directions. *Home Health Care Services Quarterly, 30*(3), 119–132. https://doi.org/10.1080/01621424.2011.592413

Chui, C. H. K., Arat, G., Chan, K., & Wong, P. W. C. (2020). Growing old as a member of an ethnic minority in Hong Kong: Implications for an inclusive long-term care policy framework. *Journal of Applied Gerontology, 39*(5), 463–471. https://doi.org/10.1177/0733464819873504

Choi, S. P. P., Yeung, C. C. Y., & Lee, J. K. L. (2018). A phenomenological study of the work environment in long-term care facilities for the older adults. *Journal of Applied Gerontology, 39*(6), 651–659. https://doi.org/10.1177/0733464818776786

Chu, C. H., Wodchis, W. P., & McGilton, K. S. (2014). Turnover of regulated nurses in long-term care facilities. *Journal of Nursing Management, 22*(5), 553–562. https://doi.org/10.1111/jonm.12031

Clarke, M., & Ravenswood, K. (2019). Constructing a career identity in the aged care sector: Overcoming the "taint" of dirty work. *Personnel Review, 48*(1), 76–97. https://doi.org/10.1108/PR-08-2017-0244

Culp, K., Ramey, S., & Karlman, S. (2008). Iowa certified nursing assistants study: Self-reported ratings of the nursing home work environment. *Research in Gerontological Nursing, 1*(2), 87–96. https://doi.org/10.3928/19404921-20080401-01

Deery, S., Kolar, D., & Walsh, J. (2019). Can dirty work be satisfying? A mixed method study of workers doing dirty jobs. *Work, Employment and Society, 33*(4), 631–647. https://doi.org/10.1177/0950017018817307

Dick, P. (2005). Dirty work designations: How police officers account for their use of coercive force. *Human Relations, 58*(11), 1363–1390. https://doi.org/10.1177/0018726705060242

Douglas, M. (1966). *Purity and danger: An analysis of concepts of pollution and taboo*. Routledge and Kegan Paul.

Fisher, L. T., & Kang, M. (2013). Reinventing dirty work: Immigrant women in nursing homes. In N. Flores-Gonzalez, A. R. Guevarra, M. Toro-Morn, & G. Chang (Eds.), *Immigrant women workers in the neoliberal age* (pp. 164–185). University of Illinois Press.

He, A. J., & Chou, K. L. (2019). Long-term care service needs and planning for the future: A study of middle-aged and older adults in Hong Kong. *Ageing & Society, 39*(2), 221–253. https://doi.org/10.1017/S0144686X17000824

Hong Kong Economic Journal. (2017, May 26). *2 years after Cambridge Home incident: Poor quality of private residential care home*. https://www2.hkej.com/instantnews/current/article/1572680/

Huang, S., Yeoh, B. S. A., & Toyota, M. (2012). Caring for the elderly: The embodied labour of migrant care workers in Singapore. *Global Networks, 12*(2), 195–215. https://doi.org/10.1111/j.1471-0374.2012.00347.x

Hughes, E. C. (1951). Work and the self. In J. H. Rohrer & M. Sherif (Eds.), *Social psychology at the crossroads* (pp. 313–323). Harper & Brothers.

Hughes, E. C. (1958). *Men and their work*. Free Press.

Hughes, E. C. (1962). Good people and dirty work. *Social Problems, 10*, 3–11. https://doi.org/10.2307/799402

Labour and Welfare Bureau. (2013, October 27). *Increasing younger manpower for service for the elderly*. https://www.lwb.gov.hk/tc/blog/post_27102013.html

Labour and Welfare Bureau and Education Bureau. (2019, June 25). *Manpower for the elderly care service sector*. The Legislative Council Commission. https://www.legco.gov.hk/yr18-19/english/panels/mp/papers/mp20190625cb2-1674-6-e.pdf

Law, K., & Aranda, K. (2010). The shifting foundations of nursing. *Nurse Education Today, 30*(6), 544–547. https://doi.org/10.1016/j.nedt.2009.11.006

Lee, S. K., & Au Yeung, K. K. (2013, June 14). *Elderly service industry is in crisis*. http://paper.wenweipo.com/2013/06/14/FI1306140037.htm

Legislative Council Secretariat. (2013, November 13). *Official record of proceedings: Wednesday, 13 November 2013*. Legislative Council. https://www.legco.gov.hk/yr13-14/english/counmtg/hansard/cm1113-translate-e.pdf

Legislative Council Secretariat. (2014, June 12). *Official record of proceedings: Thursday, 12 June 2014*. Legislative Council. https://www.legco.gov.hk/yr13-14/english/counmtg/hansard/cm0612-translate-e.pdf

Legislative Council Secretariat. (2016, February 18). *Official record of proceedings: Thursday, 18 February 2016*. Legislative Council. https://www.legco.gov.hk/yr15-16/english/counmtg/hansard/cm20160218-translate-e.pdf

Lofstrand, C. H., Loftus, B., & Loader, I. (2016). Doing "dirty work": Stigma and esteem in the private security industry. *European Journal of Criminology, 13*(3), 297–314. https://doi.org/10.1177/1477370815615624

Mendonca, A., & D'Cruz, P. (2021). Workplace bullying, emotional abuse and harassment in the context of dirty work. In P. D'Cruz, E. Noronha, L. Keashly, & S. Tye-Williams (Eds.), *Special topics and particular occupations, professions and sectors* (pp. 551–584). Springer.

Miller, W. I. (1997). *The anatomy of disgust*. Harvard University Press.

Miller, E. A., Livingstone, I., & Ronneberg, C. R. (2016). Media portrayal of the nursing homes sector: A longitudinal analysis of 51U.S. newspapers. *The Gerontologist, 57*(3), 487–500. https://doi.org/10.1093/geront/gnv684

Mok, D., & Ngo, J. (2016, May 27). Hong Kong police probe care home for leaving elderly naked in open air. *South China Morning Post*. https://www.scmp.com/news/hong-kong/law-crime/article/1810017/hong-kong-police-probe-care-home-leaving-elderly-naked-open

Ngo, J., & Lai, Y. K. (2015, May 29). Hong Kong elderly home faces loss of licence after naked abuse scandal. *South China Morning Post*. https://www.scmp.com/news/hong-kong/education-community/article/1812045/hong-kong-nursing-home-regrets-leaving-elderly

Olwig, K. F. (2018). Female immigration and the ambivalence of dirty care work: Caribbean nurses in imperial Britain. *Ethnography, 19*(1), 44–62. https://doi.org/10.1177/1466138117697744

Ostaszkiewicz, J., Oconnell, B., & Dunning, T. (2016). 'We just do the dirty work': Dealing with incontinence, courtesy stigma and the low occupational status of carework in long-term aged care facilities. *Journal of Clinical Nursing, 25*(17–18), 2528–2541. https://doi.org/10.1111/jocn.13292

Population Division. (2015). *World population ageing 2015*. Department of Economic and Social Affairs, United Nations. http://www.un.org/en/development/desa/population/theme/ageing/WPA2015.shtml

Population Division. (2020). *World population ageing 2020 highlights*. Department of Economic and Social Affairs, United Nations. https://www.un.org/development/desa/pd/sites/www.un.org.development.desa.pd/files/files/documents/2020/Sep/un_pop_2020_pf_ageing_10_key_messages.pdf

Radio Television Hong Kong. (2017, October 6). *Importing foreign workers will change the salary structure of local elderly service workers.* https://app3.rthk.hk/special/pau/article.php?aid=2727

Radio Television Hong Kong. (2018, July 16). *Repulsive work.* eTVonline. http://www.liberalstudies.hk/daily_concepts/?word=1598

Sanders, C. R. (2010). Working out back: The veterinary technician and "dirty work." *Journal of Contemporary Ethnography, 39*(3), 243–272. https://doi.org/10.1177/0891241610366711

Social Welfare Department. (2021a, June 18). *2019–20 Annual service provision and statistics.* https://www.swd.gov.hk/en/index/site_pubsvc/page_elderly/sub_elderlysps/id_rcse/

Social Welfare Department. (2021b, June 18). *Overview of residential care services for the elderly.* https://www.swd.gov.hk/en/index/site_pubsvc/page_elderly/sub_residentia/id_overviewon/

Society for Community Organisation & Elderly Rights League (Hong Kong). (2015, July 17). *Joint submission on issues relating to service quality and monitoring of private residential care homes from Elderly Rights League (H.K.) and Society for Community Organization.* The Legislative Council Commission. https://www.legco.gov.hk/yr14-15/chinese/panels/ws/papers/ws20150723cb2-1906-5-c.pdf

The Government of the Hong Kong Special Administrative Region. (2017, November 29). *LCQ7: Manpower shortage in elderly service sector.* https://www.info.gov.hk/gia/general/201711/29/P2017112900367.htm?fontSize=1

United Nations. (2021). *Ageing.* https://www.un.org/en/global-issues/ageing

Wong, W. (2018, February 27). Encourage building old-aged home during land sale. *Hong Kong Economic Journal.* https://www2.hkej.com/commentary/finanalytics/article/1776525/

Wong, K., & Yeung, M. (2019, January). *Population ageing trend of Hong Kong.* Office of the Government Economist. https://www.hkeconomy.gov.hk/en/pdf/el/el-2019-02.pdf

World Health Organization. (2015, September 29). *World report on ageing and health.* https://ahpsr.who.int/publications/i/item/world-report-on-ageing-and-health

World Health Organization. (2016, February 16). *Health workforce for ageing populations.* https://www.who.int/publications/i/item/health-workforce-for-ageing-populations

World Health Organization. (2018a, February 2018). *Ageing.* https://www.who.int/news-room/facts-in-pictures/detail/ageing

World Health Organization. (2018b, February 5). *Ageing and health.* https://www.who.int/news-room/fact-sheets/detail/ageing-and-health

World Health Organization. (2021, April 30). *Decade of healthy ageing: Baseline report—Summary.* https://www.who.int/publications/i/item/9789240023307

Zou, M., & Lee, J. (2016, February 2016). With a lack of carers in Hong Kong, who will look after us as we grow older? *South China Morning Post.* https://www.scmp.com/comment/insight-opinion/article/1913467/lack-carers-hong-kong-who-will-look-after-us-we-grow-older

Chapter 6
Palliative Care in Selected Economies in Asia: Taiwan, Singapore and Hong Kong

Hilary H. L. Yee and Vincent Tin Sing Law

Abstract People are living longer nowadays. Medical advancement has helped to prolong lives and a lot of diseases are curable. However, patients with life-limiting and terminal illnesses still suffer. Palliative care is an approach to relieve pain and other distressing symptoms and gives psychological and spiritual support to patients, as well as their families. Patients who have received palliative care have a significant decrease in readmission rate and better quality of life. In Asia, Hong Kong, Singapore, Taiwan and South Korea are the developed economies once titled the "Four Asian Dragons". They ranked differently in the 2015 Quality of Death (QOD) Index due to different development in end-of-life care. In this chapter, Taiwan, Singapore and Hong Kong, which ranked at number 6, 12 and 22, respectively, in the QOD Index, are selected to compare their resources on palliative services, advance directives (AD) policy and public awareness on palliative care. Taiwan has outperformed both Singapore and Hong Kong due to the government's sufficient support in resources, diversified education opportunities to professionals and continuous efforts on improving legislations to protect patients' autonomy. Singapore is following closely behind Taiwan's progress in expanding palliative care services. Hong Kong is relatively lagging behind for failing to have comprehensive policies and legislation to increase public awareness and protect patients' right on medical decisions. With the launched public consultation regarding AD legislation and expansion of end-of-life care, Hong Kong is targeting to follow closely with Singapore and Taiwan soon, and achieving a higher position in the QOD Index in the future. While dying in place is becoming an indicator of QOD, dying at home may not be suitable for every patient in terms of available resources at home and variation of patients' needs. In parallel, rapid technology advancement facilitates the integration of palliative care and technology such as smartphone recording app and tracking bracelet. While keeping psychological and

H. H. L. Yee
Department of Rehabilitation Sciences, The Hong Kong Polytechnic University, Hong Kong, China
e-mail: hiulam.yee@polyu.edu.hk

V. T. S. Law (✉)
School of Professional Education and Executive Development, College of Professional and Continuing Education, The Hong Kong Polytechnic University, Hong Kong, China
e-mail: vincent.law@cpce-polyu.edu.hk

V. T. S. Law and B. Y. F. Fong (eds.), *Ageing with Dignity in Hong Kong and Asia*, Quality of Life in Asia 16, https://doi.org/10.1007/978-981-19-3061-4_6

spiritual support as core components in palliative care, application of emerging technology to care and treatment could increase efficiency of care by conducting real-time assessment and preparation for more supportive services.

Keywords Palliative care · Quality of Death Index · Resources on palliative care · Advance directives · Legislation · Public awareness · Patient autonomy · Technology

6.1 Introduction

The problem of ageing population has become a global phenomenon. With advanced medical care, people live longer. The number of older populations is predicted to be doubled by 2050, reaching nearly 2.1 billion worldwide (United Nations, 2017). Many governments have sensed the need to adopt new policies that could improve citizens' quality of life, especially for the older persons who are very likely to have complex and multiple diseases including cardiovascular diseases, diabetes, dementia and cancers at the same time (World Health Organization, 2011). People who suffer from these diseases need long-term physical and mental care. Their families and caregivers would also experience problems throughout the course of illnesses and need support. However, people living longer does not mean they are living in good health conditions or with quality of life.

For people who are at the end-of-life stage, their conditions may be untreatable or terminal. Palliative care is appropriate to relieve pain and suffering for the patients and their family, as well as to provide them with a dignified demise, but has been neglected by the general public. Palliative care service is defined as "an approach that improves the quality of life of patients (adult and children) and their families facing the problems associated with life-threatening illness through the prevention and relief of suffering by means of early identification and impeccable assessment and treatment of pain and other problems, physical, psychosocial, or spiritual" (World Health Organization, 2019). Patients who have received palliative care have significant clinical improvement in depression, dyspnoea and lower readmission rate due to less symptom burden and better quality of life (Kavalieratos et al., 2016; Wong et al., 2016).

In Asia, Hong Kong, Singapore, Taiwan and South Korea are known as the "Four Asian Dragons" that have high levels of economic growth and kept up with high development rates since the 1960s (Dangayach & Gupta, 2018). Despite of their advancement in economy, provision of adequate palliative care to citizens remains a challenge for the governments and policymakers to consider carefully on the healthcare environment, availability of care, human resources, affordability of care, quality of care and community engagement (The Economist Intelligence Unit, 2015). Hong Kong, South Korea, Singapore and Taiwan ranked 22, 18, 12 and 6, respectively, in the 2015 Quality of Death (QOD) Index (The Economist Intelligence Unit, 2015). As Taiwan comes first, Singapore ranks the second and Hong Kong is at the bottom, this chapter compares their resources on palliative services, related legislation and public awareness with an aim to know what have contributed to these three "Asian Dragons" in such ranking.

6.2 Resources of Palliative Care Services

6.2.1 Capacity of Hospice Beds

In Taiwan, the number of palliative hospice care hospitals has been increasing steadily since the establishment of Hospice Palliative Care Promotion Team in 1995. By 2017, there were 62 hospitals in Taiwan with inpatient wards, 101 hospitals with hospice homecare programmes, 200 hospitals that provided collective community hospice care and 142 hospitals that offered collective hospice care (Cho, 2018). As of February, 2020, there were 81 hospice wards according to the Taiwan Academy of Hospice Palliative Medicine (TAHPM). These included government sponsored hospitals and hospitals established by religious groups such as Protestant, Buddhist and Catholic groups. The adequate provision of services led to 423,956 successful applications from 2006 to 2017.

Compared to Taiwan, Singapore has better progress in expanding the provision of palliative services. There were only 137 hospice beds in 2011 but had grown to around 230 beds in 2017 provided by 6 inpatient hospices, and had targeted to reach the capacity of 360 beds by 2020 (Arivalagan & Gee, 2019; Lien Foundation, 2015). Based on the population of 5.61 million (Department of Statistics Singapore, 2017), there were around 4.1 inpatient hospice beds per 100,000 populations in 2017. In recent years, most of them have dedicated clinical teams responsible for taking care of dementia persons and rehabilitation activities such as occupational, speech and music therapies. There are nine home palliative care providers that offer 24-h on-call homecare services to help patients with advanced illnesses, by a multidisciplinary team comprising nurses, doctors, medical social workers and trained volunteers. Three established day care services are available for those who have controlled symptoms and are able to access the centres without 24-h nursing assistance. Such services provide patients with the chance of socialising by engaging them in different activities.

In Hong Kong, there are 16 hospitals under the Hong Kong Hospital Authority (HA) with over 360 beds to provide comprehensive palliative care such as symptom control and psychological counselling for terminally ill patients and their family (Hospital Authority, 2017). Compared to Singapore, Hong Kong had a population of 7.41 million in 2017 (Census & Statistics Department, 2019), there were around 4.8 inpatient hospice beds per 100,000 of the Hong Kong population, slightly more than those of Singapore. Non-government organisations (NGOs) involved in hospice care include the Haven of Hope Christian Service (HOHCS), Hong Kong Anti-Cancer Society (HKACS) and Society for the Promotion of Hospice Care (SPHC). HOHCS provides 124 beds for palliative and hospice care services, while the 30-bed Jockey Club Home for Hospice (JCHH) offers part-public and part-private services under SPHC. The Hong Kong Anti-Cancer Society Jockey Club Cancer Rehabilitation Centre (JCCRC) provides 180 beds to cancer patients or seriously ill patients (The D. H. Chen Foundation, 2015).

6.2.2 *Palliative Care Professionals*

Both Singapore and Taiwan have made into top 10 in the category of "Human Resources" in the 2015 QOD Index due to comprehensive and diversified education and training opportunities for all allied professionals. In Singapore, palliative care has become a compulsory module in the curriculum of all medical and nursing undergraduate courses. A Postgraduate Course in Palliative Medicine and a Graduate Diploma in Palliative Medicine are especially designed for qualified physicians who are interested in working in the palliative care field (Goh, 2018). For registered nurses, Specialist Diploma in Palliative Care Nursing, Advance Diploma in Nursing (Palliative Care), etc., are provided. There are 51 registered palliative care specialists and 784 registered nurses trained in palliative care (Lien Foundation, 2015). Lien Centre for Palliative Care has developed blended certificate level learning courses in palliative care not only for nurses, but also for medical social workers and pharmacists. To support the pathways for professional development, year-round training opportunities for all allied palliative care professionals, including arts and music therapists, occupational therapists, physiotherapists, psychologists, volunteers and caregivers are provided by the Palliative Care Centre for Excellence in Research and Education in Singapore.

Similar to Singapore, Taiwan has developed a successful hospice and palliative care accreditation system of certifications for palliative care since the set-up of Hospice Foundation of Taiwan in 1990 and the TAHPM in 2001. The former provides a variety of educational training courses including spirituals and wellness care, oncology volunteer training, pre-registered and advanced medical care consultants training, etc., for physicians, nurses and other allied professionals. The latter includes 26 hospitals that provide a training capacity of 567 for palliative medicine specialists (Taiwan Academy of Hospice Palliative Medicine, 2019). A very unique professional development in Taiwan is the application of Buddha dharma in spiritual care (Cheng et al., 2016). As over 70% of Taiwanese are Buddhists, Taiwan has promoted clinical Buddhist chaplains (CBC) as core members of palliative care team. They have to complete a CBC Training Programme which consists of 62.5 h of lectures, 80 h of hospice's bedside practice and 600 h of training course in hospice wards. The duty of CBCs is different from general physicians as they lead patients to "cultivate Buddha nature", "nurture compassion", "let go of possession" and "transmute the common knowledge of this transmigration-word into Buddha-knowledge" (Chen, 2012). There are 33 qualified CBCs working in 44 palliative care and hospice units in Taiwan and it is hoping to further expand across the territory (Chen, 2017).

The specialty of palliative care in Hong Kong focuses more on nurses. Up to 2011, there were around 300 nurses engaged in the provision of palliative care (Chan et al., 2017). Unlike Singapore, palliative care is not a compulsory module in medical courses in Hong Kong. Nurses who are interested in working in the field need to take postgraduate courses or diplomas including a specialty Nursing Programme in Palliative Care provided by the Institute of Advanced Nursing Studies of the Hospital Authority, Diploma in Oncology and Palliative Care for Healthcare Professionals, Higher Diploma in Community Healthcare for Senior Citizens, etc. There are several structured palliative care training workshops provided to nurses as well as other healthcare workers by institutions such as the HKACS, SPHC and the Federation of Medical Societies of Hong Kong (Food & Health Bureau, 2019). For registered doctors, there are 49 specialist palliative care physicians in Hong Kong (Yamaguchi et al., 2017). Palliative medicine is considered as a subspecialty and there are currently only 22 registered specialists in palliative medicine (The Medical Council of Hong Kong, 2018). To promote a multidisciplinary palliative care team, clinical psychologists and medical social workers were also added in public healthcare sector since 2012 to support the psychosocial needs of patients and their families (Legislative Council, 2016). The Food and Health Bureau has also recognised the need to enhance related workforce in the latest consultation report on end-of-life, and advocated that training on initiating Advance Care Planning (ACP) should not be restricted to palliative medicine specialists, but also doctors and nurses of most specialties (Food & Health Bureau, 2020).

6.2.3 Government Subsidy and Supports

Taiwan's National Health Insurance (NHI) system requires everyone to enrol in the system within two months after birth and everyone uses NHI certificate (NHI card) when visiting any clinic or hospital for medical treatment and consultation. The system only covered patients with cancers originally but had been extended to subsidised hospice home care, inpatient hospice care and hospital shared care in 1996, 2000 and 2011, respectively (Shao et al., 2017). Starting from 2009, NHI also covers patients suffering from amyotrophic lateral sclerosis, AIDS and all major organ failures including brain, heart, lung, liver and kidney failures (Chen, 2016). The cost of hospital hospice varies depending on the days of admission. The admission cost will be cheaper when the patient is admitted for a longer period (Lee et al., 2010). The Taiwanese government also funds local non-profit organisations such as Hospice Foundation of Taiwan and Buddhist Lotus Hospice Care Foundation to train hospice care professionals and volunteers, to promote hospice services. The system helps to make palliative care services affordable to citizens and has contributed to Taiwan in achieving the ranking of number 6 in the category of "Affordability of care" in 2015 QOD Index (The Economist Intelligence Unit, 2015).

Same as Taiwan, Singapore also ranked at number 6 in the category of "Affordability of care". The government subsidises intermediate and long-term care services through the Ministry of Health (MOH). To promote home care services, MOH fully funds the services provided by HCA Hospice Care and provides a grant for its premises' rental. MOH has funded inpatient hospice care since 1994 and uses the means test to determine the amount of subsidy a patient can get (Goh, 2018). The subsidy ranges from 30 to 80%, considering the gross income of the patients, the spouse and other family members living together in the same household, and the total number of persons in the same household (Ministry of Health, 2019). MediSave, a territory-wide compulsory medical savings scheme, also covers inpatient hospice care and hospice home care. The government has increased the withdrawal limits for palliative care to $2,500 per patient for day hospice and home care. There will not be any withdrawal limit if the day hospice and adult home palliative care patient is diagnosed with terminal cancer or end stage organ failure (Ministry of Health, 2019).

There is no mandatory medical savings scheme in Hong Kong but the Food and Health Bureau (FHB) has launched the Voluntary Health Insurance Scheme (VHIS) to encourage citizens to purchase at least a Standard Plan with basic health insurance coverage. The VHIS scheme also encourages people to purchase additional "Flexi Plan" which covers the cost of palliative care. Hospice centres under Hong Kong HA are all subsidised by the government and charge the same price as normal inpatient fee which is $100 per day (Hospital Authority, 2019). Private hospices, like Haven of Hope Sister Annie Skau Holistic Care Centre and the Jockey Club Home for Hospice, have varied charges but both of them offer subsidised scheme based on income and total net asset limits of recipients. HA has cooperated with charities such as the Li Ka Shing Foundation (LKSF) and Hong Kong Jockey Club Charitable Trust Fund to expand end-of-life care and contributed 10 hospitals hospice centres under the cooperated "Heart of Gold" programme. The Hong Kong Government has also granted a land to SPHC to build the first independent hospice care centre, the Jockey Club Home for Hospice, which was opened in early 2016.

6.3 Advance Directive Policy

Advance directive (AD) is a legal document, usually in writing, in which a person signed in advance to indicate that he or she does not want extraordinary life-sustaining treatment to prolong life when he or she is no longer mentally competent (Food & Health Bureau, 2019; Singapore Legal Advice, 2019). The purpose of setting an AD is to safeguard a person's will and preference for future medical or personal care. AD is voluntary and optional. It benefits people to receive suitable palliative care services and improve their quality of life.

6.3.1 Legislation of Advance Directive in Singapore and Taiwan

Singapore passed the Advance Medical Directive (AMD) Act in 1996. Under the law, terminally ill patients who are unconscious or lacking capacity to make decision on extraordinary life-sustaining treatment and at imminent death have to be certified by attending physician and two other doctors. Note that out of the three medical practitioners, at least two of them have to be recognised specialists in order to conduct an effective AMD (Menon, 2017). Anyone aged 21 or above can make an AMD voluntarily. Singapore encourages healthy citizens to make Advance Care Planning (ACP), which records their specific health treatment and care preferences to prepare for future healthcare decisions. ACP is not a legal document and doctors should carry out an AMD that takes precedence over an ACP.

Similarly, Taiwan has legalised AD made by anyone aged 20 or above through ACP. Taiwan has further improved its law protection to patients' right to autonomy by passing of Natural Death Act in 2000 which guarantees patients' right to request "do not rescue", to a newly passed law called the Patient's Right to Autonomy Act (PRAA) on 6 January 2019. Unlike Singapore, which mainly rely on physician's professional duty and assistance in finalising the decision on AD, PRAA of Taiwan completely protects a person's medical autonomy (Chen, 2019). It is the first specialised law in Asia that ensures patients are adequately informed of their health status and information is disclosed to patients' family only after approval by the patients. This safeguards patients' right to receive the necessary treatment options and to truly participate in making an AD. PRAA is not only administered to terminally ill patients but has also expanded to cover those in irreversible comas, permanent vegetative states, severe dementia and other incurable diseases. This Act is different from legal stipulations of other Asian countries or regions like Singapore, which only allow terminally ill patients to forgo life-sustaining treatment.

6.3.2 Development of Advance Directive in Hong Kong

Compared to Singapore and Taiwan, Hong Kong is comparatively slow in developing a comprehensive legislation regarding AD and dying in place. But the latest consultation report in 2019 had moved the AD legislation a step forward. The concept of AD had been promoted in a non-legislative approach under the existing common law framework since the report made by Law Reform Commission of Hong Kong in 2006 (Food & Health Bureau, 2019). Currently, Hong Kong relies on the common law framework and the guidelines made by the HA to carry out ACP and a valid AD with patient's consent to receiving health treatment. In the light of the legal uncertainties regarding AD, health professionals are under difficult situations to follow or unfollow an AD which may create conflicts with patient's will and right to refuse treatment. The Hong Kong Government therefore launched a public consultation in September 2019 to consult the public on legislation of AD and dying in place.

The Centre for Ageing and Healthcare Management Research (CAHMR) at the School of Professional Education and Executive Development (SPEED) of The Hong Kong Polytechnic University (PolyU) conducted a mini study in response to the Hong Kong government's consultation. By conducting online questionnaire with a total of 59 responses and two focus group discussions with 23 participants, results showed that respondents at large are ready to accept the concept of AD but they agreed that people in general were not familiar with AD due to lack of promotion and education (CAHMR, 2019). Doubts on the role of witnesses, format and modification, validity and applicability of an AD were mostly reflected during the discussion sessions. Participants also held mixed views on whether to allow healthy individuals to make an AD. They agreed to amend the Corners Ordinance so as to follow patients' will on dying in place and promote better end-of-life.

The findings were similar to the 607 responses made by individuals and organisations to the consultations. Most respondents showed a supportive attitude towards initials legislative proposals. Having considered the collected public views, the government proposed some key refinements on the original proposal: (1) a person who is mentally competent and is not under undue influence can make, modify or revoke an AD, (2) a medical practitioner witness should be satisfied that the person has the capability to make an AD and is informed of the nature, effect and consequences of the AD, (3) a second witness is required for verbal revocation of an AD but no witness is required for a written one and (4) a statutory Do-Not-Attempt Cardiopulmonary Resuscitation form is needed in order to facilitate an AD outside the hospital setting. The consultation concluded that ongoing legislative initiatives would be supplemented, with efforts on public education on life and death issues, healthcare workforce training, and care for older adults.

6.4 Public Awareness

6.4.1 Life and Death Education in Taiwan

Hospice Foundation of Taiwan, Buddhist Lotus Hospice Care Foundation and Taiwan Hospice Organization were developed in the 1990s and have actively putting effort in promoting hospice care, counselling, as well as life and death education. In addition, Taiwan is the first territory in Asia to introduce and standardise death education in mainstream schools for students from primary 5 to high school (Lor, 2018). The curriculum is integrated with Character and Citizenship Education. Students can learn the concept of end-of-life options and hospices, as well as self-awareness and the way to appreciate value of life. Teachers are also encouraged to integrate life and death education in other subjects such as history and language in order to make it a core component in the education system (Lor, 2018; Muto et al., 2011). To learn beyond textbooks, experiential learning opportunities are provided through field trips to hospices and interviews with relatives to let students gain deeper insights first-hand. For younger students, activities like observing the life cycles of animals and plants in parks and zoos can help to bring out the concept of death being a natural life process, and to shape perceptions of a "good death". Together with regular community promotion activities such as life and death talks, elderly programmes, essay writing and death cafes activities, Taiwan takes the lead to promote and raise public awareness on end-of-life concept within its community, from primary schools through universities.

6.4.2 Public Engagement Activities in Singapore

Unlike Taiwan, Singapore has not included life and death curriculum in her education system but focused on organising public promotion activities. Although Singapore is still yet to catch up with Taiwan's lead on public awareness, efforts have been shown to diversify the way of promoting life and death issue and palliative care. Singapore has made use of the social media in developing the nationwide advance care planning programme called "Living Matters" in 2011 to guide readers to discover one's beliefs, values and care presence online step-by-step (SingHealth, 2019). There are also local art-based engagement programmes and activities on living and dying, well organised by the Lien Foundation and Both Sides, which encourage people to speak about life and death issues through the medium of art works, music, photography, performance activities, etc. Another online platform "The Last Outfit" encourages people to talk about death and dying by changing their ideal last outfit before the end-of-life (Life Before Death, 2019). Nowadays, 53.3% of Singaporeans are more willing and comfortable to discuss end-of-life matters, compared to only 36% in 2014, as shown by a collaborated study by Singapore Management University (SMU) and Singapore Hospice Council (Singapore Hospice Council, 2019; Singapore Management University, 2019). The public (62%) are also more aware and better informed of the details of palliative care (Singapore Management University, 2019).

6.4.3 Public Promotions in Hong Kong

The Education Bureau in Hong Kong has provided the 'Health Management and Social Care' as an elective subject in some senior forms in secondary schools, which focuses more on respecting and cherish life but not death education. The Food and Health Bureau considers that targeting a group of audience, including those older adults and patients with chronic diseases and onset of terminal illnesses, their families and carers, is a good way to directly promote end-of-life care. It also seeks additional resources and assistance from NGOs to facilitate public promotion in the community (Food & Health Bureau, 2020). For community activities, as compared to Singapore, traditional ways of promotions such as regular talks and seminars on ageing, end-of-life and bereavement are more common. The Elderly Health Service of the Department of Health carries out talks in Residential Homes for the Elderly (RCHEs) and elderly centres to guide elders to express their wishes regarding their future care options openly to their families (Food & Health Bureau, 2019). The Society for Life and Death Education and SPHC are independent charitable organisations which organise different activities and events, including talk series for adults and youngsters on life and death education, Latter Life Forum, Life On The Train Exhibition, Light Up a Life Christmas Concert, etc., with the aim to affirm life's value and heighten public awareness of living and dying.

On the other hand, the Hong Kong Jockey Club Charitable Trust Fund funded and launched an official six-year project called "Jockey Club End-of-life Community Care Project" (JCECC) in 2016 to improve and promote end-of-life care. It partners with seven other institutions and regularly organises symposiums and public talks on life and death perspectives and encourages the public to plan ahead for end-of-life care. SPHC and Hong Kong PolyU's School of Nursing have conducted a study, in which about 90% of 1,015 Hong Kong respondents indicated their willingness to discuss about end-of-life issues with their family members, with over 30% of them already having discussed about the issues (Pang, 2011). The awareness and understanding towards end-of-life care and palliative care had increased to 45.6% and 39%, respectively, in 2018. However, there were still more than 60% of the public who do not know about the terms, as shown by the research by the Social Sciences Research Centre of the University of Hong Kong from 2017 to 2018 (JCECC, 2019). For the motivation to participate in end-of-life education activities, the public responses to "yes" increased to 54.3% in 2018, compared to just 40.3% in 2016.

6.5 Discussion

6.5.1 Government Funding and Subsidy

Development of palliative care has progressed the furthest in Taiwan, compared to Singapore and Hong Kong. Taiwan has sufficient availability of palliative care services by steadily increasing the number of hospice beds, training diversified allied professionals and making palliative care affordable. These achievements are due to government funding and subsidy. Financial resources are important to the development and expansion of palliative and hospice care as they determine the infrastructures, provision of human resources and affordability of services. Governments should take the lead to promote hospice care by first ensuring palliative care services affordable by local citizens. Many developing countries fail to initiate palliative care due to the lack of financial incentives from local governments and they solely rely on fund raising and voluntary donations from NGOs. Taiwan, Singapore and Hong Kong take the advantage of being high-income regions which allow them to share the financial responsibility with citizens' co-payments to palliative care. The national mandatory medical insurance systems in Taiwan and Singapore seem to maintain a balance between government expenses and citizens' out-of-pocket payments.

Followed by government's direct subsidy to citizens, cooperation with NGOs by providing land grant and project funding is also important in capacity building, providing training opportunities to allied professionals, attracting volunteers and raising public awareness. Funding can also be allocated to universities for research purposes. Spiritual needs and personal beliefs are areas that worth more investigation on, especially in Singapore and Hong Kong. With sufficient subsidy from the governments, patients can then have affordable palliative services and the professionals can have more opportunities to get involved in this field. Stable funding of projects and programmes organised by NGOs can also help maintain a healthy fundraising climate. Therefore, governments have to ensure stable and sufficient funding is provided to the development of palliative and end-of-life care.

6.5.2 Death Taboo

Cultural taboo is another concern when implementing polices on end-of-life care. This is also a root problem to be overcome by policymakers across all countries as people in different countries have their own cultures, beliefs and customs. Most people especially the older generations living in Taiwan, Singapore and Hong Kong are influenced by traditional Chinese religious teaching and cultures such as Taoism, Confucianism and Buddhism (Hsu et al., 2009). They regard death and dying as taboo topics because people believe discussion of death would bring bad luck. This leads to the avoidance to discuss or active preparation for death. Moreover, Asians treasure getting together as a group more than individuals and this gives family members an influential role in medical decisions. As some of them would like to hide the true conditions of the patients and believe it would be better for the patients not to know the truth. Opinions of family members are more likely to be followed rather than that of the patient (Glass et al., 2010). This may lead to choosing an option in contrary to the best approach of healthcare decision. In Hong Kong, some people may even consider dying at home would affect property price and the neighbours would have negative feelings towards them (Hong et al., 2010).

It is a challenge for governments to strike a balance between implementing effective polices and maintaining culturally acceptable individual behaviours and community actions. Taiwan is leading the way to break down cultural taboo against avoiding death discussion among family members in Asia. Taiwan makes progress on changing people's traditional mindset that dying without CPR is not filial (The Economist Intelligence Unit, 2015). To fulfil the responsibility of being filial, Taiwanese are now encouraged and educated to emphasise more on supporting their family members when suffering from terminal illnesses by staying with them at their end-of-life. Meanwhile, since majority of the Taiwan citizens are Buddhists, the developed profession on CBC has also helped to guide patients and their family to open up death discussion and acceptance of death by providing spiritual support which has received very positive responses from patients and also their family.

Death taboos are fading in both Singapore and Hong Kong. More people are more ready to make their own decision in the end-of-life approach and discuss about life and death issues, but this does not truly reflect whether people really express their views when approaching their final stage of life. Moreover, without sufficient professional guidance, some people may still feel embarrassed or awkward to talk about death and dying. The CBC professional development in Taiwan is an example to show how professionals play an essential role in providing spiritual support to patients and their family members, and guiding them to enhance spiritual status. As people treasure family relationships and prefer a familial-oriented approach (Wong et al., 2019), professional development and training in spiritual care supports in Hong Kong and Singapore may enhance group counselling and facilitate the creation of family memorable moments. This helps alleviate stress and tension between patients and their family, leading them to discuss more openly about death. Integrating cultural characteristics to palliative care service and breaking death taboo remain a challenge for Singapore and Hong Kong.

6.5.3 Dying at Home

Dying in place is one of the indicators of the quality of end-of-life as more people prefer dying in a familiar environment rather than in hospitals, especially intensive care units (Sadler et al., 2014). More individuals wish to spend their final days at home or at least in a comfortable home-like place, including RCHE (Gomes et al., 2013). Studies have shown that more than 70% of Singaporeans wish to be cared and die at home while over 80% of the older adults of Hong Kong prefer end-of-life care in their homes, RHCE or hospice, with only 17% of them would choose hospitals (Food & Health Bureau, 2019; Lien Foundation, 2014). However, dying in place was still not common in Singapore and Hong Kong. Compared to 40% in Taiwan, there were 39% of Singaporean patients died at home or elderly homes while there was only 10% of Hong Kong patients died outside the hospitals (Chung, 2017).

Unlike hospitals, home settings are not designed for dying in place. Studies have criticised home deaths as not always realistic due to insufficient space, limited support from healthcare professionals, and burdens to family members who take up the role of being informal caregivers. Family members also have to face the challenges of having the "appropriate equipment and home adaptations" and managing "medications and symptoms management", as well as resolving their emotional sufferings (De Roo et al., 2014; Mogan et al., 2018). Surveys on attitude on dying at home have also been criticised for just simply asking participants' preference on dying places and lacking of details such as anticipation on their death (Pollock, 2015). In fact, changes of preference have been noted throughout an illness, with the hope to be cared at home is greater than dying at home (Gomes et al., 2013). In addition, some dying people think that minimising the burden to families, relieving from strain and pain and accompanying by loved ones are more important issues (Broom & Kirby, 2013; Steinhauser et al., 2000).

Therefore, dying at home may not always be the first priority or applicable to every individual. When facilitating patients' dying at home, it is important that the palliative care team and the family should identify the dying person's needs such as pain and symptom control, and adequacy of support at home. Not dying at home does not mean death occurring in a wrong place (Pollock, 2015). On the other hand, RCHE is an appropriate alternative for dying in place with better care and support. The government should ensure adequate resources are allocated and relevant laws are enacted to allow for and to facilitate dying in place.

6.5.4 Technology Innovation

Technology can help facilitate communication between individuals, family members, caregivers and the palliative care team. Although psychological and spiritual support are still the core elements in palliative care, emerging technology in health care and treatment can assist in performing real-time assessment and facilitate the preparation of supportive services. As an example, Tzuchi University Hospital in Taiwan has piloted an online platform that enables the palliative team to monitor patients remotely using smartphones and tablets and using Skype to communicate with caregivers (The Economist Intelligence Unit, 2015). The platform includes online care instructions in six different languages. It can help tracking patient's medical conditions and make immediate assessment without waiting for the visit by medical care team. Such wireless tracking technology facilitates the development of home care and looks after those with limited access to palliative care due to mobility problems. In Switzerland, a study has investigated mHealth technologies to detect early predicted deterioration of health status in palliative care patients by equipping them a mobile phone and tracking bracelets (Theile et al., 2017). Mobile phone is installed with an application that asks patients about their visual pain and distress level while the bracelet records heart rate, blood oxygen, skin temperature, etc. This is a development of an effective remote monitoring system through wearable devices.

During the COVID-19 pandemic, healthcare facilities and services have prevented visitors in all care settings. The restriction of allowing only one visitor at a time has forced the using of telehealth in palliative care, compelling the use of Facetime, Zoom or Skype technology to carry out real-time healthcare support (Bettini, 2020; Calton et al., 2020). Some studies documented the effective communication and care with cancer patients and caregivers at home and acute care setting via video conferencing app during the pandemic (Chávarri-Guerra et al., 2021; Lee et al., 2020). A paper had documented how Zoom platform was utilised in facilitating decision-making at end-of-life for an infant (Bettini, 2020). However, some reported challenges in the capacity to utilise technology for telehealth and difficulty to communicate without face-to-face interaction (Bettini, 2020; Chávarri-Guerra et al., 2021). At the same time, healthcare staff may also have limited experience with using the technology to interact with family members while the patients remain in hospice (Calton et al., 2020). Although telehealth is not perfectly equal to palliative care that is being carried out in face-to-face, it minimises isoaltaiona and provides some support during the pandemic. Future use of telehealth in palliative care is promising, when there are more efforts in increasing technology literacy and telehealth services.

6.6 Conclusion

As countries have different geodemographic characteristics, there is no single perfect system or approach that fits all. In contrast to the emphasis on individualism and autonomy in Western countries such as the United Kingdom and Australia, cultures in most Eastern societies including Taiwan and Hong Kong treasure more on collectivism. In United Kingdom, "Each person is seen as an individual" is the first ambition in the Palliative and End-of-Life Care National Framework, while Australia government also put "A person-centred approach" as the first guiding principle in its National Palliative Care Strategy (Australian Government Department of Health, 2018; National Palliative and End-of-Life Care Partnership, 2015).

Culture and religion affect how people perceive life and death as people have different definitions of death and expectations of the places of death. The disparities may not only happen among countries but also within countries. Singapore is one of the most religious and racial diverse countries. People comprise of Chinese, Malaysian, Indian, Eurasian, etc. Therefore, providing palliative care with cultural and religious appropriateness is important and it has been recommended that professionals need to be "race-conscious" and sensitive to individual's cultural background in order to meet their needs in healthcare setting (Arivalagan & Gee, 2019). Although Western countries dominated the top 10 in the 2015 QOD Index, it may not be appropriate to adopt the same standards and guidelines of Western countries to another country. Policymakers should always consider cultural norms and differences and be aware that suitable improvement and advancements in palliative care could continue.

In conclusion, Taiwan has outperformed Singapore and Hong Kong on the overall development of palliative and end-of-life care due to its sufficient allocated resources, well developed education system and continuous refinement on legislation to protect patients' autonomy. There are similarities and differences in the approaches to promote palliative care among these three places. From the above comparison, Taiwan would need to maintain a good standard on palliative care while both Singapore and Hong Kong should step up their efforts in breaking the death taboo and increasing public awareness. Hong Kong has only positioned at a fair to middle level on the development of palliative care but being one of the "Four Asian dragons", it is expected to reach Singapore and Taiwan soon, and edge closer to top the list in future QOD Index. Last but not least, dying at home may not improve all patients' quality of death due to different individual's needs and adequacy of resources in home settings. The governments should allocate resources and impose relevant legal provisions to facilitate the environment in RCHEs for dying in place. The governments are also encouraged to follow the trend of technology advancement and integrate it with palliative care in order to facilitate home care development and improve efficiency on care delivery.

Acknowledgements The work described in this paper was partially supported by a grant from the Research Grants Council of the Hong Kong Special Administrative Region, China (Project Reference No.: UGC/IDS24/18).

References

Arivalagan, Y., & Gee, C. (2019). *Leaving well: End-of-life policies in Singapore.* https://lkyspp.nus.edu.sg/docs/default-source/ips/ips-exchange-series_no-13_leaving-well-end-of-life-policies-in-singapore_web.pdf

Australian Government Department of Health. (2018). *National Palliative Care Strategy 2018.* https://www.safetyandquality.gov.au/sites/default/files/2019-06/national_palliative_care_strategy_2018.pdf

Bettini, E. A. (2020). COVID-19 pandemic restrictions and the use of technology for pediatric palliative care in the acute care setting. *Journal of Hospice & Palliative Nursing, 22*(6), 432–434. https://doi.org/10.1097/NJH.0000000000000694

Broom, A., & Kirby, E. (2013). The end of life and the family: Hospice patients' views on dying as relational. *Sociology of Health & Illness, 35*(4), 499–513. https://doi.org/10.1111/j.1467-9566.2012.01497.x

Calton, B., Abedini, N., & Fratkin, M. (2020). Telemedicine in the time of coronavirus. *Journal of Pain and Symptom Management, 60*(1), e12–e14. https://doi.org/10.1016/j.jpainsymman.2020.03.019

Census and Statistics Department. (2019). *Population estimates.* https://www.censtatd.gov.hk/hkstat/sub/sp150.jsp?tableID=001&ID=0&productType=8

Centre for Ageing and Healthcare Management Research. (2019). *Submission to the Food and Health Bureau of the HKSAR Government on the public consultation of the consultation document on end-of-life care: Legislative proposals on advance directives and dying in place* (private communication).

Chan, H. Y. L., Lee, D. T. F., Woo, N., & Yi, H. (2017). *A study on the development of palliative and end-of-life care services in Hong Kong.* https://www.pico.gov.hk/doc/en/research_report(PDF)/2016_A4_022_16C_Final_Report_Prof_Chan.pdf

Chávarri-Guerra, Y., Ramos-López, W. A., Covarrubias-Gómez, A., Sánchez-Román, S., Quiroz-Friedman, P., Alcocer-Castillejos, N., del Pilar Milke-García, M., Carrillo-Soto, M., Morales-Alfaro, A., Medina-Palma, M. and Aguilar-Velazco, J.C., Morales-Barba, K., Razcon-Echegaray, A., Maldonado, J., & Soto-Perez-de-Celis, E. (2021). Providing supportive and palliative care using telemedicine for patients with advanced cancer during the COVID-19 pandemic in Mexico. *The Oncologist*, *26*(3), e512–e515. https://doi.org/10.1002/onco.13568

Chen, C. H. (2019). Legislating the right-to-die with dignity in a confucian society Taiwan's Patient Right to Autonomy Act. *Hastings International and Comparative Law Review, 42*(2), 485.

Chen, R. C. (2016). A personal journey in Taiwan's hospice palliative care movement, 2. *BAOJ Pall Medicine, 2*, 019.

Chen, R. C. (2017). Clinical Buddhist chaplaincy training program: History of the development of Taiwan's clinical Buddhism. *Journal of Scientific Discovery, 1*(1), 17005. https://doi.org/10.24262/jsd.1.1.17005

Chen, Y. C. (2012). Clinical Buddhist chaplain based spiritual care in Taiwan. *Taiwan Journal of Hospice Palliative Care, 17*(3), 300–309.

Cheng, S. Y., Chen, C. Y., & Chiu, T. Y. (2016). Advances of hospice palliative care in Taiwan. *The Korean Journal of Hospice and Palliative Care, 19*(4), 292–295.

Cho, C. Y. (2018). From cure to care: The development of hospice care in Taiwan. *Hospice & Palliative Medicine International Journal, 2*(5), 286–287. https://doi.org/10.15406/hpmij.2018.02.00108

Chung, R. (2017). *Overview of end-of-life care in Hong Kong now and to the future.* PowerPoint presented at the JCECC Conference: Collaboration in Creating Compassionate Holistic End-of-Life Care for the future, Hong Kong.

Dangayach, Y., & Gupta, A. (2018). Four Asian dragons-evolution and their growth. *International Journal of Advance Research, Ideas and Innovations in Technology, 3*(1), 158–162.

De Roo, M. L., Miccinesi, G., Onwuteaka-Philipsen, B. D., Van Den Noortgate, N., Van den Block, L., Bonacchi, A., Donker, G. A., Lozano Alonso, J. E., Moreels, S., Deliens, L., & Francke, A. L. (2014). Actual and preferred place of death of home-dwelling patients in four European countries: Making sense of quality indicators. *PLoS ONE, 9*(4), 9. https://doi.org/10.1371/journal.pone.0093762

Department of Statistics Singapore. (2017). *Population trends 2017.* https://www.singstat.gov.sg/-/media/files/publications/population/population2017.pdf

Food and Health Bureau. (2019). *Public consultation on end-of-life care legislative proposals launched (with video).* https://www.info.gov.hk/gia/general/201909/06/P2019090500543.htm

Food and Health Bureau. (2020). End-of-life care: Legislative proposals on advance directives and dying in place. https://www.fhb.gov.hk/download/press_and_publications/consultation/190900_eolcare/e_EOL_consultation_report.pdf

Glass, A. P., Chen, L. K., Hwang, E., Ono, Y., & Nahapetyan, L. (2010). A cross-cultural comparison of hospice development in Japan, South Korea, and Taiwan. *Journal of Cross-Cultural Gerontology, 25*(1), 1–19. https://doi.org/10.1007/s10823-009-9108-8

Goh, S. S. L. (2018). Singapore takes six steps forward in 'The Quality of Death Index' rankings. *Asia-Pacific Journal of Oncology Nursing, 5*(1), 21.

Gomes, B., Calanzani, N., Gysels, M., Hall, S., & Higginson, I. J. (2013). Heterogeneity and changes in preferences for dying at home: A systematic review. *BMC Palliative Care, 12*(1), 7. https://doi.org/10.1186/1472-684X-12-7

Hong, T. C., Lam, T. P., & Chao, D. V. K. (2010). Barriers for primary care physicians in providing palliative care service in Hong Kong—Qualitative study. *The Journal of Hong Kong College of Family Physicians, 32*(1), 3–9.

Hospital Authority. (2017). *Strategic service framework for palliative care.* http://www.ha.org.hk/haho/ho/ap/PCSSF_1.pdf

Hospital Authority. (2019). *Fee and charges.* https://www.ha.org.hk/visitor/ha_visitor_index.asp?Parent_ID=10044&Content_ID=10045&Ver=HTML

Hsu, C. Y., O'Connor, M., & Lee, S. (2009). Understandings of death and dying for people of Chinese origin. *Death Studies, 33*(2), 153–174. https://doi.org/10.1080/07481180802440431

JCECC. (2019) *Evaluation on knowledge & skill transfer.* http://foss.hku.hk/jcecc/en/evaluation-on-knowledge-skill-transfer/

Kavalieratos, D., Corbelli, J., Zhang, D. I., Dionne-Odom, J. N., Ernecoff, N. C., Hanmer, J., Hoydich, Z. P., Ikejiani, D. Z., Klein-Fedyshin, M., Zimmermann, C., Morton, S. C., Arnold R. M., Heller, L., & Schenker, Y. (2016). Association between palliative care and patient and caregiver outcomes: A systematic review and meta-analysis. *Journal of the American Medical Association, 316*(20), 2104–2114. https://doi.org/10.1001/jama.2016.16840

Lee, A. K., Cho, R. H., Lau, E. H., Cheng, H. K., Wong, E. W., Ku, P. K., Chan, J. Y., & Yeung, Z. W. (2020). Mitigation of head and neck cancer service disruption during COVID-19 in Hong Kong through telehealth and multi-institutional collaboration. *Head & Neck, 42*(7), 1454–1459. https://doi.org/10.1002/hed.26226

Lee, C. Y., Komatsu, H., Zhang, W., Chao, Y. F., Kim, K. K., Kim, G. S., Cho, Y. H., & Ko, J. S. (2010). Comparison of the hospice systems in the United States, Japan and Taiwan. *Asian Nursing Research, 4*(4), 163–173. https://doi.org/10.1016/S1976-1317(11)60001-7

Legislative Council. (2016, March 16). *Palliative care services for terminally ill patients.* http://www.info.gov.hk/gia/general/201603/16/P201603160553.htm

Lien Foundation. (2014). *77% of Singaporeans wish to die at home.* http://lienfoundation.org/sites/default/files/Death%20survey%20Presser%20Final%20-%20Combined_0.pdf

Lien Foundation. (2015, October). *Singapore ranks 12th in the global 2015 quality of death index.* http://www.lienfoundation.org/sites/default/files/SG%20QOD%202015%20Lien%20Fdn%20Press%20Release%20Final.pdf

Life Before Death. (2019). *Last outfit.* http://lifebeforedeath.com/last-outfit/

Lor, J. (2018, August). *Death education is life education.* https://www.ipscommons.sg/death-education-is-life-education/

Menon, S. (2017). Advance decision-making in Singapore. In J. Chin, N. Berlinger, M. C. Dun & M. K. Gusmano (Eds.), *A Singapore bioethics casebook volume 2.* Singapore: National University of Singapore, 2017. http://www.bioethicscasebook.sg/backgrounder/advance-directives/

Ministry of Health. (2019). *Subsidy for government-funded intermediate long-term care services.* https://www.moh.gov.sg/cost-financing/healthcare-schemes-subsidies/subsidies-for-government-funded-intermediate-long-term-care-services

Mogan, C., Lloyd-Williams, M., Harrison Dening, K., & Dowrick, C. (2018). The facilitators and challenges of dying at home with dementia: A narrative synthesis. *Palliative Medicine, 32*(6), 1042–1054. https://doi.org/10.1177/0269216318760442

Muto, T., Nakahara, T., & Nam, E. W. (2011). *Asian perspectives and evidence on health promotion and education.* Springer. https://doi.org/10.1007/978-4-431-53889-9

National Palliative and End of Life Care Partnership. (2015). *Ambitions for palliative and end of life care: A national framework for local action 2015–2020.* https://www.eolc.co.uk/uploads/Ambitions-for-Palliative-and-End-of-Life-Care.pdf

Pang, S. (2011). *Death taboo fades in Hong Kong.* https://sn.polyu.edu.hk/en/news_events/features/death_taboo_fades_in_hong_kong/index.html

Pollock, K. (2015). Is home always the best and preferred place of death? *BMJ, 351*, h4855. https://doi.org/10.1136/bmj.h4855

Sadler, E., Hales, B., Henry, B., Xiong, W., Myers, J., Wynnychuk, L., Tagger, R., Heyland, D., & Fowler, R. (2014). Factors affecting family satisfaction with inpatient end-of-life care. *PLoS ONE, 9*(11), e110860. https://doi.org/10.1371/journal.pone.0110860

Shao, Y. Y., Hsiue, E. H. C., Hsu, C. H., Yao, C. A., Chen, H. M., Lai, M. S., & Cheng, A. L. (2017). National policies fostering hospice care increased hospice utilization and reduced the invasiveness of end-of-life care for cancer patients. *The Oncologist, 22*(7), 843–849. https://doi.org/10.1634/theoncologist.2016-0367

SingHealth. (2019). *Living matters—Advance care planning.* https://www.singhealth.com.sg/rhs/live-well/Advance-Care-Planning

Singapore Hospice Council. (2019). *Palliative care services.* https://singaporehospice.org.sg/services/

Singapore Legal Advice. (2019). *Advance medical directives in Singapore.* https://singaporelegaladvice.com/law-articles/advance-medical-directives-in-singapore/

Singapore Management University. (2019, October). *SMU study shows Singaporeans are more comfortable discussing end-of-life matters.* https://news.smu.edu.sg/news/2019/10/05/smu-study-shows-singaporeans-are-more-comfortable-discussing-end-life-matters

Steinhauser, K. E., Christakis, N. A., Clipp, E. C., McNeilly, M., McIntyre, L., & Tulsky, J. A. (2000). Factors considered important at the end of life by patients, family, physicians, and other care providers. *JAMA, 284*(19), 2476–2482. https://doi.org/10.1001/jama.284.19.2476

Taiwan Academy of Hospice Palliative Medicine. (2019). *Anning palliative medicine specialist training hospital.* http://www.hospicemed.org.tw/ehc-tahpm/s/w/conEduOrg/ConEduOrg

The D. H. Chen Foundation. (2015). *Supporting palliative and hospice care services in Hong Kong.* https://dhchenfoundation.com/initiatives/supporting-palliative-and-hospice-care-services-in-hong-kong/

The Economist Intelligence Unit. (2015). *The 2015 quality of death index: Ranking palliative care across the world*. Lien Foundation.

The Medical Council of Hong Kong. (2018). *Licensing examination*. https://leip.mchk.org.hk/EN/dexam_III.html

Theile, G., Klaas, V., Tröster, G., & Guckenberger, M. (2017). mHealth technologies for palliative care patients at the interface of in-patient to outpatient care: Protocol of feasibility study aiming to early predict deterioration of patient's health status. *JMIR Research Protocols, 6*(8), e142. https://doi.org/10.2196/resprot.7676

United Nations, Department of Economic and Social Affairs (UN BESA), Population Division. (2017). *World population ageing 2017—Highlights* (ST/ESA/SER.A/397). https://www.un.org/en/development/desa/population/publications/pdf/ageing/WPA2017_Highlihts.pdf

Wong, E. Y., Mak, P. M., Fong, H. C., & Chan., L. W. (2019). Changing minds and communities: The use of innovative strategies in community engagement for end-of-life care in Hong Kong. In K. N. Chan, H. C. Fong, W. Q. Lou & L. W. Chan (Eds.), *The foundation of community-based end-of-life care in Hong Kong* (pp. 232–248). http://www.socsc.hku.hk/JCECC/case_book/HKU_SS_JCECC_book.pdf

Wong, F. K. Y., Ng, A. Y. M., Lee, P. H., Lam, P., Ng, J. S. C., Ng, N. H. Y., & Sham, M. M. K. (2016). Effects of a transitional palliative care model on patients with end-stage heart failure: A randomised controlled trial. *Heart, 102*(14), 1100. https://doi.org/10.1136/heartjnl-2015-308638

World Health Organization. (2011). *Global health and aging*. https://www.who.int/ageing/publications/global_health.pdf

World Health Organization. (2019). *WHO definition of palliative care*. https://www.who.int/cancer/palliative/definition/en/

Yamaguchi, T., Kuriya, M., Morita, T., Agar, M., Choi, Y. S., Goh, C., Lingegowda, K. B., Lim, R., Liu, R. K., MacLeod, R., Ocampo, R., & Tsuneto, S. (2017). Palliative care development in the Asia-Pacific region: An international survey from the Asia Pacific Hospice Palliative Care Network (APHN). *BMJ Supportive and Palliative Care, 7*(1), 23–31. https://doi.org/10.1136/bmjspcare-2013-000588

Chapter 7
Vaccines for the Elderly

Daniel C. S. Chiu

Abstract The elderly population is particularly susceptible to infectious diseases because of the declining immune response with age. The risk is even higher for elders with co-morbidities such as chronic lung diseases, diabetes mellitus, stroke and cancer. Furthermore, an increase in life expectancy in the elderly population results in an increase in adults residing in long stay care homes where cross infection and infectious disease outbreaks occur more frequently. Vaccination is the most effective strategy to prevent infections. Therefore, the elderly is an important target group for vaccination. Vaccination strategies vary among different countries. Nonetheless, most authorities recommend vaccination for the elderly against COVID-19, pneumococcus infection, seasonal influenza and herpes zoster. Some countries also recommend vaccination against diphtheria, tetanus and pertussis. In this chapter, we will review the justifications, efficacy, side effects and contraindications of these vaccines. Many people after retirement like to travel abroad. Vaccines against hepatitis A, encephalitis and meningococcus infection might be necessary and vaccination schedule should be individually modified for elders with cancer and other chronic diseases. Current vaccines are less immunogenic and effective for the elderly when compared with the younger adult population. We will discuss the challenges faced in improving the immune response and enhancing the coverage rate.

Keywords Elderly vaccine · Immunosenescence · COVID-19 · Influenza · Pneumococcus · Herpes Zoster · Travel vaccines

7.1 Introduction

The pace of population ageing is much faster than in the past. World Health Organization (WHO) estimates the world's population increase for the population over 60 years will nearly double from 12 to 22% by 2050 (World Health Organization

D. C. S. Chiu (✉)
Faculty of Community Health Emergency Management, Hong Kong College of Community Health Practitioners, Hong Kong, China
e-mail: danielchiucs@gmail.com

V. T. S. Law and B. Y. F. Fong (eds.), *Ageing with Dignity in Hong Kong and Asia*, Quality of Life in Asia 16, https://doi.org/10.1007/978-981-19-3061-4_7

[WHO], 2021a). Unfortunately, the advancement in life expectancy is not fully paralleled by the improvement in the health parameters (Ciabattini et al., 2018). Infectious diseases are still common even in this era of modern antibiotics and advanced intensive care medical technology, and account for a significant proportion of hospital admissions and even up to one-third of deaths in the critically ill elderly (Esme et al., 2019). In 2020, infectious disease including COVID-19 was the third leading cause of death in the United States just after heart disease and cancer (Ahmad & Anderson, 2021).

The severity of many infections is higher in the elderly compared to younger adults (Gavazzi & Krause, 2002). These infectious diseases are frequently associated with long-term complications and permanent handicap (Janssens, 2005; Lopez-Leon et al., 2021). This is partly due to immunosenescence, a term that means declining immune system associated with ageing (Allen et al., 2020). Both the innate and adaptive immune systems are involved during ageing (Derhovanessian & Pawelec, 2012), and the changes include T cell reduction from thymic involution, less effective antigen presentation through monocytes, reduced $CD4^+$ and $CD8^+$ functions, reduced phagocytosis and superoxide production in neutrophils and macrophages (Bella et al., 2007), as well as age-related alterations in toll-like receptors and defects in class switching (Agrawal & Gupta, 2011).

For elders with co-morbidities and cancer, the incidence of infection is even higher (Centers for Disease Control and Prevention [CDC], 2021a). It may be due to the dampened immunity as a result of the disease, but it can also result from the neutropenia and immune suppression caused by the immunosuppressive agents employed in the treatment. Furthermore, the rapid increase in life expectancy of the elderly leads to more old adults residing in long-term care facility, where cross infection and outbreaks of infectious diseases occur frequently.

To protect the elderly population and to promote healthy ageing, good nutrition, appropriate exercise, sleep and optimal psychological care are essential. To prevent infections, vaccination is the most efficient measure, resulting in a reduction of the incidence of bronchopneumonia, hospital admissions and overall mortality. Benefits are more consistent in the 65–74 years age group, though less in the age group above 85 years (Nichol et al., 2007). In addition, vaccination has also important public health and socioeconomic implications (Colzani, 2019).

This chapter aims to summarise the current recommendations for vaccination of the elderly in most developed countries, review immunogenicity and efficacy data for vaccines currently used, and provide an outlook on the challenges in vaccinating this age group.

7.2 Vaccines Specifically Recommended for the Elderly

Most countries have guidelines for vaccination for adults, but many countries do not have specific guidelines for the elderly (Kim et al., 2017). Table 7.1 summarises current vaccine recommendations for older adults in most developed countries.

Table 7.1 Vaccine schedules of selected countries for the elderly

	COVID-19	Influenza	Pneumococcus	Herpes Zoster
Australia	Yes	All adults	≥70; PCV13	70–79; ZVL
Canada	Yes	All adults	>–65; PPSV23	>50; RVZ/ZVL
China HKSAR	Yes	All adults (Government subsidy >50)	PCV13/PPSV23	>50; ZVL (self finance)
France	Yes	>65	PCV13 + PPSV23	65–74
Germany	Yes	>60	>60; PPSV23	–
Japan	Yes	>65	>65; PPSV23	–
Singapore	Yes	>65	PCV13/PPSV23	>50; ZVL (self finance)
UK	Yes	>50	>65; PPSV23	70–79; ZVL
US	Yes	All adults	>65; PCV13 ± PPSV23	>60; RZV

Sources Department of Health, Australia (2020, 2021), Government of Canada (2021), Centre for Health Protection (2021), CDC (2021b), European Centre for Disease Prevention and Control (2021), Infectious Disease Surveillance Center (2016), Ministry of Health (2021), National Health Service (2021b)
Abbreviations 50 = 50 years old; 60 = 60 years old; 65 = 65 years old; 70 = 70 years old; PCV13 = Pneumococcal Conjugate Vaccine; PPSV = Pneumococcal PolySaccharide Vaccine; ZVL = Zoster Vaccine Live (vaccine); RZV = Recombinant Zoster Vaccine

7.2.1 COVID-19 Vaccine

COVID-19 stands for **CO**rona**VI**rus **D**isease 20**19**, which was declared as an epidemic by the WHO in February 2020 (WHO, 2020). It is caused by a highly infectious novel virus coined SARS-CoV-2. As of 12 August 2022, more than 585 million cases were reported worldwide leading to over 6.4 million deaths. The infection is still ongoing and at least 4 variants of concern (VOC) are active (Johns Hopkins, 2021). The elderly is at special risk as the mortality due to COVID-19 increases rapidly with age after 55 years old (Woolf et al., 2021).

To reduce transmission of the infection, personal measures, physical distancing and avoiding close contacts as well as crowded and poorly ventilated places are of paramount importance. To minimise the outbreaks, stringent measures of containment, mitigation as well as rapid and comprehensive testing are needed. To prevent infection, hospitalisation and death, vaccination is considered the most promising approach (Institute for Health Metrics & Evaluation, 2021).

The primary antigenic target for COVID-19 vaccines is the surface spike protein. These vaccines are being developed unprecedently fast using several different platforms. Some of these use traditional approaches, such as inactivated virus or live attenuated virus platforms; some take up newer approaches, such as vector vaccines, recombinant proteins, mRNA and DNA vaccines (Nagy & Alhatlani, 2021). As of August 2021, WHO has granted Emergency Utilization Authorization (EUA) for 7 vaccines (WHO, 2021b), the characteristics and efficacy of which are shown in Table 7.2. Many more COVID-19 vaccines using different platforms are under preclinical and clinical trials. Notably recombinant protein subunit vaccine (NVX-COV2373) and inhalation/intranasal vaccines are the most promising candidates (Wu et al., 2021).

All the data in Table 7.2 are pooled data and should be interpreted with great caution as the target age groups studied are mostly adults between 18 and 60 years old, who have higher immune responses after vaccination. Besides, the studies are very heterogeneous, comprising Phase III clinical trials as well as real-world data. In addition, these studies were done using different protocols targeting different populations in different countries under different circumstances. Furthermore, vaccine efficacy is greatly affected by the prevailing or emerging VOCs and the data published are always lagging behind the real-world situation.

In general, it was found that all these vaccines have satisfactory protection against hospitalisation and death. Therefore, all older adults without contraindications are recommended to get vaccination. The choice of which vaccine is based mainly on local availability. There have been no large-scale double-blind head-to-head comparative studies among these vaccines, and all of these have demonstrated effectiveness in symptomatic diseases and diminishing spread (Krammer, 2020). Difference in the efficacy reported may be due to differences in the study population and location, study periods, study design and the prevalence of the VOCs at that period. In Hong Kong, people are fortunate to have a free choice of either CoronaVac or BioNTech mRNA vaccine. Both have been shown to induce a rise of neutralising antibody. A small local study showed that vaccination with BNT162b2 induced stronger humoral responses than CoronaVac while CoronaVac induced higher $CD4^+$ and $CD8^+$ T cell responses to the structural protein than BNT162b2 (Mok et al., 2021).

The contraindications to COVID-19 vaccination include known anaphylaxis to vaccine components and severe or immediate allergic reactions after receiving the first dose. Reactions after mRNA COVID-19 vaccines are very common. Most are local and systemic reactions, including pain at the injection site, fever, fatigue and headache (Chapin-Bardales et al., 2021). These events are mild and transient, occurring for 2–3 days with spontaneous resolution. In general, side effects from the inactivated vaccines are much lower (Saeed et al., 2021; Zhu et al., 2020). Nonetheless, all people after COVID-19 vaccination should be closely monitored for Bell's palsy (Wan et al., 2021), Guillain–Barre syndrome and transverse myelitis (European Medicines Agency, 2021), myocarditis (Gargano et al., 2021) and thrombocytopenic thrombotic events (Greinacher et al., 2021).

Although over 5,000 million COVID-19 vaccines have been administered worldwide, many gaps in knowledge still exist. The duration of humoral immunity, T cell immunity and long-term protection remains to be determined. There is no universally agreed correlate of protection. VOCs are keep emerging and their effect on vaccine efficacy is still not clear. Also, the impact of the vaccines on subclinical disease and transmission is not fully understood. Breakthrough infections after vaccinations have been reported (CDC, 2021d) and the need for booster doses, particularly for

Table 7.2 Characteristics of selected COVID-19 vaccines WHO approved for elders

Name	BNT162b2 Pfizer/BioNTech	mRNA-1273 Moderna	Ad26-COV2.S Janssen/J&J	AZD1222 Astra Zeneca	BBIBP-CorV Sinopharm/Beijing China	Coronavac Sinovac Beijing China
Platform	mRNA	mRNA	RIAV 26	RIAV chimpanzee	Vero cell inactivated	Vero cell inactivated
Doses and intended interval	2 doses (3 weeks apart)	2 doses (4 weeks apart)	1 dose	2 doses (4 to 12 weeks apart)	2 doses (4 weeks apart)	2 doses (4 weeks apart)
Indication	All elders without contraindications					
Storage	−70 °C	−20 °C	2–8 °C	2–8 °C	2–8 °C	2–8 °C
Efficacy at preventing disease						
Ancestral & alpha	92–95	94.1	86	85	73	50–91
Beta, Gamma, delta	90	93	85	83	63	43–59
Prevent symptomatic disease						
Ancestral & alpha	86	89	72–82	52–70	65	44–80
Beta, Gamma, delta	42–96	66–95	56–67	57	56	38–69.5
Prevent hospitalization	95–98	94–98	64–93	86–92	93	87–88
Prevent death	91.3–100	100	95	75–99	94	85–100

Sources CDC (2021c), Cerqueira-Silva et al. (2021), Connors et al. (2021), Institute for Health Metrics and Evaluation (2021), Kang et al. (2021), Li et al. (2021), National Health Service (2021a), WHO (2021c)

Abbreviation used RIAV (recombinant incompetent adenovirus vector)

subpopulations including elderly or immunocompromised persons, is still under hot debate (Center for Infectious Disease Research & Policy, 2021).

In summary, most authorities opined that the overall benefits of the COVID-19 vaccine outweigh the risk. However, vaccination for the frail and very old elderly should be individualised and their co-morbidity and medication should be taken into consideration. As vaccination prevents mainly severe infection rather than transmission of the virus, non-pharmaceutical measures such as wearing mask, washing hands, keeping safe social distancing as well as avoiding crowded and poorly ventilated spaces must be observed till herd immunity is attained or the epidemic is over.

7.2.2 Influenza (Seasonal)

Influenza is an acute respiratory disease caused mainly by influenza A or B viruses. The virus circulates in all parts of the world and initiates epidemics almost every few years, mainly in a seasonal pattern. Worldwide, these epidemics are estimated to result in about 3 to 5 million cases of severe illness and about 290,000 to 650,000 deaths annually; the greatest impact occurs in persons aged 65 or older (WHO, 2021d).

Vaccination is a very effective way to prevent seasonal influenza. Safe and effective vaccines have been used for over half a decade. The classical vaccines against influenza are inactivated vaccines and contain three different strains (A/H1N1, A/H3N2, B), coined as trivalent inactivated influenza vaccine (TIIV). As influenza virus has high mutation rate, the selection of the influenza strains to be incorporated in the vaccine has to be decided each year by WHO based on surveillance data. In many years, two different B lineages are found to co-circulate; therefore, quadrivalent inactivated influenza vaccines (QIIV) are manufactured to broaden the coverage (Shaw et al., 2002). For the elderly, only the inactivated influenza vaccines (IIV) are recommended. Live nasal attenuated influenza vaccine (LAIV) is contraindicated for adults over the age of 50 (CDC, 2021e). In recent years, a new high-dose recombinant influenza vaccine (RIV) is also available for the elderly in some countries (Dunkle et al., 2017).

Goodwin et al. (2006) reported that the elderly had lower hemagglutination inhibition antibody concentrations and lower rates of seroconversion after vaccination. Yao et al. (2011) reported that efficacy was even lower when there are co-morbidities and frailty. In the elderly, the quality of antibody responses is altered (Wang & Stollar, 1999) and cell-mediated immunity after vaccination is lower when compared with young adults (Murasko et al., 2002). Despite all these, influenza vaccination is still found to be effective in reducing influenza-related hospitalisation and death (Nichol et al., 2007).

To enhance vaccine efficacy, extensive research has been done (Weinberger, 2018). Some of these measures elicit slightly higher antibody responses (Nichol et al., 2007), and the risk of hospitalisation for influenza or pneumonia has decreased by

25% (Goodwin et al., 2006), the effect being more significant effect in older adults with respiratory and cardiovascular disease (Gravenstein et al., 1994). The high-dose preparation has claimed greater immune response in adults 65 years of age and older (Falsey et al., 2009). However, more intensive research needs to be conducted before full implementation can be recommended.

Despite all promotional campaigns, vaccine coverage is quite variable among different countries (Mereckiene et al., 2008). In the face of COVID-19 epidemic, vaccination for seasonal influenza in most countries and Hong Kong is often neglected and the vaccination rates are appallingly low. Currently, WHO and most countries are recommending ***annual*** IIV vaccination for the elderly because of the emergence of new mutants almost every year and the immunity from previous vaccination wanes over time. Elders with co-morbidity and those dwelling in long-term care facilities are listed in the priority group. In general, side effects after IIV vaccination are usually mild and transient. Severe adverse effects such as Guillain–Barre are rare even for high-dose formulation (Perez-Vilar et al., 2021). QIIV is preferred over TIIV as it provides wider scope of protection (Department of Health & Social Care, 2021; European Centre for Disease Prevention & Control, 2020). When QIIV is not readily available, one should administer TIIV as early as possible from early fall onwards. A high-dose preparation is also available for the elderly (Falsey et al., 2009) and a recombinant quadrivalent influenza vaccine (RIV) with greater immunogenicity (Dunkle et al., 2017), but no increase in side effects (Cowling et al., 2020) has recently been approved by US Food and Drug Administration (FDA) though unfortunately it is available only in a few countries. LAIV is not recommended for people >50 years of age and vaccination should be deferred in acute phase of diseases or fever. Also, a personalised scheme should be devised for those with bleeding tendencies, anaphylaxis and chronic illness (CDC, 2021e).

7.2.3 Pneumococcal Vaccine

Pneumococcal infection accounts for 25–35% of bacterial pneumonias requiring hospitalisation (CDC, 1997). It can also cause invasive diseases such as bacteraemia and meningitis (Melagaro et al., 2006). Both the incidence of pneumococcal disease and the mortality rate increase after age 50 and more sharply after age 65 (Fung & Monteagudo-Chu, 2010).

There are two types of vaccines available to prevent pneumococcal infections:

a. **Pneumococcal PolySaccharide Vaccine (PPSV)**. PPSV23 incorporates 23 purified capsular polysaccharide serotype antigens and has been used for many years for older adults. It induces only T cell-independent IgM-dominated antibody responses without adequate immunological memory. A meta-analysis study shows a reduction of the risk of invasive pneumococcal disease (OR 0.26) and all-cause pneumonia (OR 0.71) in adults (Moberley et al., 2013). However, efficacy of PPSV against pneumococcal pneumonia in the older adult is less convincing (Maruyama et al., 2010), and serotype-specific antibody concentrations are lower in the elderly and in individuals with underlying disease (Kumar & Burns, 2008). Although antibody levels fall after about 5 years, a repeat PPSV dose is not routinely recommended as there is no data showing sufficient benefits after giving the booster (CDC, 2012).

b. **Pneumococcal Conjugate Vaccine (PCV).** PCV13 comprises 13 capsular polysaccharide antigens covalently bonded to a nontoxic protein similar to diphtheria toxin. It has been demonstrated to be very effective in children, leading to indirect protection for the elderly as an effect of herd immunity effect (Lexau et al., 2005). For the older adults, PCV13 was demonstrated to be effective in preventing vaccine-type pneumococcal (45.6%) and vaccine-type invasive pneumococcal disease (75%) but not in preventing community-acquired pneumonia from any cause. Efficacy persisted for 3.97 years, the duration of the trial (Bonten et al., 2015). Though PCV13 is more immunogenic for the vaccine-specific serotypes, this study does not show PCV13 is more efficacious than PPSV 23 in adults. Also, the study does not show whether giving PCV13 in addition to PPSV23 adds value for older adults without at-risk factors.

Vaccination recommendations for pneumococcal vaccines are heterogeneous. This is partially related to vaccine availability and cost-effectiveness of the programme in various countries. In general, pneumococcal vaccination is recommended for all adults $\geq$65 years old and adults <65 years old who are at risk for pneumococcal infection or severe complications from pneumococcal infection. Whether both PCV13 and PPSV23 are indicated and whether revaccination with PPSV23 is indicated should be based on patient age and risk status (CDC, 2012). When both PCV13 and PPSV23 are indicated, they should be given at separate sessions to help ensure protective antibodies to each vaccine develop. When possible, PCV13 should be given before PPSV23. For adults who have already received PPSV23, PCV13 should be given $\geq$1 year following PPSV23. Injection site reactions are the most common adverse effects associated with pneumococcal vaccination in adults and are typically mild. Most are self-limiting and resolve within a few days of vaccination. Vaccination is contraindicated for patients who have a history of anaphylaxis to either pneumococcal vaccine or any of its components (e.g. diphtheria toxoid).

An untoward effect of the widespread use of pneumococcal conjugate vaccines has been serotype replacement, with the emergence of Serotype 19A and Serotype 3. New vaccines such as Prevenar 20 and Prevenar 15 have been approved by FDA in United States, aiming to minimise this problem (Løchen et al., 2020). Whether further new serotypes will emerge to cause hazards still await to be seen.

7.2.4 Herpes Zoster

Herpes zoster (shingles) results from reactivation of varicella-zoster virus (VZV) latent in sensory ganglia. It can lead to unilateral painful skin eruption as well as debilitating complications such as postherpetic neuralgia, encephalitis, myelitis and nerve palsies. Herpes zoster affects about 30 per cent of individuals over their lifetime. The risk of contracting the disease rises after 50 years of age, and the risk is 8–10 times more for aged 60 years or older (Schmader, 2001). This may be due to a decline in VZV-specific T cell-mediated immunity (immunosenescence) in older adults (Oxman, 2009).

There are two types of zoster vaccines approved for adults over 50 years old to increase their immunity against herpes zoster reactivation.

a. **Live attenuated Zoster Vaccine (ZVL):** This vaccine contains a high-dose attenuated varicella-zoster virus Oka-strain. It has been shown to induce antibody and T cell responses in the elderly (Levin et al., 2008) and a reduction of herpes zoster and postherpetic neuralgia by 51.3% and 66.5%, respectively (Oxman et al., 2005). However, the efficacy was only 37.6% in persons over 69 years. ZVL is generally well tolerated. The most common adverse reactions include soreness, redness, swelling and itching at the injection site and headache (Cunha, 2014). This vaccine is widely used in countries where recombinant zoster vaccine is not available. It is contraindicated for elders with anaphylaxis to the vaccine components and for elders at high risk of immune deficiency for fear of disseminated zoster infection.
b. **Recombinant Zoster Vaccine (RZV):** RZV is more than 90% efficacious against shingles across all age groups and there is no evidence of waning efficacy over a 4-year follow-up (Cunningham et al., 2016). The absolute risk of herpes zoster infection following immunisation over three and a half years decreases from 3.54% to 0.28% while the risk of postherpetic neuralgia decreases from 0.34% to 0.06% (Therapeutics Initiative, 2018). Adverse effects of RZV are more common than ZVL. The common ones include pain, redness and swelling at the injection site and myalgia, fatigue, headache, shivering, fever and gastrointestinal symptoms (Dooling et al., 2018). Serious effect such as Guillain–Barre is rare. However, it should not be given to persons allergic to the vaccine components.

Recommendations of vaccine schedules differ greatly among different countries and depend on vaccine availability, cost-effectiveness, population characteristics as well as government policies. The vaccination schedule and strategy depend on the type of vaccine to be given. In general, zoster vaccines are recommended to all elders without contraindications from 60 years of age irrespective of any history of herpes zoster or chickenpox. For adults ≥50 years, especially those immunocompromised or with co-morbidities, they are encouraged to get vaccinated with RZV. For adults ≥60 years, RZV is preferred to ZVL because it provides better and longer lasting protection. In the absence of RZV, ZVL should also be offered to those at risk of infection. However, for both RZV and ZVL, it should not be given to those adults with a history of anaphylaxis to a vaccine component or after previous vaccination. In addition, ZVL should not be offered to adults with immunodeficiency. For those with severe acute illness or taking specific antivirals, vaccination should be deferred, and medical advice should be sought. For those who have had ZVL before or those planning for immunosuppressive therapy, vaccination schedule of the RZV should be individualised (CDC, 2021f).

7.3 Vaccination for Special Groups

Vaccine recommendation for adults in general needs to be evaluated in older elders. It is mainly due to the waning immunity with age (Hainz et al., 2005). Also, the risk of infection and pattern of lifestyles are different for thc elderly.

7.3.1 Tetanus, Diphtheria and Pertussis

Many elders got vaccination against tetanus, diphtheria and pertussis in their childhood. The immunity drops with time and protective antibodies, say against diphtheria, are not attained even after single boosters (Weinberger, 2017). In many countries, elderly adults are advised to get vaccination against tetanus and diphtheria (with or without pertussis) every 10 years. For families expecting to have new babies, pertussis booster vaccination for all adults (elders included) is recommended at least 2 weeks before the birth of baby as it was found to protect not only the adults, but also offer indirect protection for the newborn babies (CDC, 2021g).

7.3.2 Travel Vaccines

More adults travel worldwide nowadays due to improved health and mobility of this age group (Hill, 2000). Subsequently, they will be exposed to the new potential infections not prevalent in their hometowns. Unfortunately, their immunity is waning and their ability to deal with novel infection is limited. Elders are advised to review their own routine immunisation record and to make up for any missing dose. If they travel to endemic or high risk area, additional vaccine types should be considered to offer them extra protection. The choice of these vaccines depends on the destination, the duration of stay, the travel pattern (camping or staying in hotels) and their own health status. Table 7.3 summarises the common vaccines elders should consider before they travel. These vaccines, if needed, should be given early enough, say 6–8 weeks, before travelling to allow for the development of an adequate antibody response and for booster vaccination if needed. Some countries might need valid certificates of vaccination, particularly yellow fever and meningococcal vaccine, upon entry. All elders are reminded to check periodically for updated information before, during and after travelling (CDC, 2021h; HealthLinkBC, 2021; National Health Service, 2021c; U.S. Department of Health & Human Services, 2021a; WHO, 2021e).

Table 7.3 Vaccines to be considered for elder planning to travel

Cholera Vaccine Cholera is a life-threatening infection caused by bacteria, which transmits the disease through contaminated food or drink. Elders travelling to endemic areas should consider taking the vaccine which comes in liquid form
Hepatitis A Vaccine Hepatitis A is a disease caused hepatitis A virus, which is transmitted through contaminated food, particularly shell food. Elders are advised to take hepatitis A vaccine if they have not taken it in the past and will be going to areas where hepatis A is prevalent
Hepatitis B Vaccine Hepatitis B is a disease caused by hepatitis B virus, which spreads by unprotected sexual intercourse or infected needle or blood products. It can cause liver damage and liver cancer. Elders are to take the vaccine if they plan to stay for 6 months or longer in an endemic country, especially if they expect to have sexual relations or blood contact with local residents. The vaccine is in the form of injections and 3 shots are required for life long protection
Japanese Encephalitis Vaccine Japanese encephalitis is a serious and life-threatening infection caused by a virus, which spreads by the bite of infected mosquitoes. Elders are recommended to take 2 doses of the vaccine (7–28 days apart) if they plan to live or camp in rural areas in endemic countries
Meningococcal Infection Vaccine Meningococcal infection is a serious and life-threatening infection caused by meningococcal bacteria. The infection spreads by coughing, sneezing or saliva and close face-to-face contact. Elders are recommended if they travel to endemic areas especially Africa and Middle East. Vaccination certificate is a requirement for travelling to Mecca (for the annual "Hajj")
Polio Vaccine Polio is a viral disease transmitted by taking food or drink contaminated by virus-loaded faeces. Elders are advised take a dose of inactivated polio vaccine if they have not been fully vaccinated in the past and will be going to areas where polio is prevalent
Rabies Vaccine Rabies is an infection of the brain caused by a virus that spreads through the bite or scratch of an infected animal. Elders are recommended to take the vaccine if they travel to areas at risk of exposure to rabies. Examples include parts of Latin America, South East Asia, India and Africa
Tick-borne encephalitis Vaccine Ticks can cause severe viral infections of the nervous system (encephalitis). Elders are recommended to take this vaccine if they plan to go to endemic areas. Examples are eastern, central, northern and increasingly western European countries, and in northern China, Mongolia, and the Russian Federation
Typhoid Fever Vaccine Typhoid Fever is a serious infection caused by typhoid bacteria, which is transmitted through food or drinks contaminated with feces. Elders travelling to endemic areas should consider taking the vaccine which exists in oral or injection forms
Yellow Fever Vaccine Yellow Fever is a serious and life-threatening infection caused by a virus, which spreads by the bite of infected mosquitoes. Elders are recommended to take the vaccine if they travel to areas at risk. Examples include tropical areas of Africa, Central and South America. The vaccine comes in one dose and must be taken at least 10 days before you travel to a tropical area. Some countries require an "International Certificate of Vaccination Against Yellow Fever" as an entry requirement

7.3.3 Special Elderly Subgroups

Elderly adults are prone to have co-morbidities such as chronic lung diseases, stroke, cancer, cirrhosis, chronic nephritis, autoimmunity disorders and diabetes mellitus. As a result, their immunity is low. In addition, elders with cancer or after splenectomy or organ transplantation are in a worse immune status because of the immunosuppressive drugs and radiation used. Therefore, at-risk elderly persons should be considered to receive vaccine as chemoprophylaxis if they are at risk of exposure to infectious diseases. When they are planning to undergo surgery or chemotherapy, vaccination should be included as one part of the pre-treatment planning (CDC, 2021a).

7.3.4 Special Precautions

Some elderly adults might be too frail or are not suitable for vaccination because of health conditions. No live attenuated vaccines should be given to adults over 50 years of age. If the elders have acute infections, vaccination should be deferred and medical advice should be sought. Vaccination schedule might need modification as regards dosage, route of administration and timing to tailor to the individual needs (CDC, 2021i; U.S. Department of Health & Human Services, 2021b).

7.4 Challenges and the Future

The current vaccines against common elderly infectious disease have achieved great contribution in reducing infection-related morbidity and mortality. Also they have great impact on the socioeconomic and public health system (Colzani, 2019). Despite these, there remain many limitations and challenges to tackle.

a. **Suboptimal efficacy for the elderly.** In general, the efficacy of most vaccines is lower in elderly than younger adults or children. This is partly due to immunosenescence as described above. Rauch et al. (2018), van Riel and de Wit (2020) and Pollard and Bijker (2021) have recently published reviews of the new vaccine platforms and developments. Table 7.4 enlists the current strategies under research and clinical trials to enhance vaccine efficacy.

b. **Incomplete scope of protection.** Elders are particularly prone to contract pneumococcal infection, which can be caused by almost 100 serotypes of Streptococcus Pneumoniae. Current PPVS vaccine confers only mild

Table 7.4 New generation strategies to enhance vaccine efficacy

1. Increasing antigen dosages (Cate et al., 2010)
2. Adjuvants such as MF59 (Tregoning, 2018; CDC, 2021j)
3. liposome-based adjuvants AS01B (Chlibek et al., 2013)
4. Virosomal vaccines (de Bruijn et al., 2006)
5. Toll like receptor (Duggan et al., 2011)
6. Viral vector vaccines (Williams, 2014)
7. mRNA vaccines (Pardi et al., 2018)
8. DNA vaccine (Kutzler & Weiner 2008; WHO, 2021f)
9. $CD4^+$ and $CD8^+$ T cell enhancement (Berthoud et al., 2011)
10. Universal vaccine (Wiersma et al., 2015)
11. Booster schedules (Cools et al., 2009)
12. Intradermal influenza vaccination (Nicolas & Guy, 2008)
13. Antigen impregnated in micro-needles (Zhu et al., 2009)
14. Intranasal COVID 19 and influenza vaccine (HKU, 2021)
15. Inhalational covid vaccine (Wu et al., 2021)

to moderate protection against 23 serotypes, and the conjugate vaccine PCV13 is targeting only 13 serotypes. Expanding the scope of protection for the most virulent serotypes is essential. The recent approval by FDA of PCV15 and PCV20 marks a great progress, but there is still a large gap to fill and cannot alleviate the possible emergence of new serotypes replacement.

c. **Ongoing mutation and variants.** COVID-19 vaccines target mainly against the spike protein, which is constantly mutating and generating many new VOCs. Current influenza vaccines focus mainly on haemagglutinin and neuraminidase antigens, which are also notorious to mutate. New vaccines incorporating the new mutant genes can be manufactured and given annually or periodically, but that means there is always a few months lagging behind the epidemic. Current research for a universal vaccine targeting at the more conserved structure of the virus, say M protein in influenza virus, has gained some success (Wiersma et al., 2015). A similar line of research for COVID-19 might help to curb the epidemic.

d. **Failure to protect viruses at the point of pathogen invasion**. COVID-19 vaccines produce antibodies against the spike proteins in the blood circulation. However, the virus replicates at the nasopharynx and the airway before entering the lung and blood stream. As a result, transmission of the disease and emergence of VOCs keep occurring even in fully vaccinated adults. Intranasal (Clinical Trial Centre, The University of Hong Kong, 2021) and inhalational vaccines (Wu et al., 2021) are under clinical trials, aiming to curb the epidemic by generating sufficient IgA to nib the virus at first frontier of invasion.

e. **Some current vaccines are not suitable to the elderly**. Live attenuated vaccine is generally not recommended for the elderly for fear of serious side effects, especially those who are immunocompromised and have co-morbidities. As a result, intranasal influenza live attenuated vaccine is not recommended for adults over 50 years old. Fortunately, the newly developed RIV shows promising result for the elderly with no increase in side effects. Another example is for herpes zoster, when ZVL is not recommended for this reason (Hales et al., 2014). In 2020, a new 2-dose RZV has been licensed in US and can safely produce over 90% protection even in persons older than 80 years (Cunningham et al., 2016). Regrettably, this vaccine is available only to a fcw wealthier countries for the time being.
f. **Many infectious diseases are not covered by current available vaccine**s. Respiratory syncytial virus (RSV), which affects the frail elders and individuals with underlying co-morbidities, results in excess hospitalisation and death every year (Fleming et al., 2015). Bacterial infections such as Staphylococcal aureus, Klebsiella pneumoniae, Escherichia Coli and Clostridium are highly detrimental to the elderly as antibiotic resistance is a growing problem. Current success in producing vaccines against these infections is still limited (Fowler et al., 2013; Swanson et al., 2015) and this should be targets for vaccine development. Furthermore, new developments are needed to tackle new foreseeable novel epidemics (Rauch et al., 2018).
g. **Storage and transportation problems.** Most current vaccines need to be transported and stored in strict cold-chain environment. In particular, mRNA COVID-19 vaccines have to be stored at −50 to −70C. This is a great handicap for underdeveloped countries. New development should be directed to develop effective vaccines for the elderly with more desirable properties including single-dose, no cold-chain and non-injectable delivery system.
h. **Adverse events following immunisation**. Though most current vaccines produce acceptable side effects. Serious complications such as anaphylaxis, Guillain–Barre syndrome, myocarditis and thrombosis, though rarely, do occur. In addition, many vaccines suffer from side effects such as fever, chills, malaise and pain caused frequently in mRNA vaccines. Research should be directed to identify and alleviate all the risk factors to minimise undue sufferings.
i. **Low vaccine coverage**. Despite extensive promotion, the vaccine coverage is low for the elderly population (US Pharmacist, 2021). As a result, building up an efficient herd immunity is a haunting target for highly infectious diseases. The low coverage rate is partly due to the inadequate knowledge of the elders about the vaccines. Many elders fear side effects and doubt the efficacy of the vaccines. More promotional exercises need to be organised to rebut these myths. In addition, practical and customer friendly implementation strategies are needed (CDC, 2021j; Immunization Action Coalition, 2017). Otherwise, guidelines without implementation strategies will end up in unsatisfactory vaccination coverage and exist only as theoretical benefits (European Centre for Disease Prevention & Control, 2017). Mandatory vaccination is always a debatable

subject though small-scale herd immunity through mass vaccination of healthcare workers in hospitals and long-term care facilities has been shown to provide indirect protection for the elderly (Cortes-Penfield, 2014).

j. **Insufficient global coordination of research and data sharing**. Data sharing about diseases, prevalence, effectiveness and adverse effects after vaccination is of paramount importance to provide optimal care for the elderly. Also, the problem of vaccine equity should be addressed. Failure to do so will leave epidemics lingering on for a long time and more VOCs will emerge. WHO and developed countries should take the lead to coordinate different governments to develop efficient plans to curb the epidemics, which include both data and knowledge sharing, expertise and financial support, effective vaccination strategy and distribution equity.

7.5 Conclusion

Older adults are at high risk for infectious diseases, and vaccination is an important preventive measure to prevent infection and facilitate healthy ageing. Major advances in the field of vaccinology over the last decades have saved many lives and reduce sufferings especially for the elders. Nonetheless, there are still arenas for improvement.

At the research level, further work has to be done to probe into the basics of immunosenescence, to facilitate the development of a single-dose, safe, needle-free affordable vaccine with higher efficacy, long-term protection and least reactogenicity vaccines for the elderly. Also, vaccines with broader scope of protections should be developed to meet the emergence of new pathogens and resurge of older pathogens.

At the government level, in conjunction with other measures of preventing infections, dedicated vaccination guidelines should be drawn and properly implemented for the elderly for her own country, considering all the epidemiological and socioeconomic factors. Practical promotional strategy should be devised to enhance vaccine coverage. This does not only save lives but also alleviates healthcare costs and socioeconomic losses. For the developed countries, more funding should be invested for vaccine research.

At a global level, WHO can coordinate research and data sharing among all countries. Guidelines at a global perspective are essential particularly for the less privileged countries, who need also financial, knowledge and expertise support. The problem of vaccine equity must be addressed because "*No one is safe until everyone is safe*" (UNICEF, 2021).

Finally, the least an individual can do is to get protected through appropriate vaccines at the right time. However, it must be stressed that vaccination is only one of the measures to prevent infections. All other non-pharmaceutical interventions such as personal and environmental hygiene, early identification and containment of infection as well as measures to interrupt the spread of pathogens are of equal importance, especially in the prevailing phase of epidemics or outbreaks.

References

Agrawal, A., & Gupta, S. (2011). Impact of aging on dendritic cell functions in humans. *Ageing Research Reviews, 10*(3), 336–345. https://doi.org/10.1016/j.arr.2010.06.004

Ahmad, F., & Anderson, R. (2021). The leading causes of death in the US for 2020. *JAMA, 325*(18), 1829–1830. https://doi.org/10.1001/jama.2021.5469

Allen, J., Toapanta, F., Chen, W., & Tennant, S. (2020). Understanding immunosenescence and its impact on vaccination of older adults. *Vaccine, 38*(52), 8264–8272. https://doi.org/10.1016/j.vaccine.2020.11.002

Bella, D., Bierti, L., Presicce, P., Arienti, R., Valenti, M., Saresella, M., Vergani, C., & Villa, M. (2007). Peripheral blood dendritic cells and monocytes are differently regulated in the elderly. *Clinical Immunology, 122*(2), 220–228. https://doi.org/10.1016/j.clim.2006.09.012

Berthoud, T., Hamill, M., Lillie, P., Hwenda, L., Collins, K., Ewer, K., Milicic, A., C. Poyntz, H., Lambe, T., Fletcher, H., Hill, A., & Gilbert, S. (2011). Potential CD8+ Tcell immunogenicity in humans of a novel heterosubtypic influenza A vaccine. MVA-NP+M1. *Clinical Infectious Diseases, 52*, 1–7.

Bonten, M. J., Huijts, S. M., Bolkenbaas, M., Webber, C., Patterson, S., Gault, S., van Werkhoven, C. H., van Deursen, A. M. M., Sanders, E. A. M., Verheij, T. J. M., Patton, M., McDonough, A., Moradoghli-Haftvani, A., Smith, H., Mellelieu, T., Pride, M. W., Crowther, G., Schmoele-Thoma, B., Scott, D. A., ... & Grobbee, D. E. (2015). Polysaccharide conjugate vaccine against pneumococcal pneumonia in adults. *The New England Journal of Medicine, 372*(12), 1114–1125. https://doi.org/10.1056/NEJMoa1408544

Cate, T. R., Rayford, Y., Nino, D., Winokur, P., Brady, R., Belshe, R. et al. (2010). A high dosage influenza vaccine induced significantly more neuraminidase antibody than standard vaccine among elderly subjects. *Vaccine, 28*, 2076–2079.

CDC. (1997). *Prevention of pneumococcal disease: Recommendations of the Advisory Committee on Immunization Practices (ACIP).* https://www.cdc.gov/mmwr/preview/mmwrhtml/00047135.htm

CDC. (2012). *Licensure of 13-valent pneumococcal conjugate vaccine for adults aged 50 years and older.* https://www.cdc.gov/mmwr/preview/mmwrhtml/mm6121a3.htm

CDC. (2021a). *Preventing infections in cancer patients.* https://www.cdc.gov/cancer/dcpc/resources/features/preventinfections/index.htm

CDC. (2021b). *Immunization schedules.* https://www.cdc.gov/vaccines/schedules/index.html

CDC. (2021c). *Vaccines for COVID-19.* https://www.cdc.gov/coronavirus/2019-ncov/vaccines/index.html

CDC. (2021d). *The possibility of COVID-19 after vaccination: Breakthrough infections.* https://www.cdc.gov/coronavirus/2019-ncov/vaccines/effectiveness/why-measure-effectiveness/breakthrough-cases.html

CDC. (2021e). *Immunogenicity, efficacy, and effectiveness of influenza vaccines.* https://www.cdc.gov/flu/professionals/acip/immunogenicity.htm

CDC. (2021f). *Shingrix recommendations.* https://www.cdc.gov/vaccines/vpd/shingles/hcp/shingrix/recommendations.html

CDC. (2021g). *Pertussis: Summary of vaccine recommendations.* https://www.cdc.gov/vaccines/vpd/pertussis/recs-summary.html

CDC (2021h). *Vaccines. Medicines. Advice.* https://wwwnc.cdc.gov/travel

CDC. (2021i). *Who should not get vaccinated with these vaccines?.* https://www.cdc.gov/vaccines/vpd/should-not-vacc.html

CDC. (2021j). *Strategies for increasing adult vaccination rates.* www.cdc.gov/vaccines/hcp/adults/for-practice/increasing-vacc-rates.html.

Center for Infectious Disease Research and Policy. (2021). *Israeli advisors back COVID vaccine boosters for older people.* https://www.cidrap.umn.edu/news-perspective/2021/07/israeli-advisors-back-covid-vaccine-boosters-older-people

Centre for Health Protection. (2021). *Vaccination schemes.* https://www.chp.gov.hk/en/features/17980.html

Cerqueira-Silva, T., Oliveira, V. A., Pescarini, J., Júnior, J. B., Machado, T. M., Ortiz, R. F., Penna, G., Ichihara, M., de Barros, J., Boaventura, V., Barreto, M., Werneck, G., & Barral-Netto, M. (2021). The effectiveness of Vaxzevria and CoronaVac vaccines: A nationwide longitudinal retrospective study of 61 million Brazilians (VigiVac-COVID19). *medRxiv.* https://doi.org/10.1101/2021.08.21.21261501

Chlibek, R., Bayas, J., Collins, H., Pinta, M., Ledent, E., Mols, J., & Heineman, T. (2013). Safety and immunogenicity of an AS01-adjuvanted varicella-zoster virus subunit candidate vaccine against herpes zoster in adults >=50 years of age. *Journal of Infectious Diseases, 208*, 1953–1961.

Chapin-Bardales, J., Gee, J., & Myers, T. (2021). Reactogenicity following receipt of mRNA-based COVID-19 vaccines. *JAMA, 325*(21), 2201–2202. https://doi.org/10.1001/jama.2021.5374

Ciabattini, A., Nardini, C., Santoro, F., Garagnani, P., Franceschi, C., & Medaglini, D. (2018). Vaccination in the elderly: The challenge of immune changes with aging. *Seminars in Immunology, 40*, 83–94. https://doi.org/10.1016/j.smim.2018.10.010

Clinical Trial Centre, The University of Hong Kong. (2021). *[Now News] Phase 1 clinical trial of HKU intranasal COVID-19 vaccine has commenced (May 15, 2021).* https://public.hkuctc.com/en/news/category

Cools, H., Gussekloo, J., Remmerswaal, J., Remarque, E., & Kroes, A. (2009). Benefits of increasing the dose of influenza vaccine in residents of long-term care facilities: A randomized placebo-controlled trial. *Journal of Medical Virology, 81*, 908–914.

Colzani, E. (2019). Beyond morbidity and mortality: The burden of infectious diseases on healthcare services. *Epidemiology and Infection, 147*, e251. https://doi.org/10.1017/S0950268819001298

Connors, M., Graham, B., Lane, H., & Fauci, A. (2021). SARS-CoV-2 vaccines: Much accomplished, much to learn. *Annals of Internal Medicine, 174*(5), 687–690. https://doi.org/10.7326/M21-0111

Cortes-Penfield, N. (2014). Mandatory influenza vaccination for health care workers as the new standard of care: A matter of patient safety and nonmaleficent practice. *American Journal of Public Health, 104*(11), 2060–2065. https://doi.org/10.2105/AJPH.2013.301514

Cowling, B., Thompson, M., Ng, T., Fang, V., Perera, R., Leung, N., Chen, Y., So, H., Ip, D., & Iuliano, A. comparative reactogenicity of enhanced influenza vaccines in older adults. *The Journal of Infectious Diseases, 222*(8), 1383–1391. https://doi.org/10.1093/infdis/jiaa255

Cunha, J. (2014). *Zostavax side effects center.* https://www.rxlist.com/zostavax-side-effects-drug-center.htm

Cunningham, A., Lai, H., Kovac, M., Chlibek, R., Hwang, S., Diez-Domingo, J., Godeaux, O., Levin, M., McElhaney, J., Puig-Barberà, B., Abeele, C., & Vesikari, T. (2016). Efficacy of the herpes zoster subunit vaccine in adults 70 years of age or older. *The New England Journal of Medicine, 375*(11), 1019–1032. https://doi.org/10.1056/NEJMoa1603800

de Bruijn, I., Nauta, J., Gerez, L., & Palache, A. (2006). The virosomal influenza vaccine Invivac: immunogenicity and tolerability compared to an adjuvanted influenza vaccine (Fluad) in elderly subjects. *Vaccine, 24*, 6629–6631.

Department of Health, Australia. (2020). *National immunisation program schedule 1 July 2020.* https://www.health.gov.au/sites/default/files/documents/2020/06/national-immunisation-program-schedule-for-all-non-indigenous-people_0.pdf

Department of Health, Australia. (2021). *Immunisation for adults.* https://www.health.gov.au/health-topics/immunisation/immunisation-throughout-life/immunisation-for-adults.

Department of Health & Social Care. (2021). *JCVI interim advice: Potential COVID-19 booster vaccine programme winter 2021 to 2022.* https://www.gov.uk/government/publications/jcvi-interim-advice-on-a-potential-coronavirus-covid-19-booster-vaccine-programme-for-winter-2021-to-2022/jcvi-interim-advice-potential-covid-19-booster-vaccine-programme-winter-2021-to-2022

Derhovanessian, E., & Pawelec, G. (2012). Vaccination in the elderly. *Microbial Biotechnology, 5*(2), 226–232. https://doi.org/10.1111/j.1751-7915.2011.00283.x

Dooling, K., Guo, A., Patel, M., Lee, G., Moore, K., Belongia, E., & Harpaz, R. (2018). Recommendations of the advisory committee on immunization practices for use of Herpes Zoster vaccines. *MMWR Morbidity and Mortality Weekly Report, 67*(3), 103–108. https://www.cdc.gov/mmwr/volumes/67/wr/mm6703a5.htm

Duggan, J., You, D., Cleaver, J., Larson, D., Garza, R., Pruneda, F., Tuvim, M., Zhang, J., Dickey, B., & Evans, S. (2011) Synergistic interactions of TLR2/6 and TLR9 induce a high level of resistance to lung infection in mice. Journal of Immunology, *186*, 5916–5926.

Dunkle, L., Izikson, R., Patriarca, P., Goldenthal, K., Muse, D., Callahan, J., & Cox, M. (2017). Efficacy of recombinant influenza vaccine in adults 50 years of age or older. *The New England Journal of Medicine, 376*(25), 2427–2436. https://doi.org/10.1056/NEJMoa1608862

Esme, M., Topeli, A., Yavuz, B., & Akova, M. (2019). Infections in the elderly critically-ill patients. *Frontiers in Medicine, 6*, 118. https://doi.org/10.3389/fmed.2019.00118

European Centre for Disease Prevention and Control. (2017). *Seasonal influenza vaccination in Europe—Vaccination recommendations and coverage rates in the EU member states for eight influenza seasons: 2007–2008 to 2014–2015.* https://www.ecdc.europa.eu/sites/portal/files/documents/influenza-vaccination-2007%E2%80%932008-to-2014%E2%80%932015.pdf

European Centre for Disease Prevention and Control. (2020). *Systematic review of the efficacy, effectiveness and safety of newer and enhanced seasonal influenza vaccines.* https://www.ecdc.europa.eu/en/publications-data/seasonal-influenza-systematic-review-efficacy-vaccines

European Centre for Disease Prevention and Control. (2021). *Vaccine schedule in all countries in the EU/EEA.* https://vaccine-schedule.ecdc.europa.eu/

European Medicines Agency. (2021). *COVID-19 Vaccine Janssen: Guillain-Barré syndrome listed as a very rare side effect.* https://www.ema.europa.eu/en/news/covid-19-vaccine-janssen-guillain-barre-syndrome-listed-very-rare-side-effect

Falsey, A., Treanor, J., Tornieporth, N., Capellan, J., & Gorse, G. (2009). Randomized, double-blind controlled phase 3 trial comparing the immunogenicity of high-dose and standard-dose influenza vaccine in adults 65 years of age and older. *The Journal of Infectious Diseases, 200*(2), 172–180. https://doi.org/10.1086/599790

Fleming, D., Taylor, R., Lustig, R., Schuck-Paim, C., Haguinet, F., Webb, D., Matias, G., & Taylor, S. (2015). Modelling estimates of the burden of respiratory Syncytial virus infection in adults and the elderly in the United Kingdom. *BMC Infectious Diseases, 15*, 443. https://doi.org/10.1186/s12879-015-1218-z

Fowler, V., Allen, K., Moreira, E., Moustafa, M., Isgro, F., Boucher, H., Corey, G., Carmeli, Y., Betts, R., Hartzel, J., Chan, I., McNeely, T., Kartsonis, N., Guris, D., Onorato, M., Smugar, S., DiNubile, M., & Meulen, A. (2013). Effect of an investigational vaccine for preventing Staphylococcus Aureus infections after cardiothoracic surgery: A randomized trial. *JAMA, 309*(13), 1368–1378. https://doi.org/10.1001/jama.2013.3010

Fung, H., & Monteagudo-Chu, M. (2010). Community-acquired pneumonia in the elderly. *The American Journal of Geriatric Pharmacotherapy, 8*(1), 47–62. https://doi.org/10.1016/j.amjopharm.2010.01.003

Gargano, J., Wallace, M., Hadler, S., Langley, G., Su, J., Oster, M., Broder, K., Gee, J., Weintraub, E., Shimabukuro, T., Scobie, H., Moulia, D., Markowitz, L., Wharton, M., McNally, V., Romero, J., Talbot, H., Lee, G., Daley, M., & Oliver, S. (2021). Use of mRNA COVID-19 vaccine after reports of myocarditis among vaccine recipients: Update from the advisory committee on immunization practices—United States, June 2021. *MMWR Morbidity and Mortality Weekly Report, 70*(27), 977–982. https://www.cdc.gov/mmwr/volumes/70/wr/mm7027e2.htm

Gavazzi, G., & Krause, K. (2002). Ageing and infection. *The Lancet Infectious Diseases, 2*(11), 659–666. https://doi.org/10.1016/s1473-3099(02)00437-1

Goodwin, K., Viboud, C., & Simonsen, L. (2006). Antibody response to influenza vaccination in the elderly: A quantitative review. *Vaccine, 24*(8), 1159–1169. https://doi.org/10.1016/j.vaccine.2005.08.105

Government of Canada. (2021). *Immunization of adults: Canadian Immunization Guide.* https://www.canada.ca/en/public-health/services/publications/healthy-living/canadian-immunization-guide-part-3-vaccination-specific-populations/page-2-immunization-of-adults.html

Gravenstein, S., Drinka, P., Duthie, E., Miller, B., Brown, C., Hensley, M., Circo, R., Langer, E., & Ershler, W. (1994). Efficacy of an influenza hemagglutinin-diphtheria toxoid conjugate vaccine in elderly nursing home subjects during an influenza outbreak. *Journal of the American Geriatrics Society, 42*(3), 245–251. https://doi.org/10.1111/j.1532-5415.1994.tb01746.x

Greinacher, A., Thiele, T., Warkentin, T., Weisser, K., Kyrle, P., & Eichinger, S. (2021). Thrombotic thrombocytopenia after ChAdOx1 nCov-19 vaccination. *The New England Journal of Medicine, 384*(22), 2092–2101. https://doi.org/10.1056/NEJMoa2104840

Hainz, U., Jenewein, B., Asch, E., Pfeiffer, K., Berger, P., & Grubeck-Loebenstein, B. (2005). Insufficient protection for healthy elderly adults by tetanus and TBE vaccines. *Vaccine, 23*(25), 3232–3235. https://doi.org/10.1016/j.vaccine.2005.01.085

Hales, C., Harpaz, R., Ortega-Sanchez, I., & Bialek, S. (2014). Update on recommendations for use of herpes zoster vaccine. *MMWR Morbidity and Mortality Weekly Report, 63*(33), 729–731. https://www.cdc.gov/mmwr/preview/mmwrhtml/mm6333a3.htm

HealthLinkBC. (2021). *Travel immunizations for adults.* https://www.healthlinkbc.ca/healthlinkbc-files/travel-immunizations-adults

Hill, D. (2000). Health problems in a large cohort of Americans traveling to developing countries. *Journal of Travel Medicine, 7*(5), 259–266. https://doi.org/10.2310/7060.2000.00075

Immunization Action Coalition. (2017). *Strategies to improve adult vaccination coverage.* https://www.immunize.org/catg.d/p2050.pdf

Institute for Health Metrics and Evaluation. (2021). *COVID-19 vaccine efficacy summary.* http://www.healthdata.org/covid/covid-19-vaccine-efficacy-summary

Janssens, J. (2005). Pneumonia in the elderly (geriatric) population. *Current Opinion in Pulmonary Medicine, 11*(3), 226–230. https://doi.org/10.1097/01.mcp.0000158254.90483.1f

Infectious Disease Surveillance Center. (2016). *Routine/voluntary immunization schedule in Japan (October 1, 2016).* https://www.niid.go.jp/niid/images/vaccine/schedule/2016/EN20161001.pdf

Johns Hopkins. (2021). *COVID-19 dashboard.* https://coronavirus.jhu.edu/map.html

Kang, M., Yi, Y., Li, Y., Sun, L., Deng, A., Hu, T., Zhang, J., Liu, J., Cheng, M., Xie, S., Luo, M., Jiang, J., Jiang, Y., Tang, S., & He, J. (2021). Effectiveness of inactivated COVID-19 vaccines against COVID-19 pneumonia and severe illness caused by the B.1.617.2 (Delta) variant: Evidence from an outbreak in Guangdong, China. *SSRN.* https://doi.org/10.2139/ssrn.3895639

Kim, D., Riley, L., Harriman, K., Hunter, P., & Bridges, C. (2017). Advisory Committee on Immunization Practices recommended immunization schedule for adults aged 19 years or older-United States, 2017. *MMWR Morbidity and Mortality Weekly Report, 66*(5), 136–138. https://doi.org/10.15585/mmwr.mm6605e2

Krammer, F. (2020). SARS-CoV-2 vaccines in development. *Nature, 586*(7830), 516–527. https://doi.org/10.1038/s41586-020-2798-3

Kumar, R., & Burns, E. (2008). Age-related decline in immunity: Implications for vaccine responsiveness. *Expert Review of Vaccines, 7*(4), 467–479. https://doi.org/10.1586/14760584.7.4.467

Kutzler, M., & Weiner, D. (2008). DNA vaccines: Ready for prime time? *Nature Reviews Genetics, 9*, 776–788. https://doi.org/10.1038/nrg2432

Levin, M., Oxman, M., Zhang, J., Johnson, G., Hayward, S., Caulfield, M., Irwin, M., Smith, J., Clair, J., Chan, I., Williams, H., Harbecke, R., Marchese, R., Gershon, S., & Weinberg, A. (2008). Varicella-zoster virus-specific immune responses in elderly recipients of a herpes zoster vaccine. *The Journal of Infectious Diseases, 197*(6), 825–835. https://doi.org/10.1086/528696

Lexau, C., Lynfield, R., Danila, R., Pilishvili, T., Facklam, R., Farley, M., Harrison, L., Schaffner, W., Reingold, A., Bennett, N., Hadler, J., Cieslak, R., Whitney, C., & Active Bacterial Core Surveillance Team. (2005). Changing epidemiology of invasive pneumococcal disease among older adults in the era of pediatric pneumococcal conjugate vaccine. *JAMA, 294*(16), 2043–2051. https://doi.org/10.1001/jama.294.16.2043

Li, X., Huang, Y., Wang, W., Jing, Q., Zhang, C., Qin, P., Guan, W., Gan, L., Li, Y., Liu, W., Dong, H., Miao, Y., Fan, S., Zhang, Z., Zhang, D., & Zhong, N. (2021). Efficacy of inactivated SARS-CoV-2 vaccines against the Delta variant infection in Guangzhou: A test-negative case-control real-world study. *Emerging Microbes & Infections*. https://doi.org/10.1080/22221751.2021.1969291

Løchen, A., Croucher, N., & Anderson, R. (2020). Divergent serotype replacement trends and increasing diversity in pneumococcal disease in high income settings reduce the benefit of expanding vaccine valency. *Scientific Report, 10*, 18977. https://doi.org/10.1038/s41598-020-75691-5

Lopez-Leon, S., Wegman-Ostrosky, T., Perelman, C., Sepulveda, R., Rebolledo, P., Cuapio, A., & Villapol, S. (2021). More than 50 long-term effects of COVID-19: A systematic review and meta-analysis. *Scientific Report, 11*, 16144. https://doi.org/10.1038/s41598-021-95565-8

Maruyama, T., Taguchi, O., Niederman, M. S., Morser, J., Kobayashi, H., Kobayashi, T., & Gabazza, E. (2010). Efficacy of 23-valent pneumococcal vaccine in preventing pneumonia and improving survival in nursing home residents: Double blind, randomised and placebo controlled trial. *BMJ, 340*. https://doi.org/10.1136/bmj.c1004

Melegaro, A., Edmunds, W., Pebody, R., Miller, E., & George, R. (2006). The current burden of pneumococcal disease in England and Wales. *Journal of Infection, 52*(1), 37–48. https://doi.org/10.1016/j.jinf.2005.02.008

Mereckiene, J., Cotter, S., Nicoll, A., Levy-Bruhl, D., Ferro, A., Tridente, G., Zanoni, G., Berra, P., Salmaso, S., & O'Flanagan, D. (2008). National seasonal influenza vaccination survey in Europe, 2008. *Eurosurveillance, 13*(43), 19017.

Ministry of Health. (2021). *Nationally recommended vaccines*. https://www.moh.gov.sg/resources-statistics/nationally-recommended-vaccines

Moberley, S., Holden, J., Tatham, D., & Andrews, R. (2013). Vaccines for preventing pneumococcal infection in adults. *Cochrane Database of Systematic Reviews, 1*. https://doi.org/10.1002/14651858.CD000422.pub3

Mok, C., Cohen, C., Cheng, S., Chen, C., Kwok, K., Yiu, K., Chan, T., Bull, M., Ling, K., Dai, Z. and Ng, S., Lui, G., Wu, C., Amarasinghe G., Leung, D., Wong, S., Valkenburg, S., Peiris, M., & Hui, D. (2021) Comparison of the immunogenicity of BNT162b2 and CoronaVac COVID-19 vaccines in Hong Kong. *Respirology*. https://doi.org/10.1111/resp.14191

Murasko, D., Bernstein, E., Gardner, E., Gross, P., Munk, G., Dran, S., & Abrutyn, E. (2002). Role of humoral and cell-mediated immunity in protection from influenza disease after immunization of healthy elderly. *Experimental Gerontology, 37*(2–3), 427–439. https://doi.org/10.1016/S0531-5565(01)00210-8

Nagy, A., & Alhatlani, B. (2021). An overview of current COVID-19 vaccine platforms. *Computational and Structural Biotechnology Journal, 19*, 2508–2517. https://doi.org/10.1016/j.csbj.2021.04.061

National Health Service. (2021a). *Coronavirus (COVID-19) vaccines*. https://www.nhs.uk/conditions/coronavirus-covid-19/coronavirus-vaccination/coronavirus-vaccine/

National Health Service. (2021b). *NHS vaccination schedule*. https://www.nhs.uk/conditions/vaccinations/nhs-vaccinations-and-when-to-have-them/

National Health Service. (2021c). *Overview travel vaccinations*. https://www.nhs.uk/conditions/travel-vaccinations/

Nichol, K., Nordin, J., Nelson, D., Mullooly, J., & Hak, E. (2007). Effectiveness of influenza vaccine in the community-dwelling elderly. *New England Journal of Medicine, 357*(14), 1373–1381. https://doi.org/10.1056/NEJMoa070844

Nicolas, J., & Guy, B. (2008). Intradermal, epidermal and transcutaneous vaccination: From immunology to clinical practice. *Expert Review of Vaccines, 7*(8), 1201–1214. https://doi.org/10.1586/14760584.7.8.1201

Oxman, M. (2009). Herpes zoster pathogenesis and cell-mediated immunity and immunosenescence. *Journal of Osteopathic Medicine, 109*(s62), 13–17. https://doi.org/10.7556/jaoa.2009.20009

Oxman, M. N., Levin, M. J., Johnson, G. R., Schmader, K. E., Straus, S. E., Gelb, L. D., Arbeit, R. D., Simberkoff, M. S., Gershon, A. A., Davis, L. E., Weinberg, A., Boardman, K. D., Williams, H. M., Hongyuan Zhang, J., Peduzzi, P. N., Beisel, C. E., Morrison, V. A., Guatelli, J. C., Brooks, P. A., ... & Silber, J. L. (2005). A vaccine to prevent herpes zoster and postherpetic neuralgia in older adults. *New England Journal of Medicine, 352*(22), 2271–2284. https://doi.org/10.1056/NEJMoa051016

Pardi, N., Hogan, M., Porter, F., & Weissman, D. (2018). mRNA vaccines—A new era in vaccinology. *Nature Reviews Drug Discovery, 17*(4), 261–279. https://doi.org/10.1038/nrd.2017.243

Perez-Vilar, S., Hu, M., Weintraub, E., Arya, D., Lufkin, B., Myers, T., Woo, E.J., Lo, A.C., Chu, S., Swarr, M., Liao, J., Wernecke, M., MaCurdy, T., Kelman, J., Anderson, S., Duffy, J., & Forshee, R. A. (2021). Guillain-barré syndrome after high-dose influenza vaccine administration in the United States, 2018–2019 Season. *The Journal of Infectious Diseases, 223*(3), 416–425. https://doi.org/10.1093/infdis/jiaa543

Pollard, A. J., & Bijker, E. M. (2021). A guide to vaccinology: From basic principles to new developments. *Nature Reviews Immunology, 21*(2), 83–100. https://doi.org/10.1038/s41577-020-00479-7

Rauch, S., Jasny, E., Schmidt, K., & Petsch, B. (2018). New vaccine technologies to combat outbreak situations. *Frontiers in Immunology, 9*, 1963. https://doi.org/10.3389/fimmu.2018.01963

Saeed, B., Al-Shahrabi, R., Alhaj, S., Alkokhardi, Z., & Adrees, A. (2021). Side effects and perceptions following Sinopharm COVID-19 vaccination. *International Journal of Infectious Diseases.* https://doi.org/10.1016/j.ijid.2021.08.013

Schmader, K. (2001). Herpes zoster in older adults. *Clinical Infectious Diseases, 32*(10), 1481–1486. https://www.jstor.org/stable/4482574

Shaw, M. W., Xu, X., Li, Y., Normand, S., Ueki, R. T., Kunimoto, G. Y., Hall, H., Klimov, A., Cox, N. J., & Subbarao, K. (2002). Reappearance and global spread of variants of influenza B/Victoria/2/87 lineage viruses in the 2000–2001 and 2001–2002 seasons. *Virology, 303*(1), 1–8. https://doi.org/10.1006/viro.2002.1719

Swanson, K. A., Schmitt, H. J., Jansen, K. U., & Anderson, A. S. (2015). Adult vaccination: Current recommendations and future prospects. *Human Vaccines & Immunotherapeutics, 11*(1), 150–155. https://doi.org/10.4161/hv.35858

Tregoning, J., Russell, R., & Kinnear, E. (2018). Adjuvanted influenza vaccines. *Human Vaccines & Immunotherapeutics, 14*(3), 550–564. https://doi.org/10.1080/21645515.2017.1415684

Therapeutics Initiative. (2018). *Shingrix: A new vaccine for Shingles.* https://www.ti.ubc.ca/2018/10/10/114-shingrix-a-new-vaccine-for-shingles/

UNICEF. (2021). *No-one is safe until everyone is safe—Why we need a global response to COVID-19.* https://www.unicef.org/press-releases/no-one-safe-until-everyone-safe-why-we-need-global-response-covid-19

U.S. Department of Health & Human Services. (2021a). *Vaccines for travelers.* https://www.hhs.gov/immunization/who-and-when/travel/index.html

U.S. Department of Health & Human Services. (2021b). *Who and when.* https://www.vaccines.gov/who_and_when/health_conditions

US Pharmacist. (2021). *Even before COVID-19 outbreak, U.S. adult vaccination rates remained low.* https://www.uspharmacist.com/article/even-before-covid19-outbreak-us-adult-vaccination-rates-remained-low

van Riel, D., & de Wit, E. (2020). Next-generation vaccine platforms for COVID-19. *Nature Materials, 19*(8), 810–812. https://doi.org/10.1038/s41563-020-0746-0

Wan, E. Y. F., Chui, C. S. L., Lai, F. T. T., Chan, E. W. Y., Li, X., Yan, V. K. C., Gao, L., Yu, Q., Lam, I. C. H., Chun, R. K. C., Cowling, B.J., & Wong, I. C. K. (2021). Bell's palsy following vaccination with mRNA (BNT162b2) and inactivated (CoronaVac) SARS-CoV-2 vaccines: A case series and nested case-control study. *The Lancet Infectious Disease.* https://doi.org/10.1016/S1473-3099(21)00451-5

Wang, X., & Stollar, B. (1999). Immunoglobulin VH gene expression in human aging. *Clinical Immunology, 93*(2), 132–142. https://doi.org/10.1006/clim.1999.4781

Weinberger, B. (2017). Adult vaccination against tetanus and diphtheria: The European perspective. *Clinical & Experimental Immunology, 187*(1), 93–99. https://doi.org/10.1111/cei.12822

Weinberger, B. (2018). Vaccines for the elderly: Current use and future challenges. *Immunity & Ageing, 15*(1), 1–8. https://doi.org/10.1186/s12979-017-0107-2

WHO. (2020). *Director-General's remarks at the media briefing on 2019-nCoV on 11 February 2020.* http://www.who.int/dg/speeches/detail/who-director-general-s-remarks-at-the-media-briefing-on-2019-ncov-on-11-february-2020

WHO. (2021a). *Ageing and health.* https://www.who.int/news-room/fact-sheets/detail/ageing-and-health

WHO. (2021b). COVID 19 vaccine tracker. (2021b). *7 Vaccines approved for use by WHO.* https://covid19.trackvaccines.org/agency/who/

WHO. (2021c). *COVID-19 vaccines.* https://www.who.int/emergencies/diseases/novel-coronavirus-2019/covid-19-vaccines

WHO. (2021d). *Influenza (Seasonal).* https://www.who.int/news-room/fact-sheets/detail/influenza-(seasonal)

WHO. (2021e). *Vaccines.* https://www.who.int/travel-advice/vaccines

WHO. (2021f). *DNA vaccines.* https://www.who.int/teams/health-product-policy-and-standards/standards-and-specifications/vaccines-quality/dna

Wiersma, L., Rimmelzwaan, G., & de Vries, R. (2015). Developing universal influenza vaccines: Hitting the nail, not just on the head. *Vaccines, 3*(2), 239–262. https://doi.org/10.3390/vaccines3020239

Williams, J. (2014). Improving DNA vaccine performance through vector design. *Current Gene Therapy, 14*(3), 170–189. https://doi.org/10.2174/156652321403140819122538

Woolf, S., Chapman, D., & Lee, J. (2021). COVID-19 as the leading cause of death in the United States. *JAMA, 325*(2), 123–124. https://doi.org/10.1001/jama.2020.24865

Wu, S., Huang, J., Zhang, Z., Wu, J., Zhang, J. L., Hu, H., Zhu, T., Zhang, J., Luo, L., Fan, P., Wang, B., Chen, C., Chen, Y., Song, X., Wang, Y., Si, W., Sun, T., Wang, X., Hou, L., & Chen, W. (2021). Safety, tolerability, and immunogenicity of an aerosolised adenovirus type-5 vector-based COVID-19 vaccine (Ad5-nCoV) in adults: Preliminary report of an open-label and randomised phase 1 clinical trial. *The Lancet Infectious Disease.* https://doi.org/10.1016/S1473-3099(21)00396-0

Yao, X., Hamilton, R., Weng, N., Xue, Q., Bream, J., Li, H., Tian, J., Yeh, S., Resnick, B., Xu, X., Walston, J., Fried, L., & Leng, S. (2011). Frailty is associated with impairment of vaccine-induced antibody response and increase in post-vaccination influenza infection in community-dwelling older adults. *Vaccine, 29*(31), 5015–5021. https://doi.org/10.1016/j.vaccine.2011.04.077

Zhu, F. C., Guan, X. H., Li, Y. H., Huang, J. Y., Jiang, T., Hou, L. H., Li, J. X., Yang, B. F., Wang, L., Wang, W. J. and Wu, S. P., & Chen, W. (2020). Immunogenicity and safety of a recombinant adenovirus type-5-vectored COVID-19 vaccine in healthy adults aged 18 years or older: A randomised, double-blind, placebo-controlled, phase 2 trial. *The Lancet, 396*(10249), 479–488. https://doi.org/10.1016/S0140-6736(20)31605-6

Zhu, Q., Zarnitsyn, V., Ye, L., Wen, Z., Gao, Y., Pan, L., Skountzou, I., Gill, H., Prausnitz, M., Yang, C., & Compans, R. (2009). Immunization by vaccine-coated microneedle arrays protects against lethal influenza virus challenge. *Proceedings of the National Academy of Sciences, 106*(19), 7968–7973. https://doi.org/10.1073/pnas.0812652106

Chapter 8
Effectiveness of Elderly Health Care Voucher Scheme and Private Healthcare Providers in Hong Kong

Hilary H. L. Yee and Vincent Tin Sing Law

Abstract Facing the problem of ageing population, the Department of Health of Hong Kong launched an Elderly Care Voucher Pilot Scheme in 2009 and it has become a regular programme called Elderly Health Care Voucher Scheme (EHCVS) since 2014. In 2019, vouchers that worth HK$2000 were given to elders aged 65 or above and the accumulation limit was $8000. It aims at easing the current heavy reliance on public healthcare services and encouraged elders to choose private healthcare services with the partial subsidy. However, despite the older adults have high awareness of the voucher scheme and vouchers utilisation rate has reached 90%, they still tend to spend vouchers on acute disease treatment. This shows that EHCVS is still ineffective in changing the behaviour of older adults in using vouchers for disease management and preventive care in the private sector. It may be due to inadequate knowledge of the use of vouchers among recipients and ineffective promotion of the aim of the scheme. This chapter reviews and analyses the factors affecting the use of elderly health care vouchers and suggests feasible recommendations to the government in order to sustain the effectiveness of the scheme.

Keywords Elderly Health Care Voucher Scheme · Public healthcare services · Private healthcare services · Preventive care · Effectiveness

H. H. L. Yee
Department of Rehabilitation Sciences, The Hong Kong Polytechnic University, Hong Kong, China
e-mail: hiulam.yee@polyu.edu.hk

V. T. S. Law (✉)
School of Professional Education and Executive Development, College of Professional and Continuing Education, The Hong Kong Polytechnic University, Hong Kong, China
e-mail: vincent.law@cpce-polyu.edu.hk

V. T. S. Law and B. Y. F. Fong (eds.), *Ageing with Dignity in Hong Kong and Asia*, Quality of Life in Asia 16, https://doi.org/10.1007/978-981-19-3061-4_8

8.1 Introduction

According to the statistics of the Census and Statistics Department (2014), there were 76% of elderly aged 70 or above suffering from at least one type of chronic diseases. The prevalence of multimorbidity increases with age, and elderly aged 85 or above have greater than 80% prevalence of multimorbidity (Salive, 2013). A cross-sectional national survey in China revealed that 69.1% of elderly aged 65 or above suffered from at least 14 common chronic diseases, while 43.6% of them suffered from multimorbidity (Zhang et al., 2019). This reflects that health problems among the ageing population in Hong Kong are also quite serious and have created a heavy burden to the public healthcare sector. In order to alleviate the pressure of the public healthcare system, the Hong Kong Government has launched a scheme for the elderly called 'Elderly Health Care Voucher Scheme' (EHCVS). The main objective of this scheme is to act as an incentive to the elderly by partially subsidising them to purchase primary healthcare services from the private sector. The need of relying on public sector is expected to be lowered as the older adults are able to choose both public and private healthcare services (Wong et al., 2015). Another aim is to encourage the elderly to receive preventive care services.

The vouchers are applicable to various kinds of health services provided by medical practitioners, Chinese medicine practitioners, dentists, chiropractors, registered nurses and enrolled nurses, physiotherapists, occupational therapists, radiographers and optometrists (Health Care Voucher, 2019b). The vouchers can also be used in all the preventive care, curative and rehabilitative services provided by enrolled healthcare providers. However, the vouchers are prohibited for the purchase of medication in pharmacy, prosthesis, medical items, and public healthcare services that are already being subsidised, including those private services purchased by the Hospital Authority (HA).

In 2011, the Food and Health Bureau conducted a comprehensive interim review of the effectiveness of the EHCVS and found that the Scheme was ineffective in increasing the utilisation of preventive care services or private healthcare (Liu et al., 2013). Although the cumulative number of older adults who had used vouchers increased from 1,294,000 in 2019 to 1,350,000 in 2020, visits for management of acute episodic conditions remained high while visits of preventive care service increased moderately between 2010 and 2017 (Department of Health, 2019; Food & Health Bureau, 2019; The Government of the Hong Kong Special Administrative Region [HKSAR], 2020). After several quality improvements, EHCV is strengthening the relationship between the older adults, private healthcare providers and the government (Pun & Elliott, 2020). But changing health-seeking behaviour of the elderly (i.e. shifting from public to private healthcare) remains a constraint for EHCVS to reach its intended full potential.

8.2 Implementation of EHCVS

8.2.1 Adjustment of Measures

When the EHCVS was first introduced as a pilot scheme in 2009, five vouchers valued at $50 each were given to each elderly citizen aged 70 or above annually. The Hong Kong Government increased the voucher amount to $500 and $1,000 in 2012 and 2013, respectively, after conducting an Interim Review in 2011, and had eventually converted the scheme into a recurrent programme from 2014.

Adjustments have been made throughout the years to improve the EHCVS. The total annual value of vouchers has been adjusted to $2,000, with the face value of each voucher lowered to $1 and maximum accumulation limit of unspent vouchers doubled to $4,000 (Health Care Voucher, 2019a). The eligible age for the scheme was also lowered from 70 to 65 in 2017. An additional one-off voucher amount of $1,000 was deposited to eligible older adults on 8 June 2018 and 26 June 2019. The accumulation limit of the vouchers was further raised to $8,000 in 2018. Moreover, voucher value of $2,000 was allowed for use on optometry services every two years (Health Care Voucher, 2019a). Apart from using the vouchers in Hong Kong, eligible older adults can also use the vouchers for designed outpatient services provided by the Hong Kong University-Shenzhen Hospital (HKU-SZ Hospital) in Shenzhen, which is next door to Hong Kong, since 26 June 2019. The hospital is managed by the University of Hong Kong and invested by the Shenzhen Government. The fees would be converted from renminbi (RMB) to Hong Kong dollars and rounded to three decimal places.

8.2.2 Utilisation of Vouchers

An interim review was conducted in 2011 and showed a total of 300,292 accounts had made voucher claims in 2010. The number of new voucher accounts has been steadily increasing after the various enhancements. The ratio of account to claim transaction made was almost equal to 1:1. The review conducted in phases between 2015 and 2018 indicated that the utilisation rate of EHCV had dramatically increased from 28% in 2009 to 94% in 2018, with an annual voucher claim of 2.8 billion Hong Kong dollars (Department of Health, 2019). Another noticeable statistic was the increase in the number of enrolled healthcare professionals, from 2,540 in 2009 to 7,941 in 2018, with a corresponding increase in service sites from 3,202 in 2009 to 18,725 in 2018. More private healthcare providers had enrolled in the scheme in 2016 with optometrists being the highest (67%), followed by dentists (44%) and medical practitioners (42%).

It is promising to see that participants surveyed in the 2011 review agreed that the voucher scheme had encouraged them to seek private primary healthcare. However,

90% of the respondents said they had mainly spent the vouchers on acute episodic care services. There was a small change in the utilisation pattern between 2011 and 2018. The visit rate of management of acute episodic conditions decreased from 69% in 2009 to 54% in 2017 and it still remained high (Food & Health Bureau, 2019). Visits to medical practitioners and Chinese medicine practitioners were the highest and the third highest voucher claim transactions, respectively, in 2018 (Department of Health, 2019). There was only a modest increase in using vouchers for follow-up or monitoring of long-term conditions, from 26% in 2010 to 36% in 2017. Voucher claims on visits to optometrists accounted for 27% of healthcare services. Overall, EHCVS is yet to bring significant impacts to the utilisation of public healthcare service and preventive care.

8.3 From Public Health Services to Private Healthcare

Despite the progressive increase in expenditure on the voucher scheme and utilisation of vouchers, the scheme did not significantly increase the use of private primary services for disease management and health prevention by the elderly. The scheme is ineffective in serving the intended purposes to bring down the visits to public hospitals and ease the overloading problem, as well as to encourage the use of private healthcare services. 66.2% of elderly who were eligible voucher users agreed that the voucher scheme did not change their behaviours of consulting public or private healthcare services (Yam et al., 2011). The situation aligned with the results of the survey conducted by the Hong Kong Medical Association in 2015, which showed that only a minority of elderly would receive preventive care with the vouchers. In a more recent interview study, healthcare professionals also agreed that the vouchers had failed to encourage the use on chronic disease management (Fung et al., 2020). The price gap between public and private sector, understanding of the use of voucher, and disproportion of voucher use were barriers in changing health-seeking practice from public to private healthcare among the older population.

8.3.1 Unwillingness to Pay for Expensive Private Healthcare Services

The elderly's willingness to pay for private healthcare, particularly for chronic conditions and preventive care, remains low (Liu et al., 2013). The 2011 interim review showed that the older adults generally preferred to use the vouchers for acute episodic diseases more than preventive care. Participants were asked three questions in this review: (1) maximum amount of money willing to pay for private healthcare service without subsidy; (2) maximum amount of money willing to co-pay for private healthcare service with the government voucher; and (3) minimum amount of subsidy that would encourage the change of behaviour on the use of primary healthcare service. Respondents indicated that the mean subsidy amount requested for chronic conditions ($511) and preventive care including health check ($336) and dental check ($222) were higher than average money they were willing to pay, respectively, at $222, $208 and $161. Such findings had revealed that the respondents were only willing to pay for preventive care such as health and dental check below market price in the private sector. The respondents requested higher amount of subsidy on preventive care.

Private healthcare services are expensive to the elderly, particularly to those who need multiple consultations for chronic diseases (Fung et al., 2020). The majority of them have limited income and budget, and hence they remain heavy users of public health services when there is no significant reduction in price in private services (Liu et al., 2013). The average cost of single visit to dentist is around $884 and optometrist costs around $1,769, respectively, which consume a large proportion of the annual voucher amount (Research Office of Legislative Council Secretariat, 2018). Older adults are more willing to pay for one-off curative treatment in private healthcare like influenza and acute diseases (Fung et al., 2020; Liu et al., 2013). Furthermore, consumers would not go for the expensive ones when the outcome of treatment from public and private clinics is similar. As a result, older people are comfortable with the existing public healthcare system as the services are both at low charges and 'good quality' in terms of referral and follow-up visits (Lai et al., 2017).

8.3.2 Lack of Trust in Private Healthcare Providers

There were 240 complaints about voucher defrauding and professional misconduct against private services from 2014 to 2018, and most of the complaints were against medical practitioners and optometrists (Chiu, 2019; Food & Health Bureau, 2019). Improper voucher claims and service charges were the major issues. There is no limitation on the voucher amount to be spent each time and some service providers exploit this chance to maximise profits. Individual cases included persuading the elderly to purchase expensive dried seafood products at Chinese Medicine clinics, buying corrective spectacles and doing unnecessarily eye tests at optical stores, etc. Inappropriate voucher claims were particularly apparent in optometry services, as reflected by the disproportion in total claims to the numbers of enrolled optometrists. This had affected the trust in private services, leading the elderly to doubt the service standards in the private market (Liu et al., 2013). It is difficult for older adults to search and identify which service providers have good reputation, and hence they continue to visit the public ones for reasons of confidence, trust and quality assurance.

8.3.3 Inadequate Knowledge on the Purposes of EHCVS

More older adults are aware of the scheme and know about the new measures such as the increase of annual voucher amount and accumulation limit, but not the main purpose of the scheme (Legislative Council, 2019a; Liu et al., 2013). They perceived the scheme as a social welfare, not an initiative to choose private healthcare services on top of the existing public primary healthcare. It is noticed that the EHCVS was not promoted in a way to encourage the utilisation on disease prevention and management in the private sector (Lai et al., 2017). The use of vouchers was perceived as a way of seeking services from private doctors, and not specifically for disease prevention or screening. Although there were over ten areas of medical services enrolled in the scheme from 2015 to 2018, the elderly might not have the knowledge to choose the service that was the best for them and thus ending up saving the vouchers for future use on acute medical treatment (Department of Health, 2019).

To avoid exceeding the voucher accumulation limit, some older adults might spend the vouchers for unnecessary health services and products. In the study conducted by Lai et al. (2017), interviewees confessed that they spent the vouchers for one-off purposes such as expensive magnetic resonance imaging scan, expensive prescription spectacles and dental service. The increasing use of vouchers on optometrists reveals a question on the appropriate use of vouchers as this may divert the elderly to a 'shopping' nature rather than a health precaution purpose. Therefore, inadequate health knowledge among the older adults has hindered them to make good use of the vouchers by spending on disease management and other primary care prevention.

8.3.4 Disproportion of Voucher Use on Private Healthcare Services

As mentioned, inappropriate voucher claims on optometry service have been observed. However, it turns out that some optometrists are dominating the private healthcare sector in EHCVS and causes an unhealthy voucher utilisation on private healthcare services. This lowers the effectiveness in promoting the use of vouchers in a variety of private primary healthcare. The median amount of voucher claim on optometrists was the highest since 2015 (Food & Health Bureau, 2019). 76% of voucher claims above $4000 were spent on optometry services. Under the revamped arrangement, the intended purpose of allowing voucher value of $2,000 to be spent on optometry services every two years is to divert the utilisation more to other primary healthcare.

8.4 Recommendations

8.4.1 Educate the Public to Use and Manage Vouchers Wisely

There is an immense need to enhance the public's knowledge of the background of EHCVS so as to encourage the utilisation of private primary healthcare, including preventive care. As the general public regard using the vouchers as a mean to visit doctors for acute disease only, the concept of prevention healthcare should be emphasised and strengthened. Examples of different preventive health services such as body check, screening and vaccination should be promoted in the community. The variety of healthcare professionals including physiotherapists, chiropractors and radiographers who are less known by the public should be introduced. The older adults need to understand how the vouchers act as an extra household resource and incentive to help purchase of additional quality healthcare (Chui et. al., 2016).

The 18 Visiting Health Teams from Department of Health should organise regular talks to update the elderly on details and advice such as updated eligible age, new additional voucher amount, etc. It is also important to remind the older adults to avoid spending vouchers on unnecessary healthcare or other services, and they should ask the service providers about details of healthcare products before giving consent. The older adults cannot plan ahead for their health precaution if they are unable to manage their account efficiently. There were 182,000 elders who had voucher amounts forfeited because of exceeding the accumulation limit (The Government of the Hong Kong Special Administrative Region, 2020). Therefore, workshops should be organised to teach the older adults how to manage their vouchers accounts regularly and review the claims on healthcare services. Some older adults are unfamiliar with the technology and fail to manage their accounts by themselves through the online platform called eHealth System. The workshops can remind the elderly to check their account balance via an Interactive Response System or ask for a printed record of their account balance after each visit to the healthcare providers. In fact, the target audience should not only be restricted to the elderly. Their family members should be encouraged to be actively taking care of the health of the elderly and get familiar with EHCVS, so that they can convey health knowledge and messages to them. Therefore, apart from health talks, brochures and leaflets can be sent to residential mailboxes regularly to remind people about the purposes of the scheme.

8.4.2 Promotion of Private Healthcare Services

It is important to raise public awareness of private healthcare services in EHCVS through different sources of promotion. Apart from relying on television and radio broadcasts, highlights of the promotional materials should focus more on health prevention in the private sector and should be available in public clinics, hospitals and community centres. As studies have shown that eligible older adults remain regular consumers of public services, eye-catching posters can be posted on the wall while leaflets can be distributed through public facilities.

Meanwhile, the setting-up of District Health Centres (DHCs) is expected to enhance primary healthcare within each of the 18 districts of Hong Kong through medical-social collaboration and public–private partnership. The first centre was set up in Kwai Tsing District in September 2019 and the scope of services includes health promotion, health assessment, chronic disease management and community rehabilitation (District Health Centres, 2019). The second and third district health centres located in Sham Shui Po and Wong Tai Sin would commence operations in 2021 and 2022, respectively. DHCs are supported by a network of private healthcare practitioners who should help guiding the elderly to use the vouchers for chronic disease management and prevention in the private sector. The expansion of DHCs would be a stepping stone to change the public's general behaviour and mindset from being treatment-oriented to prevention-focused, and help improving the efficiency of the EHCVS.

Some older adults may prefer reading hard copies. The elderly community centres could print and distribute updated list of enrolled private healthcare service providers to the elders (Legislative Council, 2019b). The list should categorise the providers in terms of professions and districts. For example, an elderly who lives in the Western District and want to have a body check can look up the list conveniently. The list can update elders on the availability of private healthcare services and where to purchase suitable services near their home.

8.4.3 Build Trust Between Consumers and Healthcare Service Providers

To minimise inappropriate practices of some enrolled providers, the Health Care Voucher Division set up by the Department of Health should conduct more regular and random inspections. From 2009 to 2018, only 358,000 claim transactions which accounted for 2% of the total claim were checked by the department. The inspection team should strengthen the monitoring on the pattern of unusual transactions in voucher accounts and investigate suspicious cases. With the advancement of monitoring system, it is easier to identify abnormal voucher transaction and potential defraud cases in the eHealth system (Legislative Council, 2019a). Warnings can then be issued to service providers suspected of possible malpractice.

Moreover, enrolled providers who have committed serious misconduct or violated the terms in the Scheme Agreement should be discharged from the Scheme. They could enrol again after meticulous examination and assessment by the Health Care Voucher Division with satisfaction and confidence. This can ensure the enrolled services providers are conforming to the requirements of the Scheme and providing quality services. With fewer complaints and reports concerning the misuse of vouchers, the public will build up trust on private services and the elderly will be encouraged to subscribe to them.

The Health Care Voucher website can include positive personal feedbacks from recipients who have chosen private healthcare services so that people can know how useful and effective the scheme is in private primary healthcare service. It can encourage the older adults to change their behaviour by building trust on private healthcare and it is worth paying for private services but not just public services.

8.4.4 Promote Concept of Family Doctors

The concept of family doctors is not well established in Hong Kong. Most people think family doctors are for treating acute disease but not for managing chronic diseases or preventive care (Mercer et al., 2010). Some people think family doctors are unnecessary as cold and flu are not that frequent, while some people worry about the quality of the doctors. One way to increase the effectiveness of the EHCVS is to develop a health-seeking behaviour in the community for having personal family doctors as they should be the ones who clearly understand patients' health background and provide personal medical services. By developing a closer relationship between the patients and family doctors, the elderly can seek suitable care from their family doctors and thus help promote the proper use of vouchers and primary healthcare. To adopt the model of family doctor needs longer term planning as it will require a comprehensive registration system, training and qualification in family medicine and promotion to the general public (Food & Health Bureau, 2010). The government should adopt and further promote the policy on the city-wide practice of having family doctors in order to make full use of the voucher scheme.

8.4.5 Expand Service Points to Greater Bay Area

Apart from encouraging more local private providers to enrol in the scheme, along with the regularised scheme at the Hong Kong University—Shenzhen (HKU-SZ) Hospital, the government may consider further expanding the voucher scheme to other cities of the Greater Bay Area (GBA) such as Guangzhou and Zhuhai. The pilot scheme recorded 3,400 elders who had used their vouchers at the HKU-SZ Hospital from 2015 to 2018. There has been demand for healthcare services provided by Mainland hospitals (Legislative Council, 2019a). Therefore, collaboration between hospitals in GBA and providers in Hong Kong should be explored. For example, The Chinese University of Hong Kong has ongoing academic and research collaboration with hospitals across the border such as the Shenzhen Traditional Chinese Medicine Hospital and No. 2 Affiliated Hospital of Guangzhou University of Chinese Medicine. Collaborating healthcare facilities and providers in the GBA which are conveniently located and accessible by the express railway can be developed in a bigger scale and wider scope to provide the elderly with a retiring option in neighbouring locations where the EHCV can be redeemed. More pilot schemes should be initiated in the GBA.

8.4.6 Review the Voucher Amount

A comprehensive study should be conducted to examine the willingness of older adults to pay for various types of healthcare in private sector. This may help to explore what kind of care services are perceived to be more important to the elderly and which services they would be more willing to pay for. This also helps to rationalise the spending of public money and increase the effectiveness of EHCVS. For example, additional amount designated for dental service can be established. Since single visit of dentist is around $900, the additional amount on dental service could be $1,000 to $1,500 every two years.

8.5 Conclusion

The EHCVS aims to create a sustainable primary healthcare system to tackle partly the problems of the ageing population. It is a good initiative to promote primary healthcare service and to divert excessive pressure from the public sector to the private sector. After years of implementation, the voucher claims and enrolled private healthcare professionals have increased. These reflect that the scheme has encouraged recipients to use more healthcare services. However, the scheme is ineffective in meeting its main objectives as the number of visits to public clinics and hospitals for acute diseases remains high and the elderly still prefer not to use the vouchers for preventive health services.

The government has introduced enhanced measures such as increasing the total voucher allowance, raising the accumulation limit and providing additional one-off vouchers. However, adjustments and improvements are still needed to improve and sustain the effectiveness of the scheme in order to meet the objectives of encouraging the elderly to use more private care services and ease the overloading of public hospitals and clinics. It is recommended that the government should enhance public awareness, improve promotion materials, facilitate the older adults to manage their voucher accounts, monitor healthcare providers, further promote the family doctor concept, and expand service points in the Greater Bay Area. A comprehensive review of the scheme is recommended.

Acknowledgements The work described in this paper was partially supported by a grant from the Research Grants Council of the Hong Kong Special Administrative Region, China (Project Reference No.: UGC/IDS24/18).

References

Census and Statistics Department. (2014). *Persons with disabilities and chronic diseases (Special Topics Report No. 62).* https://www.censtatd.gov.hk/hkstat/sub/sp380.jsp?productCode=FA100059

Chiu, P. (2019). *Hong Kong's health voucher scheme for the elderly has been running for a decade—So why are curbs on usage being imposed and what effect will they have?.* https://www.scmp.com/news/hong-kong/health-environment/article/3001592/hong-kongs-health-voucher-scheme-elderly-has-been

Chui, E., Law, C. K., Bai, X., Dai, D., Lai, D., Ma, C., & Tsien T. (2016). *Feasibility study on introducing a voucher scheme on residential care services for the elderly.* https://www.elderlycommission.gov.hk/en/download/library/Report%20on%20RCS%20Vou cher_2016(ENG).pdf

Department of Health. (2019). *Review on the elderly health care voucher scheme.* https://www.legco.gov.hk/yr18-19/english/panels/hs/papers/hs20190318cb2-962-1-e.pdf

District Health Centres. (2019). *Background.* https://www.dhc.gov.hk/en/general_public.html

Food and Health Bureau. (2010). *Our partner for better health.* https://www.fhb.gov.hk/download/press_and_publications/otherinfo/101231_primary_care/e_strategy_doc.pdf

Food and Health Bureau. (2019). *Report on the review of the elderly health care voucher scheme.* https://www.hcv.gov.hk/files/pdf/Review_Report_English.pdf

Fung, V. L. H., Lai, A. H. Y., Yam, C. H. K., Wong, E. L. Y., Griffiths, S. M., & Yeoh, E. K. (2020). Healthcare vouchers for better elderly services? Input from private healthcare service providers in Hong Kong. *Health & Social Care in the Community, 00*, 1–13. https://doi.org/10.1111/hsc.13203

Health Care Voucher. (2019a). *Background of elderly health care voucher scheme.* https://www.hcv.gov.hk/en/hcvs/background.html

Health Care Voucher. (2019b). *Healthcare service provider.* https://www.hcv.gov.hk/en/hcvs/target_group.html

Lai, A. H. Y., Kuang, Z., Yam, C. H. K., Ayub, S., & Yeoh, E. K. (2017). Vouchers for primary healthcare services in an ageing world? The perspectives of elderly vouchers recipients in Hong Kong. *Health and Social Care in the Community, 26*(3), 374–382. https://doi.org/10.1111/hsc.12523

Legislative Council. (2019a). *Review on the elderly health care voucher scheme.* https://www.legco.gov.hk/yr18-19/english/panels/hs/papers/hs2019a0318cb2-962-1-e.pdf

Legislative Council. (2019b). *Updated background brief prepared by the Legislative Council Secretariat for the meeting on 18 March 2019b.* https://www.legco.gov.hk/yr18-19/english/panels/hs/papers/hs2019b0318cb2-964-5-e.pdf

Liu, S., Yam, C. H., Huang, O. H., & Griffiths, S. M. (2013). Willingness to pay for private primary care services in Hong Kong: Are elderly ready to move from the public sector? *Health Policy and Planning, 28*(7), 717–729. https://doi.org/10.1093/heapol/czs112

Mercer, S. W., Siu, J. Y., Hillier, S. M., Lam, C. L., Lo, Y. Y., Lam, T. P., & Griffiths, S. M. (2010). A qualitative study of the views of patients with long-term conditions on family doctors in Hong Kong. *BMC Family Practice, 11*(1), 46. https://doi.org/10.1186/1471-2296-11-46

Pun, J. W., & Elliott, L. (2020). A systematic review to assess the impact of the Elderly Health Care Voucher Scheme (EHCVS) and the feasibility to fully adopt in Hong Kong elder care services. *Research Square.* https://doi.org/10.21203/rs.3.rs-48276/v1

Research Office of Legislative Council Secretariat. (2018, February 27). *Elderly health care voucher scheme.* https://www.legco.gov.hk/research-publications/english/1718issh14-elderly-health-care-voucher-scheme-20180227-e.pdf

Salive, M. E. (2013). Multimorbidity in older adults. *Epidemiologic Reviews, 35*(1), 75–83. https://doi.org/10.1093/epirev/mxs009

The Government of the Hong Kong Special Administrative Region. (2020). *LCQ18: Elderly health care voucher scheme.* [Press release]. https://www.info.gov.hk/gia/general/202101/13/P2021011300557.htm?fontSize=1

Wong, E. L., Yeoh, E., Chau, P. Y., Yam, C. H., Cheung, A. W., & Fung, H. (2015). How shall we examine and learn about public-private partnerships (PPPs) in the health sector? Realist evaluation of PPPs in Hong Kong. *Social Science & Medicine, 147*, 261–269. https://doi.org/10.1016/j.socscimed.2015.11.012

Yam, C. H., Liu, S., Huang, O. H., Yeoh, E., & Griffiths, S. M. (2011). Can vouchers make a difference to the use of private primary care services by older people? Experience from the health care reform programme in Hong Kong. *BMC Health Services Research, 11*(1), 255. https://doi.org/10.1186/1472-6963-11-255

Zhang, R., Lu, Y., Shi, L., Zhang, S., & Chang, F. (2019). Prevalence and patterns of multimorbidity among the elderly in China: A cross-sectional study using national survey data. *British Medical Journal Open, 9*(8), e024268. https://doi.org/10.1136/bmjopen-2018-024268

Chapter 9
Dignified Ageing in Place Using Electronic Health Records as a Backbone: A Medico-Legal Perspective

Kar-wai Tong

Abstract Population ageing has become a global issue and triggered off societies to make new plans and tactics to face challenges arising from the phenomenon. Among various initiatives, electronic health records play an important role to help older persons to live in communities in a dignified manner. In this chapter, the author discusses briefly dignity in general, dignity in healthcare, and dignity of older persons. The author also examines the roles of and the legal risks inherent in electronic health records as a fundamental element of telehealth in facilitating dignified ageing in place, with an attempt to share some regional and international references from the medico-legal perspective with healthcare professionals and institutes.

Keywords Dignified ageing in place · Telehealth · Electronic health records · Medico-legal risks

9.1 Introduction

Population ageing is an inexorable trend. The Department of Economic and Social Affairs of the United Nations (UN) (2020) has projected that the global number of people aged 65 years and above would jump from 727 million in 2020 (9.3% worldwide) to more than 1.5 billion by 2050 (16.0%), representing an increase of over 200%, and by then, one in six of the global population would be 65 years old or over, with longer life expectancy of female. In Asia–Pacific countries, the lifespans of people in low- / lower-middle income and upper-middle / high-income countries have increased respectively by nearly 6 and 4 years since 2000, and in 2050, the population at the age of 65 and older in low- / lower-middle income countries has been projected to grow by approximately 250%, with 14.1% being female and 11% male, whereas the respective female and male proportions of people of at least 65 years old would become 23.1% and 19.4% in upper-middle income countries, and

K. Tong (✉)
City University of Hong Kong, Hong Kong, China
e-mail: karwtong2@cityu.edu.hk

V. T. S. Law and B. Y. F. Fong (eds.), *Ageing with Dignity in Hong Kong and Asia*, Quality of Life in Asia 16, https://doi.org/10.1007/978-981-19-3061-4_9

32.6% and 27.5% in high-income countries (Organisation for Economic Cooperation and Development, 2021). The ageing trend also arises in less developed regions like African countries, where the number of Africans at the age of 60 and over would be tripled from 46 million in 2015 to 147 million by 2050 (World Health Organisation (WHO) Regional Office for Africa, 2021). In view of the challenges by virtue of population ageing, societies have been exploring development strategies to sustain the provisions of adequate healthcare and other services such as social welfare, housing, transportation, and family support (Oosterhof, 2018). In the formulation of ageing policies and programmes, the authorities have to take the dignity of older persons into full account (UN General Assembly, 1991, Article 14).

9.2 Dignity

What is dignity? It may not be easy to define this word (Social Care Institute for Excellence, 2020). People have diverse and sometimes contradictory comprehension of human dignity (Li, 2021). Such disparity may be due to substantial cultural differences (Koehn & Leung, 2008). Nordenfelt (2004) discussed four notions of dignities in the European context, namely the universal human dignity, as well as the dignities of merit, moral stature, and identity. Häyry (2004) examined five plausible interpretations of dignity, respectively from the Catholic, Kantian, genetic, utilitarian, and anti-egalitarian aspects, and he found that no perspective should be dominated over others in moral disputes. In China, 'dignity' is not a term apparent in Confucius's ethics, and the Confucian concept comprises the inner values of human life as the universal dignity and of the respect to interpersonal relationships as the personal dignity (Li & Li, 2017). The word 'dignity' is in fact rooted from the Latin, *dignitas*, but the drafters of the Universal Declaration of Human Rights have used this word as embodying a non-Western and universally recognisable concept (Hughes, 2011).

9.3 Dignity in Healthcare

There are no clear definitions of 'dignity in healthcare' (Tadd et al., 2002) or universal interpretations of 'dying with dignity' (Hemati et al., 2016), either. In practice, patients' dignity may not always be preserved (Lothian & Philp, 2001). A president commission in the United States (US) noted that a number of people misperceived a 'right to die with dignity' as a guarantee for a 'peaceful and aesthetically appealing death', but in reality, deaths with distressful symptoms like being confused, nauseated, vomiting, bleeding, etc. might not be avoidable, and 'dignified death' was only a slogan (President's Commission for the Study of Ethical Problems in Medicine and Biomedical and Behavioral Research, US, 1983, p. 24). A professor of medical ethics also echoed such a view and argued, 'Dignity is a useless concept in medical ethics and can be eliminated without any loss of content' (Macklin, 2003, p. 1420).

That said, dignity is still one of the universal values, as enshrined in the preamble of the Charter of the United Nations, the founding treaty of the UN, 'We the peoples of the [UN] determined … to reaffirm faith in fundamental human rights, in the dignity and worth of the human person …' (UN, 1945). More than that, dignity is a fundamental human right and the word 'dignity' appears five times in the Universal Declaration of Human Rights (UN General Assembly, 1948) as an essential component of human rights. Decades after the promulgation of the Charter of the UN, dignity continues to be a contemporary international concern. In 2006, the UN adopted the Convention on the Rights of Persons with Disabilities and its Optional Protocol to promote the respect for the basic dignity of people with disabilities (UN General Assembly, 2006, Article 1).

Dignity is deepened at the heart of healthcare. The World Health Organisation (WHO, 1994) announced in A Declaration of the Promotion of Patients' Rights in Europe that it is a human right for patients to receive diagnosis, treatments, and care with dignity and die in dignity. The WHO also promotes and advocates patients' dignity in specialist care such as mental health (Singh, 2015) as well as maternal, newborn and child health (WHO, 2018). Courts have given similarly due weight to dignity in healthcare. In the United Kingdom (UK), in *Nursing and Midwifery Council v Iestyn Bryant* [2021] EWHC 1064 (Admin), Mrs Justice Eady sitting on the Queen's Bench of the High Court said at paragraph 16, 'I … accept that dignity and respect are at the heart of nursing practise [*sic*] …'. In *Chester v Afshar* [2004] UKHL 41, [2005] 1 AC 134, a case heard before the House of Lords, Lord Steyn said at paragraph 18,

> A rule requiring a doctor to abstain from performing an operation without the informed consent of a patient serves two purposes. It tends to avoid the occurrence of the particular physical injury the risk of which a patient is not prepared to accept. It also ensures that due respect is given to the autonomy and dignity of each patient.

In *R v Ashworth Hospital Authority (Now Mersey Care National Health Service Trust)* [2005] UKHL 58, [2006] 2 AC 148, Lord Brown sitting on the House of Lords gave comments at paragraph 118 on the long-term seclusion of mental patients by the appellant hospital as a compromise of patients' dignity (with Lord Hope and Lord Scott dissenting at paragraphs 98–100 and 101–104 respectively as to whether the practice of seclusion in the appellant hospital was unlawful),

> It is unthinkable that a mental patient can be subjected to seclusion, particularly on a long-term basis as is often the case at [the appellant hospital], without good reason and, in the language of [A]rticle 8(2) [of the European Convention on Human Rights], without such interference with his rights being 'in accordance with the law.' … [S]eclusion is always an interference with the patient's right to private life, … there are bound to be occasions when the patient's 'personal autonomy' or 'moral integrity' … are undermined, occasions when his 'human dignity' (and, indeed, important elements also of his residual 'human freedom') are compromised.

In Hong Kong, the Court of First Instance in *Re NLS* HCMH 4/2020, [2021] HKCFI 2203 emphasised in paragraph 74 that under the Mental Health Ordinance (Cap 136), the court has to respect the personality and dignity of a mentally incapacitated person and it would intervene only if such a person has had no mental capacity to make a decision about his or her welfare and interests such as financial affairs.

9.4 Dignity of Older Persons

In view of the population ageing, older persons' dignity has aroused international attention. Dignity is a genuine matter when one gets older, as every older person has the fear of vulnerability, being scared of 'becoming less than ourselves in the last stage of life' (Moody, 1998, p. 14). In 1991, the UN General Assembly (1991) adopted the UN Principles for Older Persons. Its Article 17 states, 'Older persons should be able to live in dignity and security and be free of exploitation and physical or mental abuse'. In 2002, the UN further promulgated the Political Declaration and Madrid International Plan of Action on Ageing, which states, 'We are determined to enhance the recognition of the dignity of older persons and to eliminate all forms of neglect, abuse and violence' (UN, 2002a, 'Political Declaration', Article 5). In this document, the UN expressed clearly, 'The aim of the International Plan of Action is to ensure that persons everywhere are able to age with security and dignity and to continue to participate in their societies as citizens with full rights' (2002a, see 'Madrid International Plan of Action on Ageing', paragraph 10).

Dignity of older persons is not just a theoretical concept but a practical issue (Heggestad et al., 2015). Jacobson (2007) suggested that dignity in the context of care for older persons and other vulnerable people focus on the substance and the style of care to identify appropriate approaches to sustain the integrity and self-pride of both patients and healthcare professionals. However, there may be gaps between the understanding of the term 'dignity' from the older persons' perspectives and from the angles of nurses (Karimi et al., 2019; Šaňáková & Čáp, 2019) and other healthcare professionals (Cairns et al., 2013), as healthcare professionals can only 'try their best' under constraints and challenges like staff shortages, working environments and ward layouts, etc. and healthcare may occasionally override or dominate the reality of happening (Gantley et al., 2020, p. 2).

Notwithstanding dignity being a noticeable concern of older people (Woolhead et al., 2004), the number of studies on the dignity and ageing of older persons in the context of daily living is limited (Black & Dobbs, 2014). In the current literature, various themes of older persons' dignity have been identified. In the UK, for instance, Webster and Bryan (2009) interviewed ten patients aged 73–83 at home and noticed a few potential factors to promote dignity, namely patients' privacy, cleanliness, independence, and ability of patients to exercise control, staff having enough time, their attitudes to older persons, and communication. In Australia, Kerr et al. (2020) revealed three themes of dignity through interviews with a sample of 24 patients (at least 65 years old) and 12 relatives: involving patients in decisions about their care and treatment, keeping them safe when they are vulnerable, and treating them as an individual with respect. In Taiwan, Lin et al. (2011) surveyed 40 patients of a teaching hospital at the average age of 57.5 and they found six themes strengthening their dignity: patients' perception of control and autonomy, respecting patients as a person, indecent body exposure, nursing staff's care, patient confidentiality, and timeliness to meet patient needs. In the South-eastern US, Black and Dobbs (2014) conducted a study on community-dwelling older persons' perceptions of dignity, having engaged 51 older persons in focus groups and 216 respondents in an electronic survey, with respective mean ages of 79.4 and 75.9, and they reported three cores of dignity: autonomy (e.g. self-choice), relational dignity (e.g. respectful treatment of self and others), and self-identity (e.g. self-acceptance and appreciation).

9.5 Dignified Ageing in Place

To integrate elderly care through promoting deinstitutionalisation and strengthening community-based care is considered one of the ways out to tackle the foreseeable population ageing (Johri et al., 2003). To put this deinstitutionalised community-based care into practice, ageing in place supported by telehealth has been proposed among other tactics to enhance older people's quality of life in the community (Tong, in press; Tong, 2021). Older persons prefer ageing in place (Feldman et al., 2004; Hwang et al., 2011; Kendig et al., 2017; Lum et al., 2016), which means 'the ability to live in one's own home and community safely, independently, and comfortably, regardless of age, income or level of capacity' (WHO, 2015, p. 225). An illustration of ageing in place with the support of telehealth is the legislative passage of House Bill 3308 in Illinois, which became effective from July 2021 (Illinois General Assembly, US, 2021). With this enactment, Illinois has become one of the first American states that have expanded access to telehealth permanently, and its Governor, J. B. Pritzker said, 'We are taking great strides to make sure that where [citizens] live no longer impacts how long [they] live … Thanks to this new law, we are one step closer to that reality today' (cited in Jercich, 2021). In the UK, the East Sussex County Council has also provided 'Telecheck' services to support the vulnerable including older persons to age in place safely, securely, and for longer by making personal telephone service to send welfare checks and reminders for food, water, medication, etc. in a proactive manner (East Sussex County Council, 2021; Local Government Association, UK, 2016). Although telephone call is a traditional and simplest form of telehealth among diversified digital initiatives (Wootton, 1996), it still plays an important role for the communication between healthcare professionals and patients (Queirós et al., 2017).

Dignified ageing in place relies on the full respect of older persons' dignity and their functional independence in housing (Heumann & Boldy, 1993). As spelt out in the UN Principles for Older Persons (UN General Assembly, 1991, Article 14),

> Older persons should be able to enjoy human rights and fundamental freedoms when residing in any shelter, care or treatment facility, including full respect for their dignity, beliefs, needs and privacy and for the right to make decisions about their care and the quality of their lives.

In practice, there are challenges for older persons to age in place (Connelly et al., 2014). Some governments have made use of legislative and executive means to support dignified ageing in place. In Norway, the Regulations on Dignified Care for the Elderly (Dignity Guarantee) have entered into force since 1 January 2011, with a purpose to ensure that municipal nursing and care services are to be delivered in a manner to facilitate 'a dignified, safe and meaningful old age' (Rule 1), with respect to older people's right to self-determination, self-worth, and way of life and, in particular, their medical needs, such as continuous healthcare follow-up and treatment, habilitation and rehabilitation, palliative care, and a dignified death (Rule 8) (Ministry of Health and Care Services, Norway, 2010). In Finland, Section 14 of the Act on Supporting the Functional Capacity of the Older Population and on Social and Health Care Services for Older Persons, effective from 1 July 2013, stipulates that long-term care and attention for older persons be provided primarily in their private homes or other home-like accommodations, and exceptionally in institutions only when such arrangements are medically necessary or justified for older persons' dignified life and safe care (Ministry of Social Affairs and Health, Finland, 2012). In Denmark, paragraph 2 of the Executive Order on Dignity Policies for Elderly Care came into effect on 1 February 2019, requiring the municipal council to make dignity policies for older persons in areas of, among others, quality of life, quality and continuity of care, supporting those with loneliness, and a dignified death (Ministry of Social Affairs and Health, Denmark, 2019). In Malaysia, the mass media has reported that the government would enact a new piece of legislation to protect older persons' rights to dignified ageing (*The Star*, 2019). In Europe, the European Economic and Social Committee (2019), an advisory body of the European Union, has advocated to recognise dignified ageing as a fundamental human right, with digital tools such as telehealth and electronic health records (EHR) to help older people's ageing in place.

9.6 Electronic Health Records and Dignified Ageing in Place

The success of dignified ageing in place with telehealth requires a common platform of health information technology, as the mode of care will be changed from 'one to one' to 'many to one' (Chau & Leung, 2017, p. 134). The lack of information sharing among healthcare professionals and institutes has been reported as one of the barriers to the integration (Lau et al., 2018), and there have been calls for the adoption of digital technologies to share patients' data and records in a common platform of health information technology among healthcare institutes, social care organisations, other concerned agencies and individuals to expedite better integration of elderly care, so that healthcare professionals may work at any locations at any time (He & Tang, 2021; NHS Confederation, 2016). In Hong Kong, the 'Electronic Health Record Sharing System' developed by the government provides a practical example to enable two-way EHR sharing among healthcare institutes and professionals in local public and private sectors and to facilitate healthcare public–private partnership (Electronic Health Record Office, Hong Kong, 2020).

EHR is in fact one of the basics in a common platform of health information technology. There is no universal definition of EHR (Jha et al., 2006). The use of the term EHR may mean different records in institutions or countries, and there are various terms such as automated health records, computer-based patient records, electronic medical records, and EHR to signify the shift from a hardcopy system to an electronic system in general (WHO Regional Office for the Western Pacific, 2006). The terms of 'electronic medical records' and EHR, for instance, may sound similar to each other, as both aim at improving patient safety, healthcare quality and efficiency, as well as saving healthcare costs, but Garets and Davis (2006) have argued that the use of them interchangeably is not appropriate as they are important but different concepts, where electronic medical records generated through hospital and ambulatory care are the data sources of EHR to empower the latter to share patients' healthcare information in different kinds of care among stakeholders, such as various disciplines of healthcare professionals, employers, insurance companies and governments. That said, knowing the differences between electronic medical records and EHR (WHO, 2016), the WHO Global Observatory for eHealth still deliberately used these two terms interchangeably to conduct the third global survey on eHealth in 2015 and reported that out of 125 member states under survey, 57 countries (47%) had put a national EHR system in place, and for those without a national coverage, they had some form of local or regional systems in use.

EHR is one of the keys to the successful implementation of telehealth (Kluge, 2011). It is 'the backbone of all major international eHealth developments currently taking place internationally' (Sheikh et al., 2011, p. 22). The use of EHR has become a global trend, as Kauger J sitting on the Supreme Court of Oklahoma in *Johnson v Hillcrest Health Centre, Inc.* 70 P.3d 811, 2003 OK 16 (Okla. 2003) noted at Footnote 12, 'We recogni[s]e that medical literature reflects and supports the advent of electronic medical records and even advocates the movement towards the elimination of handwritten clinical data in the foreseeable future'. EHR has had a number of advantages, such as providing accurate, up-to-date and complete patient information at the point of care in an efficient and coordinated manner, enabling healthcare information exchange with different healthcare professionals, and reducing medical errors and costs (Office of the National Coordinator for Health Information Technology, US, 2019). EHR may also better elderly care, as exemplified in the finding of a study across eight countries that the Netherland did especially best in the area of patient access, as its EHR systems, together with its strong primary care system and physicians' cooperatives, facilitated Dutch chronic patients to have expeditious healthcare access even after practice hours of healthcare professionals, leading to the least casualty visits or coordination issues among the countries under study (Schoen et al., 2008). EHR systems may further provide necessary patient data to allow computer algorithms to analyse prognostic factors and predict patients' risk of recurrence (Knight et al., 2018).

9.7 Medico-Legal Risks Inherent in EHR

The use of EHR is subject to potential legal liabilities. Court cases have illustrated medico-legal risks inherent in EHR. A few of the risks are shared below, which are by no means exhaustive.

9.7.1 Ownership of EHRs

Patients may not own their healthcare records absolutely at common law (Yeo, 2004). In Australia, the High Court in *Breen v Williams* [1995] HCA 63, (1996) 43 ALD 481 dismissed the appellant's appeal and ruled that doctors do not have a contractual or fiduciary duty to provide patients with a right of access to their medical records, that documents prepared by professional persons during their services are their own properties, not those of clients, and that there is no general common law right of access to medical records with reference to Australian law.

In Canada, the Supreme Court in *Mclnerney v MacDonald* [1992] 2 SCR 138 held that in the absence of legislation, a patient is allowed to examine and copy his records upon request, but such access does not apply to records generated outside the doctor-patient relationship. However, a patient's right of access to medical records is not absolute, as physical medical records belong to doctors. A doctor may refuse a patient's request to access his or her medical records if the former believes reasonably that it is not in the patient's best interest to see the records. On the other hand, the patient may apply for the court's jurisdiction against the doctor's decision. The burden rests upon the doctor to justify the denial.

In the UK, the patient applicant in *R v Mid Glamorgan Family Health Services Authority Ex p. Martin* [1995] 1 WLR 110 had a history of psychological problems. He had made recurring requests to access his medical records since the late 1960s. As his records were made before 1991, they were not subject to the Data Protection Act 1984[1] or the Access to Health Records Act 1990. The trial judge in proceedings for judicial review ruled that the applicant did not have the right of access to his medical records at common law and that the health authorities' decisions to turn down his requests were not in breach of Article 8 of the Convention for the Protection of Human Rights and Fundamental Freedoms. Upon appeal, the Court of Appeal held that a health authority, being the owner of medical records, can refuse a patient's access to the records if it is in the best interests of the patient to do so. The patient's petition for leave to appeal was dismissed.

The prevalent use of EHR has further complicated the issues on the ownership of healthcare records. For example, Barrows and Clayton (1996) raised concerns

[1] The Data Protection Act 1984 in the UK was repealed by the Data Protection Act 1998 (House of Lords, UK, 2017, paragraph 55), which was further replaced by the Data Protection Act 2018 to make data protection 'fit for the digital age' (Department for Digital, Culture, Media & Sport, UK, 2018, p. 1).

about data ownership, data owners' obligations and the delegation of data owners' powers. Cohen (2021, p. 19) argued that with the bright future of healthcare brought by artificial intelligence, the existing EHR systems should be wrenched off from the 'antiquated pillars' to allow patients to own their personal healthcare data, which in turn better the protection of patient privacy and create a functioning market for healthcare data.

9.7.2 *Data Privacy and Confidentiality*

The use of EHR may increase medico-legal risks in data privacy and confidentiality, as any infringement in the electronic environment may expose many patients at risk of being exploited (Chiruvella & Guddati, 2021). For instance, it was reported that a security infringement at MyHeritage, a family networking and genealogy website, had leaked a total of 92 million clients' data in 2018 (Reuters Staff, 2018). Privacy risks may come from user access and authentication (Datta & Dunlop, 2009), as unauthorised persons may download health data for malicious or inquisitive purposes, including but not limited to 'identity theft to embarrassment to prurient interest in the life of a celebrity or neighbour' (Department of Health and Human Services, US, 2000, p. 82,465). In Hong Kong, in *HKSAR v Tsun Shui Lun* HCMA723/98, [1999] 3 HKLRD 215, the appellant worked as a hospital technical assistant. He had been allowed only to access an EHR system by password to conduct research, but he logged in the system and leaked purposely the radiological records of the then Secretary for Justice to the mass media. The Court of First Instance dismissed the appellant's appeal for conviction but set aside the original sentence of 6-month imprisonment for a community service order of 100 hours.

9.7.3 *Electronic Signatures*

Electronic signature is defined as 'data in electronic form in, affixed to or logically associated with, a data message, which may be used to identify the signatory in relation to the data message and to indicate the signatory's approval of the information contained in the data message' (UN, 2002b, p. 1, Article 2(a)). A number of jurisdictions have enacted electronic signature laws, such as the Electronic Transactions Act 1999 in Australia, the Electronic Transactions Act 2002 in New Zealand, the Electronic Communications Act 2000 in the UK, the Electronic Signature Law in China, and the Electronic Transactions Ordinance (Cap 553) in Hong Kong. To ratify the UNCITRAL Model Law on Electronic Transferable Records 2017 (UN, 2018), Singapore further amended its Electronic Transactions Act (Cap 88), which became effective on 19 March 2021.

Not all jurisdictions see electronic signatures in the same manner (Gitlin, 1997). For instance, courts in Singapore and the UK have had different views as to whether it is legally sufficient if an email appends no name at the end of the mail but there is a name generated automatically appearing adjacent to the email address of the sender at the 'from' column. The High Court of Singapore in *SM Integrated Transware Pte Ltd v Schenker Singapore (Pte) Ltd* [2005] SGHC 58 did not find that Section 4 of the Electronic Transactions Act (Cap 88) had barred any electronic communications for the satisfaction of Section 6 of the Civil Law Act 1994 (Cap 43) (CLA) and that it all depended on how Section 6 of the CLA would be construed. The court found that the concept of 'signature' at common law does not necessitate a handwritten signature for the purpose of Section 6(d) of the CLA, and a typewritten or printed signature would suffice. It held that the name automatically generated is sufficient to meet the statutory requirements of writing and signing as stipulated in Section 6(d) of the CLA and that the lease agreement in question was binding between the parties. In the UK, the position may not be the same. The High Court (Chancery Division) in *J Pereira Fernandes SA v Mehta* [2006] EWHC 813 (Ch) held that the automatic inclusion of the sender's email address by an Internet service provider after a document had been sent did not amount to a signature satisfying sufficiently the purposes of Section 4 of the Statute of Frauds Act 1677, where Pelling J said at paragraph 31,

> [The Electronic Communications Act 2000] empowers the appropriate minister to issue statutory instruments in order to modify any other stature [*sic*] or statutory instrument in order to facilitate electronic communications. My understanding is that this Act was enacted in order to give effect to the Directive on European Electronic Commerce (Council Directive 2000/31/EC). No relevant statutory instrument made under this Act has been drawn to my attention. … [T]he Law Commission's view in relation to this Directive is that no significant changes are necessary in relation to statutes that require signatures because whether those requirements have been satisfied can be tested in a functional way by asking whether the conduct of the would be signatory indicates an authenticating intention to a reasonable person. … [I]f a party or a party's agent sending an e-mail types his or her or his or her principal's name to the extent required or permitted by existing case law in the body of an e-mail, then in my view that would be a sufficient signature for the purposes of section 4 [of the Statute of Frauds Act 1677]. However that is not this case.

The two cases above were not relevant to healthcare, but as a prudent approach, it seems advisable for healthcare professionals and institutes to typewrite or sign their names in full in any healthcare records and record-related communication exchanges to avoid unnecessary disputes on electronic signatures.

9.7.4 Maintenance of EHR Systems

Tong (2019) discussed a case in Michigan heard before the US District Court (Eastern), *Allen v Shawney* (an unreported case; Westlaw citation number: 2014 WL 1089618). The claimant alleged that her constitutional rights were infringed when she was in custody, as correctional facilities were indifferent to her healthcare needs as evidenced by repeated changes of dates of telehealth consultations with excuses of infrastructure breakdowns, such as malfunctions of EHR system, failures of either telemedical network or system, and suspension of power supply. Despite that the claimant was not successful in her claim, such system failures have led to an avoidable lawsuit.

9.7.5 Management of EHR

R (on the application of Morris) v Parliamentary and Health Service Ombudsman [2019] EWHC 1603 (Admin) was a case heard before the Queen's Bench (Administrative Court) in England. The claimant's daughter died in 2011. She sought judicial review of the report of the defendant Ombudsman on her complaint of maladministration against a National Health Service (NHS) trust, arising from the fact that the trust failed to locate all the medical records of the deceased. The Ombudsman received the claimant's first complaint against the trust in 2012 and decided not to pursue an investigation as the opportunity to find the missing records was slim. Upon the trust's further investigations, some of the missing records were traced in 2013 and 2014, having spotted its weaknesses in the medical record management. Upon receipt of the claimant's second complaint, the Ombudsman agreed to make an investigation and finalised the report in 2017. He upheld the complaint and recommended the trust to give a written apology and make a payment of £1,000 for the claimant's anxiety, frustration, and distress, but he did not suggest that the trust do extra searches for the records of the deceased on the grounds that the chance was small to locate new records and that it would be disproportionate. The Ombudsman did not agree to pay the claimant's legal costs or recommend the trust to make her legal costs. The claimant submitted that the 2017 report of the Ombudsman was unlawful on various grounds. After hearing, the court dismissed the claim for judicial review. This case has highlighted the resultant medico-legal risks as a consequence of poor medical record management.

9.7.6 Quality of Images

Quality of healthcare records may affect a witness's reliability in court. A heavier weight may be accorded in court to written healthcare records than to a witness's memory (Yeo, 2004). Lord Pearce sitting on the House of Lords in *Toohey v Metropolitan Police Commissioner* [1965] AC 595 said at page 609, 'Medical evidence is admissible to show that a witness suffers from some disease or defect or abnormality of mind that affects the reliability of his evidence'.

Quality of images stored in EHR systems may also affect their evidential weights in court. In England, *OCC v B, C, A (by her children's guardian)* [2018] 7 WLUK 166 was a family case. In this case, the judge pointed out that the quality of images would have an impact on the weight of evidence in court. One of the issues before the court was whether the child respondent had bruises at the material time. A consultant paediatrician (Dr. J) saw the child in April 2018 and he found no bruises on examination, but after seeing photographs taken by the child's mother a few days earlier on her phone, Dr. J gave a conclusion that the 'marks' appeared thereon were consistent with bruises. Among others, Dr. J testified the following in court at paragraph 23(iv):

a. The photos were transferred to another smartphone through a messaging application named 'WhatsApp' and they were then emailed to the hospital internet system for storage into the EHR of the child;
b. The quality of the images may have been affected during such transfer and reproduction;
c. For clinical purposes, photographs were taken by the use of specialised camera in good light;
d. His description of the marks on the photos was not reliable as he had only looked at the smartphone images, in which there was no scale ruler, and he had not measured the size of the marks; and
e. He could not undergo physical tests such as touch and measurement of the influenced area by looking at the images only.

As endorsed by the judge, legal representatives of the parties also had similar observations at paragraphs 37–38 that photographic images not taken at professional level may misrepresent the facts and that other elements such as light exposure and device used may influence the reliability of photographic images. The judge commented at paragraph 29 that while Dr. J could hold his professional view that the marks looked like bruises, the court considered the substantial weight of the evidence differently as, inter alia, the quality of the images presented to the court varied and no bruises were seen in all clinical examinations in person, except through the diagnosis of the smartphone photographs.

In California, *Chabra v Southern Monterey County Memorial Hospital* (an unreported case; Westlaw citation number: 1994 WL 564566), the concern on the quality of image was also raised, where the plaintiff radiologist alleged at paragraph 6 that excessive transmission of non-emergency radiological films through teleradiology to a venue away from the defendant hospital resulted in poorer film quality and poorer correlation between radiological studies and pathological results. The court ordered the plaintiff to amend his claims and had not dealt with this allegation.

9.7.7 Staff Training

R (on the application of Wiggins) v HM Assistant Coroner for Nottinghamshire [2015] EWHC 2841 (Admin) was a case heard before the Queen's Bench (Divisional Court) in England. The claimant is the mother of a late prisoner who was found hanging in the prison in 2013. A coroner's inquest was held and the jury reached an 'uncertain' conclusion as to the intention of the deceased to end his life. The claimant sought to quash the conclusion of the inquest. Her concern was not to challenge the jury's verdict but on the failure of the Prison Service and particular officers in the provision of medical care and in the assessment of suicide risk. Although the court dismissed the claimant's application finally, there is a lesson to learn from this case. Before the coroner's inquest, the Prisons and Probation Ombudsman (PPO) investigated the case and prepared a report, which the court considered at paragraph 9 'an important report for the arguments about the scope of the inquest'. The PPO identified that in the initial health screen at the time of reception of the deceased, nurses of the prison in question did not have access to the deceased's EHR from the preceding prison in which he had served before the transfer, where a recent history of his deliberately cutting wrists was recorded. The PPO worried about the lack of full assessment of the known suicidal risks of newly arrived prisoners and recommended accessing EHR once after the completion of the reception health screen. At the coroner's inquest, the healthcare officer in charge of the prison in question testified that not all staff at the time of the deceased's reception would have had the knowledge about how to get access to prisoners' previous records from the EHR system, as the retrieval of past records required some technical knowhow in using the system, and that the risk of self-harm might have left unheeded if a prisoner at reception did not mention any issues about self-harm and such risk was not revealed through standard questions. The healthcare officer in charge continued to explain the subsequent staff training and improvements after the mishap. This case has demonstrated the need for effective training for healthcare staff to understand and make good use of EHR systems and the need to assign access rights to appropriate levels of staff.

9.7.8 Procurement of EHR Systems

Healthcare institutes and professionals should be vigilant to the selection of capable contractors and better plan the procurement processes of EHR systems. In England, the parties in *Royal Devon and Exeter NHS Foundation Trust v ATOS IT Services UK Ltd* [2017] EWHC 3168 (TCC) entered into a contract to design, deliver, install, test, implement, and maintain an EHR system to store and manage medical records. The claimant NHS trust alleged that the defendant's system was insufficiently designed, commissioned, and managed, in addition to other claims that it was too slow to be employed by clinicians, bug-ridden, undependable, and uncertain as to patients' safety. The defendant argued that the claimant caused the problems, as it did not take sufficient ownership of the EHR system, did not administer it properly, and did not accept the defendant's offer for a managed service. Upon the claimant's application, the court ruled that the defendant should disclose certain source code of the system to the claimant.

In the Northern Ireland, the claimant in *CSC Computer Sciences Ltd (trading as DXC Technology) v Business Services Organisation* [2019] NIQB 18 was a tenderer in a public procurement exercise of an EHR system. It failed to enter into the second phase of the exercise. The defendant organised the exercise with an aim to identify a suitable candidate to work with the Health and Social Care Northern Ireland to commission an EHR system across health and social care services throughout the territory. The court considered at paragraph 40 that it was in the public interest to have a territory-wide EHR system to integrate 'all of the disparate elements' of healthcare services and that the claimant had delayed for three months without justifiable explanation to apply for an injunction. The court refused the claimant's application for an interim injunction to stop the defendant's procurement process.

In Scotland, in *Elekta Ltd v Common Services Agency* [2011] CSOH 107, the defendant is Common Services Agency, also known as the NHS National Services Scotland. It arranged a procurement exercise in late 2010 in support of five Scottish health boards to look for a contractor to supply, install and maintain a series of equipment for incorporation into the existing radiotherapy management system and provide staff training accordingly. The claimant alleged that the defendant's procurement exercise was discriminatory, as one of the mandatory tender terms requiring the new system to be compatible with the radiotherapy management system in use, which was manufactured by a third-party, had deterred it from submitting an offer. The claimant also argued that the defendant had a duty to ensure equal treatment and not to discriminate and to devise tender requirements in a manner to allow effective competition to enable potential tenderers other than the said manufacturer to bid. The Outer House of the Court of Session ruled that it did not violate the principles of equality and non-discrimination for a contracting authority like the defendant to include tender criteria that could be only met by a single tenderer, unless the authority could not provide objective justifications for such criteria.

9.8 Conclusion

The global ageing population has posed real challenges to the traditional modes of hospital-based and institutional-based healthcare, on top of other considerations such as the sustainability of social welfare systems and economic developments. To manage the growing needs of older persons, ageing in place is recognised internationally one of the viable options. It being a conceptual slogan, ageing in place is however not adequate. The dignity of older persons has to be considered as a crucial element in practice.

Telehealth reinforces dignified ageing in place to bolster older persons' independence and well-being. Notwithstanding it being a state-of-the-art healthcare technology, telehealth is not legal-risk free. In particular, EHR as one of its basic but vital components faces various potential medico-legal risks. It cannot be emphasised enough that healthcare institutes and professionals better check possible medico-legal risks in the design and management of any EHR systems.

9.9 Limitations

With the support of a few court cases in the common law context, some potential medico-legal risks of EHR are discussed generally. The court cases mentioned in this chapter may not be authoritative in the legal and judicial senses, but they share practical lessons with healthcare professionals and institutes. Owing to resource constraints, the author has only cited cases from several jurisdictions as examples. Such discussion is in no way encyclopaedic. Court judgments in jurisdictions practising civil law are not addressed at all. Potential risks of EHR in the boom of artificial intelligence have not been explored, either. The risks discussed in this chapter may vary under the laws of different jurisdictions and may not be generalised or applicable to specific litigious disputes. To the author's best knowledge, the law mentioned in this chapter is current as of late July 2021.

References

Allen v Shawney. Case number: 11–10942. Not reported in F.Supp.3d. Westlaw citation number: 2014 WL 1089618 (District Court, E.D. Michigan, Northern Division, 2014), United States.

Barrows, R. C., & Clayton, P. D. (1996). Privacy, confidentiality and electronic medical records. *Journal of the American Medical Informatics Association, 3*(2), 139–148. https://doi.org/10.1136/jamia.1996.96236282

Black, K., & Dobbs, D. (2014). Community-dwelling older adults' perceptions of dignity: Core meanings, challenges, supports and opportunities. *Ageing & Society, 34*(8), 1292–1313. https://doi.org/10.1017/S0144686X13000020

Breen v Williams [1995] HCA 63, (1996) 43 ALD 481 (High Court), Australia.

Cairns, D., Williams, V., Victor, C., Richards, S., Le May, A., Martin, W., & Oliver, D. (2013). The meaning and importance of dignified care: Findings from a survey of health and social care professionals. *BMC Geriatrics, 13*(1), 28. https://doi.org/10.1186/1471-2318-13-28

Chabra v Southern Monterey County Memorial Hospital. Civ. No. C 94–20335 EAI. Not Reported in F.Supp. Westlaw citation number: 1994 WL 564566 (District Court of California, 1994), United States.

Chau, C. W., & Leung, E. (2017). Health informatics and technology for integrated elderly care in the context of Hong Kong: A case study. *Studies in Health Technology and Informatics, 241*, 134–144. https://doi.org/10.3233/978-1-61499-794-8-134

Chester v Afshar [2004] UKHL 41, [2005] 1 AC 134 (House of Lords), United Kingdom.

Chiruvella, V., & Guddati, A. K. (2021). Ethical issues in patient data ownership. *Interactive Journal of Medical Research, 10*(2), e22269, 9 pages. https://doi.org/10.2196/22269

Cohen, J. (2021). The path to better health: Give the people their data. *Issues in Science and Technology, 37*(2), 19–21.

Connelly, K., ur Rehman Laghari, K., Mokhtari, M., & Falk, T. H. (2014). Approaches to understanding the impact of technologies for aging in place: A mini-review. *Gerontology, 60*(3), 282–288. https://doi.org/10.1159/000355644

CSC Computer Sciences Ltd (trading as DXC Technology) v Business Services Organisation [2019] NIQB 18 (Queen's Bench [Northern Ireland]), United Kingdom.

Datta, M., & Dunlop, K. O. (2009). Privacy of electronic health information. In L. D. Fleisher & J. C. Dechene (Eds.), *Telemedicine and e-health law* (Release 9; [2004] - <2009>). Law Journal Press.

Department for Digital, Culture, Media & Sport, United Kingdom. (2018). *Data protection act 2018: Factsheet – overview*. https://assets.publishing.service.gov.uk/government/uploads/system/uploads/attachment_data/file/711162/2018-05-23_Factsheet_1_-_Act_overview.pdf

Department of Health and Human Services, United States. (2000). Standards for privacy of individually identifiable health information. *Federal Register, 65*(250), 82239–82878.

East Sussex County Council. (2021). *Leaflet: Do you look after someone?* (2021/22 edition (IL04)). https://new.eastsussex.gov.uk/social-care/getting-help-from-us/asc-leaflets/leaflet-do-you-look-after-someone?print=true

Electronic Communications Act 2000, United Kingdom.

Electronic Health Record Office, Hong Kong. (2020). *Electronic health record sharing system*. https://www.ehealth.gov.hk/en/whats-ehealth/index.html

Electronic Signature Law of the People's Republic of China.

Electronic Transactions Act (Cap 88), Singapore.

Electronic Transactions Act 1999, Australia.

Electronic Transactions Act 2002, New Zealand.

Electronic Transactions Ordinance (Cap 553), Hong Kong.

Elekta Ltd v Common Services Agency [2011] CSOH 107 (Court of Session [Outer House]), United Kingdom.

European Economic and Social Committee. (2019). *Opinion of the European Economic and Social Committee on 'economic, technological and social changes in advanced health services for the elderly' (own-initiative opinion)* (2019/C 240/03). https://eur-lex.europa.eu/legal-content/EN/TXT/HTML/?uri=CELEX:52018IE4518&from=EN

Feldman, P. H., Oberlink, M. R., Simantov, E., & Gursen, M. D. (2004). *A tale of two older Americas: Community opportunities and challenges*. Center for Home Care Policy and Research. http://www.civicengagement.org/agingsociety/links/two_americas.pdf

Gantley, N., Bradshaw, C., & Doody, O. (2020). Healthcare professionals' perceptions of privacy and dignity afforded to palliative care patients in an acute hospital setting: A qualitative descriptive study. *Nursing and Palliative Care, 5*, 1–5. https://doi.org/10.15761/NPC.1000215

Garets, D., & Davis, M. (2006). *Electronic medical records vs. electronic health records: Yes, there is a difference* (HIMSS Analytics, Chicago, United States). https://www.aao.org/asset.axd?id=8e9b1f20-0ed6-4d2b-92f8-e28fbaf378ec&t=634962799822530000

Gitlin, J. N. (1997). Teleradiology. In R. L. Bashshur, J. H. Sanders, & G. W. Shannon (Eds.), *Telemedicine: Theory and practice* (pp. 111–178). Charles C Thomas Publisher.

Häyry, M. (2004). Another look at dignity. *Cambridge Quarterly of Healthcare Ethics, 13*(1), 7–14. https://doi.org/10.1017/S0963180104131034

He, A. J., & Tang, V. F. Y. (2021). Integration of health services for the elderly in Asia: A scoping review of Hong Kong, Singapore, Malaysia, Indonesia. *Health Policy, 125*(3), 351–362. https://doi.org/10.1016/j.healthpol.2020.12.020

Heggestad, A. K. T., Nortvedt, P., & Slettebø, Å. (2015). Dignity and care for people with dementia living in nursing homes. *Dementia, 14*(6), 825–841. https://doi.org/10.1177/1471301213512840

Hemati, Z., AllahBakhshian, M., Pourfarzad, Z., Shirani, F., Safazadeh, S., Ziyaei, M., Varzeshnejad, M., Hashemi, M., & Taleghani, F. (2016). Dying with dignity: A concept analysis. *Journal of Clinical Nursing, 25*(9–10), 1218–1228. https://doi.org/10.1111/jocn.13143

Heumann, L. F., & Boldy, D. P. (1993). The basic benefits and limitations of an aging-in-place policy. In L. F. Heumann & D. P. Boldy (Eds.), *Aging in place with dignity: International solutions relating to the low-income and frail elderly* (pp. 1–8). Praeger.

HKSAR v Tsun Shui Lun HCMA723/98, [1999] 3 HKLRD 215 (Court of First Instance), Hong Kong.

House of Lords, United Kingdom. (2017). Data Protection Bill [HL]: Explanatory notes. https://publications.parliament.uk/pa/bills/lbill/2017-2019/0066/18066en.pdf

Hughes, G. (2011). The concept of dignity in the Universal Declaration of Human Rights. *Journal of Religious Ethics, 39*(1), 1–24. https://doi.org/10.1111/j.1467-9795.2010.00463.x

Hwang, E., Cummings, L., Sixsmith, A., & Sixsmith, J. (2011). Impacts of home modifications on aging-in-place. *Journal of Housing for the Elderly, 25*(3), 246–257. https://doi.org/10.1080/02763893.2011.595611

Illinois General Assembly, United States. (2021). *Bill status of HB3308: 102nd General Assembly*. https://www.ilga.gov/legislation/BillStatus.asp?DocNum=3308&GAID=16&DocTypeID=HB&SessionID=110&GA=102

J Pereira Fernandes SA v Mehta [2006] EWHC 813 (Ch) (High Court [Chancery Division]), United Kingdom.

Jacobson, N. (2007). Dignity and health: A review. *Social Science & Medicine, 64*(2), 292–302. https://doi.org/10.1016/j.socscimed.2006.08.039

Jercich, K. (2021, July 26). *Illinois permanently expands access to telehealth*. Healthcare IT News. https://www.healthcareitnews.com/news/illinois-permanently-expands-access-telehealth

Jha, A. K., Ferris, T. G., Donelan, K., DesRoches, C., Shields, A., Rosenbaum, S., & Blumenthal, D. (2006). How common are electronic health records in the United States? A summary of the evidence. *Health Affairs (Millwood), 25*(6), 496–507. https://doi.org/10.1377/hlthaff.25.w496

Johnson v Hillcrest Health Centre, Inc. 70 P.3d 811, 2003 OK 16 (Okla. 2003) (Supreme Court of Oklahoma), United States.

Johri, M., Beland, F., & Bergman, H. (2003). International experiments in integrated care for the elderly: A synthesis of the evidence. *International Journal of Geriatric Psychiatry, 18*(3), 222–235. https://doi.org/10.1002/gps.819

Karimi, H., Ajorpaz, N. M., & Aghajani, M. (2019). Older adults' and nurses' perception of dignity in the setting of Iranian hospitals: A cross-section study. *Central European Journal of Nursing and Midwifery, 10*(4), 1134–1142. https://doi.org/10.15452/CEJNM.2019.10.0025

Kendig, H., Gong, C. H., Cannon, L., & Browning, C. (2017). Preferences and predictors of aging in place: Longitudinal evidence from Melbourne, Australia. *Journal of Housing for the Elderly, 31*(3), 259–271. https://doi.org/10.1080/02763893.2017.1280582

Kerr, D., Crone, R., & Dunning, T. (2020). Perspectives about dignity during acute care for older people and their relatives: A qualitative study. *Journal of Clinical Nursing, 29*(21–22), 4116–4127. https://doi.org/10.1111/jocn.15438

Kluge, E.-H.W. (2011). Ethical and legal challenges for health telematics in a global world: Telehealth and the technological imperative. *International Journal of Medical Informatics, 80*(2), e1–e5. https://doi.org/10.1016/j.ijmedinf.2010.10.002

Knight, A., Fouyaxis, J., Jarrad, G., Beski, K., Cho, G., & Bidargaddi, N. (2018). Systems to harness digital footprint to elucidate and facilitate ageing in place. In M. E. L. van den Berg & A. J. Maeder (Eds.), *Telehealth for our ageing society* (pp. 91–101). IOS Press. https://doi.org/10.3233/978-1-61499-845-7-91

Koehn, D., & Leung, A. (2008). Dignity in western versus in Chinese cultures: Theoretical overview and practical illustrations. *Business and Society Review, 113*(4), 477–504. https://doi.org/10.1111/j.1467-8594.2008.00329.x

Lau, J.Y.-C., Wong, E.L.-Y., Chung, R. Y., Law, S. C. K., Threapleton, D., Kiang, N., Chau, P., Wong, S. Y. S., Woo, J., & Yeoh, E.-K. (2018). Collaborate across silos: Perceived barriers to integration of care for the elderly from the perspectives of service providers. *International Journal of Health Planning and Management, 33*(3), e768–e780. https://doi.org/10.1002/hpm.2534

Li, Y. (2021). The Confucian concept of human dignity and its implications for bioethics. *Developing World Bioethics*. https://doi.org/10.1111/dewb.12312

Li, Y., & Li, J. (2017). Death with dignity from the Confucian perspective. *Theoretical Medicine and Bioethics, 38*(1), 63–81. https://doi.org/10.1007/s11017-016-9383-7

Lin, Y.-P., Tsai, Y.-F., & Chen, H.-F. (2011). Dignity in care in the hospital setting from patients' perspectives in Taiwan: A descriptive qualitative study. *Journal of Clinical Nursing, 20*(5–6), 794–801. https://doi.org/10.1111/j.1365-2702.2010.03499.x

Local Government Association, United Kingdom. (2016). *Transforming social care through the use of information and technology*. https://www.local.gov.uk/sites/default/files/documents/Transforming%20Social%20Care%20through%20Information%20and%20Technology.pdf

Lothian, K., & Philp, I. (2001). Care of older people: Maintaining the dignity and autonomy of older people in the healthcare setting. *British Medical Journal, 322*(7287), 668–670. https://doi.org/10.1136/bmj.322.7287.668

Lum, T. Y. S., Lou, V. W. Q., Chen, Y., Wong, G. H. Y., Luo, H., & Tong, T. L. W. (2016). Neighborhood support and aging-in-place preference among low-income elderly Chinese city-dwellers. *The Journals of Gerontology: Series B, 71*(1), 98–105. https://doi.org/10.1093/geronb/gbu154

Macklin, R. (2003). Dignity is a useless concept. *British Medical Journal, 327*(7429), 1419–1420. https://doi.org/10.1136/bmj.327.7429.1419

Mclnerney v MacDonald [1992] 2 SCR 138 (Supreme Court), Canada.

Ministry of Health and Care Services, Norway. (2010). Regulations on Dignified Care for the Elderly (Dignity Guarantee) (*Forskrift om en verdig eldreomsorg (verdighetsgarantien)*). https://www.regjeringen.no/no/dokumenter/Forskrift-om-en-verdig-eldreomsorg-verdighetsgarantien/id624655/

Ministry of Social Affairs and Health, Denmark. (2019). Executive Order on Dignity Policies for Elderly Care (*Bekendtgørelse om værdighedspolitikker for ældreplejen*). https://www.elov.dk/bekendtgorelse-om-vaerdighedspolitikker-for-aeldreplejen/

Ministry of Social Affairs and Health, Finland. (2012). *Act on Supporting the Functional Capacity of the Older Population and on Social and Health Care Services for Older Persons* (No. 980/2012). https://www.finlex.fi/fi/laki/kaannokset/2012/en20120980_20120980.pdf

Moody, H. R. (1998). Why dignity in old age matters. *Journal of Gerontological Social Work, 29*(2–3), 13–38. https://doi.org/10.1300/J083V29N02_02

NHS Confederation. (2016). *Stepping up to the place: The key to successful health and care integration.* https://www.nhsconfed.org/sites/default/files/media/Stepping%20up%20to%20the%20place_Br1413_WEB.pdf

Nordenfelt, L. (2004). The varieties of dignity. *Health Care Analysis, 12*(2), 69–81. https://doi.org/10.1023/B:HCAN.0000041183.78435.4b

Nursing and Midwifery Council v Iestyn Bryant [2021] EWHC 1064 (Admin) (Queen's Bench), United Kingdom.

OCC v B, C, A (by her children's guardian) [2018] 7 WLUK 166 (Family Court), United Kingdom.

Office of the National Coordinator for Health Information Technology, United States. (2019). *What are the advantages of electronic health records?* https://www.healthit.gov/faq/what-are-advantages-electronic-health-records

Oosterhof, P. D. (2018). *Ageing related policies and priorities in the implementation of the 2030 agenda for sustainable development: As reported in the voluntary national reviews of 2016, 2017 and 2018.* https://www.un.org/development/desa/ageing/wp-content/uploads/sites/24/2019/07/Analysis-Ageing_VNRs_Final28122018.pdf

Organisation for Economic Cooperation and Development. (2021). *Ageing*. https://www.oecd-ilibrary.org/sites/1ad1c42a-en/index.html?itemId=/content/component/1ad1c42a-en

President's Commission for the Study of Ethical Problems in Medicine and Biomedical and Behavioral Research, United States. (1983). *Deciding to forego life-sustaining treatment: A report on the ethical, medical, and legal issues in treatment decisions.* U.S. Government Printing Office. https://repository.library.georgetown.edu/bitstream/handle/10822/559344/deciding_to_forego_tx.pdf?sequence=1&isAllowed=y

Queirós, A., Pereira, L., Dias, A., & Rocha, N. P. (2017). Technologies for ageing in place to support home monitoring of patients with chronic diseases. In E. L. van den Broek, A. Fred, H. Gamboa, & M. Vaz (Eds.), *Proceedings of the 10th International Joint Conference on Biomedical Engineering Systems and Technologies – Volume 5: HEALTHINF, (BIOSTEC 2017)* (pp. 66–76). https://doi.org/10.5220/0006140000660076

R v Ashworth Hospital Authority (Now Mersey Care National Health Service Trust) [2005] UKHL 58, [2006] 2 AC 148 (House of Lords), United Kingdom.

R v Mid Glamorgan Family Health Services Authority Ex p. Martin [1995] 1 WLR 110 (Court of Appeal), United Kingdom.

R (on the application of Morris) v Parliamentary and Health Service Ombudsman [2019] EWHC 1603 (Admin) (Queen's Bench (Administrative Court)), United Kingdom.
R (on the application of Wiggins) v HM Assistant Coroner for Nottinghamshire [2015] EWHC 2841 (Admin) (Queen's Bench (Divisional Court)), United Kingdom.
Re NLS HCMH 4/2020, [2021] HKCFI 2203 (Court of First Instance), Hong Kong.
Reuters Staff. (2018, June 6). *Security breach at MyHeritage website leaks details of over 92 million users*. Reuters. https://www.reuters.com/article/us-myheritage-privacy-idUSKCN1J1308
Royal Devon and Exeter NHS Foundation Trust v ATOS IT Services UK Ltd [2017] EWHC 3168 (TCC) (Queen's Bench [Technology & Construction Court]), United Kingdom.
Šaňáková, Š, & Čáp, J. (2019). Dignity from the nurses' and older patients' perspective: A qualitative literature review. *Nursing Ethics, 26*(5), 1292–1309. https://doi.org/10.1177/0969733017747960
Schoen, C., Osborn, R., How S. K. H., Doty, M. M., & Peugh, J. (2008). In chronic condition: Experiences of patients with complex health care needs, in eight countries. *Health Affairs, 27*(Supp. 1), w1–w16. https://doi.org/10.1377/hlthaff.28.1.w1
Sheikh, A., McLean, S., Cresswell, K., Pagliari, C., Pappas, Y., Car, J., Black, A., Hemmi, A., Nurmatov, U., Mukherjee, M., McKinstry, B., Procter, R., & Majeed, A. (2011). *The impact of ehealth on the quality and safety of healthcare: An updated systematic overview & synthesis of the literature—Final report for the NHS Connecting for Health Evaluation Programme (NHS CFHEP 001)*. The University of Edinburgh. https://moam.info/the-impact-of-ehealth-on-the-quality-and-safety-of-_59f051ae1723dd1d8d71a63e.html
Singh, P. K. (2015). *Dignity in mental health*. WHO Regional Office for South-East Asia. https://www.who.int/southeastasia/news/detail/08-10-2015-dignity-in-mental-health
SM Integrated Transware Pte Ltd v Schenker Singapore (Pte) Ltd [2005] SGHC 58 (High Court), Singapore.
Social Care Institute for Excellence. (2020). *Defining dignity in care*. https://www.scie.org.uk/dignity/care/defining
Tadd, W., Bayer, T., & Dieppe, P. (2002). Dignity in health care: Reality or rhetoric. *Reviews in Clinical Gerontology, 12*(1), 1–4. https://doi.org/10.1017/S095925980201211X
The Star. (2019, January 10). Protecting seniors' right to dignified ageing. https://www.thestar.com.my/lifestyle/family/2019/01/10/right-to-dignified-ageing
Tong, K.-w. (2019). Telehealth as a double-edged sword: Lessons from court cases to gain understanding of medico-legal risks. *Medicine and Law: World Association for Medical Law, 38*(1), 85–106.
Tong, K.-w. (2021). Community care: To "tele", or not to "tele"? Considerations from the medico-legal and operational perspectives. In B. Y. F. Fong & M. C. S. Wong (Eds.), *Routledge handbook of public health and the community*. Routledge.
Tong, K.-w. (In press). Population ageing, ageing in place, telehealth and its legal concerns. In K. N-K. Fong, & K.-w. Tong (Eds.), *Ageing care in the community: Current practices and future directions*. City University of Hong Kong.
Toohey v Metropolitan Police Commissioner [1965] AC 595 (House of Lords), United Kingdom.
United Nations. (1945). *United Nations charter*. https://www.un.org/en/about-us/un-charter/full-text
United Nations. (2002a). *Political Declaration and Madrid International Plan of Action on Ageing*. Second World Assembly on Ageing in Madrid, Spain on 8–12 April 2002a. https://www.un.org/esa/socdev/documents/ageing/MIPAA/political-declaration-en.pdf
United Nations. (2002b). *UNCITRAL model law on electronic signatures with guide to enactment 2001*. United Nations publication. https://uncitral.un.org/sites/uncitral.un.org/files/media-documents/uncitral/en/ml-elecsig-e.pdf
United Nations. (2018). *UNCITRAL model law on electronic transferable records*. United Nations publication. https://uncitral.un.org/sites/uncitral.un.org/files/media-documents/uncitral/en/mletr_ebook_e.pdf

United Nations Department of Economic and Social Affairs. (2020). *World population ageing 2020 highlights*. https://www.un.org/development/desa/pd/sites/www.un.org.development.desa.pd/files/files/documents/2020/Sep/un_pop_2020_pf_ageing_10_key_messages.pdf

United Nations General Assembly. (1948). *Universal Declaration of Human Rights*. https://www.un.org/sites/un2.un.org/files/udhr.pdf

United Nations General Assembly. (1991). *United Nations Principles for Older Persons* (A/RES/46/91). https://www.ohchr.org/en/professionalinterest/pages/olderpersons.aspx#:~:text=17.,independently%20of%20their%20economic%20contribution

United Nations General Assembly. (2006). *Convention on the Rights of Persons with Disabilities and its Optional Protocol* (A/RES/61/106). https://www.un.org/esa/socdev/enable/rights/convtexte.htm

Webster, C., & Bryan, K. (2009). Older people's views of dignity and how it can be promoted in a hospital environment. *Journal of Clinical Nursing, 18*(12), 1784–1792. https://doi.org/10.1111/j.1365-2702.2008.02674.x

Woolhead, G., Calnan, M., Dieppe, P., & Tadd, W. (2004). Dignity in older age: What do older people in the United Kingdom think? *Age and Ageing, 33*(2), 165–170. https://doi.org/10.1093/ageing/afh045

Wootton, R. (1996). Telemedicine: A cautious welcome. *British Medical Journal, 313*(7069), 1375–1377. https://doi.org/10.1136/bmj.313.7069.1375

World Health Organisation. (1994). *A declaration of the promotion of patients' rights in Europe* (ICP/HLE 121). https://www.who.int/genomics/public/eu_declaration1994.pdf

World Health Organisation. (2015). *World report on ageing and health*. Geneva, Switzerland. http://apps.who.int/iris/bitstream/handle/10665/186463/9789240694811_eng.pdf;jsessionid=8319553806154EE9B136071BE8C5D668?sequence=1

World Health Organisation. (2016). *Global diffusion of eHealth: Making universal health coverage achievable. Report of the third global survey on eHealth*. World Health Organisation. https://apps.who.int/iris/rest/bitstreams/1071614/retrieve

World Health Organisation. (2018). *Quality, equity, dignity: The network to improve quality of care for maternal, newborn and child health – Strategic objectives*. https://apps.who.int/iris/bitstream/handle/10665/272612/9789241513951-eng.pdf

World Health Organisation Regional Office for Africa. (2021). *The time to ensure a healthy and dignified ageing for Africans is now*. https://www.afro.who.int/regional-director/regional-director-commentaries/time-ensure-healthy-and-dignified-ageing-africans

World Health Organisation Regional Office for the Western Pacific. (2006). *Electronic health records: Manual for developing countries*. https://iris.wpro.who.int/bitstream/handle/10665.1/5533/9290612177_eng.pdf

Yeo, K. Q. (2004). Medical records and confidentiality. In K. Q. Yeo, L. Chew, L. G. Goh, T. Kaan, B. T. Kuah, & E. Tong (Eds.), *Essentials of medical law* (pp. 209–241). Sweet & Maxwell Asia.

Chapter 10
Age-Friendly City Movement

Fiona C. M. Yuen and Chesney P. Y. Wong

Abstract Recent trend of demography gives a clear view of ageing population worldwide. The significant increase in ageing population brings an overwhelming challenge to both Asian and European countries. Meanwhile, globalisation, advanced technology, social stigmas and complex city structures make elderly live with barriers. How to live with dignity is always a complicated and controversial topic. Luckily, the reflections and comparisons between Asian and European countries provide opportunities for countries in the world to learn from each other about how to provide holistic care to old adults to live with social respect. Moreover, some successful age-friendly communities reveal that the modification of community to be an age-friendly place may be a way out for the regions or countries. An age-friendly city with comprehensive community support and positive attitude towards elderly is a key to discrimination-free city. This chapter provides an analysis of the negative labels and potential opportunities for elderly. Strategies from different aspects to shape an age-friendly city will be discussed in detail. Lastly, the discussion and comparison between Asian and European age-friendly cities with two examples will be demonstrated by integrating information and sources of successful programmes by some outstanding countries. This article provides an impulse for further studies of age-friendly city in the future.

Keywords Age-friendly city · Active ageing · Social connectivity · Ageism · Social participation · Life-long learning · Gerontotechnology

F. C. M. Yuen
Department of Oncology, Princess Margaret Hospital, Hospital Authority, Hong Kong, China
e-mail: cmyuen@ha.org.hk

C. P. Y. Wong (✉)
Department of Surgery, Queen Mary Hospital, Hospital Authority, Hong Kong, China
e-mail: wpy685@ha.org.hk

V. T. S. Law and B. Y. F. Fong (eds.), *Ageing with Dignity in Hong Kong and Asia*, Quality of Life in Asia 16, https://doi.org/10.1007/978-981-19-3061-4_10

10.1 Introduction

There is a Chinese proverb saying that 'An old person is like a treasure to a family' to describe how precious an elderly person is. Undoubtedly, older adults who have seen a great deal of life with wisdom are a treasure to the society and their contribution to society should not be forgotten. However, the ways to develop a discrimination-free city with supportive social services and facilities can be a big challenge to a country with an ageing population.

Population ageing is taking place worldwide. There is no universally accepted definition of ageing process. It is mostly described as the type of ageing on the top of the population pyramid which has been prevailing because of the slow growth rate of the young population and low death rate of the older population, as well as change of marriage pattern and decline in fertility (Dufek & Minařík, 2009; Viña et al., 2007). Ageing is also contributed by advances in health care and technology but it also leads an increased susceptibility of trauma, diseases and other forms of stress. According to the United Nations (2020), the world population of people aged 65 or over reached 727 million in 2020, and it was projected to be larger than double, approximately over 1.5 billion in 2050. This is an unavoidable challenge to countries, particularly in Asia, Europe and the Mediterranean etc. Facing with population ageing, an age-friendly city fitted with the specific culture, society and city structure of a country is a way to benefit both the old age group and society.

According to the active ageing framework of the World Health Organization (WHO) and its framework for age-friendly cities, an 'ideal' age-friendly city has the capacity to optimise opportunities for participation, health and security so as to enhance the quality of life of the elderly. There are some main approaches to achieve a successful age-friendly city: recognising capacities and resources among old adults, anticipating flexibly to their needs and preferences, promotion of the elderly's contribution to community life, and protecting vulnerable elderly and respecting their own lifestyle choices (World Health Organization [WHO], 2002, 2007).

10.2 Ageing Without Dignity

10.2.1 Physical and Mental Limitations

There are no Asian countries exempt from the trend of ageing cities. Urbanisation and community development policies are beneficial to sustainable city development. However, it brings an unfamiliar and challenging living environment to the elderly.

Advanced age brings significant decline in physical and cognitive functions to the elderly, who experiences decreased strength, ambulatory ability and physical activity due to change in muscle strength and body functions. Cancers, diabetes, strokes, loss of balance and decreased range of motions of the limbs bring significant disablement to the older adults (Motl & McAuley, 2010). These are all the activity-limiting changes which restrict their performance on Activity of Daily Living (ADL). The participants in a Korean study in 2019 revealed that such frailties had prevented the elderly from having independent lifestyle, good self-management and barrier-free daily life, and, at the same time, increased risk of falls. The older adults even admitted that they had suffered from depression, stress and gloom because of the limited physical strength (Lee & So, 2019). Poor social connection would result from limited mobility and travel constraints especially in condensed living environments in Asia (Hung et al., 2016).

Depression and elderly suicide became two main problems among the geriatric population. A study about depression among Hong Kong and Singapore elderly in 2020 revealed that 7.8% and 15.6% of the old adults had depressive symptoms, respectively (Lam et al., 2020). It might indicate insufficient social support to cater for the needs of elderly. Dementia and loss of memory can also bring disastrous impact to the quality of life of the elderly and their communication with the younger generation (Stough, 2013). The above factors also induce.

10.2.2 Poor Social Connection

Ageing brings another inexorable challenge to the elderly. Poor social connection and social isolation appear to be prevalent among older members in developing and developed countries (Chen & Schulz, 2016). Social isolation means an individual has poor sense of belonging, poor relationships with other social members and inadequate social engagements. The loss of companionship induces subjective and negative feeling, loneliness and emotional isolation (Dury, 2014). A Taiwanese study has defined the social position of an individual based on the social hierarchy, occupation and income (Chang & Yen, 2011). It explained that retirement would bring social withdrawal and decreased self-esteem to the old adults. The retirement age in Asian countries is mostly around 60 to 65. Some Asian countries, including Japan, are raising the retirement age from 65 to 70. Moreover, the death of friends and spouses and the lack of technology knowledge also hinder their participation in social activities (Beckett et al., 2002). Lastly, losses of social roles, function and opinion expressing channels lead to the withdrawal of the elderly, and hence, their needs and thoughts are always being neglected (Şahin et al., 2019). They can easily become an invisible group in the community. Therefore, accessibility of social service centres and facilities becomes a key factor in an age-friendly city.

10.2.3 Ageism

In 1969, the first Director of the National Institute on Ageing in the United States, Robert N. Butler, introduced the concept of 'ageism'. It was a socially created product under urbanisation which affected the quality of life of the elderly. It was an ultimate prejudice which includes negative attitude and behaviours towards the elderly. Ageism is linked the concept of 'growing old' with disability and decline (Butler, 1980). Once this stigma is attached, an individual would be viewed as lazy and unproductive due to disability and low workforce participation. Eventually, ageism builds a wall to isolate the ageing population from the mainstream society (Levy & Macdonald, 2016). The social image of elderly and youth-obsessed culture has thus created an atypical and negative label on the elderly. The change of body shape and other visible signs of ageing become unacceptable to the younger age groups, who may have a concept of 'fear of growing old' (Widrick & Raskin, 2010). Geriatric depression, social isolation and discrimination eventually become the 'side products' of ageism.

10.3 Mental Health of the Elderly

Longevity is a blessing to a person in his or her life and is commonly known as one of the Five Blessings in the Asian culture. The golden age is meaningful and precious to older adults in the rest of their life journey. The elderly ought to have the right to enjoy the time and to live it better. But how can we create a positive atmosphere to support them? It is inevitable the older adults are encountering difficulties: loss of social network, impoverishment, involuntary relocation, cognitive decline, frailty and debilitate illness (The Lancet, 2005). Kassebaum et al. (2016) stated depression as one of the leading causes which increase disability adjusted life years (DALYs), and they also found that ageing and changing in population growth could contribute to increased DALYs owing to non-communicable diseases. It was shown that depression was a risk factor for excess morbidity and mortality and negatively affected the overall health of the elderly and their quality of life (Hall & Reynolds-Iii, 2014).

A significant relationship between geriatric depression, and multiple descriptive variants and health-related factors, for example, living alone, marital status, chronic pain, vision problem and financial difficulties etc. (Chi et al., 2005). Sun et al. (2012) conducted a community-based prospective cohort study in Hong Kong, and 7.2% and 11% of 56,000 Chinese men and women participants who got depressive symptoms, which were common among those with lower income or poorer health status. In addition, in a cross-sectional study carried out in Chachoengsao Province in eastern Thailand in 2018 found that being a female, or having illiteracy, smoking or imbalanced family were strongly associated with geriatric depression (Charoensakulchai et al., 2019).

To promote healthy ageing, the primary health care sector, with the related stakeholders and institutions, for example, doctors, nurses, social workers, government, non-government organisations (NGOs), nursing homes etc. play a central role in health promotion and disease prevention. They focus on improving mental health service for the elderly in the community as collaborative consultation in primary care setting could improve user satisfaction and adherence to treatment (Gillies et al.,

2015). For instance, Chang and Yen (2011) conducted an elderly suicide prevention programme in Hong Kong on cases presented to regional mental health service by public hospitals in collaboration with the psychogeriatric consultation liaison service team. There was a significant reduction in suicidal rate in the intervention group as the programme offered an early screening and intervention for the at-risk elderly, provided treatment of depression, gatekeeper training and used the community oriented psychiatric care management model to provide aftercare for suicide attempters. More importantly, mental wellness of the elderly should be acknowledged to advocate their dignity and autonomy in daily life and in making health decision.

10.4 Shaping Age-Friendly Cities

The creation of age-friendly cities is not only for the older adults in the society, but also for different groups to maintain social harmony and community participation in sustainable development. Echoed by the World Health Organization, active ageing is a life-long process, and the elderly is a social resource for their families, communities and economies in supportive, inclusive and enabling community environments, conducive for health participation and security in late life. In 2007, WHO issued a guide to promote age-friendly cities with an emphasis on humanity and quality of life as people age through structures and services accessible to the elderly (WHO, 2007).

A successful age-friendly city identifies the needs of the old age population, and then improves the community conditions by meeting their needs, and also creates living space with rich opportunities for active ageing (Fitzgerald & Caro, 2017).

10.4.1 Community Support and Social Participation

In most of the Asian countries, especially China, carers for the elderly are mainly the spouse, children and extended family members. It imperceptibly becomes a normative duty for them. Under the influence of urbanisation, globalisation and social and economic changes in Asian countries, there appears a need of social support to the elderly as it is not common for the whole family to live under one roof. There is an increasing trend of institutionalisation for older adults. Moreover, transportation and personal disability limit the elderly to reach social services. Equitable allocation of community care service is affecting the engagement in social interaction of the older adults and their self-empowerment (Wu & Tseng, 2018). Community-based elderly care centres can encourage the elderly in reaching for social support and connectivity. Accessibility also encourages the gathering of the old age groups to share their interests, experiences and worries. The combination of convenient community services with accessible modes of public transportation and accessory infrastructures such as outdoor seats, public toilets and level-access sidewalks facilitate the delivery of community supports (Van Hoof et al., 2018).

Social participation entails contributing and receiving societal resources in different format and levels of involvement which shape social belonging and network embeddedness (Rainer, 2014). Improving the quality of life of old age groups, especially for those with physical and cognitive disabilities, by encouraging them to participate and contribute to the society, as well as forming their own social group, is a key to active ageing. A holistic, smart and visionary town planning is desirable for age-friendly cities with focuses on integrated community and associated infrastructures like green open spaces, barrier-free facilities and comprehensive transportation network. A supportive neighbourhood environment with easy-access infrastructures is the first step for the elderly to step out of their living space, not only allowing older adults optimal liveability but also more active time in the community with the objectives of quality of life and healthy living environment (Lam et al., 2021).

Furthermore, favourable neighbourhoods with good interpersonal environments will encourage individual elderly to participate in social interactions, and this will bring a long-term impact on their health (Kim & Kawachi, 2017). In most of the Asian countries, the beneficial effects of compacted housing allow for accessible and affordable care at community centres to provide a platform for the elderly to express their needs via social interactions. Moreover, restaurants, parks and sport facilities also provide incentive venues for older adults to enjoy themselves in accordance to their own behavioural habits and living styles. They will also form their own peer group as a way to increase social participation and adaptation. Formal and informal participation in group activities with people of similar age facilitates the sharing of experiences and wisdom and this is conducive to their health and well-being. It also helps them by gaining respect, recognition and building self-confidence (Zheng et al., 2019). Activities like sport games, health talks, interest classes (such as tai chi, qigong class) and movie sharing can be organised by community centres to encourage the formation of social groups within the old population and facilitate their social participation.

In addition, volunteer activity is an option for the older adults to work and interact with others via cooperation. It also promotes the contribution by them to the community because the elderly can also be service providers. A study in Japan revealed that volunteer groups gained both self and mutual help-relationship among members and maintained independent lives. They also provided the older adults a means to collect information for self-development and learning (Chan et al., 2021). Recruitment of elderly as members of the volunteer team by community centres is a practical approach to an age-friendly city.

10.4.2 Employment and Retirement

Workforce is always linked with social status and self-contribution, especially for men. A study in Australia presented an interesting conclusion about the effects of retirement for men and women. It was found that women tended to increase the time spent in volunteering and household activities, and they also would try to engage in social activities including joining community clubs. However, men felt reluctant to participate in social activities or mental exercise. Eventually, it increases the risk of decline in 'intelligence' and memory (Atalay et al., 2019). Delay in retirement or transition from the labour force into social engagement can promote cognitive maintenance and rewarding retirement. A study in Taiwan supported delayed retirement could bring happiness and self-satisfaction (Chang & Yen, 2011). It is beneficial for the elderly to establish confidence and healthy living when retirement is fit for their physical strength. The promotion of rewarding retirement by encouraging them to participate in social interactions is a way for the elderly to live their fruitful life. The labels of 'weak', 'burden' and 'lack of contribution' linked with retirement should be removed. Governments should encourage companies to recruit capable older adults to contribute to the labour market or in the role of consultants.

10.4.3 Life-Long Learning

As Henry Ford (n.d.), an American industrialist, has said *'Anyone who stops learning is old, whether at twenty or eighty. Anyone who keeps learning stays young. The greatest thing in life is to keep young mind young'*. However, phrases like 'cognitive decline', 'dementia', 'neurodegenerative diseases', 'poor memory' are commonly used to describe the elderly. Does it really mean to be so? Or is it possible for the elderly to learn new skills? It is noted the older adults are less inclined to practice self-initiated learning compared with the young adults. This may be one of the main reasons for the memory decline during the learning process (Kenney et al., 2019). There should be ways for the elderly to pick up new skills, for example, new technology, language or slangs to 're-connect' with the society and to become more functionally independent. Leanos et al. (2020) found the working memory and episode memory of elderly participants were significantly increased after 3-months learning multiple real-world skills simultaneously, like painting, Spanish and using the iPad. This indicated the elderly could benefit from learning different new skills in boosting their cognitive function and independence. Some participants stated their confidence being enhanced with the technological devices and were able to teach their grandchildren to use the iPad (Leanos et al., 2020). Learning promotes continuous physical and cognitive functioning for the elders, benefits their performance of ADLs and IADLs (instrumental activities of daily living) and enhances their confidence as well (Hui, 2005; Vaughan et al., 2016). The elders should be encouraged to participate in life-long learning.

10.4.4 Respect and Social Connectivity

Respect is a basic construct in interpersonal relationship regardless of age, race, gender or ethnicity. There is a rising concern over the stereotypes about ageing which could negatively influence one's experience of ageing, self-efficacy, physical and mental health, productivity, the social dynamics and even the quality of healthcare received (Burnes et al., 2019; Donizzetti, 2019). Indeed, it is essential to unpack and transform the biases towards ageing, shift the perception of ageing from negative to positive and expand the knowledge about ageing with the aim to promote equality among the generations, and to advocate the dignity of the elderly, feeling respected by others. In addition, Ko et al. (2021) found that age discrimination and negligence from caregivers or family members were significantly associated with suicidal ideation and attempts among Korean elders. Their suicide rate among those aged over 65 years old was 3 times higher than that of the Organization for Economic Co-operation and Development (OECD) countries. It was suggested that negative effects of social exclusion and discrimination leads to limited access to social and health information.

Anti-ageism interventions to effectively reduce ageism is the crux for the society to think about. Burnes et al. (2019) suggested education and intergenerational contact were effective, feasible and at low-cost. They promoted the right attitude towards ageing, knowledge, and comfort with elderly among the youth and adults. For example, an interesting Life Story Encounter Programme (LSEP), including elements of biographical-narrative and reminiscence therapy, was conducted in Germany and the programme offered a platform for the youth and older people to have meaningful dialogue which targeted to reduce ageism and promote cross-generational interaction (Kranz et al., 2021).

10.5 Movement of Age-Friendly Cities

10.5.1 Hong Kong

Hong Kong is a special administrative region located at the south coast of China, and it is Asia's financial and travel hub that is proximally connected to Mainland China and the international community. It is also a place full of hustle and bustle, densely populated with high-rise commercial buildings, shown in Figs. 10.1, 10.2 and 10.3.

It is expected the ageing population of Hong Kong will rise sharply from 1.32 million in 2019 to 2.52 million in 2039 and will reach 2.58 million in 2069. With decline in the number of births, the dependency ratio is expected to increase from 441 in 2019 to 853 in 2066. Dependency ratio is defined as {(No. of persons aged <15 + aged >65) /No. of persons aged 15–64} *1000 e.g. there were 441 people dependent on every 1000 of the working population in 2019 (Census and Statistics Department, 2020). The workforce is shrinking and the number of caregivers is reducing. The demand for long-term care services will also rise sharply in the long run. Therefore,

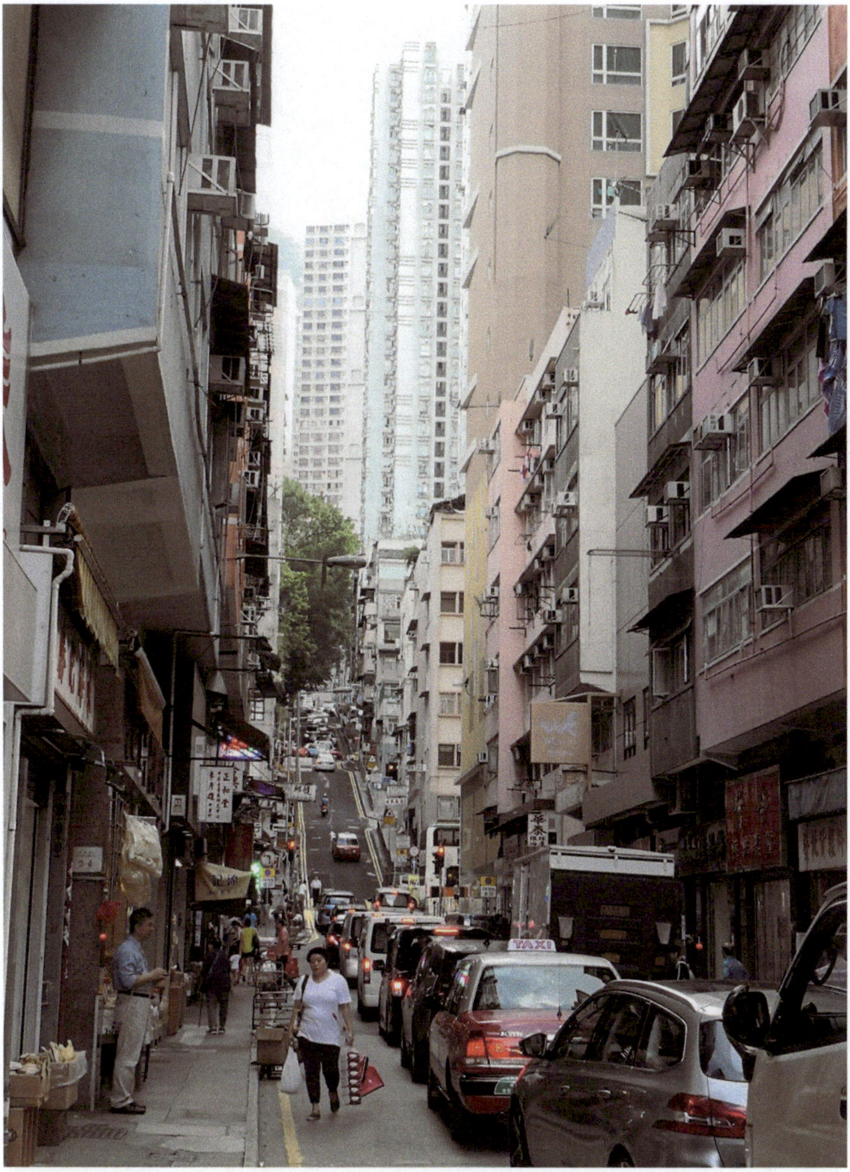

Fig. 10.1 Sai Ying Pun, one of old-school charm in western of Hong Kong Island

it is imperative for the Hong Kong government to lead and promote elderly care service in the community. In 2014, the Elderly Commission established an Elderly Services Programme Plan (ESPP) with the aims to support the spirit of respecting, loving and caring for the elderly (Elderly Commission, 2017).

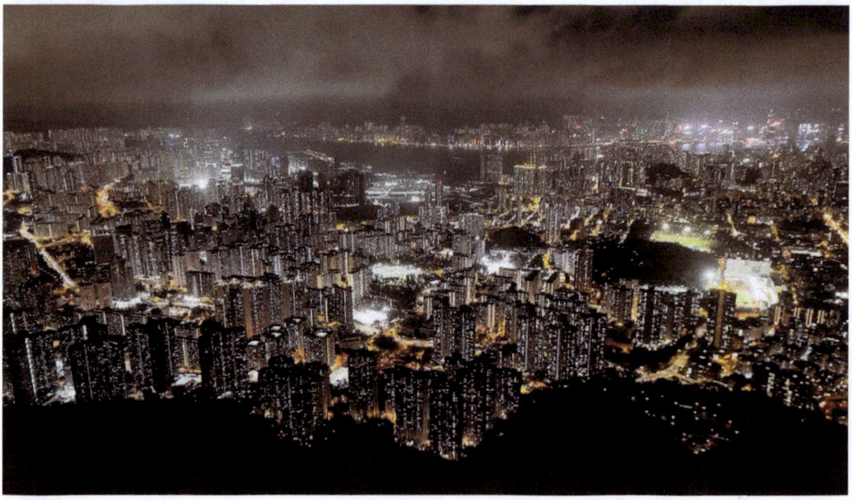

Fig. 10.2 'Concrete jungle', taken from the top of Lion Rock Mountain, Hong Kong

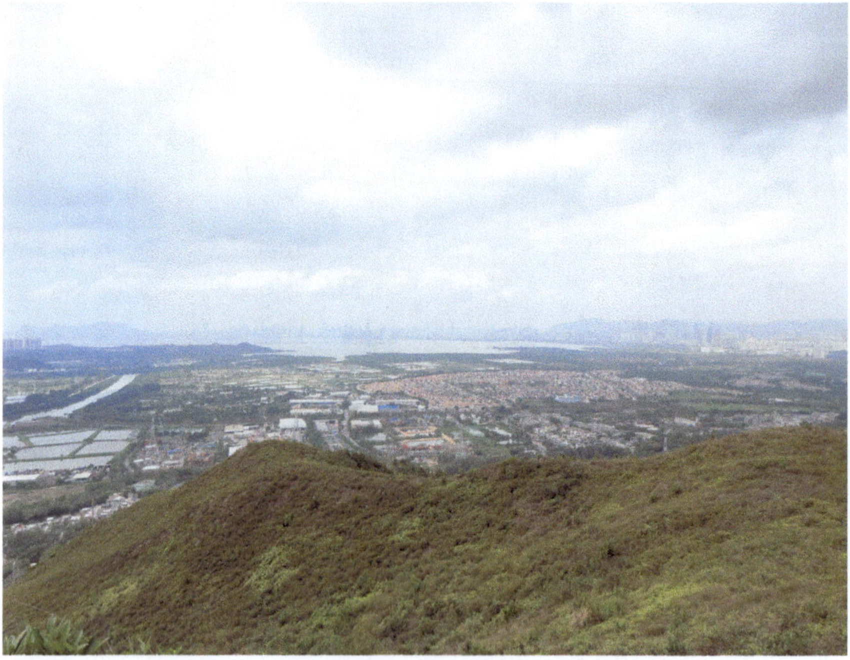

Fig. 10.3 Country areas in Sheung Shui, New Territories near Shenzhen, China

10.5.1.1 Supporting 'Ageing in Place'

The 'Ageing in place' scheme has been promoted by the Hong Kong Housing Society since 2012 with partnership with healthcare providers, welfare organisations and the government, targeting those aged 60 and above. There are 20 rental housing estates in total for the qualified senior citizens. The tenants can enjoy different services. For example, 'Jolly Place', one of the rental housing estates, provides home care, volunteer visit, clubhouse for the residents, rehabilitation room etc. (Hong Kong Housing Society, 2019, 2020). The scheme aims to reduce the institutionalisation rate and promotes well-being of the older adults so that they can live in a familiar place and maintain their quality of life. Moreover, community care service is one of the highlights of ageing policies in Hong Kong. There are different types of service and facilities provided by the Social Welfare Department, for instance, Day Care Centre for the Elderly, Pilot Scheme on Community Care Service Voucher for the Elderly and Enhanced Home and Community Care Services etc. (Social Welfare Department, 2021).

10.5.1.2 Promoting the Sense of Ageing Friendliness

The Hong Kong Jockey Club Charities Trust (HKJCCT) initiated a city-wide project to promote the network of Age-Friendly Cities of the World Health Organization in 2015 with an aim to mitigate health inequalities among the elderly. Local networks politicians, enterprise and the older adults at the district level were engaged and the concept was found in the 2016 Policy Address of the Chief Executive of the Hong Kong Government (Woo et al., 2021). HKJCCT, together with the Institute of Active Ageing of The Hong Kong Polytechnic University, conducted an age-friendly city project in Kwun Tong district which is one of 'old districts' in Hong Kong. The project aimed to enhance community participation and the age-friendliness of the district. The researchers firstly obtained the baseline information such as sociodemographic and sense of age-friendliness of the residents. They conducted field visits and identified the problems, and then formulated a framework of continual improvement of an age-friendly community (The Hong Kong Jockey Club Charities Trust, 2017). The Hong Kong Jockey Club (HKJC) has also inaugurated various campaigns and conferences with entrepreneurs, the government and NGOs to promote the sense of respect, connectivity and public awareness on ageing (The Hong Kong Jockey Club, 2018). More recently, HKJC supported NGOs to conduct several district-based progrmammes in training volunteers, regardless of age, to become 'Elderly Care Ambassadors' who would deliver the message of age-friendliness to the community, including house modification like installation of handrails (Jockey Club Age-friendly City, 2021). The hard work in supporting the age-friendly city movement by the NGOs, institutions and citizens is appreciated. However, there should be timely evaluation of the interventions to assess whether they are cost effective, feasible to the specific area and achievable to the needs of the locals with the objective to identify the limitations of the movement. Thence, the community-based interventions could be further modified and the needs of the residents of the district were prioritised from time to time, to allow for flexible planning in the promotion of age-friendliness. The CUHKJockey Club Institute of Ageing at The Chinese University of Hong Kong (CUHK) evaluated the impact of initiatives of the age-friendly cities to monitor trend of changes in various areas and to assess the effectiveness of policies and community efforts in promotion. They proposed to have an 'age-friendly theme' included in the policy of government departments, such as income security in the form of allowances for the elderly since there was no pension system for all residents in Hong Kong (Woo et al., 2021).

10.5.2 Switzerland

Far away from Asia, there is a glacier paradise in central Europe. Switzerland a landlocked country with an extensive and high Alpine Mountain range, deep valleys, small villages, farms and prosperous cities; shown in Figs. 10.4, 10.5 and 10.6. The population is similar to that of Hong Kong, around 8.6 million (Federal Statistical Office, 2020).

Although the gross domestic product (GDP) per capita of Switzerland is the second highest in the world, and it is top-ranked in the Global AgeWatch Index, the government and local organisations are actively preparing for the ageing population

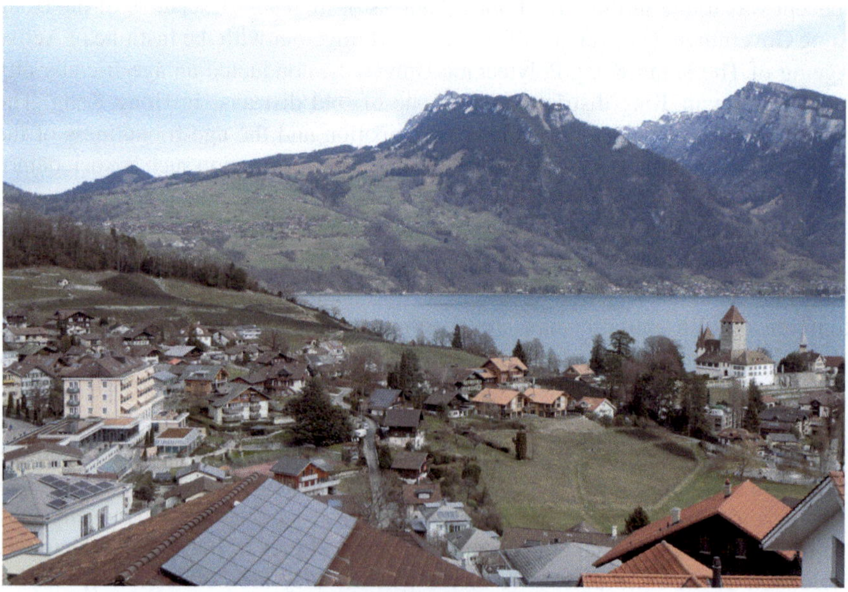

Fig. 10.4 Villages near Lake Brienz, Interlaken, Switzerland

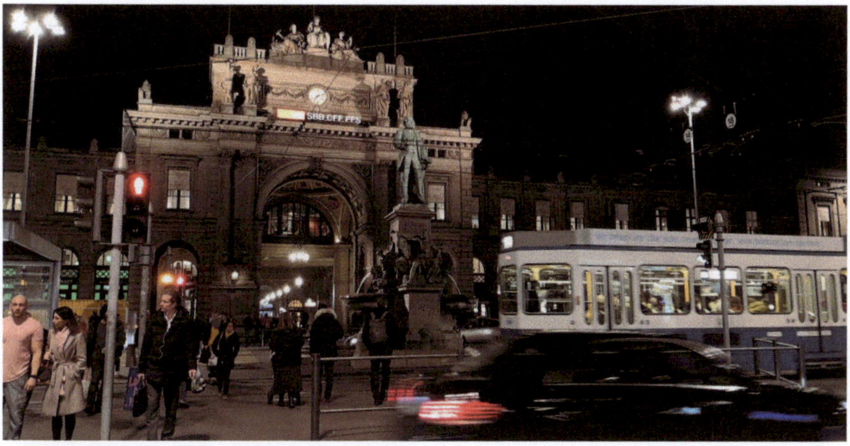

Fig. 10.5 Main street in Zurich, Switzerland

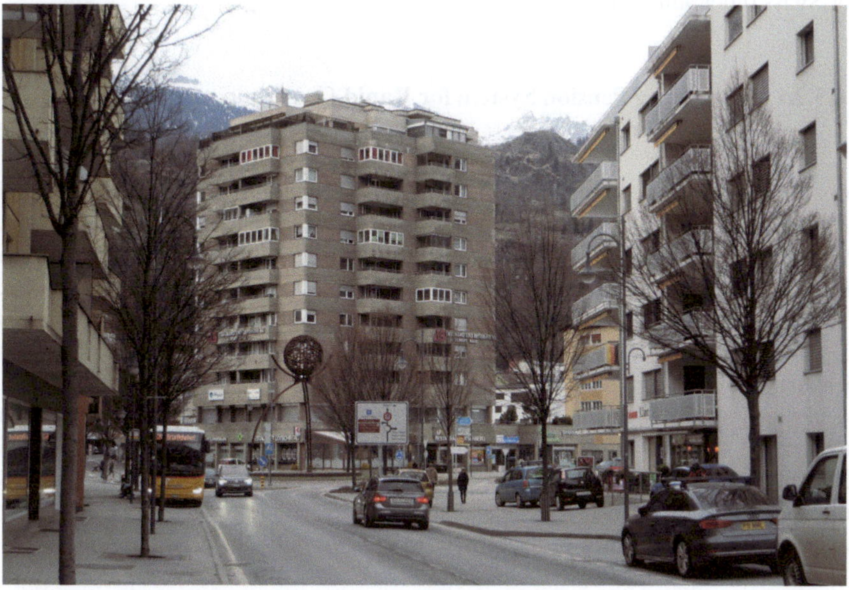

Fig. 10.6 Brig, a town in Valais, Switzerland

to preserve the high living standard for the elderly, as the population of aged 65 and above is expected to increase to 30% of the population in 2050 (HelpAge International, 2015; Organization for Economic Co-operation and Development, 2019; The Federal Council, 2020). Life expectancy of Swiss men and women are around 80 years which is longer than the average of 69 years in the world. The government

Table 10.1 Summary of Swiss pension system

	First pillar	Second pillar	Third pillar
Types of pensions	State pension, including old age and survivor's insurance, disability insurance and income compensation allowance	Occupational pension plan	Private pension plan
Coverage	Mandatory and is legal minimum for the Swiss working population to contribute	Mandatory for all Swiss employee and employer to contribute	Not compulsory to join
Goal	Provide basic monthly income for retirement	As additional capital	As additional capital

Sources Crédit Agricole Next Bank (2021) and Lewis and Ollivaud (2020)

has policies on healthy ageing and an increase in long-term care health expenditure for Swiss older adults (Bonk, 2016).

10.5.2.1 Preparing Pension System for Rapid Growth in Ageing Population

It is inevitable the income at retirement age has a great difference than that earned at working age. This is one of the challenges the older adults need to encounter. A well-developed pension system and well-planned retirement plan are essential to help the elderly to maintain the living standard and to ensure their quality of life. The Swiss pension system is relatively ably among those of other OECD countries (Lewis & Ollivaud, 2020). It consists of three pillars: state pension, occupational pension plan and private pension plan (Table 10.1).

In addition, the Swiss government finds it necessary to reform the pension system to prepare for the rapid growth of ageing population. In 2019, The Swiss National Council announced the conversion rate of occupational pension is reduced from 6.8 to 6% which aims to ensure the sustainability of pension provision in long run by redistribution of the capital of the retirees (SWI swissinfo.ch, 2020).

10.5.2.2 Supporting an Age-Friendly Environment

The Swiss government supports the creation of age-friendly environment, for example, by implementing various research and projects of designing and planning the public spacing like 'Urbaging: Designing urban space for an ageing society' in 2009. The goals of the project were to identify and analyse public space and services, transportation system, geographical data then match the data with the distribution of senior citizens population. The qualitative and quantitative data from the research work could be a model or reference for the government and stakeholders to develop the strategies with priorities, for instance, focusing more on the specific needs and obstacles of the elderly in public space (Acebillo, 2009). For example, the older adults in Lugano were interviewed about the most favourite outdoor places to go to and the reasons. It was found easy accessibility, greenery and quiet environment were important. The elderly like to meet up friends and families in public spaces like the parks and café shops. In addition, urban green space is regarded as a public good and the local government is responsible to create more such spaces for the residents. This can be achieved by reconciling the needs and interests of the different stakeholders and the implementation of urban landscape and design projects, to frame an 'ideal' vision of the age-friendly environment and, at the same time, to utilise the scarce land resources effectively and wisely for the long-term benefits of the population (Tappert et al., 2018).

10.6 Limitations

There is no one way to solve the problems arising from the ageing, and it is necessary to review the current policy continuously, intensify the information exchange with different stakeholders like having dialogue with district representatives, NGOs, researchers, entrepreneurs, urban planners and senior citizens etc. to encourage active community participation in promoting age-friendly issues, learn the experience from other countries and have a better and effective planning with specific goals.

Before starting the planning of ageing policy, the preparation work should include detailed and accurate data collection. Recently, active senior citizens participation in framing the ageing policy is emphasised (Dizon et al., 2020). For instance, Falanga et al. (2020) found the well-being and quality of life of older adults could be improved through joining the voting and decision-making on the policies especially regarding the pension schemes and social care under different NGOs like HelpAge International, International Federation on Ageing and The European Federation of Older Persons etc. Besides, the participation could positively influence the policymaking at local, regional and international levels.

Whether creating an age-friendly city with senior citizens' active participation could be carried out effectively to improve the public health measures and solve the challenges from ageing issues or not, it is never too late to revise the strategic direction, to acknowledge the needs and values of elderly, and conduct sustainable research for the innovative solutions to achieve a better health of the population.

10.7 Innovation and Digital Technology in Shaping Age-Friendly Cities

Skyrocketing advancement in information technology greatly facilitates people in various aspects of daily life, like communication, healthcare services, transportation etc. According to WHO (2020), healthy ageing is about creating the environments and chances where allow the elderly to be and do what they value. Technology plays a vital role in healthy ageing. Bixter et al. (2019) mentioned the social communication technology like Facebook, Twitter, WhatsApp, Zoom etc. could benefit the elderly to communicate with family and friends and maintain relationship despite geographical distance and so as to foster their sense of connectedness. Moreover, technology improves the quality and efficacy of primary healthcare services for the elderly. Haufe et al. (2019) conducted a participatory action research in the Netherlands to develop a new gerontechnology matchmaking tool which added value to the elderly who were ageing in place independently. The tool could provide more personalised needs to both the elderly and the caregivers. However, it was suggested to identify needs of the elderlies and study about their acceptance, willingness, adoption of the gerontechnology to promote the generalisability of the tool.

10.8 Towards Healthy Ageing in the Age-Friendly World

The concept of age-friendly cities is actually well-known in European countries and is coming to Asian countries. The advocacy of the actual actions in constructing healthy ageing in the society at the local level is a key step forward in promoting active and healthy ageing with dignity. Having every citizen embracing the concept of respecting ageing and removing the stigma and fear of growing old should be the ultimate goals in every society. However, expanding this concept beyond the theoretical level is not without limitations or barriers. Moreover, the sustainability of age-friendly cities is an emerging issue which deserves further discussion and research, as well as the attention of the policy makers. With reference to some successful countries such as the Netherlands, advanced technology and a strong database about the implementation of age-friendly policy, an age-friendly city development is a hope and a possible solution. Future study and research on implementation of proactive policy and programme are significant in providing more diverse perspectives and insights to healthy ageing in the age-friendly world. A lot can be accomplished if every citizen collaborates sincerely and builds a strong partnership in facing the challenges of ageing population together. Eventually, ageing is no longer a fear to all members of the global population.

References

Acebillo, J. (2009). *Urbaging: Designing urban space for an ageing society*. https://www.urbaging.ch/fr/files/NRP54_FSReport_16-02_DEF.pdf

Atalay, K., Barrett, G. F., & Staneva, A. (2019). The effect of retirement on elderly cognitive functioning. *Journal of Health Economics, 66*, 37–53. https://doi.org/10.1016/j.jhealeco.2019.04.006

Beckett, M., Goldman, N., Weinstein, M., Lin, I. F., & Chuang, Y. L. (2002). Social environment, life challenge, and health among the elderly in Taiwan. *Social Science & Medicine, 55*(2), 191–209. https://doi.org/10.1016/S0277-9536(01)00161-7

Bixter, M. T., Blocker, K. A., Mitzner, T. L., Prakash, A., & Rogers, W. A. (2019). Understanding the use and non-use of social communication technologies by older adults: A qualitative test and extension of the UTAUT model. *Gerontechnology: International Journal on the Fundamental Aspects of Technology to Serve the Ageing Society, 18*(2), 70–88. https://doi.org/10.4017/gt.2019.18.2.002.00

Bonk, M. B. (2016). *Policies on ageing and health: A selection of innovative models*. Multisectoral action for a life course approach to healthy ageing. Swiss Federal Office of Public Health.

Burnes, D., Sheppard, C., Henderson, C. R., Jr., Wassel, M., Cope, R., Barber, C., & Pillemer, K. (2019). Interventions to reduce ageism against older adults: A systematic review and meta-Analysis. *American Journal of Public Health, 109*(8), e1–e9. https://doi.org/10.2105/AJPH.2019.305123

Butler, R. N. (1980). Ageism: A foreword. *Journal of Social Issues, 36*(2), 8–11. https://doi.org/10.1111/j.1540-4560.1980.tb02018.x

Census and Statistics Department. (2020). *Hong Kong population projections 2020–2069*. https://www.censtatd.gov.hk/en/data/stat_report/product/B1120015/att/B1120015082020XXXXB0100.pdf

Chang, H. H., & Yen, S. T. (2011). Mental health and employment of the elderly in Taiwan: A simultaneous equation approach. *Pacific Economic Review, 16*(4), 504–519. https://doi.org/10.1111/j.1468-0106.2011.00560.x

Chan, W., Chui, C., Cheung, J., Lum, T., & Lu, S. (2021). Associations between volunteering and mental health during COVID-19 among chinese older adults. *Journal of Gerontological Social Work, 64*(6), 599–612. https://doi.org/10.1080/01634372.2021.1904079

Charoensakulchai, S., Usawachoke, S., Kongbangpor, W., Thanavirun, P., Mitsiriswat, A., Pinijnai, O., ... & Kaewput, W. (2019). Prevalence and associated factors influencing depression in older adults living in rural Thailand: A cross-sectional study. *Geriatrics and Gerontology International, 19*(12), 1248–1253. https://doi.org/10.1111/ggi.13804

Chen, Y. R. R., & Schulz, P. J. (2016). The effect of information communication technology interventions on reducing social isolation in the elderly: A systematic review. *Journal of Medical Internet Research, 18*(1), e18. https://doi.org/10.2196/jmir.4596

Chi, I., Yip, P. S. F., Chiu, H. F. K., Chou, K. L., Chan, K. S., Kwan, C. W., Conwell, Y., & Caine, E. (2005). Prevalence of depression and its correlates in Hong Kong's Chinese older adults. *The American Journal of Geriatric Psychiatry, 13*(5), 409–416. https://doi.org/10.1097/00019442-200505000-00010

Crédit Agricole Next Bank. (2021). *The Swiss pension system*. https://www.ca-nextbank.ch/en/en/expat-switzerland/insurance/how-does-retirement-work-in-switzerland.html

Dizon, L., Wiles, J., & Peiris-John, R. (2020). What is meaningful participation for older People? An analysis of aging policies. *The Gerontologist, 60*(3), 396–405. https://doi.org/10.1093/geront/gnz060

Donizzetti, A. R. (2019). Ageism in an aging society: The role of knowledge, anxiety about aging, and stereotypes in young people and adults. *International Journal of Environmental Research and Public Health, 16*(8), 1329. https://doi.org/10.3390/ijerph16081329

Dufek, J., & Minařík, B. (2009). Age of population and the development of population ageing in the regions of the Czech Republic. *Agricultural Economics, 55*(6), 259–270.
Dury, R. (2014). Social isolation and loneliness in the elderly: An exploration of some of the issues. *British Journal of Community Nursing, 19*(3), 125–128. https://doi.org/10.12968/bjcn.2014.19.3.125
Elderly Commission. (2017). *Elderly Services Programme Plan.* https://www.elderlycommission.gov.hk/en/download/library/ESPP_Final_Report_Eng.pdf
Falanga, R., Cebulla, A., Principi, A., & Socci, M. (2020). The participation of senior citizens in policy-making: Patterning initiatives in Europe. *International Journal of Environmental Research and Public Health, 18*(1), 34. https://doi.org/10.3390/ijerph18010034
Federal Statistical Office. (2020). *Population.* https://www.bfs.admin.ch/bfs/en/home/statistics/population/effectif-change/population.html
Fitzgerald, K. G., & Caro, F. G. (2017). *International perspectives on age-friendly cities.* Routledge.
Ford, H. (n.d.). *Henry Ford—Quotes and phrases.* https://www.henry-ford.net/english/quotes.html
Gillies, D., Buykx, P., Parker, A. G., & Hetrick, S. E. (2015). Consultation liaison in primary care for people with mental disorders. *The Cochrane Database of Systematic Reviews, 2015*, 9. https://doi.org/10.1002/14651858.CD007193.pub2
Hall, C. A., & Reynolds-Iii, C. F. (2014). Late-life depression in the primary care setting: Challenges, collaborative care, and prevention. *Maturitas, 79*(2), 147–152. https://doi.org/10.1016/j.maturitas.2014.05.026
Haufe, M., Peek, S. T. M., & Luijkx, K. G. (2019). Matching gerontechnologies to independent-living seniors' individual needs: Development of the GTM tool. *BMC Health Services Research, 19*(1), 26. https://doi.org/10.1186/s12913-018-3848-5
HelpAge International. (2015). *Global rankings table.* https://www.helpage.org/global-agewatch/population-ageing-data/global-rankings-table/
Hong Kong Housing Society. (2019). *Jolly place.* https://hkhs.com/en/housing_archive/id/45
Hong Kong Housing Society. (2020). *Ageing-in-Place scheme.* https://www.un.org/development/desa/pd/sites/www.un.org.development.desa.pd/files/undesa_pd-2020_world_population_ageing_highlights.pdf
Hui, S. S. (2005). *Lifelong learning for older persons in Hong Kong* (Master's thesis, Lingnan University, Hong Kong). https://commons.ln.edu.hk/cgi/viewcontent.cgi?article=1016&context=soc_etd
Hung, K., Bai, X., & Lu, J. (2016). Understanding travel constraints among the elderly in Hong Kong: A comparative study of the elderly living in private and in public housing. *Journal of Travel & Tourism Marketing, 33*(7), 1051–1070. https://doi.org/10.1080/10548408.2015.1084975
Jockey Club Age-friendly City. (2021). *District-based Programmes.* https://www.jcafc.hk/en/Project-Components/Comprehensive-Support-Scheme-For-Districts/District-Based-Programmes.html
Kassebaum, N. J., Arora, M., Barber, R. M., Bhutta, Z. A., Brown, J., Carter, A., ... & Biryukov, S. (2016). Global, regional, and national disability-adjusted life-years (DALYs) for 315 diseases and injuries and healthy life expectancy (HALE), 1990–2015: A systematic analysis for the Global Burden of Disease Study 2015. *The Lancet, 388*(10053), 1603–1658. https://doi.org/10.1016/S0140-6736(16)31460-X
Kenney, J. P. M., Ward, C., Gallen, D., Roche, R. A. P., Dockree, P., Hohensen, N., Cassidy, C., Keane, M. A., & Hogan, M. J. (2019). Self-initiated learning reveals memory performance and electrophysiological differences between younger, older and older adults with relative memory impairment. *European Journal of Neuroscience, 50*(11), 3855–3872. https://doi.org/10.1111/ejn.14530
Kim, E. S., & Kawachi, I. (2017). Perceived neighborhood social cohesion and preventive healthcare use. *American Journal of Preventive Medicine, 53*(2), e35–e40. https://doi.org/10.1016/j.amepre.2017.01.007

Ko, Y., Han, S. Y., & Jang, H. Y. (2021). Factors influencing suicidal ideation and attempts among older Korean adults: Focusing on age discrimination and neglect. *International Journal of Environmental Research and Public Health, 18*(4), 1852. https://doi.org/10.3390/ijerph18041852

Kranz, D., Thomas, N. M., & Hofer, J. (2021). Changes in age stereotypes in adolescent and older participants of an Intergenerational Encounter Program. *Frontiers in Psychology, 12*, 658–797. https://doi.org/10.3389/fpsyg.2021.658797

Lam, C. Y. H., Lee, J. W. Y., & Chan, T. T. C. (2021). Town planning and community development—Healthy and happy housing. In B. Y. F. Fong & M. C. S. Wong (Eds.), *Routledge handbook of public health and the community* (pp. 186–195). Routledge. https://www.routledge.com/The-Routledge-Handbook-of-Public-Health-and-the-Community/Fong-Wong/p/book/9780367634193

Lam, W. W., Loo, B. P., & Mahendran, R. (2020). Neighbourhood environment and depressive symptoms among the elderly in Hong Kong and Singapore. *International Journal of Health Geographics, 19*(1), 1–10. https://doi.org/10.1186/s12942-020-00238-w

Leanos, S., Kürüm, E., Strickland-Hughes, C. M., Ditta, A. S., Nguyen, G., Felix, M., Yum, H., Rebok, G. W., & Wu, R. (2020). The impact of learning multiple real-world skills on cognitive abilities and functional independence in healthy older adults. *The Journals of Gerontology: Series B, 75*(6), 1155–1169. https://doi.org/10.1093/geronb/gbz084

Lee, K., & So, W. Y. (2019). Differences in the levels of physical activity, mental health, and quality of life of elderly Koreans with activity-limiting disabilities. *International Journal of Environmental Research and Public Health, 16*(15), 2736. https://doi.org/10.3390/ijerph16152736

Levy, S. R., & Macdonald, J. L. (2016). Progress on understanding ageism. *Journal of Social Issues, 72*(1), 5–25.

Lewis, C., & Ollivaud, P. (2020). *Policies for Switzerland's ageing society.* https://www.oecd.org/officialdocuments/publicdisplaydocumentpdf/?cote=ECO/WKP(2020)8&docLanguage=En

Motl, R. W., & McAuley, E. (2010). Physical activity, disability, and quality of life in older adults. *Physical Medicine and Rehabilitation Clinics, 21*(2), 299–308. https://doi.org/10.1016/j.pmr.2009.12.006

Organization for Economic Co-operation and Development. (2019). *Switzerland: Prepare for population ageing to maintain high living standards.* https://www.oecd.org/economy/switzerland-prepare-for-population-ageing-to-maintain-high-living-standards.htm

Rainer, S. (2014). Social participation and social engagement of elderly people. *Procedia-Social and Behavioral Sciences, 116*, 780–785. https://doi.org/10.1016/j.sbspro.2014.01.297

Şahin, D. S., Özer, Ö., & Yanardağ, M. Z. (2019). Perceived social support, quality of life and satisfaction with life in elderly people. *Educational Gerontology, 45*(1), 69–77. https://doi.org/10.1080/03601277.2019.1585065

Social Welfare Department. (2021). *Community care and support services for the elderly.* https://www.swd.gov.hk/en/index/site_pubsvc/page_elderly/sub_csselderly/

Sun, W. J., Xu, L., Chan, W. M., Lam, T. H., & Schooling, C. M. (2012). Depressive symptoms and suicide in 56,000 older Chinese: A Hong Kong cohort study. *Social Psychiatry and Psychiatric Epidemiology, 47*(4), 505–514. https://doi.org/10.1007/s00127-011-0362-z

Stough, L. (2013). *Population segments with disabilities.* https://oaktrust.library.tamu.edu/bitstream/handle/1969.1/153151/Population%20segments%20with%20disabilites.pdf?sequence=1

SWI swissinfo.ch. (2020). *Government hopes for 'first successful pension reforms' of the century.* https://www.swissinfo.ch/eng/government-hopes-for--first-successful-pension-reforms--of-the-century/46185336

Tappert, S., Klöti, T., & Drilling, M. (2018). Contested urban green spaces in the compact city: The (re-)negotiation of urban gardening in Swiss cities. *Landscape and Urban Planning, 170*, 69–78. https://doi.org/10.1016/j.landurbplan.2017.08.016

The Federal Council. (2020). *Swiss economy—Facts and figures.* https://www.eda.admin.ch/aboutswitzerland/en/home/wirtschaft/uebersicht/wirtschaft---fakten-und-zahlen.html

The Hong Kong Jockey Club Charities Trust. (2017). *Jockey club age-friendly city project: Baseline assessment report for Kwun Tong district.* https://extranet.who.int/agefriendlyworld/wp-content/uploads/2017/02/Kwun-Tong-District-baseline-assessment.pdf

The Hong Kong Jockey Club. (2018). *Club launches partnership scheme to encourage community support in building an age-friendly city.* https://charities.hkjc.com/charities/english/community-contributions/activities/article.aspx?in_file=charities_2018060701848.html&current_category=4

The Lancet. (2005). Countering the difficult aspects of ageing. *The Lancet, 365*(9475), 1904. https://doi.org/10.1016/S0140-6736(05)66633-0

United Nations. (2020). *World population ageing.* https://www.un.org/development/desa/pd/sites/www.un.org.development.desa.pd/files/undesa_pd-2020_world_population_ageing_highlights.pdf

Van Hoof, J., Kazak, J. K., Perek-Białas, J. M., & Peek, S. (2018). The challenges of urban ageing: Making cities age-friendly in Europe. *International Journal of Environmental Research and Public Health, 15*(11), 2473. https://doi.org/10.1016/j.archger.2019.103915

Vaughan, L., Leng, X., LaMonte, M. J., Tindle, H. A., Cochrane, B. B., & Shumaker, S. A. (2016). Functional independence in late-life: Maintaining physical functioning in older adulthood predicts daily life function after age 80. *The Journals of Gerontology. Series A, Biological Sciences and Medical Sciences, 71* (Suppl. 1), S79–S86. https://doi.org/10.1093/gerona/glv061

Viña, J., Borrás, C., & Miquel, J. (2007). Theories of ageing. *IUBMB life, 59*(4–5), 249–254. https://doi.org/10.1080/15216540601178067

Widrick, R. M., & Raskin, J. D. (2010). Age-related stigma and the golden section hypothesis. *Aging & Mental Health, 14*(4), 375–385. https://doi.org/10.1080/13607860903167846

Woo, J., Leung, D., Yu, R., Lee, R., & Wong, H. (2021). Factors affecting trends in societal indicators of ageing well in Hong Kong: Policies, politics and pandemics. *The Journal of Nutrition, Health & Aging, 25*, 325–329. https://doi.org/10.1007/s12603-020-1488-z

World Health Organization. (2002). *Active ageing: A policy framework (No. WHO/NMH/NPH/02.8).* World Health Organization. https://apps.who.int/iris/handle/10665/67215

World Health Organization. (2007). *Global age-friendly cities: A guide.* World Health Organization.

World Health Organization. (2020). *Ageing: Healthy ageing and functional ability.* https://www.who.int/westernpacific/news/q-a-detail/ageing-healthy-ageing-and-functional-ability

Wu, H. C., & Tseng, M. H. (2018). Evaluating disparities in elderly community care resources: Using a geographic accessibility and inequality index. *International Journal of Environmental Research and Public Health, 15*(7), 1353. https://doi.org/10.3390/ijerph15071353

Zheng, Z., Chen, H., & Yang, L. (2019). Transfer of promotion effects on elderly health with age: From physical environment to interpersonal environment and social participation. *International Journal of Environmental Research and Public Health, 16*(15), 2794. https://doi.org/10.3390/ijerph16152794

Part II
Holistic and Humanistic Care for Elderly

Chapter 11
Monitoring Elderly Healthcare and Social Services

Billy S. H. Ho, Kenneth H. H. Chui, and Ben Yuk Fai Fong

Abstract High demand for elderly healthcare and social services is a major policy issue in many countries facing with increasing ageing populations. The community and the older adults are more likely seeking to pursue quality healthcare delivery in medical treatments and age-friendly environments. To alleviate public concerns, governments should design and promulgate integrated care standards to maintain high-quality, holistic and humanistic services in healthcare practices to allow for ageing with dignity. This chapter examines measures and strategies to monitor the utilisation of the large social resources effectively, efficiently and flexibly in the healthcare system and social services for the elderly. Performance indicators include external accountability and internal quality improvement. However, there are barriers to successful implementation, including poor collaboration between professional agencies and the government, failure to involve stakeholders, underfunding and lack of government commitment. Similar measures have been established by various countries and they are associated with the higher standards of quality, services and convenience and ensuring that the service areas are responsive to the target groups and clients. The performance standards can be further developed and enhanced by taking references from policies and strategies in other countries. This means the quality of health services would become better monitored and assured. Practically, it will not only benefit the older adults but also the whole community, aiming to provide quality professional services. In essence, monitoring elderly healthcare and social services in a more humane and comfortable way should be the goal of all societies. Policy makers, politicians and government bureaucrats should be making continuing improvement in healthcare and social services, facilities and delivery conditions for

B. S. H. Ho (✉)
School of Professional Education and Executive Development, The Hong Kong Polytechnic University, Hong Kong, China
e-mail: 6768879@gmail.com

K. H. H. Chui
Hong Kong College of Community Health Practitioners, Hong Kong, China

B. Y. F. Fong
College of Professional and Continuing Education, The Hong Kong Polytechnic University, Hong Kong, China

V. T. S. Law and B. Y. F. Fong (eds.), *Ageing with Dignity in Hong Kong and Asia*, Quality of Life in Asia 16, https://doi.org/10.1007/978-981-19-3061-4_11

the older adults in the promotion of ageing with dignity and safety because health is essential and vital for the whole community.

Keywords Performance indicators · Quality of life · Income security · Capacity to care · Health literacy · Accountability

11.1 Evaluation of Elderly Care

11.1.1 Gaps in Elderly Healthcare and Social Services

Elderly care has caught the attention of the global society. The Hong Kong Monthly Digest of Statistics inferred that the proportion aged over 65 will rise from 17% in 2016 to 31% in 2036, and the population is expected to continue. More specifically, there will be one out of three people aged 65 or above in the coming 20 years (Census and Statistics Department, 2017). The demand for the healthcare system is rapidly increasing due to the ageing population. Older adults have been the major group incurring medical expenditure. The research office of the Legislative Council Secretariat (2019) indicated that the percentage of the government expenditure on the elderly service had increased from 16.5% in 2012 to 20.8% in 2019. On the other hand, increased life expectancy and declining fertility would put a lot of pressure and dependency on the medical, social and healthcare systems.

The elderlies are living with chronic illnesses, physical disabilities and other co-morbidities, leading to higher health costs worldwide (Centers for Disease Control and Prevention, 2021). In Hong Kong, over 70% of the elderly suffer from one or more chronic illnesses (Elderly Health Service, 2018). However, there is a lack of coordination in healthcare and social services. Elderly health services, residential care home for the elderly, daycare centres, etc. are not under one policy bureau in Hong Kong. Specifically, the Department of Health and the Hospital Authority each operate health centres, while the Social Welfare Department and the Department of Health, and even nurse clinics within the Hospital Authority, provide health education, health screening, risk assessment and physical therapy services. Furthermore, the Social Welfare Department and the Hospital Authority also provide on-site health services. This lack of uniform and coordinated care, with duplicated services in the community cause waste of resources. The quality of care for the elderly is compromised. Similarly, in Singapore, despite the availability of a variety of financial assistance schemes, low-income elders remain vulnerable due to insufficient publicity and a complex application process, healthcare self-efficacy is undermined. Like Hong Kong and some Asian societies, the Singapore healthcare system is overly dependent on specialist care, and there is a lack of coordinated action and consensus among care providers (Lee et al., 2020).

11.1.2 Quality of Life for Older Adults

Measuring quality of life is a complex and comprehensive process. Since 2017, the Chinese University of Hong Kong began to refer to the Global Age Observation Index suggested by the World Health Organization to design the Hong Kong Quality of Life Index (HKEQOL), with 22 indicators and four categories including income security, health status, capacity and enabling environment (CUHK Jockey Club Institute of Ageing, 2020).

The gradual degradation of physical function, loss of economic independence and lack of life goals after retirement affect the mentality of the elderly. In addition, the lack of timely and appropriate psychological counselling will also increase the possibility of depression and suicide (Radicic & Rivardo, 2019). It is not surprising to note that Hong Kong ranks first in life expectancy but comes 79th in terms of mental health (CUHK Jockey Club Institute of Ageing, 2018). The number of suicide deaths among the elderly in Hong Kong accounts for about 30% of the total, which is twice the average of all age groups (Centre for Suicide Research and Prevention, 2021).

On the other hand, high property prices, an overly dense and crowded living environment and air pollution have reduced the quality of life of the elderly. Housing is essential to safety and well-being. An age-friendly environment and public buildings have a major impact on the mobility, independence, and quality of life of the elderly and affect their ability to 'age in place'. A study in Singapore has found that elderly living in public rental housing have poorer health conditions and higher prevalence of depression and cognitive impairment. They are usually unwilling to participate in health screening, causing delays in treatment (Chan et al., 2018).

Income security means the ability to receive continuously stable income to fulfil medical and other needs. In Hong Kong, Old Age Allowance (OAA) or Comprehensive Social Security Assistance (CSSA) are available to older adults. However, the eligibility age for CSSA was raised from 60 to 65 in 2019, leaving some elderlies aged 60 to 65 in financial trouble. According to the Hong Kong Poverty Situation Report (Census and Statistics Department, 2020), approximately 32 per cent of residents aged 65 and above lived in poverty. It has been shown that there is a positive correlation between health and socioeconomic status (SES), and elderly with low SES are more likely to get sick. A study in the United States (Huguet et al., 2008) found that people with higher household income levels have higher overall functional health. Older adults are often the underprivileged group, but they may have difficulty to reduce their health risks by improving their living environment and adopting a healthy lifestyle (Wang et al., 2018).

The capacity to care and person and family-centred service provision are keys to maintain high-quality, holistic and humanistic services in healthcare practices (D'Avanzo et al., 2017). In Hong Kong, it is generally difficult for the vulnerable elderly population to obtain high-quality primary medical care services. For example, the older adults with lower SES are more likely to be hospitalised due to avoidable medical problems (Schoeb, 2016). Nonetheless, employment rate of the elderly has significantly increased and the number of working elders in Hong Kong had nearly tripled, from 42,600 in 2008 to 139,300 in 2018 (Census and Statistics Department, 2020). The elderly is willing to continue to work after retirement age for a stable income. However, age discrimination commonly exists in workplace. South Korea or Singapore have adopted different measures to require companies to extend the retirement age and provide subsidies to employers to retain older workers at low wages (Chan & Yip, 2019).

11.1.3 Governments Should Do More

The development of integrated care is essential to maintain the health of older people. Integrated care is a collection of approaches and models based on various financial, administration, organization and service delivery levels. Care coordination, person-centred care, governance and accountability are crucial elements of effective integrated care implementation (International Foundation for Integrated Care, n.d.). Moreover, it ensures effective coordination and collaboration in the multiple services related to diagnosis, rehabilitation, and health promotion. Quality of care and quality of life, as well as the efficiency of systems, can be improved (World Health Organization, 2016). The Hong Kong Government has an irreplaceable role to play in formulating a comprehensive elderly policy to promote comprehensive healthcare services for the elderly. A local study found that integrated care and discharge support (ICDS) for older patients reduced the number of accident and emergency department (AED) visits, acute admissions and hospital days (Lin et al., 2015).

The healthcare system in Japan is based on a social health insurance model. Citizens participate in compulsory long-term care insurance (LTCI), such as the Longevity Medical Care System for people aged 75 or over, allowing the elderly to access medical services at a lower cost. Working adults pay from the age of 40, and they receive services at only 10% of the cost of nursing care. In addition, local elderly will receive a needs assessment from the age of 65 by a doctor appointed by the health system to ensure that they meet the requirements for care. The government requires the elderly service sector to employ experienced dieticians to oversee the preparation of meals to ensure that appropriate dietary intakes are achieved. With the high level of interpersonal care, caregivers are also required to maintain a low ratio of hospital admissions. Overall, the Japanese government can reduce the tax burden of aged care, while maintaining high-quality, holistic, and humanistic services in healthcare practices to allow for ageing with dignity (Annear et al., 2016).

11.2 Monitoring Elderly Healthcare and Social Services

11.2.1 Evaluation of Performance

The healthcare system is built on an intricate network of care processes and pathways. The quality of care it offers is largely determined by how well the healthcare network functions and how collaborative the administrators are. Good performance indicators and diverse integrated techniques can improve the quality of treatment for the entire community with more effective application of resources. Accountability is a key to achieving high-quality healthcare and maintaining public health outcomes (Denis, 2014). The purpose of accountability is to reduce or avoid the misuse and abuse of public resources and to ensure that resources are used, and authority is exercised by due process of law, professional standards and societal values. Different types of accountability relationships exist in all health systems, with three main categories of financial, performance and political democracy (Brinkerhoff, 2004).

Lam (2017) suggested the establishment of a new and statutory agency to implement health policies and be responsible for health service management at different levels in Hong Kong. Moreover, the new organisation should be authorised to supervise and revise the relevant laws and regulations to ensure the availability of community medical services. It can provide consultations on public health and medical services to relevant departments. Through the establishment of a registration system, the transparency and the external accountability is further improved.

There are different requirements for internal quality improvement and external accountability, but the information available is not the same. Internal improvement to reduce waste, defects and errors can encourage health departments and medical institutions to learn from the differences among providers, and promote the transformation and improvement of the quality of care. Improving the reliability of the healthcare system and the clinical process is essential for quality improvement (Freeman, 2002). Collective mindfulness can increase the willingness of employees to invest time and resources to improve the system. Designing more effective systems and clinical pathways, establishing more standardised nursing procedures and using effective resources to achieve high-quality care are some common examples of quality improvement methods in the healthcare field (Chassin & Loeb, 2013). Furthermore, taking care of chronic multi-morbidity, improving public health and upgrading residential care homes for the elderly are some essential key performance indicators (KPIs) for evaluating and monitoring elderly healthcare.

11.2.2 *Barriers*

11.2.2.1 Underfunding

It is extrapolated that the number of citizens receiving elderly care will at least double in 20 years. The total population of Hong Kong will rise from 5 to 11% within 40 years, and the cost of social care in Hong Kong will increase from HK$38.8 billion in 2018 to HK$222.4 billion in 2060. Therefore, the cost of elderly care in Hong Kong is expected to be escalated and the internal growth is nearly 6 times (Asia Advisers Network, 2019). However, this developmental speed is still far behind the strong growth of long-term care (LTC) and its demand due to the ageing of the society (Legislative Council Secretariat, 2021).

11.2.2.2 Failure to Involve Stakeholders

Organisations and individuals participating in the production, consumption, management, regulation or assessment of certain health programmes, such as the governance of medical systems or the creation of health policy, are referred to as health stakeholders (Hyder et al., 2010). Older people are the main users of different forms of care and healthcare services. However, they are often in a vulnerable position when it comes to participating in and making health decisions. Studies have shown that under-involved health decision-making can lead to a high risk of devaluation and disempowerment for older people who rely on services (D'Avanzo et al., 2017). A survey showed that 79% of the elderly do not know how to use the 'eHealth' online system or telephone inquiries at all, reflecting the government's failure to involve elderly stakeholders. Furthermore, the elderly generally lack trust in private medical services and are less willing to use medical measures in public–private partnerships (PPPs) (Liu et al., 2013).

11.2.2.3 Poor Collaboration Between Professional Agencies and the Government

The private sector is in a strategic position in healthcare systems and should be more involved in policy development. However, private providers in Hong Kong are often in a passive role when promoting health plans for the elderly even in the public–private partnership scheme. This can potentially lead to mistrust and false expectations. When promoting the Elderly Health Care Voucher Scheme, the government has not provided the private suppliers technical supports such as advanced information technology systems and staff training. Hence, it is difficult for private providers and the lack of a high level of their commitment may make it challenging to promote and maintain the health of the elderly. Therefore, it is essential to strengthen cooperation between the government and the private sector to attain a full commitment from both parties (Ho & Ng, 2020).

11.3 Strategies in Utilisation of Public Resources

11.3.1 Effectiveness, Efficiency and Flexibility in the Healthcare System and Social Services

A key impact of population ageing is the increase in healthcare utilisation. However, healthcare utilisation is not the same for all older people, compounded by shortage of healthcare provisions in both high-income and low-income countries in the Asia–Pacific region. An understanding of the demographic, health and social characteristics of older people is necessary to identify the key drivers. Providing integrated care for older people requires a large number of qualified and devoted professionals with the necessary knowledge in gerontology. Therefore, governments need to develop sufficient expertise in geriatrics and provide the necessary training in integrated care services for all concerned health departments and social care workers. For example, geriatrics have been integrated into the curricula to provide a comprehensive health services programmes in Malaysia for some years already (Forsyth & Chia, 2009).

Some countries in the Asia–Pacific region have decentralised health service systems, which pose a major challenge to the comprehensive, coordinated, and continuous care provided to the elderly (Chen et al., 2018). In Hong Kong, the referral mechanism is not coordinated, and this is making limited protection to the discharge plan for the elderly. Nevertheless, primary care in family or personal medicine, geriatrics and chronic disease management is foundations for the quality of health services for the elderly. Additionally, the traditional structural barriers caused by the roles and norms of primary and secondary care should be eliminated. All providers must work together to provide seamless, effectiveness, efficiency and flexibility services (Forsyth & Chia, 2009).

Health literacy of the elderly is widely acknowledged as a key to appropriate utilisation of public resources. A study in Malaysia found that age and health literacy were negatively correlated in the elderly, and low health literacy had increased the difficulty of interpreting drug labels and health information, causing more hospitalisation. Such elderly is more likely to experience poor health and higher mortality rates because they were less likely to participate in preventive services and have poorer medication compliance. The inadequate health literacy had led to greater use of healthcare services such as counselling, outpatient visits and hospital admissions (Yunus et al., 2017).

Evidence has indicated that disease-centric and hospital-oriented health services are detrimental to elderly care. Therefore, shifting towards patient-centred and community-based health services should be strengthened (Lim et al., 2017; Ng et al., 2019). Through the coordinated efforts of policymakers, health service providers and funders and service users, the healthcare system and social services for the elderly can be improved in an effective, efficient and flexible manner.

11.3.2 Services Responsive to the Target Groups and Clients

Sustainable long-term care services require a multi-sectoral response and the involvement of a wide range of stakeholders from all sectors. In many low- and middle-income countries with limited resources and infrastructure, there is a general lack of formal and well developed long-term care services. In Goa, for example, there are no specialised dementia care homes, resulting in high levels of psychological distress for families and the elderly. The government has developed a community-based intervention programme to provide support and education to families of people suffering from dementia through appropriate local health and human resources, which help older people to achieve activities of daily living (ADLs). Similar intervention has been promulgated in Peru and Russia (World Health Organization, 2015).

The Chiayi government is actively working with universities, local research institutes and civic societies to provide enhanced services related to elderly care, including transport to activities, organising grandparents' festivals, providing vocational training courses and subsidies. In Seoul, Korea, they have set up a Policy Monitoring Group on Ageing to scrutinise and evaluate the awareness of relevant policies among the elderly through surveys and assessments. These initiatives provide opportunities for greater participation in decision-making by the elderly (Jockey Club Age-Friendly City, 2021). On the other hand, anxiety about affordability among low-income people may reduce their access to medical help such as chronic disease screening and related management programmes. In Singapore, older people of lower SES can participate in the Community Health Assistance Scheme (CHAS) to increase their access to healthcare (Community Health Assistance Scheme, n.d.).

11.4 Enhancement of Performance Standards of Care and Services

11.4.1 Policies and Strategies in Asian Countries

11.4.1.1 Policies and Strategies in Taiwan

In 1998, the Taiwan government started to improve the healthcare services for the elderly because the ageing problems became more serious. In 2007, the first Long-term Care (LTC) Plan 1.0 was launched (Ministry of Health and Welfare, 2019; Yang et al., 2020). This action plan was meant to construct a diverse local community medical system that could fulfil the various needs of residents and offer a legislative base to build up the system (Ministry of Health and Welfare, 2016). 10 years later, LTC Plan 2.0 was launched in 2016 to provide more comprehensive and suitable services to the needy population, especially the elderly (Ministry of Health and Welfare, 2019, 2020). Moreover, the supervision was also upgraded, ensuring services were maintained with satisfaction.

First, the framework of LTC organization was composed of government departments, experts and the representative of services providers and local organisations (Ministry of Health and Welfare, 2019). The purposes and authorities of district care management centre were well-defined to harmonise issues related to healthcare workers, and analysis which will be used for strategical planning was also conduct (Ministry of Health and Welfare, 2020). These two actions were completing the application of policy and system, improving the integration of policy and service and increasing the effectiveness and efficiency of LTC services.

Second, a clear definition of each kind of service, the qualifications of service workers, professional training requirements and the requirement of personnel and organization management of the healthcare service organization were pointed out in the LTC Plan 2.0 (Ministry of Health and Welfare, 2019). Healthcare providers needed to accomplish a high standard of service with no excuses. Last but not least, the care managers in the system were the goalie from the government. They attended to medical and social service matching and the monitoring of service quality. Once the services had been matched to the needy people, the care manager would review and observe the quality regularly (Yang et al., 2020).

11.4.1.2 Policies and Strategies in Singapore

Singapore has started research on ageing since 1980. They seem doing the best on the related aspect in Asia (Thang & Hong, 2015). Their healthcare system has been acclaimed as one of the top systems in the world, and they improve the services and the quality continuously. The local government offers necessary resources and government assistance to the non-governmental or voluntary welfare organisations (VWOs) rather than provide long-term care service to the citizens directly. This is because it can avoid unnecessary demand from the citizens and provide the services in more flexible manner. Furthermore, this setting can encourage more involvement and more support from the local citizens, while the government sets the direction, financing and regulation of the long-term care services (Phua et al., 2019). The strategy of decentralisation helps to reduce the burden of the government while healthcare service can be delivered more effectively. The reorganisation of government departments is also implemented to improve the service planning and sector development, which are practicable to increase the service quality (Phua et al., 2019). It can also broaden the scope of the service area and cover the whole health and social care spectrum. In addition, it is convenient for different government departments and local industries to coordinate, establish quality benchmarks, develop guidelines for healthcare sectors and enhance the quality of care (Agency for Integrated Care, 2016). In such a context, it is important for the industry-led workgroups to set up the guidelines because they understand the details of the industry better than the government.

Health informatics is another aspect that can improve and uphold healthcare service quality. The integrated health information system has been implemented in Singapore since 2011. All health records are stored in the national database. All authorised healthcare providers, from both the private and public sectors, are enabled to access patients' records via the integrated virtual system. The use of integrated technology can avoid duplication in treatment and tests, and also promote better observation of health conditions and the coordination between public and private providers (He & Tang, 2021).

11.4.1.3 Policies and Strategies in Indonesia

In 1999, Indonesia was severely hurt by the Asian financial crisis. The local government proceeded with a decentralisation reform. The health system was reorganised. The provincial and district governments were empowered to take over the health services from the Ministry of Home Affairs, one of the government departments, and responsible for the planning and managing service delivery. The relationship between the central, provincial and district governments is not hierarchical. They all have their own mandates and areas of authority. Unique schemes and strategies have been developed in some governments to ordinate, manage and regulate the health services, while the main function of the Ministry of Health (MoH) is to regulate, monitor the availability of the resources (Mahendradhata et al., 2017). In addition, the MoH is responsible for the policy formulation and standards and guidance development of healthcare services to the lower levels of government (Kadar et al., 2013).

The disconnected and fragmented health system is the result of decentralisation. The central government does not have adequate power to control the provincial and district governments (Mahendradhata et al., 2017). Policies from the central government are hard to fully execute and synchronise in the lower levels of governments, or even being ignored (Kadar et al., 2013). In addition, qualitative research reported that some elderlies were disappointed because the healthcare workers did not meet their expectations or needs in the non-coordinated environment (Pratono & Maharani, 2018). Lastly, although Indonesia has developed a national information system for the healthcare system, there is a lack of effectiveness and efficacy because of decentralisation, resulting in complex information uploading procedures. Each level of governmental organization builds its own format and style, leading to overlap and duplication of information (Mahendradhata, et al., 2017).

11.4.2 Better Monitoring of Quality of Health Services

11.4.2.1 Regulation and Legislation

In order to solve the social issues, collective decisions are required, and it depends on the power owner and player. The local government is the greatest legal organisation within a country or city, and it has the authority to make the decisions and people have to follow (Buse et al., 2012). There are several kinds of policy instruments that the government can implement to monitor and assure the quality of healthcare services such as exhortation, taxation, expenditure, regulation and public ownership (Buse et al., 2012). The government should conduct relevant research to review what should be regulated as problems are hard to be improved solely by exhortation. For example, ageing-friendly cities and holistic and humanistic care should have foundational regulations and legislations to support the quality and services provided with dignity to the elderly. In addition, in a supportive environment, healthcare providers will observe and follow the law in establishing high standards of services (Buse et al., 2012). Unfortunately, the coordination among different government departments is commonly weak and fragmentary. Therefore, it is imperative for governments and practitioners to intergrade the services and strengthen the communication and coordination for better service provision.

11.4.2.2 Health Literacy of Healthcare Service Users

Health literacy refers to a person's ability to discover, understand and apply the knowledge to determine health-related decisions for their own and others. The knowledge can help a person to solve the health problem by themselves initially and consider what actions to take. The person is also able to discuss with the professionals and participate in decision-making (Centers for Disease Control and Prevention, 2020; He & Tang, 2021). On the other hand, service users who are lack of health literacy do not understand the information provided by the healthcare service providers, and thus not making 'well-informed' decisions (Centers for Disease Control and Prevention, 2020). In general, the academic attainment of the elderly is low because of the social environment and culture in the past. They are inclined to be passive in seeking health care and face cognitive barriers in medical decisions. (He & Tang, 2021). This is significantly associated with the underused integrated healthcare services and primary care services in some Asian countries, including Hong Kong. The purpose for most people to seek medical help is for curative care but not health maintenance purposes (He & Tang, 2021).

11.4.2.3 Health Education and Training for Professionals

As the needs of the elderly are unique, and factors affecting their physical and mental health are complicated, the provision of high-quality and dignified elderly healthcare services is challenging (Borhani et al., 2014; Coghlan, 2021; Kjølseth et al., 2010; Kunsmann-Leutiger et al., 2021). Healthcare service providers play an important role and therefore, they have to offer satisfying services and keep a positive working attitude. Gerontology and geriatrics are the medical and health specialties related to the elderly and they are cross-disciplined, involving medicine, psychology, social and environmental systems (Arai et al., 2012). With sufficient training and practice, healthcare professionals are able to handle the senior patients in a better way with dignified services with their basic understanding of the perspective of the elderly.

11.4.3 Age-Friendly Policies and Services

The Indonesian government has implemented ageing-friendly policies such as foundational legislation on welfare for the elderly, and the national social security system. Government departments, commissions and organisations are working together for elderly development like the National Commission for Seniors and Local Seniors Commissions. In 2017, the new law and detailed planning were proposed for the new direction with the aims to enhance different aspects related to the elderly such as spiritual health, education and training, social welfare and protection. The government tried to create, support and encourage the elderly to participate in community events, religious activities and competitions by offering free entrance to recreation services such as the Ragunan Wildlife Park, as well as providing friendly public open spaces with accessible green space to activate the social interaction between residents of different ages in the country (Suriastini et al., 2019).

In Singapore, age-friendly surroundings are available in residential neighbourhood to keep the elderly physically active and healthy, socially active to avoid social isolation and to reinforce the duration of ageing in place. To achieve the objectives, cross-government department, cross-agency lines of responsibility, working with local organisations and extensive public consultation are mobilised to set up the Action Plan for Successful Ageing with topics such as public spaces, lifelong learning, social engagement and housing (Thang & Hong, 2015). The city is more walkable and accessible. For example, seats are provided within a short distance, and thus the elderly can get some rest during their journeys. The connectivity of public transportation and the wayfinding signs are improved as well. In addition, slip-resistant treatment, support hand bars and emergency pull-cords are examples of (home) infrastructure improvement, fully funded by the government if eligible. To promote and increase the social interaction between different age groups, the Singaporean government provides lifelong learning opportunities to activate their learning interests via an intergenerational environment (Thang & Hong, 2015).

In the past, the healthcare services seemed to be focusing only on what types of services should be provided to the elderly and how they can be implemented, but that is not enough nowadays. The findings and discussion from the site visit report by The Control Yuan (2015) of Taiwan showed that some elderly homes in Japan are good examples to demonstrate how to provide humane and comfortable services with dignity and consideration of the mental needs of the elderly. At the same time, diversified service modes can be provided in different commercial environment.

A natural environment in the surrounding of the building, creating an atmosphere of friendliness and family warmth with well-designed decoration should be common features in elderly homes (The Control Yuan, 2015). Health workers in the homes should not shout at the elderly, who are free to do what they want, just like in their own homes. Moreover, there should be sufficient activity space for each individual inside the home, respecting their rights. There should also be special facilities inside the homes, for instance, the beauty room, recreation room, mahjong room and movie theatre. The function of these elderly homes is not just providing and handling basic care but also aiming to reinforce and improve the ability of self-management and self-care of the older adults, making life meaningful for them, without any defective and inhumane care, or unprofessional workers (Hasegawa & Ota, 2019).

11.5 Implications of Holistic and Humanistic Elderly Care

The elderly is the vulnerable group but may still be one of the powerful groups in the society with great influence. Thus, the expenditure for health and social welfare services of the elderly is increasing due to ageing in the community (Arai et al., 2012; Cheng, 2020; Tiraphat et al., 2020). The older adults should be respected, loved and protected. They are powerful if their abilities and potentials are well-tapped, activated and used. For instance, the silver economy generates financial benefits by employment and consumption from the elderly (Cheng, 2020). Qualitative and quantitative research have found that spiritual needs, respect from others, affective care are key elements of humanistic care, influencing the health status (Borhani et al., 2014; Coghlan, 2021; Kunsmann-Leutigeret al., 2021). Care robots are introduced and has been applied in some countries to replace and provide affective care. They are able to respond to particular words, facial expressions and actions from the users (Coghlan, 2021). However, it does not mean that it can substitute humanistic care. Indeed, humanistic and affective care is characterised by the complicated and attentive relationship between caregivers and users (Borhani et al., 2014; Coghlan, 2021; Sadruddin, 2020).

Elderly should not be abandoned or forsook after they have spent their whole life in building up a better society for the new generations. Holistic and humanistic elderly care is a way for the society to respect and appreciate what the older adults have done and contributed. In fact, some simple actions are easy to accomplish such as the home modifications (Beard & Bloom, 2015; Hong et al., 2015). Furthermore, humanistic elderly care includes autonomy. Some elderly do not seek medical help because they do not trust the healthcare service workers and think things will be out of their control (Kjølseth et al., 2010). The elderly also want to solve the daily activities and problems such as taking a shower, sustaining anal hygiene by themselves (Arai et al., 2012; Hasegawa & Ota, 2019; Hong et al., 2015; Prachuabmoh, 2015). Well-established elderly services are important to let them live in peace in the last stage of life and then passed away peacefully.

If the ageing-friendly city can provide holistic and humanistic elderly care to the elderly, not only the elderly can obtain the benefits, the family caregivers, the government and the whole society can also gain from the advantages and outcomes. Burden of caregivers can be reduced and public resource can be rechannelled for better use. Last but not least, it is beneficial for the whole society in the long-term because health cost is decreased and the demand for healthcare services from the elderly is declined (Cheng, 2020; Prachuabmoh, 2015).

References

Agency for Integrated Care. (2016). *Introduction to Singapore healthcare.* https://partners.aic.sg/sites/aicassets/AssetGallery/HC%20Information%20Kit_book1_FA-5(online).pdf

Annear, M. J., Otani, J., & Sun, J. (2016). Experiences of Japanese aged care: The pursuit of optimal health and cultural engagement. *Age and Ageing, 45*(6), 753–756. https://doi.org/10.1093/ageing/afw144

Asia Advisers Network. (2019, May 9). *Cost of eldercare in Hong Kong projected to grow nearly six times in 40 years.* https://www.asiaadvisersnetwork.com/Article?aid=46706

Arai, H., Ouchi, Y., Yokode, M., Ito, H., Uematsu, H., Eto, F., Oshima, S., Ota, K., Saito, Y., Sasaki, H., Tsubota, K., Fukuyama, H., Honda, Y., Iguchi, A., Toba, K., Hosoi, T., & Kita, T. (2012). Toward the realization of a better aged society: Messages from gerontology and geriatrics. *Geriatrics & Gerontology International, 12*(1), 16–22. https://doi.org/10.1111/j.1447-0594.2011.00776.x

Beard, J. R., & Bloom, D. E. (2015). Towards a comprehensive public health response to population ageing. *The Lancet, 385*(9968), 658–661. https://doi.org/10.1016/S0140-6736(14)61461-6

Borhani, F., Abbaszadeh, A., & Moosavi, S. (2014). Status of human dignity of adult patients admitted to hospitals of Tehran. *Journal of Medical Ethics and History of Medicine, 7*(20). https://www.ncbi.nlm.nih.gov/pmc/articles/PMC4648216/

Brinkerhoff, D. W. (2004). Accountability and health systems: Toward conceptual clarity and policy relevance. *Health Policy and Planning, 19*(6), 371–379. https://doi.org/10.1093/heapol/czh052

Buse, K., Mays, N., & Walt, G. (2012). *Making health policy* (2nd ed.). Open University Press. https://www.bookdepository.com/Making-Health-Policy-Kent-Buse/9780335246342

Census and Statistics Department. (2017, October). *Hong Kong monthly digest of statistics.* https://www.censtatd.gov.hk/en/data/stat_report/product/FA100061/att/B71710FA2017XXXXB0100.pdf

Census and Statistics Department. (2020, December). *Hong Kong poverty situation report 2019.* https://www.povertyrelief.gov.hk/eng/pdf/Hong_Kong_Poverty_Situation_Report_2019.pdf

Centers for Disease Control and Prevention. (2020). *What is health literacy?* https://www.cdc.gov/healthliteracy/learn/index.html

Centers for Disease Control and Prevention. (2021, June 23). *Health and economic costs of chronic diseases.* https://www.cdc.gov/chronicdisease/about/costs/index.htm

Centre for Suicide Research and Prevention. (2021). *Suicide death by age group in Hong Kong 1981–2019.* https://csrp.hku.hk/statistics/#

Chan, C. Q. H., Lee, K. H., & Low, L. L. (2018). A systematic review of health status, health seeking behaviour and healthcare utilisation of low socioeconomic status populations in urban Singapore. *International Journal for Equity in Health, 17*(1), 1–21. https://doi.org/10.1186/s12939-018-0751-y
Chan, D., & Yip, D. (2019, August). *Elderly employment: Latest developments in Hong Kong and policies in international perspective.* Office of the Government Economist, The Government of the Hong Kong Special Administrative Region. https://www.hkeconomy.gov.hk/en/pdf/el/el-2019-10.pdf
Chassin, M. R., & Loeb, J. M. (2013). High-reliability health care: Getting there from here. *The Milbank Quarterly, 91*(3), 459–490. https://doi.org/10.1111/1468-0009.12023
Chen, C. Y., Gan, P., & How, C. H. (2018). Approach to frailty in the elderly in primary care and the community. *Singapore Medical Journal, 59*(5), 240–245. https://doi.org/10.11622/smedj.2018052
Cheng, F. K. (2020). From an aging person to an elegant senior: A humanistic approach to viewing older adults. *Frontiers of Nursing, 7*(3). https://doi.org/10.2478/fon-2020-0032
Coghlan, S. (2021). Robots and the possibility of humanistic care. *International Journal of Social Robotics*, 1–14. https://doi.org/10.1007/s12369-021-00804-7
Community Health Assistance Scheme. (n.d.). *Eligibility and application.* https://www.chas.sg/content.aspx?id=306
CUHK Jockey Club Institute of Ageing. (2018). *AgeWatch index for Hong Kong: Topical report on health status.* https://www.jcafc.hk/uploads/docs/AgeWatch_Index_Topical_Report_on_Health_Status.pdf
CUHK Jockey Club Institute of Ageing. (2020). *Report on Hong Kong elder quality of life index incorporating AgeWatch index for Hong Kong 2019.* https://www.jcafc.hk/uploads/docs/HKEQOL_2019_final_online(v2)-1.pdf
D'Avanzo, B., Shaw, R., Riva, S., Apostolo, J., Bobrowicz-Campos, E., Kurpas, D., Bujnowska-Fedak, M., & Holland, C. (2017). Stakeholders' views and experiences of care and interventions for addressing frailty and pre-frailty: A meta-synthesis of qualitative evidence. *PLoS ONE, 12*(7), e0180127. https://doi.org/10.1371/journal.pone.0180127
Denis, J. L. (2014). *Accountability in healthcare organizations and systems. Healthcare Policy, 10*(SP), 8–11. https://www.ncbi.nlm.nih.gov/pmc/articles/PMC4255571/
Elderly Health Service. (2018, March 5). *Coping with chronic illness.* https://www.elderly.gov.hk/english/healthy_ageing/mental_health/coping_with_chronic_illness.html
Forsyth, D. R., & Chia, Y. C. (2009). How should Malaysia respond to its ageing society? *Medical Journal of Malaysia, 64*(1), 46–50. http://www.e-mjm.org/2009/v64n1/Ageing_Society.pdf
Freeman, T. (2002). Using performance indicators to improve health care quality in the public sector: A review of the literature. *Health Services Management Research, 15*(2), 126–137. https://doi.org/10.1258/0951484021912897
Hasegawa, N., & Ota, K. (2019). Concept synthesis of dignity in care for elderly facility residents. *Nursing Ethics, 26*(7–8), 2016–2034. https://doi.org/10.1177/0969733018824763
He, A. J., & Tang, V. (2021). Integration of health services for the elderly in Asia: A scoping review of Hong Kong, Singapore, Malaysia, Indonesia. *Health Policy, 125*(3), 351–362. https://doi.org/10.1016/j.healthpol.2020.12.020
Ho, C. C. W., & Ng, T. K. C. (2020). Improvement of elderly health care voucher scheme in Hong Kong. *Asia Pacific Journal of Health Management, 15*(2), 18–22. https://doi.org/10.24083/apjhm.v15i2.387
Hong, S. L., Lee, M. J., & Han, C. K. (2015). Home modification among families with older adults with disability in Korea. *Asia Pacific Journal of Social Work and Development, 25*(4), 186–197. https://doi.org/10.1080/02185385.2015.1116192
Huguet, N., Kaplan, M. S., & Feeny, D. (2008). Socioeconomic status and health-related quality of life among elderly people: Results from the joint Canada/United States survey of health. *Social Science & Medicine, 66*(4), 803–810. https://doi.org/10.1016/j.socscimed.2007.11.011

Hyder, A., Syed, S., Puvanachandra, P., Bloom, G., Sundaram, S., Mahmood, S., Iqbal, M., Hongwen, Z., Ravichandran, N., Oladepo, O., Pariyo, G., & Peters, D. (2010). Stakeholder analysis for health research: Case studies from low- and middle-income countries. *Public Health, 124*(3), 159–166. https://doi.org/10.1016/j.puhe.2009.12.006

International Foundation for Integrated Care. (n.d.). *Specific facets of IC.* https://integratedcarefoundation.org/ific-integrated-care-search/ific-integrated-care-search-narrow

Jockey Club Age-friendly City. (2021). *AFC concept world efforts.* https://www.jcafc.hk/en/Afc-Concept/World-Efforts.html

Kadar, K. S., Francis, K., & Sellick, K. (2013). Ageing in Indonesia—Health status and challenges for the future. *Ageing International, 38*(4), 261–270. https://doi.org/10.1007/s12126-012-9159-y

Kjølseth, I., Ekeberg, O., & Steihaug, S. (2010). Elderly people who committed suicide – their contact with the health service. What did they expect, and what did they get? *Aging & Mental Health, 14*(8), 938–946. https://doi.org/10.1080/13607863.2010.501056

Kunsmann-Leutiger, E., Straßner, C., Schalhorn, F., Stolz, R., Stotz-Ingenlath, G., Buhlinger-Göpfarth, N., Bentner, M., Joos, S., Valentini, J., & Frick, E. (2021). Training general practitioners and medical assistants within the framework of HoPES3, a holistic care program for elderly patients to integrate spiritual needs, social activity, and self-care into disease management in primary care. *Journal of Multidisciplinary Healthcare, 14*, 1853–1861. https://doi.org/10.2147/JMDH.S312778

Lam, A. H. Y. (2017). *Strategies of Hong Kong's healthcare system in ageing population.* Official Conference Proceedings of The Asian Conference on Ageing & Gerontology. The University of Hong Kong, Hong Kong. http://papers.iafor.org/wp-content/uploads/papers/agen2017/AGEN2017_36030.pdf

Lee, J. M. G., Chan, C. Q. H., Low, W. C., Lee, K. H., & Low, L. L. (2020). Health-seeking behaviour of the elderly living alone in an urbanised low-income community in Singapore. *Singapore Medical Journal, 61*(5), 260–265. https://doi.org/10.11622/smedj.2019104

Legislative Council Secretariat. (2019, December 13). *Government expenditure on the elderly.* https://www.legco.gov.hk/research-publications/english/1920rt02-government-expenditure-on-the-elderly-20191213-e.pdf

Legislative Council Secretariat. (2021). *Community care services for the elderly in Germany and Japan.* https://www.legco.gov.hk/research-publications/english/2021in12-community-care-services-for-the-elderly-in-germany-and-japan-20210616-e.pdf

Lim, W. S., Wong, S. F., Leong, I., Choo, P., & Pang, W. S. (2017). Forging a frailty-ready healthcare system to meet population ageing. *International Journal of Environmental Research and Public Health, 14*(12), 1448. https://doi.org/10.3390/ijerph14121448

Lin, F. O., Luk, J. K., Chan, T. C., Mok, W. W., & Chan, F. H. (2015). Effectiveness of a discharge planning and community support programme in preventing readmission of high-risk older patients. *Hong Kong Medical Journal, 21*(3), 208–216. https://doi.org/10.12809/hkmj144304

Liu, S., Yam, C. H., Huang, O. H., & Griffiths, S. M. (2013). Willingness to pay for private primary care services in Hong Kong: Are elderly ready to move from the public sector? *Health Policy and Planning, 28*(7), 717–729. https://doi.org/10.1093/heapol/czs112

Mahendradhata, Y., Trisnantoro, L., Listyadewi, S., Soewondo, P., Marthias, T., Harimurti, P., & Prawira, J. (2017). The Republic of Indonesia Health System Review. *Health Systems in Transition, 7*(1). WHO Regional Office for South-East Asia. https://apps.who.int/iris/handle/10665/254716

Ministry of Health and Welfare. (2016). *2007–2016: Ten year long-term care plan 1.0* (in Chinese). https://1966.gov.tw/LTC/cp-3981-38770-201.html

Ministry of Health and Welfare. (2019). *The full policy of long-term care* (in Chinese). https://1966.gov.tw/LTC/cp-5198-42393-201.html

Ministry of Health and Welfare. (2020). *2017–2026: Ten year long-term care plan 2.0* (in Chinese). https://1966.gov.tw/LTC/cp-4001-42414-201.html

Ng, T. K. C., Fong, B. Y. F., & Kwong, C. K. Y. (2019). Transition of hospital acute-centric to long term care in an ageing population in Hong Kong—Is it an issue of service gap? *Asia-Pacific Journal of Health Management, 14*(1):11–15. https://doi.org/10.24083/apjhm.v14i1.207

Phua, K. H., Lee, G. G., & Mui, T. Y. (Eds.). (2019). *Ageing in Asia: Contemporary trends and policy issues*. World Scientific. https://doi.org/10.1142/10585

Pratono, A. H., & Maharani, A. (2018). Long-term care in Indonesia: The role of integrated service post for elderly. *Journal of Aging and Health, 30*(10), 1556–1573. https://doi.org/10.1177/0898264318794732

Radicic, J. S., & Rivardo, M. G. (2019). The relationships between meaning in life, spirituality, and depression. *North American Journal of Psychology, 21*(3), 525–539. http://najp.us/wp-content/uploads/2019/10/Vol.21-Issue-3.doc

Sadruddin, A. F. A. (2020). The care of "Small Things": Aging and dignity in Rwanda. *Medical Anthropology, 39*(1), 83–95. https://doi.org/10.1080/01459740.2019.1643852

Schoeb, V. (2016). Healthcare Service in Hong Kong and its Challenges. The role of health professionals within a social model of health. *China Perspectives, 2016*(2016/4), 51–58. https://doi.org/10.4000/chinaperspectives.7118

Suriastini, W., Buffardi, A. L., & Fauzan, J. (2019). What prompts policy change? Comparative analyses of efforts to create age-friendly cities in 14 cities in Indonesia. *Journal of Aging & Social Policy, 31*(3), 250–270. https://doi.org/10.1080/08959420.2019.1589889

Thang, L. L., & Hong, S. L. (2015). Ageing-in-place in studio apartments in Singapore: Maintaining independence in community living. *Asia Pacific Journal of Social Work and Development, 25*(4), 250–263. https://doi.org/10.1080/02185385.2015.1120414

The Control Yuan, Taiwan. (2015). *Report on elderly welfare organisations in Japan* (in Chinese). https://www-ws.cy.gov.tw/Download.ashx?u=LzAwMS9VcGxvYWQvQ3lPbGRGaWxlL1VwbG9hZC9LUG9zdF9Ub091dC85OTQwL%2BaXpeacrOiAgeS6uuemj%2BWIqeapn%2Bani%2BiAg%2BWvn%2BWgseWRii5wZGY%3D&n=5pel5pys6ICB5Lq656aP5Yip5qmf5qeL6ICD5a%2Bf5aCx5ZGKLnBkZg%3D%3D

Tiraphat, S., Buntup, D., Munisamy, M., Nguyen, T. H., Yuasa, M., Nyein Aung, M., & Hpone Myint, A. (2020). Age-friendly environments in ASEAN plus three: Case studies from Japan, Malaysia, Myanmar, Vietnam, and Thailand. *International Journal of Environmental Research and Public Health, 17*(12), 4523. https://doi.org/10.3390/ijerph17124523

Prachuabmoh, V. (2015). A lesson learned from community-based integrated long-term care in Thailand. *Asia Pacific Journal of Social Work and Development, 25*(4), 213–224. https://doi.org/10.1080/02185385.2015.1119526

Wang, F., Zhen, Q., Li, K., & Wen, X. (2018). Association of socioeconomic status and health-related behavior with elderly health in China. *PLoS ONE, 13*(9), e0204237. https://doi.org/10.1371/journal.pone.0204237

World Health Organization. (2015). *World report on ageing and health*. https://apps.who.int/iris/bitstream/handle/10665/186463/9789240694811_eng.pdf?sequence=1&isAllowed=y

World Health Organization. (2016, October). *Integrated care models: An overview*. https://www.euro.who.int/__data/assets/pdf_file/0005/322475/Integrated-care-models-overview.pdf

Yang, C. C., Hsueh, J. Y., & Wei, C. Y. (2020). Current status of long-term care in Taiwan: Transition of long-term care plan from 1.0 to 2.0. *International Journal of Health Policy and Management, 9*(8), 363–364. https://doi.org/10.15171/ijhpm.2019.115

Yunus, N. M., Abd Manaf, N. H., Omar, A., Omar, M. A., & Salleh, M. (2017). Determinants of healthcare utilisation among the elderly in Malaysia. *Institutions and Economies, 9*(3), 115–140. https://jummec.um.edu.my/index.php/ijie/article/view/4891/2749

Chapter 12
Longevity and Ageing of World Citizens

Fowie Sze Fung Ng, Roger Watson, and Graeme Drummond Smith

Abstract Rapidly changing demographics worldwide are evidenced by increased life expectancy and the concomitant increase in the ageing population. Longevity has recently became an important issue for the healthcare industry, especially for those working with the ageing population. Social media and popular books suggest ways in which people can stay healthy and live a long life, including enhancing psychological well-being. Economies, like Hong Kong, which already have a high life expectancy do not automatically put health-related measures in place to increase their peoples' longevity. It is envisaged that healthcare policy, especially in primary care, is important for any country to promote the concepts and health-related practices to increase the longevity of their citizens. In this chapter, the theory and biological and psychological perspectives of longevity will be addressed, including the physiological aspects of ageing, nutrition and so on. Specific attention will be given to issues surrounding frailty in older people. This will be followed by the assimilation of relevant evidence from both western and eastern perspectives. Regarding the implementation of modalities to enhance longevity, case studies will be used to highlight the policy as well as implementation issues for the way towards healthy ageing to achieve longevity of world citizens.

Keywords Longevity · Living longer · Life expectancy

F. S. F. Ng (✉)
Tung Wah College, Hong Kong, China
e-mail: fowieng@twc.edu.hk

R. Watson
Southwest Medical University, Luxhou, China

G. D. Smith
Caritas Institute of Higher Education, Hong Kong, China
e-mail: gsmith@cihe.edu.hk

V. T. S. Law and B. Y. F. Fong (eds.), *Ageing with Dignity in Hong Kong and Asia*, Quality of Life in Asia 16, https://doi.org/10.1007/978-981-19-3061-4_12

12.1 Introduction

People are living longer, as any examination of international demographics demonstrates, and we currently take this for granted, especially in the developed world. The increase was marked in the last century where the life expectancy in the west, for example, the United States was only 46 years for men and 48 years for women at the start of last century and 76 years for men and 81 years for women by the end of the century (Schanzenbach et al., 2016). On the eastern side, Hong Kong has the highest life expectancy in the world with 81.8 years for men and 87.6 years for women in 2020 and has been leading the world for the last few years (Chung & Marmot, 2020; SCMP, 2019). Japan, Singapore, South Korea are ranked as second, fourth and ninth in the ranking of longest life expectancy (Infoplease, 2021), respectively. There is an immense interest from the public, government, business as well as the scientific community to investigate how to achieve longevity with longer life which is both physically and mentally healthy.

12.2 The Biology of Longevity

The reasons for high life expectancy are complex but some of the factors involved include wider availability of healthcare, vaccinations, improved nutrition, a cleaner environment and better sanitation. Some of these factors will be explored in this chapter and elsewhere in this book. Longevity is clearly a success story, but it does have social and economic consequences, and these will also be discussed elsewhere. However, the process of ageing and the phenomenon of longevity are biologically based and the purported factors leading to longevity are acting on biological processes. Therefore, this section of this chapter will examine the biology of ageing and how these factors may have been influenced to increase longevity.

12.2.1 What Is Ageing?

From the biological perspective, ageing is the process of getting older and that process, according to the World Health Organisation (2021) is described as 'the impact of the accumulation of a wide variety of molecular and cellular damage over time'. This leads to a gradual decrease in physical and mental capacity, a growing risk of disease, and ultimately, death. But ageing is not linear and not necessarily associated with chronological age. It varies between people and some people are considered to age more 'successfully' than others (Stowe & Cooney, 2015). The biomarkers of successful again include (Mathers et al., 2012) physical capability, physiological function, cognitive function, endocrine function and immune function.

Ageing adversely affects every system of the body. Some of these effects are superficial and of little consequence in normal health, for example, the obvious ageing of the skin. But others have more important impact, for example, with ageing, the cardiovascular, respiratory and skeletomuscular system all deteriorate. Despite ageing, and in the absence of illness, people can still function perfectly well but, even with regular exercise, the older self will be less 'fit' than the younger self. Fitness here is referring to our ability, for example, to run or lift weights. However, every other system of the body is adversely affected, albeit much less noticeably, such as the endocrine system and the immune system.

12.2.2 Why Do We Age?

The above is what happens with ageing but what is less well understood is why ageing occurs and what biological process leads to ageing. The question of why ageing occurs takes us into the realm of theory and, amid a plethora of theories related to ageing, two not too dissimilar theories appear to hold most validity. These theories are the 'antagonistic pleiotropy' and 'disposable soma' theories (Kirkwood, 2011). The first proposes that some genes which are advantageous to younger organisms become harmful to older organisms. The second proposes that our primary biological purpose is to reproduce and that as we age and our reproductive ability declines the body invests less resources in maintenance, leading to ageing.

The processes that are taking place can be summarised as the eight hallmarks of ageing and these include a range of biological processes which are: genomic instability, telomere attrition, epigenetic alterations, loss of proteostasis, deregulated nutrient-sensing, mitochondrial dysfunction, cellular senescence, stem cell exhaustion and altered intercellular communication (López-Otin et al., 2013). In summary, these point, among other things, to significant changes in our genetic material, deleterious changes to proteins which serve both structural and metabolic functions, cell death and increased inflammation.

The common denominator to these processes almost certainly lies in our genes and this is powerfully expressed by López-Otin et al., (2013, p. 5) who say, 'There is extensive evidence that genomic damage accompanies aging and that its artificial induction can provoke aspects of accelerated aging'. As our genes replicate, they do not do so perfectly each time due to mutations (Partridge, 2010). In other words, while our genome remains essentially the same, it does change with time due to these mutations. Put simply, we become slightly less like our younger selves—genetically—as we age. The problem with this is twofold: as we age these mutations, some of which are harmful, accumulate. The reasons for these mutations are varied but one possible reason is the harmful effects of oxygen, which is a very toxic substance. We expend considerable energy in protecting ourselves from the harmful effects of oxygen and we become less able to do this as we age (Finkel & Holbrook, 2000).

12.2.3 So Why Are We Living Longer?

Strictly speaking, we are not living longer. The human lifespan—approximately a decade over a century—remained unchanged over the past century and seems to indicate that there is a maximum human lifespan in which the current world record was 122 years and 164 days when Jeanne Calment of France died in 1997 (Punt, 2020). 'Supercentenarians', people who live to age 110 or even longer are expected to rise slowly by the end of this century to a lifespan of 125 years, or even 130 years (UW News, 2021). A more accurate description of the situation is that more of us are living longer. The numbers of those who reach extreme old age (the 'oldest old') are, for example, centenarians, remain relatively few and are not representative of all old people (Pignolo, 2019). Nevertheless, the factors that lead them to live to extreme old age, especially those who do so without illness or disability, are worth studying. There are some possible endogenous factors, possibly genetic, that the oldest old possess. But there has been great interest in the exogenous factors: environmental, behavioural and nutritional, that contribute to longevity as these could be adopted by others.

It appears, therefore, that the oldest old can mitigate and postpone the deleterious effects of ageing. It is hard to distinguish the effects of nature or nurture here, in other words, which factors leading to successful ageing are endogenous and which are exogenous but, according to Pignolo (2019, p. 111), 'Careful observations in the oldest old offer some empirical strategies that favour increased health span and life span, including eating in moderation, regular exercise, purposeful living, and strong social support systems'. This, therefore, provides some insight into what has led to more people living longer and what may need to be done, politically, socially and from a public health perspective, to help older people age more successfully and have longer and healthier lives.

12.2.4 Does Ageing Serve a Useful Purpose?

Whatever the biological causes and consequences of ageing, the question remains, from the existential perspective, of why we age and what purpose it serves. Despite efforts to increase the human lifespan by abolishing ageing and improvements in healthcare, it is so far the case that ageing has not been abolished and, if we wait long enough, the death rate for humans is 100%. We can hypothesise that ageing may have some useful functions, for example the hypothesis that ageing in women which, inevitably, leads to loss of reproductive function, may free older women to assist with childcare of their grandchildren. However, this is highly speculative, applies only to humans and, of course, is only recently very widely significant as longevity is only relatively recently widespread. Otherwise, the reasons for ageing—an almost universal phenomenon in living organisms—remain a mystery. However, whatever the reasons, we must continue to learn how to cope as a society with increased ageing.

Especially, as years are being added to life, we must continue to learn to help add life to years with quality of life but not merely the number.

12.3 The Psychosocial Factors of Longevity

Globally, the World Health Organization estimates that number of people over the age of 60 will total two billion by 2050, up from 900,000 in 2015 (World Health Organization, 2021). The maintenance of good health status is paramount for the welfare of older people and this includes psychosocial well-being. Many older people do enjoy good levels of psychosocial health. However, with increased numbers of people living longer, it is anticipated that levels of psychosocial problems in older people will increase. Changes in psychosocial well-being may often result from deterioration in physical health status. There is a strong relationship between the physical and psychological aspects of the ageing process. Conversely, the development of psychological symptoms, like depression and anxiety, can have a negative effect on physical health and the functional capabilities of an individual. People may have to contend with many issues as they get older including, physical health problems, caring for a spouse who is unwell and grieving for loss of friends and family and loneliness. From the perspective of the healthcare professionals, it is vitally important that psychosocial problems and issues are not over-looked, and that they are managed appropriately. This section of this chapter aims to provide an overview of the most common psychological and mental health problems in older people. Although there are a multitude of factors that are associated with this topic, the latter part of this section will give specific attention issues associated with health literacy in older people.

12.3.1 Psychology of Ageing

The psychology of ageing can be viewed as the study of patterns of change throughout the life cycle. In relation to older people, understanding the psychology of ageing can provide useful insights into changes in cognition and behaviour. This area is an increasing field of clinical practice within professional psychology related to the study of ageing and the provision of care for older people and is known as 'Geropsychology', concerned with expanding the knowledge of the influence of psychological factors in the ageing process (Li, 2014). This area of study provides valuable information for those involved in the psychological care of older people to enable them to overcome issues associated with physical health deterioration, enhance a sense of well-being and quality of life in the latter stages of life. As outlined earlier, as we age there is a very close interface between physical and mental health. Older people with physical health problems, such as hypertension, can have higher levels of psychosocial distress than those who remain medically well. Equally, untreated psychological morbidity, such as depressive symptoms, in an older person with hypertension may lead to a more negative clinical outcome. Psychological symptoms can lower the immunity levels of an individual and may compromise their ability to fight infection, highlighted by the COVID-19 pandemic (Wong et al., 2020).

Until recently, the understanding of the psychological aspects of ageing has been firmly entrenched in a disease based or deficit orientated approach, primarily focusing on sub-optimal cognitive, social and emotional function. However, with the emergence of positive psychology, there is evidence to support the view that psychological well-being may act as a protective factor for health, in particular physical health. This has opened avenues for positive psychology research in older people. Older people can face many psychosocial and mental health challenges, including neurological conditions. Globally, the most common neurological disorders in older people are dementia and depression. It is alarming to note that over 15% of all adults aged over 60 years old have some form of psychosocial mental conditions (World Health Organization, 2020).

12.3.2 Dementia and Depression

Living longer life does not guarantee better quality of life. Globally, dementia in older people affects well over 50 million people. This figure is estimated to increase to over 150 million by 2050 (Alzheimer's Disease International, 2020). Although it is not specifically part of the ageing process, dementia is a condition that predominately affects older people. Dementia is a condition which is usually chronic and progressive in nature, usually causing issues of memory loss, difficulty concentrating, cognitive dysfunction and the ability to perform the most basic everyday tasks. Not only does dementia cause distress for the older person with these problems, families and informal carers are known to be under enormous physical, emotional and economic stress when living and caring for someone with dementia.

There are many risk factors that can lead to psychological and mental health issues throughout the life cycle. However, older people must deal with additional stressor, such as, progressive loss in capacity and reduction in functional abilities. From a physical perspective, they may need to contend with reduced mobility, chronic pain and other physical health problems. Therefore, it is important to address psychosocial factors as these can lead to isolation and loneliness, impairing quality of life.

Depression is another mental health problem that is commonly seen in older people. Depressive symptoms can have a major impact on health status and the quality of life of older people. There are two types of factors that are associated with the onset of depression in older people: those related to the pressure and stress of an older person's living environment, and those related to biological function in an older person. Reduced levels of neurotransmitters, such as serotonin and noradrenalin, can influence the communication between cells in the brain. The impact of a negative event in an older person's life, such as the loss of a partner, in combination with side effects of drugs that may be taken for a medical condition may lead to the development of symptoms of depression. Additionally, depression in older people increases the perception of poor health and the use of healthcare services (National Institute of Ageing, 2017).

Individuals with depressive symptoms usually have low mood, fatigue, sleep disruption and withdrawal from other people and activities that they previously enjoyed. These symptoms can go unnoticed or be viewed as a normal consequence of the ageing process. Indeed, around the world, depressive symptoms go undiagnosed and untreated, mainly as they can coexist and are associated with other age-related factors. One typical indicator of potential symptoms of depression might be the loss of interest in grandchildren. It should be noted that suffering from depressive symptoms is a significant predictor of suicide in older people. It has been estimated that up to 15% of older people with severe depression commit suicide (Mendoza, 2020). To reduce the impact of depression and the suicidal risk in older people, interventions aimed to improve mental health and psychological well-being of older people is merited. Early detection and management of depressive symptoms can reduce these self-destructive actions. Psychological well-being in older people is associated with many factors including, diet, well-being, social support and loneliness (Grønning et al., 2018).

12.4 Health Literacy in Older People

Another factor associated with psychological health in older people is the influence of health literacy. In this section, emphasis will be placed on the impact that health literacy can have in older people. Health literacy involves the use of a range of skills that can improve the ability to act on health-related information to maximise health. The skills of health literacy include writing, listening, speaking, numeracy and critical analysis. Health literacy is a fairly complex concept, which has been defined as 'the degree to which individuals have the capacity to obtain, process and understand basic health information and services to make appropriate health decision' (U.S. Department of Health and Human Services, 2010). From a psychological perspective, age-related changes in health literacy have been explained in terms of differences in cognitive abilities including, speed of thought processes, closely aligned with the traditional theories of ageing and comprehension (Wingfield & Stine-Morrow, 2000).

Older people are far more likely to have limited health literacy, compromising physical and psychological health outcomes (Paasche-Orlow et al., 2005). Low levels of health literacy are known to be a problem. In older people, poor health literacy has been associated with sub-optimal levels of health and critical health outcomes, such as compliance with treatment regimes, medication adherence and self-care capacity. In one large cohort survey study, Panagioti et al. (2018) identified several studies that directly linked limited health literacy with low health status and poor quality of life.

Unfortunately, these older people with low health literacy commonly report low health status, which is potentially problematic as they require reliable and up-to-date health information to prevent disease development and to maximise their health and wellness. Although the cognitive capacity and cognitive ageing varies from one older person to another, the higher order cognitive processes required for health literacy tend to decline with age. To be a health literate older person, the skills of understanding, comparing, reasoning, numeracy and synthesising need to be demonstrated. Worryingly, the National Assessment of Adult Literacy (NAAL) in United States reported that 71% of adults over the age of 60 years had difficulty using print materials, 80% struggled to use forms and charts and 68% had difficult with numeracy (NAAL, 2016). These figures are quite alarming, as older adults use more health services and acquire more chronic illnesses than other age groups. This problem has been exemplified by the COVID-19 pandemic, Brørs et al. (2020) raised concerns about the impact of COVID-19, particularly in older people with multiple comorbidities. Older people could easily become overwhelmed by the infodemic that has accompanied the pandemic, which could lead to greater uncertainties, distress and problems with health-related decision-making (Rathore & Farooq, 2020). Based in Hong Kong, Leung et al. (2021) advocated the importance of digital health literacy. This involves the capacity to understand and apply health-related information from electronic resources.

Getting older is not in itself an obstacle to using the internet or other forms of computer-based technology, like telemedicine services. An increasing number of older people are using the internet where vast amount of health-related information is available, although caution needs to be taken about the reliability and trustworthiness of some of this information. To enhance the use of internet and computer services, health-related websites need to be specifically developed to be accessible to older people. Providing a user-friendly resource that take into consideration age-related changes in vision and cognition. Failure to do so may affect computer use for older people in several ways including working memory, perceptual speed, text comprehension and spatial memory to deal with these issues and potentially help improve health literacy in older adults. All forms of health-related information could be made more accessible to older people by using an appropriate typeface, writing style, navigational structure and accessibility. Moreover, we should not take it for granted that touch screen can be easily used by elderly. Digital exclusion has left 5.6 million UK elderly behind due to loss of moisture from skin as touch screen requires fingers to conduct electricity (mHealth, 2021). Attention to these issues may help to counteract natural age-related changes to have digital inclusion for the aged (Ageing Better, 2021).

Caregivers, both formal and informal, should ensure that they have the skills to help to influence the health-related decisions that older people may face. Older people can encounter complex health situations that may involve some degree of trade-offs when they make decisions, as such, it is vitally important that they are adequately informed. Healthcare professionals must listen to the wishes of older people, as they may choose health options that are most suited to their personal values and beliefs.

Around the world, healthcare professionals should not only be aware of the potential problems associated with limited health literacy in older people, but they should also be able to actively try to remedy the situation. Unlike socio-demographic characteristics, like age and ethnicity, which are mostly fixed, there is good evidence to suggest that levels of health literacy can be modified in older people (Nutbeam, 2000). Health literacy interventions, like educational programmes, can directly tackle the cognitive difficulties which may limit the ability to access and understand health-related information. To date, most interventions for improving levels of health literacy in older people have focused on reducing the cognitive demands, usually involving increasing the readability of materials or to ensure that assistance is being provided by healthcare staff. All healthcare professionals working with older people should have an awareness of simple approaches that can be implemented to address health literacy deficits, including using plain terms when communicating and simplifying health-related information (Sudore & Schillinger, 2009). Providing attention to these very basic requirements may be effective to facilitate the understanding of older people, potentially enhancing empowerment (Speros, 2011). Morrow (2006) reported that older adults with limited health literacy had a greater understanding and preferred information that was designed to, where possible, reduce comprehension demands. He strongly advocated the application of a patient-centred approach to communication, when dealing with health literacy issues in older people. Patient-centred approaches focus on identifying an individual's knowledge, motivation, and skills to gain, comprehend and apply health-related information. From this perspective, low health literacy can be seen a potential barrier to patient-centred approaches. As health service providers around the world move to a more person-centred approach to care, proactive planning by healthcare professionals is essential in low health literacy associated with cognitive deterioration.

12.5 The Facilitators of Longevity

In the ancient history of mankind, different leaders of various centuries have been looking at ways how to live longer. China's first emperor Qin Shihuang of the 'Qin' Dynasty was well-known for his nationwide hunt for the mythical potion for elixir of life (BBC, 2017). Contemporary research and studies are focusing on both macro and micro level of factors to achieve longevity. Buettner (2012, 2017) analysed the lessons from people who have lived the longest and happiest people from the 'Blue Zones' including Barbagia region of Sardinia, Ikaria of Greece, Nicoya Peninsula of Costa Rica, Seventh Day Adventists in Loma Linda of California and Okinawa of Japan. Nine factors for longevity have been identified, including 'Move Naturally', 'Purpose', 'Downshift', 'The 80 Percent Rule', 'Plant Slant', 'Wine @ 5', 'Belong', 'Loved Ones First' and 'Right Tribe' in his 'Power9' model. This model stresses the importance of social relatedness and friendship which are crucial in the pursuit of happiness and longevity. A community-wide approach to improve well-being is being implemented in US cities under the Blue Zones Project (Blue Zones, 2021). Another school of thoughts have looked into micro cellular level such as how senescent cells, gut microbiome, genetics as well as fasting can contribute to the biological process to slow down the ageing processes (Dinicolantonio & Fung, 2019; Sinclair & LaPlante, 2019; van Deursen, 2014; Wilmanski et al., 2021; Young, 2021). Literature about the keywords of ‘longevity’, ‘healthy aging’, ‘productive ageing’, ‘positive ageing’ and so on are adding to the volume of knowledge on a regular basis.

Although Hong Kong has the highest life expectancy in the world, aged people are not necessarily healthy and happy. Researchers are trying to understand what are the contributing factors for longevity in Hong Kong. On one hand, the dense and compact environment with relatively easy access to healthcare facilities in primary care level and above including emergency services has contributed to save life with quick medical attention. The design of built environment of residential blocks and districts have facilitated a closer neighbourhood in community and the nature movement of exercises when they are shopping at nearby market or relaxing at nearby playgrounds with facilities for elderly. Hong Kong has also taken great measures to curb smoking and all public places such as restaurants are banned from smoking. Regarding diet, traditional Chinese diet recipes are common with steamed dishes and fresh vegetables. Chinese herbs are being used for treatment and cooking which is conducive to good health (Chung & Marmot, 2020; EIU, 2021; SCMP, 2019).

12.6 Summary

Unlimited lifespan is not a possible phenomenon of human mankind. Researchers are trying to look into the reasons why some people in some localities are living longer and healthier than the others. Scientists around the globe are investigating into products and intervention strategies to reserve ageing to archive longevity. Business corporations are tapping into the big commercial market internationally. There is still a way forward to integrate various schools of thoughts in an evidence-based manner for the benefits of the society especially in the era of the ‘New Normal’ affected by COVID-19. The integration of the traditional wisdom and new cutting-edge science seems to be the panacea of the mythical potion that Emperor Qin hunted for.

References

Ageing Better. (2021). *Digital inclusion.* https://www.ageing-better.org.uk/digital-inclusion

Alzheimer’s Disease International. (2020). *Dementia statistics.* https://www.alzint.org/about/dementia-facts-figures/dementia-statistics/

BBC. (2017). *How China’s first emperor searched for elixir of life.* https://morokbarok.ru/news/world-asia-china-42477083

Blue Zones. (2021). *Blue zones project.* https://www.bluezones.com/services/blue-zones-project/

Brørs, G., Norman, C. D., & Norekvål, T. M. (2020). Accelerated importance of eHealth literacy in the COVID-19 outbreak and beyond. *European Journal of Cardiovascular Nursing, 19*(6), 458–461. https://doi.org/10.1177/1474515120941307

Buettner, D. (2012). *Blue zones* (2nd ed.). Random House Publisher Services.

Buettner, D. (2017). *The blue zones of happiness: Lessons from the world’s happiest people.* National Geographic Partners LLC.

Chung, R. Y., & Sir Marmot, M. (2020). People in Hong Kong have the longest life expectancy in the world: Some possible explanations. NAM perspectives. *Commentary, National Academy of Medicine*. https://doi.org/10.31478/202001d

DiNicolantonio, J., & Fung, J. (2019). *The longevity solution: Rediscovering centuries-old secrets to a healthy, long life*. Victory Belt Publishing.

EIU. (2021). *Productive ageing in Hong Kong: Breaking the mould of ageing*. The Economist Intelligence Unit. https://eiuperspectives.economist.com/financial-services/productive-ageing-hong-kong-breaking-mould-ageing

Finkel, T., & Holbrook, N. J. (2000). Oxidants, oxidative stress and the biology of ageing. *Nature, 408*, 239–247. https://doi.org/10.1038/35041687

Grønning, K., Espnes, G. A., Nguyen, C., Rodrigues, A. M. F., Gregorio, M. J., Sousa, R., Canhão, H., & André, B. (2018). Psychological distress in elderly people is associated with diet, wellbeing, health status, social support and physical functioning—A HUNT3 study. *BMC Geriatrics, 18*(1), 205. https://doi.org/10.1186/s12877-018-0891-3

Infoplease. (2021). *Life expectancy for countries*. https://www.infoplease.com/world/health-and-social-statistics/life-expectancy-countries

Kirkwood, T. B. L. (2011). Systems biology of ageing and longevity. *Philosophical Transactions of the Royal Society B, 366*(1561), 64–70. https://doi.org/10.1098/rstb.2010.0275

Leung, A., Parial, L., Tolabing, M., Sim, T., Mo, P., Okan, O., & Dadaczynski, K. (2021). Sense of coherence mediates the relationship between digital health literacy and anxiety about the future in aging population during the COVID-19 pandemic: A path analysis. *Aging & Mental Health*. https://doi.org/10.1080/13607863.2020.1870206

Li, W. (2014). Geropsychology, overview. In T. Teo (Eds.), *Encyclopedia of critical psychology*. Springer. https://doi.org/10.1007/978-1-4614-5583-7_405

López-Otin, C., Blasco, M. A., Serrano, M., & Kroemer, G. (2013). The hallmarks of ageing. *Cell, 153*, 1194–1217. https://doi.org/10.1016/j.cell.2013.05.039

Mathers, J. C., Deary, I. J., Kuh, D., Lord, J. M., Khaw, K.-T., Lara, J., Nussan, J., Cooper, R., & Ginty, A. (2012). *Guidelines for biomarkers of healthy ageing*. Medical Research Council.

Mendoza, M. (2020). Why do the elderly commit suicide? *Psychology Today*. https://www.psychologytoday.com/intl/blog/understanding-grief/202001/why-do-the-elderly-commit-suicide

mHealth. (2021). *Digital exclusion: New research reveals how touchscreen future leaves 5.6 million elderly behind. The Journal of mHealth*. https://d1h06bsnqv2xsg.cloudfront.net/Images/DigitalExclusion_Report_NoIsolation_Jul2021.pdf

Morrow, D. (2006). *Mitigating the impact of low health literacy on older adults' self-care*. American Psychological Association. https://www.apa.org/science/about/psa/2006/10/morrow

NAAL. (2016). *Demographics*. National Assessment of Adult Literacy. https://nces.ed.gov/naal/kf_demographics.asp

National Institute of Ageing. (2017). *Depression and older adults*. https://www.nia.nih.gov/health/depression-and-older-adults

Nutbeam, D. (2000). Health literacy as a public health goal: A challenge for contemporary health education and communication strategies into the 21st century. *Health Promotion International, 15*(3), 259–267. https://doi.org/10.1093/heapro/15.3.259

Paasche-Orlow, M. K., Parker, R. M., Gazmararian, J. A., Nielsen-Bohlman, L. T., & Rudd, R. R. (2005). The prevalence of limited health literacy. *Journal of General Internal Medicine, 20*(2), 175–184. https://doi.org/10.1111/j.1525-1497.2005.40245.x

Panagioti, M., Skevington, S. M., Hann, M., Howells, K., Blakemore, A., Reeves, D., & Bower, P. (2018). Effect of health literacy on the quality of life of older patients with long-term conditions: A large cohort study in UK general practice. *Quality of Life Research, 27*(5), 1257–1268. https://doi.org/10.1007/s11136-017-1775-2

Partridge, L. (2010). The new biology of ageing. *Philosophical Transactions of the Royal Society B, 365*(1537), 147–154. https://doi.org/10.1098/rstb.2009.0222

Pignolo, R. J. (2019). Exceptional human longevity. *Mayo Clinic Proceedings, 94*(1), 110–124. https://doi.org/10.1016/j.mayocp.2018.10.005

Punt, D. (2020). *The world's oldest people and their secrets to a long life.* https://www.guinnessworldrecords.com/news/2020/10/the-worlds-oldest-people-and-their-secrets-to-a-long-life-632895

Rathore, F. A., & Farooq, F. (2020). Information overload and infodemic in the COVID-19 pandemic. *Journal of the Pakistan Medical Association, 70*(5), S162–S165. https://doi.org/10.5455/JPMA.38

Schanzenbach, D. W., Nunn, R., & Bauer, L. (2016). *The changing landscape of American life expectancy.* https://www.hamiltonproject.org/papers/the_changing_landscape_of_american_life_expectancy

SCMP. (2019). *Hong Kong has the highest life expectancy in the world—What is the secret behind it?* https://www.scmp.com/magazines/post-magazine/long-reads/article/3034349/hong-kong-has-highest-life-expectancy-world-what

Sinclair, D., & LaPlante, M. (2019). *Lifespan: The revolutionary science of why we age—And why we don't have to.* Atria Books.

Speros, C. (2011). Promoting health literacy: A nursing imperative. *Nursing Clinics of North America, 46*(3), 321–333. https://doi.org/10.1016/j.cnur.2011.05.007

Stowe, J. D., & Cooney, T. M. (2015). Examining Rowe and Kahn's concept of successful aging: Importance of taking a life course perspective. *The Gerontologist, 55*(1), 43–50. https://doi.org/10.1093/geront/gnu055

Sudore, R., & Schillinger, D. (2009). Interventions to improve care for patients with limited health literacy. *Journal of Clinical Outcomes Management, 16*(1), 20–29.

U.S. Department of Health and Human Services. (2010). *National action plan to improve health literacy.* Office of Disease Prevention and Health Promotion. https://health.gov/sites/default/files/2019-09/Health_Literacy_Action_Plan.pdf

UW News. (2021). *How long can a person live? The 21st century may see a record-breaker.* https://www.washington.edu/news/2021/07/01/how-long-can-a-person-live-the-21st-century-may-see-a-record-breaker/

van Deursen, J. M. (2014). The role of senescent cells in ageing. *Nature, 509*, 439–446. https://doi.org/10.1038/nature13193

Wilmanski, T., Diener, C., Rappaport, N., Patwardhan, S., Wiedrick, J., Lapidus, J., Earls, J. C., Zimmer, A., Glusman, G., Robinson, M., Yurkovich, J. T., Kado, D. M., Cauley, J. A., Zmuda, J., Lane, N. E., Magis, A. T., Lovejoy, J. C., Hood, L., Gibbons, S. M., … Price, N. D. (2021). Gut microbiome pattern reflects healthy ageing and predicts survival in humans. *Nature Metabolism, 3*, 274–286. https://doi.org/10.1038/s42255-021-00348-0

Wingfield, A., & Stine-Morrow, E. A. L. (2000). Language and speech. In F. I. M. Craik & T. A. Salthouse (Eds.), *The handbook of aging and cognition* (pp. 359–416). Lawrence Erlbaum Associates Publishers.

Wong, S., Zhang, D., Sit, R., Yip, B., Chung, R., Wong, C., Chan, D., Kwok, W., & Mercer, S. (2020). Impact of COVID-19 on loneliness, mental health, and health service utilisation: A prospective cohort study of older adults with multimorbidity in primary care. *British Journal of General Practice, 70*(700), e817–e824. https://doi.org/10.3399/bjgp20X713021

World Health Organization. (2020). *Dementia.* https://www.who.int/news-room/fact-sheets/detail/dementia

World Health Organization. (2021). *Ageing and health.* https://www.who.int/news-room/fact-sheets/detail/ageing-and-health

Young, S. (2021). *The science and technology of growing young: An insider's guide to the breakthroughs that will dramatically extend our lifespan . . . and what you can do right now.* BenBella Books, Inc.

Chapter 13
Social Determinants of Health and Dignity

Hongjiang Wu and Katy N. W. Wong

Abstract Social determinants of health are the social and economic conditions in which people are born, grow, live, work and age that affects individual's health outcomes. A wide range of social factors such as education, poverty, employment and social support have been shown to play an important role in health outcomes, although they have no direct biological connection to diseases. Social factors influence the onset and progression of diseases, and premature death through their effects on health-related behaviours, access to healthcare, and environmental exposures, all of which are considered as the upstream determinants of people's health as well as life expectancy. An inverse relationship between socioeconomic status and morbidity and mortality has been well documented. Given the long-term effects of social factors, beginning in childhood and progressively accumulating over time across the entire lifetime, the health gaps between socioeconomic groups widen with age and peak in ageing. Towards the goal of elongating life expectancy with health and dignity, it is important to understand the role of social factors in health and to determine whether health inequities can be reduced with ageing. This chapter will introduce the concept of social determinants of health, describe the mechanisms linking social factors and health outcomes with emphasis on social inequities in health among the older adults, and the key challenges and ways forward in achieving successful ageing from the perspective of social factor will be identified.

Keywords Social determinants · Health equities · Elderly · Successful ageing

H. Wu
The Chinese University of Hong Kong, Hong Kong, China
e-mail: hongjiangwu@cuhk.edu.hk

K. N. W. Wong (✉)
Hong Kong College of Community Health Practitioners, Hong Kong, China

V. T. S. Law and B. Y. F. Fong (eds.), *Ageing with Dignity in Hong Kong and Asia*, Quality of Life in Asia 16, https://doi.org/10.1007/978-981-19-3061-4_13

13.1 Concept of Social Determinants of Health and Health Inequities

In the last two decades, growing evidence has demonstrated a significant role of social factors in affecting health outcomes beyond healthcare (Lynch et al., 1997; Marmot et al., 1984). The World Health Organization established the Commission on Social Determinants of Health (CSDH) in 2005 to support countries to deal with the social factors that lead to ill health and health inequities. The CSDH defines the social determinants of health as the conditions in which people are born, grow, live, work and age (World Health Organization, 2008). These circumstances are non-medical factors that affect a variety of health, functioning and quality-of-life outcomes and risks. The social determinants of health include a wide range of social factors such as education, income, employment, physical environment, social support, health systems and services and public safety.

The concept of health inequities was initially defined by Margaret Whitehead in the early 1990s that differences in health '*are not only unnecessary and avoidable but, in addition, are considered unfair and unjust*' (Whitehead, 1992). Later, the International Society for Equity in Health defined equity in health as '*the absence of potential remediable, systematic differences in one or more aspects of health across socially, economically, demographically, or geographically defined population groups or subgroups*' (Macinko & Starfield, 2002). Nowadays, health inequities generally refer to unfair, avoidable and disparities in health status or in the distribution of health resources between different populations based on population characteristics defined socially, economically, geographically or demographically (Braveman, 2006). These characteristics can be age, gender, race/ethnicity, social and economic factors, geographic location and sexual orientation. For example, racial and ethnic minorities systematically appear to receive lower-quality healthcare and have a higher risk of morbidity and mortality than non-minorities in the United States (Bailey et al., 2017). The causes of health inequities are diverse and complex. Health inequities often arise from poor governance, corruption, or cultural exclusion and have huge adverse effects on both individuals and society (Kawachi et al., 2002).

13.2 Measures of Social Determinants of Health

The social determinants of health include many social factors. In accordance with the U.S. Department of Health and Human Services, these factors can be categorised into five broad categories, including education access and quality, healthcare access and quality, neighbourhood and built environment, economic stability, and social and community context (Fig. 13.1). These five domains of social determinants of health are interrelated and can be affected by each other.

Stability in the economy, the first domain, is the connection between a person's financial resources and his or her ability to access resources essential to a healthy

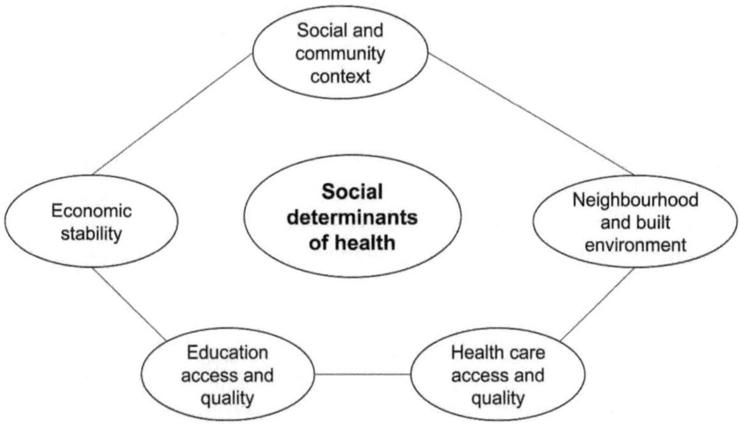

Fig. 13.1 The five domains of social determinants of health

lifestyle. It includes employment, poverty/income, food security and housing stability. Among these, employment is the key factor in the economic stability domain and is directly related to other indicators. People with better employment status often have a higher income level, have less likelihood to live in poverty and more likelihood to afford to eat properly and live safely.

The education access and quality domain include educating children at an early age, registering in higher education and advancing in language and literacy. Education has been shown as the most important modifiable social determinant of health. It predicts both future employment opportunities and earning potential and also reflects family characteristics. Many studies have shown that people with a higher educational level have better health-related behaviours, which are strongly linked to development and progression of health conditions (Wu et al., 2018).

The healthcare access and quality domain include health literacy, access to primary care, and access to healthcare. It reflects the ability to access to healthcare services, to understand and utilise health information and services to make appropriate health-related decisions and actions to improve health. There are many barriers affecting healthcare access and quality, such as lack of health insurance coverage, limited or no transportation access to healthcare providers, limited health literacy for health-related decision making.

The neighbourhood and built environment domain include access to healthy foods, crime and violence and conditions in the environment. The neighbourhoods where people live affect health and well-being of the residents because they are related to quality of air and water, pollution and other risks of health and safety.

Civic participation and discrimination are included in the domain of social and community context (e.g. racial discrimination), incarceration and social cohesion. It reflects the relationships of people's social environment and social activities with health resource allocation and health outcomes, such as social support, family circumstances and community engagement.

13.3 Relationship Between Social Factors and Health Inequities

Social determinants of health are considered as the fundamental causes of health inequities (World Health Organization, 2010). Social factors importantly contribute to wide health disparities and inequities and affect almost everyone in the society. Health and health-related outcomes follow a social gradient. There is consistent evidence that disadvantaged populations with lower socioeconomic status often have worse health outcomes in both communicable and non-communicable diseases and have poorer survival chances.

Social factors have profound effects on a wide range of non-communicable diseases, for example, cardiovascular disease (Clark et al., 2009), diabetes (Agardh et al., 2011; Wu et al., 2019), obesity (McLaren, 2007), hypertension (Leng et al., 2015), cancer (Bristow et al., 2013) and mortality (Stringhini et al., 2017), with different strengths and directions in different populations. For example, in the Prospective Urban Rural Epidemiologic (PURE) study which included participants from 20 countries, results show that compared to people received college or university education, those who received none or only primary education had 23, 59, and 123% increased risk of developing major cardiovascular events in high-income countries, middle-income countries and low-income countries, respectively (Rosengren et al., 2019). A meta-analysis including 23 studies shows that compared to people with high levels of educational level, occupation and income, those with low levels of these determinants had 41%, 31%, 40% increased risk of developing type 2 diabetes respectively (Agardh et al., 2011). In Hong Kong people with diabetes, those receive university education had 30% lower risk of all-cause mortality compared to those who only receive primary school education (Wu et al., 2018). In India, it has been reported that the infant mortality is more than two-fold higher in the poorest wealth quintile compared to those in the richest wealth quintile (Balarajan et al., 2011). Moreover, the direction of the association between social factors and some non-communicable diseases may differ across countries which are at different stages of epidemiological transition. For instance, a systematic review finds that in developing countries people with a higher socioeconomic status have a higher risk of obesity, while in developed countries those with a low socioeconomic status tends to increase the incidence of obesity (McLaren, 2007).

Social factors also greatly influence communicable diseases. During the COVID-19 pandemic, both the incidence rate of COVID-19 and morality rate due to COVID-19 in the United States were substantially higher in African American/black and Latino than white individuals (Hooper et al., 2020). Similarly, in the United Kingdom, minority groups including black and south Asian groups were also at a higher risk of COVID-19 infection compared to the white British (Niedzwiedz et al., 2020). Data from the United States show that between 1987 and 1993, the incidence rate of tuberculosis increased uniformly with the decreasing socioeconomic status measured by any of income, education, employment, poverty, public assist or crowding (Cantwell et al., 1998). Furthermore, data from Asian also show that poverty increased the risk of a number of disease including tuberculosis, malaria and HIV/AIDS particularly in low-income countries (Bishwajit et al., 2014).

Marked social gradients in health exist not only within but also between countries. From a global perspective, the life expectancy is generally higher in countries with a higher level of gross domestic product (GDP) per capita (Linden & Ray, 2017). Worldwide, the life expectancy at birth in 2019 ranged between 53 years in Central African Republic (GDP per capita = 478 US dollars) and 85 years in Hong Kong (GDP per capita = 48,713 US dollars) (The World Bank, 2020). Human Development Index, which is a composite measure of a country's education, per capita income and income, significantly predicts the under-five child mortality rates across countries (Khazaei et al., 2016). Therefore, the social determinants of health are regarded as playing a key role in determining health inequities within and between countries by the World Health Organization (World Health Organization, 2011).

13.4 Mechanisms Linking Social Factors and Health

The mechanisms linking social factors and health outcomes are complex and multi-factorial. Although no direct biological connection to disease, social factors influence health outcomes mainly through their effects on health-related behaviours, access to healthcare and environmental exposure (Adler & Newman, 2002).

Social factors are highly linked to an individual's health-related behaviours, such as smoking, drinking, diet, physical activity, health seeking behaviours and medical treatment compliance. These health-related behaviours are major risk/protective factors for non-communicable diseases, which vary substantially across people with different levels of socioeconomic status and account for about 80% of premature mortality worldwide (Lee & Paxman, 1997). Globally, the prevalence of smoking is often high among people who are unemployed, homeless, less educated and minorities (Hiscock et al., 2012). For example, a survey in 11 countries of the European Union in 1998 shows that the prevalence of smoking was 40% among people with the lowest education as compared to 22% among those with the highest education (Huisman et al., 2005). In China, studies finds that people with low levels of education or socioeconomic status were more likely to use tobacco and start smoking at a younger age (Cai et al., 2019). Data from England and Wales, United States, Canada and Poland indicate that smoking-attributed mortality is estimated to be responsible for nearly half of the social disparities in death rates among men aged 35 to 69 years (Jha et al., 2006). Greater consumption of fruit and vegetables and healthy eating habits have been observed among people with higher socioeconomic status (De Irala-Estevez et al., 2000; Rydén & Hagfors, 2011).

Social factors are important determinants of access to, use, and quality of healthcare. People in poverty are less likely to have health insurance coverage and thus are often unable to afford out-of-pocket healthcare costs. In countries, where universal health coverage has not been established, affordability has been found to be the most important reason for not seeking for healthcare among people who reported an illness (Balabanova et al., 2004). Nevertheless, financial barriers do not fully explain the differences in use of healthcare among people with ill conditions. Studies have found that better education and health literacy are associated with greater use of healthcare services, including participating in disease screening programme, routine physical examination and other preventive activities (Vandenbosch et al., 2016). In a systematic review of 96 studies, a low level of health literacy has consistently been associated with lower flu vaccine rates, poorer adherence to medical treatments, and difficulty understanding health messages (Berkman et al., 2011).

Social factors drive an individual's exposure to both health-related social and physical environment. Social environment, including network of personal social relationships and community-level social characteristics, may influence health through providing informational and tangible resources that promote adaptive behaviours or neuroendocrine responses to illness. On the other hand, social environment may also affect health through its direct cognitive, emotional, behavioural and biological effects. Mortality risk has been reported to be 50% higher among people who are socially isolated than those with better social relationships (Holt-Lunstad et al., 2010). In addition to social environment, people interact with their physical environment to affect health. More disadvantaged groups are more likely to be exposed to air and water pollution, work and live closer to toxic sites but far away from healthcare facilities.

13.5 Health Inequities in the Elderly

With the improvement in quality of healthcare and living conditions, the proportion of elderly people has increased significantly not only in high-income countries but also in some middle-and low-income counties. According to estimates that between 2015 and 2050, the number of people over 60 years old will double from 10 to 20% (World Health Organization, 2018). Asia is also ageing fast that 16% of Asian population is estimated to be older than 65 years by 2040 (United Nations, 2020).

The process of ageing is a major risk factor of poor health that the prevalence of majority non-communicable diseases increases with increasing age, such as diabetes, cancer, cardiovascular disease, Alzheimer's disease, arthritis and so on. The World Health Organization defines healthy ageing or successful ageing as 'the process of developing and maintain functional ability that enables well-being in older age' (World Health Organization, 2017). Elderly people are one of the most vulnerable groups who are significantly affected by health inequities. According to the accumulation hypothesis, health inequities in old age often reflect accumulated disadvantage (Singh-Manoux et al., 2004). The long-term effects of social factors begin in early stage of life and progressively accumulate over time across the entire lifetime. As a result, low socioeconomic conditions and ageing additively accumulate to produce poor health that the health gaps between socioeconomic groups widen with age and peak in ageing. For example, a study based on participants from British civil servants show that people from lower occupational grades had a more rapidly deterioration in physical health with ageing compared with those from higher grades (Chandola et al., 2007). In another nationally representative study in Great Britain, the results show that social inequities in health vary over the life course (Sacker et al., 2005). There were no social inequities in health detected among young people aged 21 years, but the health inequities emerged later in life with the gap between people with different levels of socioeconomic status widening between ages 40 and 59 years. A study in China using data from a nationally representative survey covering 31 provinces and including 1 million people showed that health differentials increased with age both by education and by income (Lowry & Xie, 2009). Given the divergence of health inequities with age, addressing health inequities in the elderly has been among the highest priority for the care of the ageing population and is a key indicator of successful ageing.

13.6 Key Challenges to Successful Ageing from Social Factor Perspective

13.6.1 Diversity

Many countries in the world are familiar with the fact that the population is ageing, but only a few are aware that it is becoming more diverse as a result (Fong et al., 2020; World Health Organization, 2018). It is partly due to the amount of time people have had to develop their distinctive individuality. It may also be a result of inequities that have accumulated thus far over the life span of a person which are now contributing to the disparities in later life (Daatland & Biggs, 2006). Increasing research evidences confirm that exposure to multiple factors over an individual's lifetime, including differences in health, environmental and societal factors, shapes an individual's initial health status as well as their health pathways and outcomes as they age (Sadana et al., 2016). Social disadvantages can accumulate with associated health consequences over an individual's lifetime which makes it hard to overcome (Goodman et al., 2011; Woolf & Aron, 2013).

Taking into account the diverse needs of the ageing population and the fundamental inequities developed over one's life course, it is important that policies are developed in a holistic approach that can cater the needs of individual elderly and at the same time to identify areas for action throughout the life course to address the contributing factors for enhancing healthy ageing and equity (World Health Organization, 2018).

13.6.2 Social, Biological and Behavioural Interplay

What is more is that the determinants of health are also determined by interactions between social, biological and behavioural factors (Institute of Medicine, 2001). In recent decades, increased attention has been given to the reciprocal interactions among health factors, biological factors, social risk factors and behavioural factors over time.

Nevertheless, our healthcare systems often fall into the loophole to provide solely clinical care to patients (Daniel et al., 2018). Research has revealed that segregating healthcare from its social context produces segregating outcomes in patient care. For example, the blood sugar level of a diabetic man who is under doctor's care may drop dramatically due to not having enough food, or a woman with asthma may take her medicine but end up in the hospital because the apartment she lives in is filled with mould. The examples illustrate how a disease situation may occur outside of a clinical context and thus be made worse by factors outside the normal medical training. Multiple disciplines should be coordinated and interacted to understand the influence of social determinants of health in addition to the clinical preventive efforts and medical management (Institute of Medicine, 2001).

13.6.3 Across Groups, Populations and Even Generations

An attempt was made by Sadana et al. (2016) to better understand the pathways that contribute to health inequities by taking into account four blocks of contributing factors that contribute towards differences in health between older adults, namely the natural-socioeconomic-political environment, genetic inheritance and socioeconomic status, intermediary determinants and outcomes related to healthy ageing. The framework tried to identify the root causes and explain levels and distributions observed in each block of the model for their effect contributing to health inequalities and inequities and emphasises that all underlying determinants at each level are susceptible to policy change. Over time, individuals are found to exercise a powerful impact on stratification patterns and, consequently, people's chances for health. According to Solar and Irwin (2007), the key feature of health inequities is their impact across the life course and the diversity of health across groups, populations and even generations. Consequently, the context embraces a wide range of structural, cultural, natural and functional features of a society that pose challenges to policymakers in making the right decisions to reduce health inequities.

13.6.4 Ageist Stereotypes

While it is evident that ageing is becoming more diverse and we are being forced to recognise its heterogeneous nature, countervailing attempts are being made to foster understanding and decrease stereotyping of the older population. The ageing process is accompanied by a series of social expectations that may or may not correspond to their actual circumstances or individual potentials (Daatland & Biggs, 2006). Societal perceptions of older people often include frailty, dependence or declining health, or somehow a burden on others (Daatland & Biggs, 2006). A view of such has identified ageism as a phenomenon that intersects class, gender and age, which is harming both the sense of self and the physical well-being of older people. Such a condition on negative stereotypes about ageing was described by Professor Becca Levy as a public health concern (Levy et al., 2002). There have been findings showing that elders who have negative perceptions of ageing are more likely to suffer from cardiac disease, have a shorter median life expectancy and have a lower likelihood of recovering from disability, memory, and cognition. Creating a supportive and enabling social environment for older adults is, therefore, crucial for fostering an age-friendly community (Ho, 2001; O'Brien, 2014).

13.6.5 Fair and Justice in Provision of Long-Term Care for Elderly

To reduce health inequities in old age, one of the approaches is to provide readily accessible healthcare to the old adults. This has however created the largest social challenges for the next decade to address the ageing population's increasing demands on healthcare systems, especially in providing long-term care (Zeeb et al., 2018). It is especially relevant for Hong Kong, which has the longest life expectancy across the globe. As per the latest data from the World Bank, Hong Kong females have an average life expectancy of 88 years old, and males are expected to live to 82. Thus, the quest of health equity prompts several challenges: In the first place, there are persistent inequities that are caused by a social gradient in health, while on the other hand, the limited number of resources will always lead to distributive justice challenges for society. Especially for older adults, fair and effective health and social services are of crucial importance, since they may have a more severe burden in disability than middle-aged populations. The circumstance that chronic diseases lead to most health conditions seen in older adults also underscores the importance of health prevention and promotion throughout the lifespan to alleviate the burden (Zeeb et al., 2018).

13.7 The Way Forward

Rather than simply improving the status of the well-off population, policies must target inequities as they appear across all social strata, not just those at the top or the average. Due to the way socioeconomic position impacts almost all aspects of the community, the elimination of health disparities and promotion of health equity by social determinants cannot be accomplished through a single policy or programme (Daniel et al., 2018). When it comes to solving social issues, different approaches and careful implementation are required to accommodate different demographic and socioeconomic groups. Without careful planning, actions could indirectly worsen social stigma, increase inequities and weaken solidarity. To promote healthy old age and reduce health inequities, it is necessary to: (a) take action inside, as well as outside of the health sector, including social care, environmental and economic policy; and (b) address the social determinants of health, the fundamental cause of health inequity (Sadana et al., 2016). Collaboration among key stakeholders, including doctors, health professionals, academics, politicians, taxpayers and the general public of different age groups and social backgrounds is imperative to advance the common goals and know their own roles better.

In the way forward, through identifying the components of biomedical causation, social determinants and life-course perspective, a multilevel, multidomain framework should be formed to highlight factors and pathways that are plausible as entry points to tackle health inequities. It is important to understand that health equity promotion should start as early as possible in early childhood development and education since many inequities in health are caused by the social gradient resulting in social and economic inequality since childhood. Considering data on education programmes for early childhood that supports their effectiveness for enhancing long-term health outcomes, and consideration of data on social and health outcomes, the Community Preventive Services Task Force (CPSTF) committee, U.S. Department of Health and Human Services, recommended early childhood education programmes as an entry point to promote equity and efficiency in public health (Ramon et al., 2018).

As it is well-documented that the social determinants of health evolve during the life course, physicians, who play a key role in provision of care, must develop a more in-depth awareness of social and environmental factors that influence a patient's adherence to treatment. The American College of Physicians advocates that social determinants of health and issues related to health inequities, which affect individuals, communities and systems, should be taught in medical education at all levels (Daniel et al., 2018). For better care provision and future research purposes, it is also important to incorporate social determinants of health into the health record so that researchers can conduct surveys to determine contributing factors to one's health and assess health inequities from a public health perspective for future research (Cantor & Thorpe, 2018).

The public also needs to be educated so a supportive attitude could be developed towards the elderly in order to avoid discrimination against ageing. According to Leedahl et al. (2020), addressing and improving age stereotyping should start in young adults. Improvement in attitudes and perceptions towards ageing, use of less negative descriptions and improved interest to engage in career that relates to older people in the future have been observed at the end of the participation in an intergenerational reverse mentoring programme.

One of the key factors in improving immediate health equity is through improving access to healthcare for vulnerable groups (Richard et al., 2016). In Hong Kong, financial assistance to needy patients is provided via the Samaritan Fund and Community Care Fund (Medical Assistance Programmes) with the philosophy that medical care should not be denied to anyone because of lack of means (Lee, 2019). Needy patients who are indicated for expensive medical items or new technologies that are not included by the standard fees and charges in public hospitals are entitled to apply the Funds. This significantly narrows the gap in access to healthcare in the rich and poor in the provision of expensive or standard treatment. This is however challenging for some health systems to remain publicly owned health services. For example, in Korea, there remains a challenge of healthcare access with a social insurance programme without adequate subsidies to the poor (less than 3% of the population receives medical assistance from tax-financed sources) (Jeon & Kwon, 2017). It is therefore becoming increasingly common for both developed and developing country governments to partner with the private sector in order to achieve their public policy goals. A growing body of evidence shows that these partnerships can improve healthcare access, quality, and efficiency. Partnerships should be initiated and evaluated, while the lessons should be shared widely to other countries to guide policymakers on how to apply this model effectively (Sekhri et al., 2011).

To conclude, as we move forward, the health sector must be a leader and a catalyst in various fields and contribute to align the goals and actions of other sectors. Research relating to implementation is fundamental to guiding realistic policy formulation and translating policy into tangible actions in the health sector as well as across other sectors. A great deal of work lies ahead, including agreeing on key concepts and definitions, understanding plausible pathways, as well as developing integrated multilateral and multisectoral approaches to engage older adults in healthy ageing with dignity.

References

Adler, N. E., & Newman, K. (2002). Socioeconomic disparities in health: Pathways and policies. *Health Affairs, 21*(2), 60–76. https://doi.org/10.1377/hlthaff.21.2.60

Agardh, E., Allebeck, P., Hallqvist, J., Moradi, T., & Sidorchuk, A. (2011). Type 2 diabetes incidence and socio-economic position: A systematic review and meta-analysis. *International Journal of Epidemiology, 40*(3), 804–818. https://doi.org/10.1093/ije/dyr029

Bailey, Z. D., Krieger, N., Agénor, M., Graves, J., Linos, N., & Bassett, M. T. (2017). Structural racism and health inequities in the USA: Evidence and interventions. *The Lancet, 389*, 1453–1463. https://doi.org/10.1016/S0140-6736(17)30569-X

Balabanova, D., Mckee, M., Pomerleau, J., Rose, R., & Haerpfer, C. (2004). Health service utilization in the former Soviet Union: Evidence from eight countries. *Health Services Research, 39*, 1927–1950. https://doi.org/10.1111/j.1475-6773.2004.00326.x

Balarajan, Y., Selvaraj, S., & Subramanian, S. V. (2011). Health care and equity in India. *The Lancet, 377*, 505–515. https://doi.org/10.1016/S0140-6736(10)61894-6
Berkman, N. D., Sheridan, S. L., Donahue, K. E., Halpern, D. J., & Crotty, K. (2011). Low health literacy and health outcomes: An updated systematic review. *Annals of Internal Medicine, 155*(2), 97–107. https://doi.org/10.7326/0003-4819-155-2-201107190-00005
Bishwajit, G., Ide, S., & Ghosh, S. (2014). Social determinants of infectious diseases in South Asia. *International Scholarly Research Notices, 2014*, 135243. https://doi.org/10.1155/2014/135243
Braveman, P. (2006). Health disparities and health equity: Concepts and measurement. *Annual Review of Public Health, 27*, 167–194. https://doi.org/10.1146/annurev.publhealth.27.021405.102103
Bristow, R. E., Powell, M. A., Al-Hammadi, N., Chen, L., Miller, J. P., Roland, P. Y., Mutch, D. G., & Cliby, W. A. (2013). Disparities in ovarian cancer care quality and survival according to race and socioeconomic status. *JNCI: Journal of the National Cancer Institute, 105*(11), 823–832. https://doi.org/10.1093/jnci/djt065
Cai, L., Wang, X. M., Fan, L. M., Cui, W. L., & Golden, A. R. (2019). Socioeconomic disparities in prevalence and behaviors of smoking in rural Southwest China. *BMC Public Health, 19*, 1117. https://doi.org/10.1186/s12889-019-7455-0
Cantor, M. N., & Thorpe, L. (2018). Integrating data on social determinants of health into electronic health records. *Health Affairs, 37*(4), 585–590. https://doi.org/10.1377/hlthaff.2017.1252
Cantwell, M. F., Mckenna, M. T., Mccray, E., & Onorato, I. M. (1998). Tuberculosis and race/ethnicity in the United States: Impact of socioeconomic status. *American Journal of Respiratory and Critical Care Medicine, 157*, 1016–1020. https://doi.org/10.1164/ajrccm.157.4.9704036
Chandola, T., Ferrie, J., Sacker, A., & Marmot, M. (2007). Social inequalities in self reported health in early old age: Follow-up of prospective cohort study. *BMJ, 334*, 990. https://doi.org/10.1136/bmj.39167.439792.55
Clark, A. M., Desmeules, M., Luo, W., Duncan, A. S., & Wielgosz, A. (2009). Socioeconomic status and cardiovascular disease: Risks and implications for care. *Nature Reviews Cardiology, 6*, 712–722. https://doi.org/10.1038/nrcardio.2009.163
Daatland, S. O., & Biggs, S. (2006). *Ageing and diversity: Multiple pathways and cultural migrations*. Policy Press.
Daniel, H., Bornstein, S. S., & Kane, G. C. (2018). Addressing social determinants to improve patient care and promote health equity: An American college of physicians position paper. *Annals of Internal Medicine, 168*(8), 577–578. https://doi.org/10.7326/M17-2441
De Irala-Estevez, J., Groth, M., Johansson, L., Oltersdorf, U., Prättälä, R., & Martínez-González, M. A. (2000). A systematic review of socio-economic differences in food habits in Europe: Consumption of fruit and vegetables. *European Journal of Clinical Nutrition, 54*, 706–714. https://doi.org/10.1038/sj.ejcn.1601080
Fong, B. Y. F., Law, V. T. S., & Lee, A. (2020). Primary care revisited: Interdisciplinary perspectives for a new era. *Springer Nature*. https://doi.org/10.1007/978-981-15-2521-6
Goodman, D. J. (2011). *Promoting diversity and social justice: Educating people from privileged groups*. Routledge.
Hiscock, R., Bauld, L., Amos, A., Fidler, J. A., & Munafò, M. (2012). Socioeconomic status and smoking: A review. *Annals of the New York Academy of Sciences, 1248*(1), 107–123. https://doi.org/10.1111/j.1749-6632.2011.06202.x
Ho, P. Y. A. (2001, May). *Creating A supportive environment for elderly with chronic illness* [Plenary presentation]. Healthy Ageing Convention, Hong Kong. https://www.elderlycommission.gov.hk/en/library/pdf/amy-ho.pdf
Holt-Lunstad, J., Smith, T. B., & Layton, J. B. (2010). Social relationships and mortality risk: A meta-analytic review. *PLOS Medicine, 7*(7), e1000316. https://doi.org/10.1371/journal.pmed.1000316
Hooper, M. W., Nápoles, A. M., & Pérez-Stable, E. J. (2020). COVID-19 and racial/ethnic disparities. *JAMA, 323*(24), 2466–2467. https://doi.org/10.1001/jama.2020.8598

Huisman, M., Kunst, A. E., & Mackenbach, J. P. (2005). Inequalities in the prevalence of smoking in the European Union: Comparing education and income. *Preventive Medicine, 40*(6), 756–764. https://doi.org/10.1016/j.ypmed.2004.09.022

Institute of Medicine. (2001). *Health and behavior: The interplay of biological, behavioral, and societal influences*. Washington, DC: The National Academies Press. https://doi.org/10.17226/9838

Jeon, B., & Kwon, S. (2017). Health and long-term care systems for older people in the republic of Korea: Policy challenges and lessons. *Health Systems & Reform, 3*(3), 214–223. https://doi.org/10.1080/23288604.2017.1345052

Jha, P., Peto, R., Zatonski, W., Boreham, J., Jarvis, M. J., & Lopez, A. D. (2006). Social inequalities in male mortality, and in male mortality from smoking: Indirect estimation from national death rates in England and Wales, Poland, and North America. *The Lancet, 368*(9533), 367–370. https://doi.org/10.1016/S0140-6736(06)68975-7

Kawachi, I., Subramanian, S. V., & Almeida-Filho, N. (2002). A glossary for health inequalities. *Journal of Epidemiology & Community Health, 56*, 647–652. https://doi.org/10.1136/jech.56.9.647

Khazaei, S., Ayubi, E., & Nematollahi, S. (2016). Variations of infant and under-five child mortality rates around the world, the role of human development index (HDI). *International Journal of Pediatrics, 4*(5), 1671–1677. https://doi.org/10.22038/ijp.2016.6730

Lee, P., & Paxman, D. (1997). Reinventing public health. *Annual Review of Public Health, 18*, 1–35. https://doi.org/10.1146/annurev.publhealth.18.1.1

Lee, V. F. (2019). Oncology healthcare provision in Hong Kong: Viewpoint of a clinical oncologist. *Clinical Oncology, 31*(8), 490–491. https://doi.org/10.1016/j.clon.2019.05.019

Leedahl, S. N., Brasher, M. S., Lobuono, D. L., Wood, B. M., & Estus, E. L. (2020). Reducing ageism: Changes in students' attitudes after participation in an intergenerational reverse mentoring program. *Sustainability, 12*(17), 6870. https://doi.org/10.3390/su12176870

Leng, B., Jin, Y., Li, G., Chen, L., & Jin, N. (2015). Socioeconomic status and hypertension: A meta-analysis. *Journal of Hypertension, 33*(2), 221–229. https://doi.org/10.1097/hjh.0000000000000428

Levy, B. R., Slade, M. D., Kunkel, S. R., & Kasl, S. V. (2002). Longevity increased by positive self-perceptions of aging. *Journal of Personality and Social Psychology, 83*(2), 261–270. https://doi.org/10.1037//0022-3514.83.2.261

Linden, M., & Ray, D. (2017). Aggregation bias-correcting approach to the health–income relationship: Life expectancy and GDP per capita in 148 countries, 1970–2010. *Economic Modelling, 61*, 126–136. https://doi.org/10.1016/j.econmod.2016.12.001

Lowry, D., & Xie, Y. (2009). *Socioeconomic status and health differentials in China: Convergence or divergence at older ages?* (No. 09–690). https://www.psc.isr.umich.edu/pubs/pdf/rr09-690.pdf

Lynch, J. W., Kaplan, G. A., & Shema, S. J. (1997). Cumulative impact of sustained economic hardship on physical, cognitive, psychological, and social functioning. *New England Journal of Medicine, 337*, 1889–1895. https://doi.org/10.1056/NEJM199712253372606

Macinko, J. A., & Starfield, B. (2002). Annotated bibliography on equity in health, 1980–2001. *International Journal for Equity in Health, 1*, 1. https://doi.org/10.1186/1475-9276-1-1

Marmot, M. G., Shipley, M. J., & Rose, G. (1984). Inequalities in death - Specific explanations of a general pattern? *The Lancet, 323*(8384), 1003–1006. https://doi.org/10.1016/S0140-6736(84)92337-7

Mclaren, L. (2007). Socioeconomic status and obesity. *Epidemiologic Reviews, 29*(1), 29–48. https://doi.org/10.1093/epirev/mxm001

O'brien, E. (2014). Planning for population ageing: Ensuring enabling and supportive physical-social environments–local infrastructure challenges. *Planning Theory & Practice, 15*(2), 220–234.https://doi.org/10.1080/14649357.2014.902986

Niedzwiedz, C. L., O'Donnell, C. A., Jani, B. D., Demou, E., Ho, F. K., Celis-Morales, C., et al. (2020). Ethnic and socioeconomic differences in SARS-CoV-2 infection: Prospective cohort study using UK Biobank. *BMC Medicine, 18*, 160. https://doi.org/10.1186/s12916-020-01640-8

Ramon, I., Chattopadhyay, S. K., Barnett, W. S., & Hahn, R. A. (2018). Early childhood education to promote health equity: A community guide economic review. *Journal of Public Health Management and Practice, 24*(1), e8–e15. https://doi.org/10.1097/PHH.0000000000000557

Richard, L., Furler, J., Densley, K., Haggerty, J., Russell, G., Levesque, J. F., & Gunn, J. (2016). Equity of access to primary healthcare for vulnerable populations: The impact international online survey of innovations. *International Journal for Equity in Health, 15*(64), 1–20. https://doi.org/10.1186/s12939-016-0351-7

Rosengren, A., Smyth, A., Rangarajan, S., Ramasundarahettige, C., Bangdiwala, S. I., Alhabib, K. F., et al. (2019). Socioeconomic status and risk of cardiovascular disease in 20 low-income, middle-income, and high-income countries: The Prospective Urban Rural Epidemiologic (PURE) study. *The Lancet Global Health, 7*(6), e748–e760. https://doi.org/10.1016/s2214-109x(19)30045-2

Rydén, P. J., & Hagfors, L. (2011). Diet cost, diet quality and socio-economic position: How are they related and what contributes to differences in diet costs? *Public Health Nutrition, 14*(9), 1680–1692. https://doi.org/10.1017/S1368980010003642

Sacker, A., Clarke, P., Wiggins, R. D., & Bartley, M. (2005). Social dynamics of health inequalities: A growth curve analysis of aging and self assessed health in the British household panel survey 1991–2001. *Journal of Epidemiology & Community Health, 59*(6), 495–501. https://doi.org/10.1136/jech.2004.026278

Sadana, R., Blas, E., Budhwani, S., Koller, T., & Paraje, G. (2016). Healthy ageing: Raising awareness of inequalities, determinants, and what could be done to improve health equity. *The Gerontologist, 56*(Suppl_2), S178-S193. https://doi.org/10.1093/geront/gnw034

Sekhri, N., Feachem, R., & Ni, A. (2011). Public-private integrated partnerships demonstrate the potential to improve health care access, quality, and efficiency. *Health Affairs, 30*(8), 1498–1507. https://doi.org/10.1377/hlthaff.2010.0461

Singh-Manoux, A., Ferrie, J. E., Chandola, T., & Marmot, M. (2004). Socioeconomic trajectories across the life course and health outcomes in midlife: Evidence for the accumulation hypothesis? *Internation Journal of Epidemiology, 33*(5), 1072–1079. https://doi.org/10.1093/ije/dyh224

Solar, O., & Irwin, A. (2007). *A conceptual framework for action on the social determinants of health.* https://www.who.int/social_determinants/resources/csdh_framework_action_05_07.pdf

Stringhini, S., Carmeli, C., Jokela, M., Avendaño, M., Muennig, P., Guida, F., ... & Tumino, R. (2017). Socioeconomic status and the 25 × 25 risk factors as determinants of premature mortality: A multicohort study and meta-analysis of 1.7 million men and women. *The Lancet, 389*(10075), 1229–1237. https://doi.org/10.1016/S0140-6736(16)32380-7

The World Bank. (2020). *Life expectancy at birth.* https://data.worldbank.org/indicator/SP.DYN.LE00.IN

United Nations. (2020). *World Population Ageing 2019* (ST/ESA/SER.A/444). https://www.un.org/en/development/desa/population/publications/pdf/ageing/WorldPopulationAgeing2019-Report.pdf

Vandenbosch, J., Van Den Broucke, S., Vancorenland, S., Avalosse, H., Verniest, R., & Callens, M. (2016). Health literacy and the use of healthcare services in Belgium. *Journal of Epidemiology and Community Health, 70*(10), 1032–1038. https://doi.org/10.1136/jech-2015-206910

Whitehead, M. (1992). The concepts and principles of equity and health. *International Journal of Health Services, 22*(3), 429–445. https://doi.org/10.2190/986l-lhq6-2vte-yrrn

Woolf, S. H., & Aron, L. (2013). *U.S. health in international perspective: Shorter lives, poorer health.* Washington, DC: National Academies Press. https://doi.org/10.17226/13497

World Health Organization. (2008). *Closing the gap in a generation: Health equity through action on the social determinants of health.* Commission on Social Determinants of Health Final Report. Geneva. https://www.who.int/publications/i/item/WHO-IER-CSDH-08.1

World Health Organization. (2010). *Noncommunicable disease risk factors and socioeconomic inequalities-what are the links?: A multicountry analysis of noncommunicable disease surveillance data.* Manila: WHO Regional Office for the Western Pacific. https://apps.who.int/iris/handle/10665/207601

World Health Organization. (2011). *Rio political declaration on social determinants of health.* https://cdn.who.int/media/docs/default-source/documents/social-determinants-of-health/rio_political_declaration.pdf?sfvrsn=6842ca9f_5&download=true

World Health Organization (2017). *Global strategy and action plan on ageing and health.* https://www.who.int/ageing/WHO-GSAP-2017.pdf

World Health Organization. (2018). *Ageing and health.* https://www.who.int/news-room/fact-sheets/detail/ageing-and-health

Wu, H., Bragg, F., Yang, L., Du, H., Guo, Y., Jackson, C. A., Zhu, S., Yu, C., Luk, A. O. Y., Chan, J. C. N., Gasevic, D., Li, L., Chen, Z., & Wild, S. H. (2019). Sex differences in the association between socioeconomic status and diabetes prevalence and incidence in China: Cross-sectional and prospective studies of 0.5 million adults. *Diabetologia, 62,* 1420–1429. https://doi.org/10.1007/s00125-019-4896-z

Wu, H., Lau, E. S., Kong, A. P., Ma, R. C., Ozaki, R., Cheung, K. K., Chow, E., Tsang, C. C., Lau, K. P., Hui, E. M. T., So, W. Y., Gasevic, D., Wild, S. H., Chan, J. C. N., & Luk, A. (2018). Association between educational level and cardiovascular disease and all-cause mortality in patients with type 2 diabetes: A prospective study in the Joint Asia Diabetes Evaluation Program. *Clinical Epidemiology, 10,* 1561–1571. https://doi.org/10.2147/CLEP.S177437

Zeeb, H., Rothgang, H., & Darmann-Finck, I. (2018). Ageing, health and equity—broad perspectives are needed to understand and tackle health challenges of ageing societies. *International Journal of Environmental Research and Public Health, 15*(3), 457. https://doi.org/10.3390/ijerph15030457

Chapter 14
Cultural and Spiritual Needs of Elderly in Healthcare Setting in Hong Kong

Candy Yuen Yee Tsoi and Yim Fan Chan

Abstract Hong Kong, the once British colony and now a special administrative region of China, has led the world in life expectancy since 2010 and has seen a steady increase over the past half century with 82.3 years for men and 88.1 years for women in 2019. The necessity of cultural awareness in aged care in many different components is reinforced of quality care: physiological, psychological and esteem needs. Spirituality is integrated with the body and mind and is a multidimensional concept. Other important themes include how the meaning of life is derived through relationships and connectedness, self-reflection of responsibilities and obligations fulfilled. Healthcare setting should consider meeting the cultural and spiritual needs of the elderly.

Keywords Functional ability · Spiritual needs · Cultural assessment · Spirituality · Spiritual assessment

14.1 Quality Aged Care

Hong Kong is one of the global advanced economies and cities. Facing with the gradually ageing population, the government age-care services should be planned and implemented systematically. This chapter will discuss the quality aged care, the necessity of enclosing cultural and spiritual awareness in aged care, and consideration of the cultural and spiritual needs of the elderly in healthcare settings in Hong Kong.

The challenges for aged care policy development are the graduated physiological changes that ageing occur over time. From the perspective of old age in terms of vulnerability and disengagement, aged care services should focus on the aspects

C. Y. Y. Tsoi (✉)
Hong Kong College of Education & Research in Nursing, Hong Kong, China
e-mail: candytsoi18@gmail.com

Y. F. Chan
Hong Kong College of Paediatric Nursing, Hong Kong, China

V. T. S. Law and B. Y. F. Fong (eds.), *Ageing with Dignity in Hong Kong and Asia*, Quality of Life in Asia 16, https://doi.org/10.1007/978-981-19-3061-4_14

of dependence and demands among the elderly, including the increasing healthcare demands, social services, pensions and financial burden to the society.

Dependent older people require nursing home or old age home services, and the question is quality aged care and how to assess the services. In Australia, the system of accreditation and reaccreditation achievement in residential aged care services has been implemented to improve aged services and to recognise the service gap. The Australian Aged Care Quality Agency (ACQSC) conducts yearly customer survey of residents for visits and services audits, and for accreditation and reaccreditation of quality residential aged care services, from the experiences of people living in residential aged care (Australian Government Department of Health, 2019).

From another perspective of social engagement and the contribution, older people can foster active or successful ageing. The contribution of older people to all levels of the society is greater than the social investments. From a comprehensive public health response to population ageing, the diversity of health and functional states of the older people are kept. Good health keeps both physical and mental capacities and is the key to extending these human and social resources to maintain the ability to do things of value (World Health Organization [WHO], 2015, pp. 3–24).

The common goal of healthy ageing is to build and maintain functional ability. Five key domains of functional ability are essential for older people: (i) to meet the basic needs; (ii) to learn, grow and make decisions; (iii) to be mobile; (iv) to build and maintain relationships; and (v) to contribute to society. Moreover, effective communication with older people is important, particularly when dealing with those older people with low literacy or suffering from sensory loss. Their perception and understanding of messages received can be significantly affected. The age-friendly city model is an integral part of healthy ageing. The city is required to provide basic needs to the older people and facilitate them to learn and grow. The elderly is allowed the power and opportunities to make decisions. They should be able to move from here and there and to where they want to go. They are also supported to build and maintain relationships, to contribute to the community as a member who gives a helping hand to the community (WHO, 2015, pp. 159–210). The older people are able to live in the right place safely and do what they value. Policy-makers should address community environments when setting healthy aged care programmes that keep the elderly in personal growth and retain their physical and mental health as well as maintaining the functional ability of older people.

14.2 Cultural and Spiritual Needs of the Elderly

People from different cultural backgrounds have different interpretation of health and illnesses. Culture differences are a barrier of effective communication. Public health messages are difficult to reach to older people of culturally and linguistically diverse backgrounds (Ward et al., 2018). They are limited in access to healthcare services to get management of their chronic illnesses. Misunderstanding on cultural perceptions may also result in misinterpretation of medical advice, drug dosage and instructions of health procedures.

Contemporary research has suggested that meeting a patient's spiritual needs is a fundamental part of holistic nursing care. Holistic care involves a balance between physical body, mind and spirit (Manning, 2012). The three elements are interconnected and interact with each other, keeping the motivation in older people and guiding them to explore meanings of their individual life (Narayanasamy et al., 2004).

14.3 Cultures in Hong Kong

Hong Kong, the once British colony and now a special administrative region of China, has topped the world in life expectancy since 2010. There is a steady increase over the past half century and the figures were 82.3 years for men and 88.1 years for women in 2019 (WHO, 2020).

The population of Hong Kong consists mainly of ethnic Chinese, predominantly Cantonese who were either born locally or migrated from the Chinese Mainland. The others have come from other countries, such as Britain, America, Australia, the Philippines, Indonesia, India and the Middle East, etc. Most residents speak Cantonese and English. Therefore, the Cantonese culture is the mainstream but British and Western influence can be found everywhere in the city. Hong Kong has integrated Eastern and Western cultures in the society, with food from all over the world in the city, and making Hong Kong the paradise for foodies. In addition, Hong Kong people can enjoy movies and pop music from worldwide origins.

Culture is described as history, geography and ethnicity of the individual (Bird & Bird, 2016). History is the past life experience of an individual. Geography is where the individual is brought up and pass on. Ethnicity is the social group that shares a distinctive background, living style, tradition and language (Dejman et al., 2012). Cultures are ways of thinking and behaviour that are "customerised" within the group or community. They are shaped by many factors, including social, economic and political factors, age, gender, language or dialect, social class, education, work and personality. Cultures can also be viewed from the foods, dress, languages, religions and festivals, etc. (Tam, 2017).

14.4 Cultural Considerations for the Elderly

With the vastly different backgrounds, individuals have their own ways of living. Health professionals should incorporate cultural awareness and sensitivity into the planning and provision of health care (Rawson, 2019). The multicultural diversity has also increased the challenges for the elderly in confronting the aged care settings

(WHO, 2015). A study on adaptation of older people to cross-cultural communication, adjusting diet, diverse languages and psychosocial interactions has identified strategies to support caring environment and create positive interactive relationships in planning for aged care to help the old adults in their life (Xiao et al., 2017).

Older people will lose their sense of security easily if they are moving away from their familiar physical and social environment. According to the United Nations Committee on Economic, Social and Cultural Rights, social policy for older people should include five designate imperatives. They are independence, participation, care, dignity and self-fulfilment. Older people should be provided with appropriate living environment that are culturally adequate, familiar and preferred, with privacy and dignity. Older people should be encouraged to actively participate in social life to avoid being isolated from the community. In addition, a caring environment should have neighbours and social networks nearby to provide timely and adequate health care to the older people (Chui, 2008).

Culture definitely plays an important part in aged care. The role of culture in influencing the experiences of ageing and meanings to the ageing processes can be positive or negative. The absence of cultural awareness in aged care is a significant factor of adverse patient outcomes and health inequality (Australian Government Department of Health, 2019). The National Aged Care Quality Alliances suggests the necessity of cultural awareness in quality aged care. Healthcare providers should have relevant knowledge and respect different cultural backgrounds of individuals in person-centred care. Services should be consumer driven and meet the diversity of older people according to their needs. In essence, aged care services should respect, care and support the needs of culturally and linguistically diverse residents (Royal Commission into Aged Care Quality & Safety, 2019).

14.4.1 Cultural Assessment

The common constructs of quality ageing life include feeling satisfied, living in good physical, mental and psychological health, good cognitive functions, independence, self-care and being socially active with contribution (Tam, 2017). People from different cultures value these attributes differently. Older people will share life events within groups of relevant cultural backgrounds, norms and values. They share points of view, choices and experiences within relevant cultural norms and values. They also interact with others from different societies and cultural backgrounds. In the East–West cultural debate, the views and analysis of the same event can be different. People make different choices and the deviation increases as age advances (Tam, 2017).

Cultural assessment enables organisations and professionals to provide healthcare services effectively in cross-cultural situations to different race, ethnicity, culture or language. The ABCD mnemonic is an easy-to-remember and systematic way of cultural assessment (Levett-Jones, 2016).

Attitude,
Belief,
Context,
Decision.

Attitude of the individuals and family on health, illness, traditional and western healthcare practices and death and dying is explored. Their beliefs of health, healing and death are discussed together with how they support their religious and spiritual needs. The individual's background, social and political context should be clarified, and community resources in healthcare provision, including community groups, religious leaders, translators and traditional healers should be identified. Lastly, decision-making processes of the individual and family's cultural group will be examined (Kagawa-Singer & Backhall, 2001).

The assessment helps health professionals in accomplishing better communication with older people who are lost or isolated in changing world. They will be in a good position to deliver safe person-centred healthcare with respect and dignity to older people of different cultures (Brach et al., 2019). Furthermore, health professionals should be equipped with the required knowledge and skills to provide culturally appropriate care. Such cultural competency enables the professionals to reach and satisfy the health needs of people of different cultures. Apart from the healthcare system, the society need to create a safe and respectful environment to accommodate older people from diverse culturally and linguistically backgrounds in the communities (Gupta & Tang, 2019). It appears logical that the assessment should be ABCDE with 'E' stands for Environment where the community is situated.

14.5 Spiritual Considerations for the Elderly

In the Western literature, spirituality is related to connectedness, faith and hope. It is a multidimensional concept that integrates with the body and mind (Selman et al., 2018). Spiritual care is focused on the meaning of life and healing of the soul. It is more important to the older people as they advance ageing and face with the challenges of illness and the pending death. Spirituality provides individuals with direction and energy. Individuals will discover a healthy sense of belonging, the meaning and purpose in life and the values of the life. Psychological well-being is good for healing (Culliford, 2006). A growing body of research has been studying the notion of holistic aged care and how a balance between mind, body and spirit would maintain both physical and emotional health and well-being in older people (Manning, 2012; Weber & Pargament, 2014).

The meaning of spirituality is different for different people and is individual-centred. Spirituality care in nursing includes elements of a higher power, such as feelings of connectedness, purpose and meaning in life, relationships and transcendence. Studies show spirituality helps patients in making crucial medical decisions and managing stress. Practically one of the major roles of nursing is spiritual care (Barnett & Fortin, 2006). In hospitals, religious or spiritual needs can be entertained by special diets, the availability of places to pray, the availability of chaplains to help people when facing serious or fatal illnesses and even death. Health professionals who are in close contact relationships with the older people, such as nurses, family doctors, allied health staff and social workers, are appropriate providers of spiritual care to the older people in hospitals and clinic settings (Baetz et al., 2004).

Spiritual beliefs are associated with prayer, meditation and relationship of people. People with faith in religions will get strength to manage life challenges, such as physical or mental illnesses. Research has shown evidence of the relation of spiritual needs and health well-being (Desmet et al., 2020). To support the older people in handling stressful events, health professionals should provide care incorporated with empathetic active listening, spiritual belief and faith traditions into the care plans and identify the spiritual needs of the older people. In holistic health care, health professionals address the whole person as a bio-psycho-social-spiritual well-being, i.e. the mind, body, spirit and social aspects of a human being. A health living style with adequate and healthy nutrition, sleep, exercise and medical support is to keep the body healthy. Psychotherapy helps healing the health of the mind. Religious or spiritual beliefs also relate to health and well-being, helping people to manage stress and go through life events. It is recommended that spirituality and medicine be incorporated into medical and nursing education and training (Barnett & Fortin, 2006).

14.5.1 Spiritual Assessment

In different cultures, a culturally sensitive spiritual assessment is required to address individual spiritual needs related to health care and understand the healing process of the older people from spirituality (Rao, 2005). The spiritual assessment explores the disturbance affecting mental and physical health of the older people. Professionals may then address to spiritual concerns, help the elderly to recognise the emotional spiritual distress and to find out the most effective way of treatment with the appropriate source of coping and healing to enhance rapid recovery for the elderly with the aim to maintain health (Monod et al, 2012). Spiritual belief can be used as a tool itself to help people to change their mindsets from fear to a more confident and positive approach to the world through practicing prayers, reading devotionals and meditation, which brings joy, peace and pleasure to individuals or others. Essentially, spirituality can provide comfort, improvement of quality of life, particularly when facing life difficulties. Spiritual Assessment also help professionals and service providers to build good relationship with older people with respect, trust and understanding (Musick et al., 2003).

Holistic care involves the balance between physical body, mind and spirit (Manning, 2012). Research has explored perception of clinical staffs of their role in addressing the spiritual needs of older people and found that the way they responded to spiritual needs varied. They might explore the religious beliefs and prayer practice, observe the ways patients seek connectedness, comfort and reassurance, as well as ways of healing or searching for meaning and purpose of life. The study has also identified different aspects of spiritual needs, including respect for privacy, helping patients to connect, helping patients to complete unfinished business, listening to patients' concerns, comforting and reassuring, using personal religious beliefs to assist patients and observation of religious beliefs and practices (Narayanasamy et al., 2004).

14.5.2 The Spiritual Distress Assessment Tool

The Spiritual Distress Assessment Tool (SDAT) can help to find out the unmet spiritual needs, and spiritual distress disturbing an individual. The health professionals can have more understanding on relevant issues affecting health (Monod et al., 2012).

14.5.2.1 FICA Spiritual History Tool

The FICA spiritual history tool is a clinical assessment of spirituality tool to explore spiritual history with open questions. It is useful for health professionals to understand the individual older people of their beliefs, values and needs, and to plan and provide the appropriate care to promote better health and recovery to them (Monod et al., 2012). An acronym FICA provides the framework for systematic assessment.

F is "Faith and Belief", the meaning of belief and life.

I is "Importance", importance of spiritual belief in dealing with difficulties or illness.

C is "Community", the involvement of religious community.

A is "Address in Care", the implication of spiritual issues in healthcare process.

14.6 Cultural and Spiritual Needs of the Elderly in Hong Kong

Addressing culture needs in caring older people may result in quality improvement of care and service delivery. Caring in a culture-friendly community enhances communication. The health professionals can understand the needs of the old in more details and respond to them effectively and promptly. The positive relationship in cultural care is conducive to healthy well-being of the elderly (Davy et al., 2016). Cultural aged care also helps the elderly in facing the ageing challenges. However, most of health professionals are lack of training and competency in both spiritual and cultural care (Smith, 2013). Thus, with caring without cultural or spiritual concern, the older people are easily disconnected from place, people and spirit. They become lonely and isolated, especially for those living in the cities and the fast-changing world (Ranzijn, 2010). Cultural and spiritual needs are concerned about how the meaning of life is derived through relationships and connectedness, self-reflection of responsibilities and obligations fulfilled. In the context of Hong Kong, spirituality involves a mixture of Western and Chinese religious beliefs and practices, making it unique in the world.

A qualitative study on planning of aged healthcare services explored the expectation of Chinese elderlies in the forms and sources of future personal care (Bai et al., 2020). Participants, aged 51–80 years, were recruited from 36 Hong Kong communities. The results showed that participants preferred practicing self-care in their homes and local communities, with supports from assistive technologies, family members, home-based and community services. Most of them disliked old-aged homes, which was the last choice. Older people did not want to move away from familiar people and their usual living style, environment and community. Hence, the planning should enable the "ageing in place" policies to support self-care in the own family culture of the elderly and for improvement of aged home care services that allowed ageing with dignity (Bai et al., 2020). In a different perspective, activities benefit the older adults to enjoy their leisure time after retirement. They are encouraged to be volunteers to participate in various voluntary activities. They experience a sense of satisfaction, meaningfulness and happiness. It is not only promoting positive results, such as health improvement, training up cognitive function and boosting confidence and ability in self-care but also reducing negative behavioural problems, such as those seen in demented elderly (Department of Health, 2021).

Lou (2014) and his team conducted a series of studies on spirituality in Hong Kong to examine the conceptual structure of spirituality among older people and to identify effective intervention and strategies that enhanced spirituality care to older people. They investigated the meaning of spirituality among Chinese elderly with in-depth interviews, and focus groups of older people, their family members, healthcare professionals and social workers. Two key cultural factors that affect the perception and practice of spirituality were identified. One was the collective tradition, addressing the relationship and the social life. The other one was the harmonious relationships of life with surroundings. Based on the findings, a specific assessment tool, the validated 44-item Spirituality Scale for Chinese Elders (SSCE) was developed, supplemented by manuals. It was a model of Chinese spirituality with the concepts of mutual relationships of the nature, the person and the surrounding environment. The self-help manual which was free to the older people, was intended for spiritual support and well-being of individuals. The professional intervention manual was the evidence-based practice guide for professionals. Training was provided to equip health professionals with the spiritual and cultural competence for caring Chinese older people (Lou, 2014).

Hong Kong people have a long-life expectancy for men and women, 82 years and 88 years, respectively. Hong Kong government set up "Elderly Health Services" to organise ranges of activities for the older people. To enable the older people keep living in their community, the Hong Kong government set up the "New Neighbourhood Elderly Centres (NECs)" from 2002, with the aim to provide comprehensive support services to older people and the carers in the local community.

Services include health education, developmental activities, information on community resources, referral services, volunteer work development, carer support services, dementia support programme, counselling services, reaching out and networking, social and recreational activities, meal service and drop-in service, etc. (Social Welfare Department, 2002). Such services would take into account for the cultural needs in the context of the local community, despite the fact that Hong Kong is so small and crowded.

In the end-of-life care, the Hospital Authority (2013) set up the Hospice Services Programme to provide a comprehensive service on physical, psychological, social and spiritual care for patients and families, as an expansion of services from palliative care. The Programme is managed by a team of multi-disciplinary professionals, including specialist doctors and other health professionals, such as palliative care specialists, clinical psychologist (Hospital Authority [HA], 2013). Centres provide various supportive services for relief of symptoms, counselling sessions, social activities and spiritual care in a comfortable home-liked environment to address problems of physical discomfort, emotional or psychological issues, social affairs and spiritual matters. The services also include Christian Chaplaincy, Catholic Pastoral Care, and Buddhist Teachings (HA, 2013). The team works closely together with other community partners and religious parties in the community, such as non-governmental organisations, voluntary organisations, patients' self-help groups. They provide continuous life education talks and promotion activities in palliative care to patients and the volunteers. They also organise training to patients, as well as to volunteers, to promote self-help (HA, 2013). The HA has also conducted in-depth research on palliative care with advice from local and international experts with the objectives of further improvement in providing appropriate comprehensive care services on physical, psychological, social and spiritual care for those in need (HA, 2013).

The volunteers receive training in positive concepts of quality life, meaning of living, spiritual care and counselling skills. They are equipped to act in the role of Hospice Service Ambassadors (HSA) as soulmates to accompany and support patients and families. The volunteer team organise various cultural and social activities for patients and relatives. They construct the Community Education Programme for the public to promote public awareness on palliative care. Moreover, spiritual care is introduced to the public through publicity channels and promotion activities. It helps the society to think about end-of-life issues and the caring ageing groups (HA, 2013).

Some government policy on long-term health care for the elderly is related to palliative care and end-of-life issue. Healthcare workers have the mission to help patients stay healthy in their whole life, from birth to death, from young to old. Care and services should be provided according to personal needs, preferences and in time, and to help people, particularly the elderly, live with dignity and peace in the last stages of their life journeys. Health organisations should have a systematic framework of a holistic approach to address the needs of old people from culturally and linguistically diverse backgrounds. Practice guidelines, resources and action plans to deliver quality and respectful aged care services should include cultural and spiritual considerations. Care providers should have relevant knowledge and they should respect cultural backgrounds and religious preferences of individuals. Information on different cultures helps providers to identify the individuals or groups of their cultures, in terms of where they come from, what their lives are, and their specific ethnicity, food, language, beliefs, values, religion, behaviour and other characteristics (Centre for Cultural Diversity in Ageing, 2020).

14.7 Concluding Remarks

Cultural and spiritual issues are important in the meaning of life and self-reflection. Healthcare providers should consider the cultural and spiritual needs of the elderly. In view of the rapid growth of the elderly population in Hong Kong, there is need to prepare the society for the shift in the demographics and the associated challenges to meet the promotion of healthy ageing and age-friendly cities by the World Health Organization (2015) to enable older people to age actively and productively. The Chinese culture is helpful to the productive engagement. This is because of the ethical and cultural principles of filial piety and caring engagement. Older people not only enjoy their retirement years at home with their family members, but also engage part of the caring role of their adult children to take care of the grandchildren.

When considering the healthcare settings in Hong Kong to meet the cultural and spiritual needs of the elderly for continuing improvement of the aged care services, it is imperative to understand how health professionals meets the spiritual needs of the elderly. Health professionals should be educated in cultural and spiritual issues, be trained to apply the cultural and spiritual assessment tools and be able to identify cultural and spiritual needs of patients. Cultural awareness in aged care is one of the key components of quality care. Similarly, attention to physiological, psychological, esteem and spirituality needs is equally essential. There has been recommendation to design age-care programmes to satisfy different health needs, including the maintenance of functional capability of the elderly, to initiate community education to reduce ageism and to raise policy advocacy for age-friendly community in Hong Kong (Wen, 2017). The older people should be able to live in the right place safely and do what they value, and to retain their physical and mental health. In the long-term, empirical research is needed to explore the cultural and spiritual needs of older people to guide good practice and quality education with regard to conceptual clarity and the delivery of cultural and spiritual care to older people with dignity.

References

Australian Government Department of Health. (2019). *Actions to support older culturally and linguistically diverse people—A guide for aged care providers*. https://www.health.gov.au/sites/default/files/documents/2019/12/actions-to-support-older-cald-people-a-guide-for-aged-care-providers.pdf

Baetz, M., Griffin, R., Bowen, R., & Marcoux, G. (2004). Spirituality and psychiatry in Canada: Psychiatric practice compared with patient expectations. *The Canadian Journal of Psychiatry., 49*(4), 265–271. https://doi.org/10.1177/070674370404900407

Bai, X., Lai, W. L. D., & Liu, C. (2020). Personal care expectations: Photovoices of Chinese ageing adults in Hong Kong. *Health and Social Care in the Community, 28*(3), 1071–1081. https://doi.org/10.1111/hsc.12940

Barnett, K.G., & Fortin, A.H. (2006). Spirituality and medicine a workshop for medical students and residents. *Journal of General Internal Medicine, 21*(5), 481–485. https://doi.org/10.1111/j.1525-1497.2006.00431.x

Bird, G., & Bird, J. (2016). No place like home—The human rights of women in aged-care. In J. A. Scutt (Ed.), *Women, law and culture.* Palgrave Macmillan, Cham. https://doi.org/10.1007/978-3-319-44938-8_9

Brach, C., Hall, K. K. & Fitall, E. (2019). Cultural competence and patient safety. https://psnet.ahrq.gov/perspective/cultural-competence-and-patient-safety

Centre for Cultural Diversity in Ageing. (2020). *Practice Guide-Spiritual support.* http://www.culturaldiversity.com.au/images/Practice_Guides/Spiritual_Support.pdf

Chui, E. (2008). Ageing in place in Hong Kong—Challenges and opportunities in a capitalist Chinese City. *Ageing International, 32*(3), 167–182. https://doi.org/10.1007/s12126-008-9015-2

Culliford, L. (2006). Spirituality and the healthy mind: Science, therapy and the need for personal meaning. *Journal of the Royal Society of Medicine, 99*(3), 156–157. https://www.ncbi.nlm.nih.gov/pmc/articles/PMC1383765/

Davy, C., Kite, E., Aitken, G., Dodd, G., Rigney, J., Hayes, J., Van Emden, J. (2016). What keeps you strong? A systematic review identifying how primary health-care and aged-care services can support the well-being of older indigenous peoples. *Australasian Journal on Ageing, 35*(2), 90–97. https://doi.org/10.1111/ajag.12311

Dejman, M., Forouzzn, A. S., & Ekblad, S. (2012). Adapting research to local contexts based on the model of Campinha-Bacote for cultural competence: A case scenario of 3 ethnic groups in the Islamic Republic of Iran. *Eastern Mediterranean Health Journal, 18*(11), 1166–1169.

Department of Health. (2021). *Activities and elderly.* https://www.elderly.gov.hk/english/healthy_ageing/exe_leisure_travel/activity_and_elder.html

Desmet, L., Dezutter, J., Vandenhoeck, A., & Dillen, A. (2020). Spiritual needs of older adults during hospitalization: An integrative review. *Religions, 11*(10), 529. https://doi.org/10.3390/rel11100529

Gupta, S., & Tang, C. (2019). *Our culture affects the way we look after ourselves. It should shape the health care we receive, too.* https://theconversation.com/our-culture-affects-the-way-we-look-after-ourselves-it-should-shape-the-health-care-we-receive-too-114917

Hospital Authority. (2013). *Hospice Services Program.* https://www21.ha.org.hk/smartpatient/MiniSites/en-US/lks/ServiceScope/

Kagawa-Singer, M., & Backhall, L. (2001). Negotiating cross-cultural issues at end of life. *Journal of the American Medical Association, 286*(23), 2993–3001. https://doi.org/10.1001/jama.286.23.2993

Levett-Jones. (2016). *Cultural competence and patient safety—ABCD for Cultural Assessment.* https://www.ausmed.com.au/cpd/articles/cultural-assessment

Lou, V.W.Q. (2014). *Project -Spirituality of Chinese older adults: Conceptualization, assessment, and intervention.* http://ageing.hku.hk/en/Research/Spirituality_of_Chinese_Older_Adults_Conceptualization_Assessment_and_Intervention

Manning, L. K. (2012). Spirituality as a lived experience: Exploring the essence of spirituality for women in late life. *International Journal of Aging & Human Development, 75*(2), 95–113. https://doi.org/10.2190/AG.75.2.a

Monod, S., Martin, E., Spencer, B., Rochat, E., & Bula, C. (2012). Validation of the spiritual distress assessment tool in older hospitalized patients. *BMC Geriatrics, 12*(1), 1–9. https://doi.org/10.1186/1471-2318-12-13

Musick, D. W., Cheever, T. R., Quinlivan, S., & Nora, L. M. (2003). Spirituality in medicine: A comparison of medical students' attitudes and clinical performance. *Academic Psychiatry, 27*(2), 67–73. https://doi.org/10.1176/appi.ap.27.2.67

Narayanasamy, A., Clissett, P., Parumal, L., Thompson, D., Annasamy, S., & Edge, R. (2004). Responses to the spiritual needs of older people. *Journal of Advanced Nursing, 48*(1), 6–16. https://doi.org/10.1111/j.1365-2648.2004.03163.x

Ranzijn, R. (2010). Active ageing-another way to oppress marginalized and disadvantaged elders? Aboriginal elders as a case study. *Journal of Health Psychology, 15*(5), 716–723. https://doi.org/10.1177/1359105310368181

Rao, M. S. (2005). Spirituality with psychiatry. *Psychiatry (Edgmont), 2*(9), 20–22. https://www.ncbi.nlm.nih.gov/pmc/articles/PMC2993530/

Rawson, H. (2019). *Nursing homes for all: Why aged care needs to reflect multicultural Australia.* The conversation. https://theconversation.com/nursing-homes-for-all-why-aged-care-needs-to-reflect-multicultural-australia-123373

Royal Commission into Aged Care Quality and Safety. (2019). *Interim report: Neglect.* https://agedcare.royalcommission.gov.au/sites/default/files/2019-12/interim-report-volume-2_0.pdf

Selman, L. E., Brighton, L. J., Sinclair, S., Karvinen, I., Egan, R., Speck, P., ... & InSpirit Collaborative. (2018). Patients' and caregivers' needs, experiences, preferences and research priorities in spiritual care: A focus group study across nine countries. *Palliative Medicine, 32(1),* 216–230. https://doi.org/10.1177/0269216317734954

Smith, J. (2013). *How do we meet the spiritual needs of residents in aged care facilities?* [Doctoral dissertation, Curtin University]. http://hdl.handle.net/20.500.11937/2417

Social Welfare Department. (2002). *Neighbourhood Elderly Centres.* https://www.swd.gov.hk/en/index/site_pubsvc/page_elderly/sub_csselderly/id_neighbourhood/

Tam, M. (2017). Towards a cross-cultural understanding of ageing and learning by senior adults in Hong Kong and Australia. *International Journal of Lifelong Education.* https://doi.org/10.1080/02601370.2017.1328712

Ward, M., Kristiansen, M., & Sørensen, K. (2018). Migrant health literacy in the European Union: A systematic literature review. *Health Education Journal, 78*(1), 81–95. https://doi.org/10.1177/0017896918792700

Weber, S. R., & Pargament, K. I. (2014). The role of religion and spirituality in mental health. *Current Opinion in Psychiatry, 27*(5), 358–363. https://doi.org/10.1097/YCO.0000000000000080

Wen, Z. (2017). *Age-friendly community and productive ageing in Hong Kong.* Contextualizing Productive Ageing in Asia. Singapore. https://scholars.ln.edu.hk/en/publications/age-friendly-community-and-productive-ageing-in-hong-kong

World Health Organization. (2015). *World report on ageing and health.* Geneva. http://apps.who.int/iris/bitstream/handle/10665/186463/9789240694811_eng.pdf

World Health Organization. (2020). Life expectancy and healthy life expectancy -Data by country. *Global Health Observatory data repository.* https://apps.who.int/gho/data/node.main.688

Xiao, L. D., Willis, E., Harrington, A., Gillham, D., Bellis, A. D., Morey, W., & Jeffers, L. (2017). Resident and family member perceptions of cultural diversity in aged care homes. *Nursing & Health Sciences, 19*(1), 59–65. https://doi.org/10.1111/nhs.12302

Chapter 15
Enhanced Community-Based Programmes for Elderly—Holistic Home Care

Maggie H. Y. Kwong and Carman K. M. Leung

Abstract Many Asian countries have promulgated policies and plans on the elderly community to help the older adults live more dignifiedly through the help of the community. Community involvement of the older adults and level of support and caring by the government, non-governmental organisations and the community will be crucial to promote and implement the community-based programmes for the older adults in different aspects. The issues and challenges encountered in the implementation of community-based programmes in Asia and the physical and psychological impacts on the older adults should be social priorities. In order to provide community-based programmes with more comprehensiveness and humanity, the measures should ultimately aim to enhance the dignity of the older adults when they are growing old. Such community initiatives shall include town planning, scientific and technological development, training of healthcare practitioners, social education and intergeneration connectivity.

Keywords Community involvement · Community-based programme · Social needs · Home care · Home health nurse · Intergeneration connectivity

15.1 Introduction

Getting older does not mean lowering the quality of life, and older adults need to live a better life and be respected. The authors advocate community-based programmes for the older adults with aims to discover the extent to which community programmes can make seniors live in more dignified ways. The current situation and provision for community-based programmes and demands for community service by the older adults in Asian countries will be projected to increase fairly fast. Furthermore, the practical differences between expectations of community services and service

M. H. Y. Kwong (✉) · C. K. M. Leung
The Hong Kong Polytechnic University, Hong Kong, China
e-mail: maggiekwonghoiyee@gmail.com

C. K. M. Leung
e-mail: kmcarman.leung@polyu.edu.hk

V. T. S. Law and B. Y. F. Fong (eds.), *Ageing with Dignity in Hong Kong and Asia*, Quality of Life in Asia 16, https://doi.org/10.1007/978-981-19-3061-4_15

delivery of the older adults will be on the public agenda. Community involvement of the older adults and level of support and caring by the government, non-governmental organisations and the community will be crucial in the promotion and implementation of community-based programmes for older adults in different aspects. The issues and challenges encountered in the implementation of community-based programmes in Asia and the physical and psychological impacts on the older adults should be social priorities. In order to provide community-based programmes with more comprehensiveness and humanity, the measures should ultimately be raised to enhance the dignity of the older adults when they are growing old. Such community initiatives shall include town planning, scientific and technological development, healthcare practitioners training, social education and intergenerational connectivity.

15.2 Needs of and Demand for Community-Based Elderly Programmes

Hong Kong and Japanese are the well-known longest living populations on earth. According to Census and Statistics Department (2015), the Baseline Population Projection Up to 2064 expects that 33.1% of Hong Kong's population will be 65 or above by 2064 while the 65 or above Hong Kong's population in 2014 was 14.7%. The Hong Kong government should be fully committed to the development of community health, services and programmes for older adults. It is suggested that the government should focus on providing highly personalised community-based care services, such as improving the relationship between the older adults and their family members or caregivers, thereby delaying their admission to residential care or nursing homes. Moreover, an increase in the proportion of community-based programmes and reduction of residential care will save more public dollars.

15.2.1 Programmes to Make Seniors Live in More Dignified Ways

The community care services in Hong Kong include Day Care Services and Home Care Services. Day care services funded by the government generally provide services between 8 am and 6 pm from Monday to Saturday, and the office hours of the centres are not uniform. The day care centres provide primary care services to cater for the different needs of the older adults, with the aim to reduce the stress level of caregivers and provide more diversified services to the older adults. On the other hand, home care services are available to home-bound or bed-bound older adults with limited mobility. The scope of the door-to-door home care services is extensive, including essential nursing assistance and evaluation of the home environment and safety so that the older adults enjoy the care without leaving the house (Hong Kong Family Welfare Society, 2021).

According to the Social Welfare Department (2021a) in Hong Kong, services are provided to the older adults with aims to enable them to live in dignity and to have the sense of belonging, security and worthiness. There are a total of 80 centres and 95 teams of Community Care Services for Elderly Persons, including Day Care Centres/Units for the Elderly (80 centres), Integrated Home Care Services (60 teams), Home Help Service (1 team) and Enhanced Home and Community Care Services (34 teams). In the long run, the government should develop more community-based programmes and extend the service time for the older adults to live in their own homes. The objectives of such programmes are to provide community supports and services for the elderly and their caregivers at the district and neighbourhood levels, and multifarious services at centres in the vicinity close to their homes. In the districts, various community elderly centres should collaborate and form strategic alliances to provide appropriate professional and supporting services and to build up a caring community for the older adults. By improving the relationship between the elderly and their families, and enhancing the community engagement of the older adults, the elderly can maintain their health and sustain their basic living abilities.

HOPE worldwide is a charity organisation that aims to provide programmes for single older adults to age healthily and with dignity (HOPE worldwide, 2021). HOPE worldwide established the affiliate in Hong Kong in 1993 and carried out two significant programmes: (1) Fall Prevention and (2) Fulfil a Wish Programmes. HOPE worldwide has noted that fall prevention is necessary for every older adult as its consequences can be serious when hip fractures result from falls, including reduction in mobility and hence decreasing the quality of life. The Fulfil a Wish Programme helps to meet the emotional and social needs of single older adults. They recruited 1,398 volunteers and had successfully fulfilled the wishes of 321 needy older adults. They organised outings to Disneyland, shopping for traditional Lunar New Year and singing Cantonese opera on stage. HOPE worldwide has organised events to minimise the risk of older adults in losing their basic ability of life and assist them to experience the joy of life by fulfilling a wish they may have forgotten or given up. The older adults joining these programmes can live with dignity and happiness.

15.2.2 Demands for Community Service to the Elderly

In Hong Kong, the long waiting list for subsidised community care services (CCS) for the older adults has been a serious issue for many years. There were of total of 7,005 older adults on the waitlist for CCS with an average waiting time of 5 months for subsidised long-term care services, including Integrated Home Care Services (Frail cases) or Enhanced Home and Community Care Services (4,085 applicants), and Day Care Centres or Units for the Elderly (2,920 applicants) (Social Welfare Department, 2021b).

In Mainland China, the large working population has benefited from the economic development of the country with enhanced living standards, such as improvements in medical services and public health programmes, particularly for the older adults. In the year of 2018, the number of Chinese citizens aged 60 years and above was around 250 million, almost 18% of the total Chinese population (Ogura & Jakovljevic, 2018). The demand for community-based services for the older adults has been escalating in this vast country. More than 50% of the older adults had demand on elderly care hotline, building health facilities, on-call nursing and doctor visits, medical lectures, regular medical examinations, and sporting fitness (Gu et al., 2020). Several improvement initiatives to mitigate the situation, including information to the public, more elderly service hotlines, as well as recruitment of more community health professionals, and installation of fitness equipment have been suggested. The efficiency and effectiveness of provision of community-based care service must not be overlooked in all such programmes.

15.2.3 Provision of Community-Based Programmes

Essentially, community-based programmes are designed to enhance the quality, availability and effectiveness of health and social services to the community in the general and specific care of residents, prevention of diseases and injuries, health improvement and enhancement of quality of life in the population. They are concerned about and can influence all levels of settings in the society related to chronic conditions, nutrition, physical activity, safety, injury and violence prevention, mental illnesses and behaviours, unintended pregnancy, oral health, tobacco use, substance abuse, and obesity etc. Older adults, as a 'rule' suffer from a number of physical and mental health conditions. Community-based programmes can prevent or mitigate the poor situation or relieve their stress in facing the problems.

In Hong Kong, three thematic events related to the current provision of community-based programmes were announced (Social Welfare Department, 2021a). First, the Government Property Agency allocated 20 billion of Hong Kong Dollars to purchase private premises to provide160 welfare facilities in 18 districts. The Portable Comprehensive Social Security Assistance Scheme, Guangdong Scheme and Fujian Scheme, are important for the older adults because they need the income to maintain a good quality of life outside Hong Kong after retirement. Appointees of who, due to the COVID-19, could not return to Hong Kong were permitted to withdraw the monthly allowance outside Hong Kong. Retail banks in Hong Kong had supported the scheme by special arrangement for appointees to use the ATM card without the need to return to Hong Kong in-person. Furthermore, special arrangements were made for applicants who failed to satisfy the requirement of the Comprehensive Social Security Assistance Scheme and the Social Security Allowance Scheme, and would otherwise not be eligible, in view of the influence from the pandemic.

15.3 Impacts of Home Care on the Elderly

Loneliness arising from living alone, losing family or friends, suffering from chronic illnesses and impaired physical abilities leads to social isolation among the older adults (National Academies of Sciences, Engineering, and Medicine, 2020). Many senior adults may contemplate living in residential care homes during their twilight years because the homes can provide comprehensive healthcare and social services. Studies have found that, depending on the environment, physical discomfort and other conditions, people who live in these homes are more likely to suffer from psychological illnesses such as depression, anxiety, hopelessness and social isolation than the community-dwelling counterparts (Drageset et al., 2015). As a result, home care is the alternative and has gained popularity because of its beneficial effects on the physical and psychological well-being. Holistic and humanistic care is often an integral feature of home care that allows more people to age with dignity in the home environment with excellent feeling and happiness.

Home care is a service that allows professionals and trained personnel to provide medical or supportive work in the home of the clients, instead of in a clinic or nursing home setting (Ioanna, 2010). This mode of care has been extensively applied in the past few decades, particularly in Asia. In Taiwan, a practising home health nurse is required to complete basic training courses taught by registered nurses, as well as clinical practice placements in home healthcare and at long-term care facilities. Home health nurses offer specialised healthcare care, such as nasogastric and ostomy tube replacement, and drug injections. The service is essential for older adults who have limited self-care competence, specialised medical and nursing care needs, and chronic diseases requiring long-term or continuous nursing care after hospital discharge (Chang et al., 2010). Much time, travelling and human cost is 'saved' by home care.

In Hong Kong, the number of older adults living alone increased from 13.6% in 1986 to 15.7% in 2018 (Social Indicator of Hong Kong, 2018). Comprehensive home care services are provided to these older adults to achieve the goal of 'Ageing in Place' and 'Continuum of Care'. The services not only provide basic nursing services but also physical and psychological support to the elderly (Social Welfare Department, 2021c). The professionals, including nurses, physiotherapists, occupational therapists, doctors, Chinese medicine practitioners, social workers and community health practitioners, provide healthcare services as well as counselling in a familiar and comfortable home environment, with intangible effects to make the older adults feel respected and dignified. It helps them to cope with their daily living which becomes more meaningful and cheerful. The family and caregivers also gain from home care services by sharing the care with visiting professionals. Across the sea, home care in Japan has shown that by incorporating diverse home care services for the older adults, they can delay functional decline and maintain a degree of independence (Akiyama, 2021).

15.4 Measures to Enhance the Dignity of the Elderly

The World Health Organisation (2011) has highlighted eight fundamental health conditions and resources like peace, a stable ecosystem, social justice and equity, to realise holistic health. As people get older, their emotions become unstable due to a loss of bodily functioning and a variety of psychosocial factors. Therefore, actions have been taken to improve the dignity of the older adults in the community (World Health Organisation, 1986).

15.4.1 Town Planning

To address the requirements of people, the local governments in Japan implemented a series of ageing in place policies, for instance, setting up barrier-free public facilities. They had a project named 'Silver Housing' which provided housing for the low-income older adults with on-site care services. These homes are different because railings, stairs, doors and other obstructions had been removed to provide space for wheelchairs. The house owners could call the Life Support Adviser and Welfare Service Centre in an emergency (Kikuzawa & Nakashima, 1997; Tsuchiya-Ito et al., 2019).

In dealing with the challenges of an ageing population, Singapore is another country that is well planned, especially in town planning. Five sites have been designated as ageing neighbourhoods, all of which are separated out in different directions (Tao et al., 2021). The government has long been committed to greening cities, and green infrastructure may make cities optimise their human health, reduce air pollution and become a more livable and comfortable environment for the older adults (Tan et al., 2013). In addition, the Singapore government has constructed a complex called 'Kampung Admiralty' that fulfilled the needs of older adults. It contains 100 elderly residences, a medical centre, a childcare centre, restaurants and retail shops, and a community park (Housing & Development Board, 2021). Residents can congregate in the community park to exercise, socialise or manage the farm, and there is a Community Plaza where the public and the older adults can participate in activities at their leisure (ArchDaily, 2018). In the face of growing urbanisation and ageing population, Kampung Admiralty has restored dignity for the older adults and implemented a new strategy to establish a powerful neighbourhood.

15.4.2 Scientific and Technology Development

The concept of healthcare 4.0 is based on the strategic plan of industry 4.0. Digital health, m-health, e-health and smart health are all the terms that are commonly used interchangeably (Thuemmler & Bai, 2017). Telemedicine, also known as telehealth, is an example of application in healthcare which uses telecommunications technologies to transfer the medical knowledge and information vital to hospital and clinical management, the practice of medicine and administration, the education of healthcare workers and clients, and medical sciences, free from geographical control and time restrictions.

Telemedicine is not popular in Hong Kong. During the COVID-19 pandemic, hospitals had provided limited services at the peak high-risk period that delayed follow-up consultations. Since February 2020, medical clinic at the Chinese University of Hong Kong attempted to adopt telemedicine to see patients with chronic illnesses by video calls, allowing patients to do that without leaving home and reducing the risk of contracting COVID-19 (Ming Pao, 2020). In fact, during the COVID-19 pandemic, video consultations were the major means for citizens living in remote areas to get treatment. More people, particularly the older adults, were able to use telemedicine as a channel to seek help in healthcare and other social services without leaving home during the unusual global incident.

15.4.3 Intragenerational and Intergenerational Connectivity

Caregivers should constantly pay attention to the psychosocial needs and situations of the older adults since depressive symptoms are very common in their later life. Their mental discomfort can be minimised if the family, neighbours and friends support them. Of equal concern is the mobility of the older adults will deteriorate as they age and they will require help from others. Healthy older adults may support their homebound and bed-bound older neighbours by offering home visits and general domestic and social care, which increase a two-way interaction and decrease emotional distress. At the same time, community organisations also engage volunteers in home services. With such intragenerational connectivity, the older adults also have the chance to develop a sense of belonging and competence with team members and enrich their life experiences.

Service-learning has been found to be a useful learning experience for university students to understand and analyse the health and social conditions of elderly recipients in a practical environment conducive for the study of the older adults, by combining the ideas and concepts in the activity during services in health promotion. Students plan an appropriate health promotion programme to the older adults in the elderly centre or their home. The feel respected by the young generation through close communication, teamwork among the students and activities specifically designed to the needs of the recipients. Students have identified personality and characteristics when communicating with the older adults with empathy and dignity (Fung & Fong, 2020; Yee et al., 2020).

15.5 Conclusion

Community-based programmes can benefit all older adults, minimising the chance of injuries of the aged in their homes. With the growing number of older adults, the society needs a concerted study effort to better understand the increasing demand. In the present policy and facilities, there is still potential for improvement. Based on the requirements and demands on community health services, numerous paths that focus on measures to enhance the dignity of the older adults can be identified and developed, including boosting town planning for the older adults, promoting telemedicine in the society and providing support and education to caregivers in order to preserve the quality of care, particularly for the betterment of holistic home care as a result of enhanced community-based programmes for the older adults.

References

Akiyama, H. (2021). *Resigning communities for aged society—Experience in Japan* [Webinar]. Japan House Los Angeles. https://www.japanhousela.com/events/redesigning-communities-for-an-aging-society/

ArchDaily. (2018). *Kampung admiralty / WOHA*. https://www.archdaily.com/904646/kampung-admiralty-woha

Chang, H. T., Lai, H. Y., Hwang, I. H., Ho, M. M., & Hwang, S. J. (2010). Home healthcare services in Taiwan: A nationwide study among the older population. *BMC Health Services Research, 10*(274), 1–6. https://doi.org/10.1186/1472-6963-10-274

Census and Statistics Department. (2015). *Hong Kong population projections 2015–2064*. https://www.statistics.gov.hk/pub/B1120015062015XXXXB0100.pdf

Drageset, J., Dysvik, E., Espehaug, B., Natvig, G. K., & Furnes, B. (2015). Suffering and mental health among older people living in nursing homes—A mixed-methods study. *PeerJ, 3*, e1120. https://doi.org/10.7717/peerj.1120

Fung, R., & Fong, B. Y. F. (2020). Treasure in elderly care learning: A service-learning experience at a neighbourhood centre in Hong Kong. *Asia-Pacific Journal of Health Management, 15*(2), 5–10. https://doi.org/10.24083/apjhm.v15i2.405

Gu, T., Yuan, J., Li, L., Shao, Q., & Zheng, C. (2020). Demand for community-based care services and its influencing factors among the elderly in affordable housing communities: A case study in Nanjing City. *BMC Health Services Research, 20*(241), 1–13. https://doi.org/10.1186/s12913-020-5067-0

Hong Kong Family Welfare Society. (2021). *Community care and support services for the elderly*. https://www.hkfws.org.hk/en/how-we-help/elderly-and-community-support-services

HOPE worldwide. (2021). *Needs and our approach*. https://www.hopeww.org.hk/elderly_needs_and_our_approach.php

Housing & Development Board. (2021). *Kampung admiralty*. https://www.hdb.gov.sg/

Ioanna, C. (2010). Home nursing care. *Health Science Journal, 4*(3), 127–128. https://www.hsj.gr/medicine/home-nursing-care.pdf

Kikuzawa, Y., & Nakashima, R. (1997). A study on "silver housing" in Japan: The roles of "life support advisor" and "life support services". *Journal of Home Economics of Japan, 48*(3), 235–245. https://www.jstage.jst.go.jp/article/jhej1987/48/3/48_3_235/_pdf/-char/en

Ming Pao. (2020). *'Telemedicine' follow-up promoted in clinics—Trial for public patients with chronic diseases* (in Chinese). https://news.mingpao.com/

National Academies of Sciences, Engineering, and Medicine. (2020). *Social isolation and loneliness in older adults: Opportunities for the health care system*. National Academies Press. https://doi.org/10.17226/25663

Ogura, S., & Jakovljevic, M. M. (2018). Global population aging-health care, social and economic consequences. *Frontiers in Public Health, 6*, 335. https://doi.org/10.3389/fpubh.2018.00335

Social Indicator of Hong Kong. (2018). *Percentage of elderly aged 65 and over living alone*. https://www.socialindicators.org.hk/en/indicators/elderly/31.11

Social Welfare Department. (2021a). *Integrated Home Care Services*. https://www.swd.gov.hk/en/index/site_pubsvc/page_elderly/sub_csselderly/id_618/

Social Welfare Department. (2021b). *Statistics on 'waiting list for community care services' and 'waiting time for community care services'*. https://www.swd.gov.hk/en/index/site_pubsvc/page_elderly/sub_csselderly/id_occse/

Social Welfare Department. (2021c). *Services for the elderly*. https://www.swd.gov.hk/en/index/site_pubsvc/page_elderly/

Tan, P. Y., Wang, J., & Sia, A. (2013). Perspectives on five decades of the urban greening of Singapore. *Cities, 32*, 24–32. https://doi.org/10.1016/j.cities.2013.02.001

Tao, Y., Zhang, W., Gou, Z., Jiang, B., & Qi, Y. (2021). Planning walkable neighborhoods for "aging in place": Lessons from five aging-friendly districts in Singapore. *Sustainability, 13*(4), 1742. https://doi.org/10.3390/su13041742

Thuemmler, C., & Bai, C. (2017). *Health 4.0: How virtualization and big data are revolutionizing healthcare*. Cham Switzerland: Springer International Publishing. https://doi.org/10.1007/978-3-319-47617-9

Tsuchiya-Ito, R., Iwarsson, S., & Slaug, B. (2019). Environmental challenges in the home for ageing societies: A comparison of Sweden and Japan. *Journal of Cross-Cultural Gerontology, 34*(3), 265–289. https://doi.org/10.1007/s10823-019-09384-6

World Health Organization. (1986). *Ottawa Charter for Health Promotion, 1986*. https://www.euro.who.int/__data/assets/pdf_file/0004/129532/Ottawa_Charter.pdf

World Health Organization. (2011). *Designing the road to better health and well-being in Europe*. https://www.euro.who.int/__data/assets/pdf_file/0003/152184/RD_Dastein_speech_wellbeing_07Oct.pdf

Yee, H. L., Fong, B. Y. F., NG, T. K. C., & Chow, B. S. M. (2020). Community ageing with health and dignity through a service-learning initiative. *Asia-Pacific Journal of Health Management, 15*(2), 11–17. https://doi.org/10.24083/apjhm.v15i2.399

National Academies of Sciences, Engineering, and Medicine. (2020). Social isolation and loneliness in older adults: Opportunities for the health care system. National Academies Press. [illegible]

[illegible]

[illegible]

Chapter 16
Optimal Healthy Eating for Elderly

Carina Y. H. Lam and Fuk Tan Chow

Abstract As the ageing population rapidly grows, there is a high demand for programmes, interventions and therapies with regard to nutrition. Community nutrition intervention should target not only at the frail and dependent elderly, but also the younger ageing population to lower the incidence of malnutrition. The process of ageing affects nutrition needs due to significant changes in both internal and external factors. Physiological factors including reduced taste and appetite, altered body composition and digestion issues contribute to an increased need for nutrition in the elderly. On the other hand, social and psychological issues could limit the older adults' ability to consume sufficient amount of nutrients. Therefore, the recommended intake of several nutrients including protein, vitamin D and calcium are increased in the elderly. To better equip the community with the ability to promote nutrition in elderly, it is necessary to have comprehensive, yet practical nutrition policies and programmes involving food manufacturers, policy makers, community centres, and medical and health professionals. Age-friendly food packaging, a shared elderly nutrition care protocol and food fortification policies are recommended to tackle challenges faced by the elderly.

Keywords Malnutrition · Micronutrients · Functional capacity · Food fortification · Age-friendly food packaging

16.1 Introduction

The impact of diet and lifestyle on health is well established. Malnutrition, including nutritional inadequacy or over-nutrition, is a major challenge to public health (Kalache et al., 2019). Maintaining a good diet quality is the key to reducing the risk of chronic diseases and delaying premature ageing (Acar-Tek & Karaçil-Ermumcu, 2018). As the global life expectancy increases, the elderly population is projected to grow to 31.9% by 2038 (Wong & Yeung, 2019). Many health issues that appear

C. Y. H. Lam (✉) · F. T. Chow
Hong Kong College of Community Health Practitioners, Hong Kong, China
e-mail: lamyanho.carina@gmail.com

V. T. S. Law and B. Y. F. Fong (eds.), *Ageing with Dignity in Hong Kong and Asia*, Quality of Life in Asia 16, https://doi.org/10.1007/978-981-19-3061-4_16

along the ageing process, such as sarcopenia, hypertension and diabetes mellitus, may affect body function and ultimately worsen the quality of life and nutritional status of the elderly. As such, healthy ageing is crucial to the elderly population, especially in maintaining a good nutritional status.

Evaluation of factors associated with the ageing process and early intervention to malnutrition are important in achieving a better quality of life for the elderly. Malnutrition is associated with functional and cognitive impairment, higher morbidity and reduced quality of life in older adults (Acar-Tek & Karaçil-Ermumcu, 2018). A study has analysed over 2,000 community-dwelling older adults in Hong Kong, and concluded that better diet was associated with lower frailty risk (Chan et al., 2015). The measure of quality of life includes health status, life expectancy, physical and psychological well-being, and these could be influenced by dietary factors. Therefore, the nutritional status of the elderly plays a crucial role in protecting health and improving their quality of life (Acar-Tek & Karaçil-Ermumcu, 2018). This chapter aims to (1) identify key nutrition-related health challenges in older adults, (2) summarise general nutrition requirements of this group to achieve ageing with dignity and (3) suggest nutritional strategies to address the identified challenges in holistic and humanistic aged care.

16.2 Nutrition-Related Challenges in Ageing

16.2.1 Physiological Changes

16.2.1.1 Declining Appetite

Ageing is an inevitable and irreversible process associated with functional changes. As people age, the sense of smell and taste gradually decline, which in turn lead to a decrease in appetite (Arikawa et al., 2020). Concurrently, the elderly may experience tooth loss and reduced chewing functions, which limit their food choices to soft and easy-to-chew food. The narrowed food selection may create nutrient deficiency and increase the risk of malnutrition (Febrian & Ollivia, 2020). There is a correlation between malnutrition and functional decline in older adults, such as digestive abilities, sense perception problems, chewing and swallowing difficulties (Acar-Tek & Karaçil-Ermumcu, 2018). These malfunctions would potentially change older peoples' food preferences with increased risk of malnutrition (Wong et al., 2019). For instance, some elderly may avoid chewing chunky or chewy foods such as meat and fibrous vegetables because of their functional decline. It will lead to inadequate fibre and protein intake, and ultimately lead to various diseases or malnutrition (Whitelock & Ensaff, 2018). Epidemiological studies reported that poor dentition is directly related to a decline in energy intake (Esquivel, 2017). In extreme cases, a lack of protein intake could accelerate functional decline, and lead to further deterioration of body health and the quality of life.

Older people may experience "the anorexia of ageing" due to various appetite and eating problems (Clegg & Williams, 2018). The physiological changes limit their food choice, psychological conditions may alter their food perceptions, and acute or chronic diseases, as well as taking regular medications may interfere with the appetite-controlling nervous pathway (Acar-Tek & Karaçil-Ermumcu, 2018). For example, the decline in testosterone is commonly observed in older males, and this results in an increase in leptin that suppresses appetite (Clegg & Williams, 2018). The reduction in appetite will jeopardise the total energy intake of the elderly and this translates to a compromised nutrition status. Studies have shown that malnutrition is also linked with a longer stay in hospital, which is found to increase the morbidity and mortality of older adults (Acar-Tek & Karaçil-Ermumcu, 2018; Clegg & Williams, 2018).

16.2.1.2 Less Lean Body Mass and Shrinking Bone Density

Ageing individuals commonly present with a reduction in lean body mass and bone mass, but an increased body fat percentage (Kalache et al., 2019). The decline in lean and bone mass is associated with multiple negative outcomes such as increased falls, risk of fracture and frailty (Clegg & Williams, 2018). During the ageing process, the elderly may lose muscle mass due to unintentional weight loss, reduced physical activity, poor dietary intake or long-term illnesses that increase their metabolic demands. The muscle loss is usually unnoticeable, especially in overweight individuals whose muscles are covered by a layer of subcutaneous fat, making it difficult to identify an elderly with significant lean mass loss (Na et al., 2020). On the other hand, the decreased bone mineral density in elderly could result in loss of mandibular bone mass or loss of teeth. This reduces their ability to wear dentures, and reduces the general functions and mobility of their jaws, contributing to more limited dietary options and extra eating efforts. There is a risk of poor nutritional quality in the population that requires dental attention, but this is commonly neglected in the community (Esquivel, 2017).

16.2.2 Non-Communicable Diseases

Non-communicable diseases (NCDs), including hypertension, osteoporosis, diabetes, cardiovascular diseases and cancer are key challenges associated with the elderly. The majority of the elderly have at least one or more chronic diseases (Bernstein & Munoz, 2012). However, the risk of NCDs can be reduced by lifestyle changes, and good nutrition plays an essential part. Weight reduction helps to improve insulin sensitivity, thereby reducing the risk of heart disease. Thus, energy restriction is one of the interventions recommended by physicians to control various NCDs, such as hyperlipidemia and diabetes (Goss et al., 2020). However, if the progress of weight control is not properly monitored in the elderly, the risk of suffering from sarcopenia and related health conditions will be increased, especially when lean mass loss is significant (Avgerinou, 2020). In some cases, problems of other ageing-related nutritional problems, like gastrointestinal disorders, achlorhydria and impaired absorption of Vitamin B12, may arise in older adults. They create additional burden in achieving nutrition adequacy in the elderly (Malazonia et al., 2021).

16.2.3 Deficiency of Micronutrients

Older adults need specific micronutrients for their bodies because they commonly suffer from an extended degree of chronic inflammation or altered metabolism (Marsman et al., 2018). In China, deficiencies of vitamin Bs are common, especially for folate, B6 and B12, affecting more than 80% of the people. The inadequacy is caused by low consumption of whole foods such as dairy, wholegrains, legumes, fruits and vegetables. The situation continues to worsen over the past decades as the consumption of processed food has increased in the population. As a result, water-soluble vitamin content was even lower than before (Liu et al., 2019). According to the Chinese survey CACDNS 2015, the deficiency was still common for vitamin A, vitamin Bs and calcium regardless of the income or education level, showing that the typical dietary pattern of the Chinese population could not provide enough micronutrients for elderly (Zhao et al., 2021). Dietary intake of vitamin D is particularly poor for women, and of vitamins E and folate in the whole population. Despite their longer life expectancy, older women suffer from micronutrient deficiency more commonly than men, especially of vitamins A, B12, C and D, iron and zinc. Additionally, menopause in women is an established risk factor for micronutrient deficiency. For example, vitamin C level has been found to be significantly lower in menopausal women, and this is linked to higher obesity rate. In general, sufficient intake of antioxidant-rich foods such as herbs, fruits and vegetables can help to overcome the oxidative stress created in the ageing process, as antioxidants can effectively minimise the immune dysregulation in older people (Maggini et al., 2018).

16.2.3.1 Vitamin B12

Studies have shown that the prevalence of vitamin B12 deficiency in the elderly is higher than that of the overall population (Zik, 2019). This is possibly due to malabsorption arising from the decreased gastrin secretion which increases the pH value of gastric secretion, or from decreased vitamin B12 absorption under the effects of daily medications, despite generally adequate dietary intake, except in the strict vegans (Zik, 2019). Vitamin B12 malabsorption can lead to anaemia. Deficiency of B12 is associated with dementia and polypharmacy and affects the quality of life of the elderly (Katakam & Durgaraju, 2020).

16.2.3.2 Vitamin D

Vitamin D deficiency can induce osteomalacia or osteoporosis through secondary hyperparathyroidism. Deficiency symptoms like poor muscular coordination and muscle weakness increase the risks of falls and fractures (Wimalawansa et al., 2018). While a multimodal approach is important for falls protection, vitamin D supplementation alone, or in combination with calcium, has been shown to significantly reduce the risk of falling in elderly (Marsman et al., 2018). Vitamin D production can be stimulated by sun exposure, but older adults have a reduced ability to produce sufficient amounts for daily use, possibly due to physical disabilities, reduced physiological response to ultraviolet light or compromised kidney or liver functions (Lips, 2019). As the elderly require higher amounts of vitamin D, particularly for neuromuscular coordination, the dietary vitamin D intake is commonly inadequate. Moreover, the skin of older adults has a compromised vitamin D synthesis pathway, and the process is about 75% slower than the younger population (Maggini et al., 2018).

16.2.3.3 Calcium

Osteoporosis is a silent disease and a major health concern in the ageing population. Calcium is a key nutrient in maintaining bone health, and often considered in conjunction with vitamin D as they work closely in the metabolism of bones. Calcium together with phosphate makes up the mineral component of bones, and calcium also plays a role in maintaining nerve function, muscle contraction and heart function (Reid & Bolland, 2020). Consumption of dairy products, which is the major food source of calcium, is considerably low in Chinese elderly. Thus, calcium deficiency is much more common in the Chinese population, particularly the elderly. This may be related to the high prevalence of lactose intolerance among the Chinese (Liu et al., 2019).

A Chinese study has shown that the usual dietary intakes of overall micronutrients, including calcium, are lower in older women than older men (Liu et al., 2019). The results are consistent with a similar European study, in which older women are more calcium deficient (Mensink et al., 2013). Smaller food portions and over-restricting food choice were identified as the possible reason for the poorer calcium intake in women (Liu et al., 2019).

16.2.4 Psychological Changes

From a psychological and social perspective, bereavement, depression, isolation, dementia and socioeconomic constraints are all factors that impact on the nutritional status of older adults. These factors can result in a decline in appetite, reduced ability and motivation to purchase or prepare food. As such, depression and isolation are the major contributors to weight loss in older adults (Clegg & Williams, 2018).

Moreover, life satisfaction is compromised in depressed and malnourished older adults. Optimal nutrition is found to be associated positively with self-perceived health and life satisfaction. For instance, a higher fibre intake has been strongly associated with improved mood and life satisfaction (Ghimire et al., 2018).

On the other hand, polypharmacy also contributes to compromised food intake among older adults, by changing the mood, taste perception, mouth dryness and appetite (Rahi et al., 2020). Resilient and mentally healthy older adults demonstrate healthier behaviours, such as better diet quality and more active lifestyle (Robinson, 2017).

16.2.5 Social Supports

Level of social engagement, social network and support and marital status are social factors linked to diet quality among older adults (Robinson, 2017). It means that quality of social relationships is associated with better diet quality. This may be due to positive psychological states that encourage healthier behaviours, and consistent with the positive effects of supportive social environments for health (Robinson, 2017). Lonely adults who have poor financial status, and high dependence on economic and social supports are shown to have decreased food intake (Malazonia et al., 2021). In particular, living alone is a major contributor to malnutrition because people who dine alone tend to eat less. Age-related appetite loss can be improved by increased engagement in social events, particularly for older adults who live alone (Clegg & Williams, 2018).

Food insecurity can negatively affect diet quality in an ageing population with limited food options. During times of limited resources, the elderly would attempt various strategies to maximise their food availability. For example, some elderly may attempt to restrict food portions, overeat foods available, consume primarily cheap discretionary foods or eat a monotonic diet. These strategies increase the risk of nutrition inadequacy as much ultra-processed food is included in these strategies (Esquivel, 2017).

16.3 Nutrient Requirements of Older Adults

There is much discussion in the extant literature as to the optimum nutrient requirements of older adults especially around the need for a more nutrient dense diet (Clegg & Williams, 2018). Although the recommended daily intake for the elderly indicates that even with a low energy requirement, micronutrient requirements are mostly the same. Thus, older adults have less room for energy dense or nutrient poor food (Maggini et al., 2018). Many elderly people who have chronic diseases tend to eat less and make poor food choices such as low nutrient density food and ultra-processed food. Various micronutrient deficiencies are found both in the community (vitamins A, B12, D and zinc) and in residents of aged care facilities (vitamins A, D and E). This reflects the importance of proper nutrition care and education in the elderly and their carers (Maggini et al., 2018).

16.3.1 Proteins

There are many debates regarding protein requirements in older age. Adequate dietary protein is particularly important in old age to maintain muscle mass and support body repair. One argument against increasing protein intake is that older adults may develop resistance to the stimulatory effects of dietary protein on protein synthesis, a condition termed "anabolic resistance" that limits muscle synthesis. Older adults may have higher protein needs than average adults, in order to minimise the impact of the elevated metabolism of inflammatory conditions. In healthy older adults and in a variety of diseases, protein anabolism is related to net protein intake. However, others argue that increased dietary protein is unnecessary among elderly due to reduced needs from declines in lean body mass and the association between high protein intake and impaired renal function (Clegg & Williams, 2018).

To put maintaining lean mass as the priority, a slightly higher protein intake in the elderly is desirable to achieve the best outcome. Some experts suggest that a protein intake of 1.0 g to 1.6 g/kg body weight is safe and adequate for healthy elderly. Normally, muscle protein synthesis is stimulated after consumption of high protein food or performing resistance exercise, while studies showed that ageing does not impair this ability. Therefore, some experts now recommend that elderly consume between 25 and 30 g of protein at main meals and have at least three meals per day. This is equivalent to the protein content 4 oz of meat or 300 g of firm tofu (Watson, 2017).

16.3.2 Vitamin D and Calcium

Vitamin D and calcium are the most discussed micronutrients for optimal bone health, particularly in the preservation of bone mineral density and prevention of fractures (Reid & Bolland, 2020). Studies have suggested that higher intakes of vitamin D may be required for older adults, whose ability to synthesise vitamin D in the skin is reduced and the intestinal absorption of vitamin D is compromised. Moreover, the ability of the kidney and liver to change vitamin D precursors into its bioactive form is reduced with ageing (Remelli et al., 2019). In postmenopausal women, vitamin D requirement is suggested to be even higher due to oestrogen deprivation. They are often presented with a reduced sunlight exposure for fear of hurting or darkening the skin, accelerating the reduction of serum vitamin D levels (Wimalawansa et al., 2018). In 2010, the Institute of Medicine suggested raising the vitamin D intake target from 400 to 600 IU per day in the light of the reduced sun exposure behaviour in the population. The consensus recommendation for calcium intakes is 1300 mg/day and 600–800 IU of vitamin D per day, and the safety limit of vitamin D intake is 4000 IU. However, emerging evidence is suggesting vitamin D intake less than 1000 IU may be insufficient to overcome the vitamin D deficiency in people living in countries with shorter day time (Wimalawansa et al., 2018).

In China, vegetables and legumes are the major sources of dietary calcium, and dairy products only contribute to 15% of daily calcium intake among the Chinese. This is low compared to western countries where dairy products contribute to over 50% of their daily calcium intake (Huang et al., 2018). Food choices in the Chinese population have limited their capacity in consuming enough calcium, indicated by the overall calcium intake of Chinese remaining slightly above 300 mg per day in 2015 compared to 933–1025 mg per day in America (Huang et al., 2018). Calcium supplements should be considered only when dietary sources of calcium are unable to meet requirements, for example, when the older adults have reduced appetite and physical functions. The calcium intake of the average diet in most communities is 500–800 mg/day. Therefore, community education is needed to increase dietary calcium intake to fill the calcium gap. If their intake level cannot reach the target, calcium supplements may be indicated but the dose should not exceed 600 mg/day. Ideally, the elderly should be encouraged to have calcium-rich food that also contains numerous other important nutrients (Wimalawansa et al., 2018).

16.4 Achieving Ageing with Dignity by Nutrition

Nutritional risks for older adults can be translated into physiological, socioeconomic and psychological changes. The elderly population is more vulnerable to nutritional deficiencies due to a combination of factors, from physiological changes or deterioration of body functions, such as appetite loss, changes in taste and drug-nutrient interactions, to social and economic attributes such as income, living circumstances and lifestyle (Morais et al., 2013). The loss of functional capacity is often paired with a reduction in mobility and reduced daily activities such as shopping, cooking and eating, and all these ultimately negatively affect nutritional status. Malnutrition and decreased functional capacity are two major factors contributing to the loss of independence with ageing, thus an increased public health burden (Adıgüzel & Acar-Tek, 2019).

Together with the declining activity levels, age-related reduction in food consumption is expected to occur in later life. For example, elderly aged 60 or above consume 16–20% less food than the younger population (Robinson, 2017). Other than functional capacity, the significant loss of strength and dexterity in the elderly, which attracts much less attention, yet is potentially an important determinant, can contribute to the lower energy intake. On the other hand, tough packaging materials are the major reasons for avoidance or low consumption of the packaged food (Buddeejeen & Kengpol, 2018). While many of the elderly struggle to get help from their caretakers to open packages, their food choices and thus energy intake would be reduced. In addition, poor vision in older adults would exacerbate the problem with food packaging, as the readability of the small prints on the food label is low. This limits their ability to choose healthier food items from grocery stores and affects the elderly who prefer buying food with longer shelf life (Wong et al., 2019). Moreover, older adults are at a much greater risk of becoming ill from foodborne disease due to a weakened immunity and would require more time to recover from such an infection (Clegg & Williams, 2018).

To date, regardless of the economic status of the community, the prevalence of a range of micronutrient deficiency remains high, and the elderly is one of the most vulnerable groups that tend to consume inadequate nutrients. The nutritional status and the resulting public health concerns exist as the combined results of different physiological, environmental, social and cultural factors (Mannar & Hurrell, 2018). To achieve ageing with dignity with holistic and humanistic strategies to improve the nutritional status of the elderly, multiple factors and engagement of stakeholders should be considered.

16.5 Practical Nutritional Strategies for Holistic and Humanistic Aged Care

Appropriate dietary management is an effective approach to prevent certain chronic diseases especially in the vulnerable older adults (Bernstein & Munoz, 2012). Nutrition policies and programmes that embrace the multifactorial needs of the elderly should aim at supporting individuals to achieve healthy ageing (Kalache et al., 2019).

16.5.1 Aged Care Facilities in the Community

In the community, aged care facilities and community centres play a key and practical role in providing first-hand dietary services and resources to the elderly to avoid malnutrition. Regular malnutrition or frailty screening using validated tools can be performed in the community to properly classify members into clusters according to their nutritional needs. For frail and malnourished individuals, more acute measures such as dietetic services and nutrition supplements can be implemented to improve their nutritional status. For more robust individuals, continuous empowerment and education are essential to increase their awareness in healthy eating to prevent significant decline in their nutritional status. Their skills and knowledge can be spread to a wider population by their participation in volunteer services. The community facilities also play a role in connecting the elderly with different professionals such as doctors, nurses, dietitians and social workers in a holistic and humanistic manner. Actively seeking advice from corresponding professionals are recommended to fully utilise available resources in the community. Community centres should develop a comprehensive protocol and operating system for making referrals to nutritional services and actively inviting other organisations to join the referral network. An experimental community centre was established in Hong Kong in 2009 to complete the service gap in the community setting for elderly, providing health promotion and primary care support to the elderly and their care givers using a case management approach. Over the past years, the model has been proven to improve their member's functional capacity and has attracted numerous older adults to actively improve their own health (Woo, 2017).

In the light of the ageing population condition in Hong Kong, the government has been establishing District Health Centres since 2019 as a convenient spot for health promotion activities and primary care services (Food & Health Bureau, 2018). Despite a lack of evaluation data available, the initiative can provide a positive environment and motivation for primary care practitioner and older adults to receive a more targeted nutrition intervention for improving their overall health.

16.5.2 Community Programmes

Community programmes should be planned, developed and implemented with due consideration of the specific physiological and social changes in the elderly, instead of repeating previous or routine interventions (Robinson, 2017). As the social and environmental changes rapidly in recent decades, the older adults are facing the challenges from such changes. Frailty prevention programmes composed of frailty screening and multicomponent health activities can be implemented in the community, which can improve the physical and cognitive function of older adults in Hong Kong (Yu et al., 2020). Timely and practical approach of nutritional intervention should be considered to combat their nutritional needs in a humanistic manner. For example, community programmes can focus more on the young-old population to promote early nutrition management. The earlier life course intervention of age-related diseases is found to be more influential in terms of nutritional status and improvement of awareness, as this population has a better capacity to make changes compared to the older population (Robinson, 2017). Likewise, in designing and developing nutritional programmes for the elderly members, it is imperative to consider the effect of geriatric syndromes and changing nutritional requirements of the population instead of focusing on managing single or multiple NCDs. Prioritising appropriate nutritional messages and intervention to the elderly will increase the effectiveness of community programmes in improving nutritional status. For instance, a highly restrictive diet like a low-fat diet should not be recommended to the elderly population whose dietary choices are already more limited than the general community (Ong et al., 2019). Instead, adopting healthy dietary pattern such as the Okinawan diet and MIND diet was found to reduce the all-cause mortality risk of Chinese older adults (Chan et al., 2018). From the experience of various Asian countries, education about appropriate dietary strategies and specific nutrition requirement is required to improve the effectiveness of community nutrition programmes and the quality of life of the older adults (Ong et al., 2019). To apply the concept in a wider perspective, nutritional promotion to secondary school and university students has the potential in the improvement of overall population health because they are the future driver of the society.

16.5.3 Meal Services

Home-delivered meals have the advantage of providing quality food to individuals and help them to remain living independently. Research indicates that home-delivered meals can improve both dietary intake and quality (Clegg & Williams, 2018). Such service should be encouraged and backed by nutritional experts to ensure the meals are nutritionally adequate. The greatest health benefits are achieved when home-delivered meals are distributed to the frail and dependent population or individuals with limited cooking skills and tools at home. Though not well-documented, some community centres in Hong Kong provide cooked meals for the elderly to take home as a form of social support, and this serves as an important component to safeguard the nutrition status of the older population. The meal services can result in a reduction of the number of institutionalised older adults and the associated healthcare costs (Clegg & Williams, 2018). However, in conjunction with the healthy meal services, regular workshops should be organised to improve food knowledge and cooking skills of the elderly to ensure more holistic and life-long health benefits, especially to the more robust older adults. In addition, allowing shared mealtime and providing a catering area for the aged care members can improve their overall energy intake and appetite, as well as the social and emotional needs of ageing (Lam et al., 2020).

16.5.4 Food Fortification

To effectively combat micronutrient deficiency in the elderly population, mandatory food fortification should be considered by the government. Fortified food and snacks are becoming more common in the market while there is no mandatory fortification policy in Hong Kong to safeguard the intake of important micronutrients. In a case study involving countries with mandatory fortification of folic acid in flour such as Australia, the prevalence of folate deficiency was reduced by 7% in 7 months, with only 2.1% of their population was found to have low serum folate at time of report (Mannar & Hurrell, 2018). Fortifying food with the nutrients that the elderly need, like calcium and vitamin D in daily staples, including rice, milk or tofu, can be an effective way to increase the micronutrient intake (Gayer & Smith, 2015). In Asian countries, such as India and Nepal, a fortification policy on their food supply is mandated and the response from the industry and consumer is promising. The overall micronutrient deficiency level has shown improvement over the past 10 years in these countries, indicating that mandatory fortification, if implemented well, can be an effective way to tackle micronutrient deficiency issues (Dizon et al., 2021).

Similarly, mandatory fortification in plant-based milk can also be considered. As the Chinese population is more prone to lactose or milk protein intolerance, dairy consumption for calcium intake remains low in the population (Szilagyi et al., 2019). Plant-based milk, such as soy milk and almond milk, is an alternative to cow's milk but their nutritional contents vary. Some plant-based milk products in the market do not contain as much calcium and vitamin D as milk. Mandatory fortification in these products can minimise the elderly's efforts in picking food products, and thus increases the chance of achieving nutrition adequacy. Considering the likelihood of the elderly population to significantly change their dietary habits, manipulating the nutrition content of food supplies to the elderly can be a more feasible and effective method (Gayer & Smith, 2015). For food manufacturers, solutions are needed to develop food packaging that is user-friendly for the elderly, allowing them to obtain the food with ease (Clegg & Williams, 2018).

16.6 Conclusion

Nutrition is a major determinant of health and well-being over the life course. However, there are debates with respect to the nutrient requirements and the risk of malnutrition with advancing age. Optimal nutrition and physical activity for the elderly are essential to slow down the ageing processes that bring to numerous geriatric diseases (Adıgüzel & Acar-Tek, 2019). Various physiological, social and psychological changes occur with ageing. These changes continuously impact the nutritional status of older adults. In particular, micronutrient and protein requirements are higher due to the deteriorated digestion and catabolic events in older adults. To create a more holistic environment for the elderly to achieve nutritional adequacy, nutritional policies and programmes for the elderly in conjunction with strategic plans should be implemented by the government with stakeholders in the community. Moreover, targeted education on the nutritional requirement and dietary strategies is required to reduce the negative consequences on their quality of life (Ong et al., 2019). In view of the increasing age of the population and the costs associated with health and social care, further research is needed to help combat nutrition-related problems and to define specific nutrient requirements in old age for the benefit of individuals and society as a whole (Clegg & Williams, 2018). There is still much more work to do for Hong Kong in establishing nutritional policies and programmes for the elderly.

References

Acar Tek, N., & Karaçil-Ermumcu, M. Ş. (2018). Determinants of health-related quality of life in home dwelling elderly population: Appetite and nutritional status. *The Journal of Nutrition, Health & Aging, 22*(8), 996–1002. https://doi.org/10.1007/s12603-018-1066-9

Adıgüzel, E., & Acar-Tek, N. (2019). Nutrition-related parameters predict the health-related quality of life in home care patients. *Experimental Gerontology, 120*, 15–20. https://doi.org/10.1016/j.exger.2019.02.018

Arikawa, E., Kaneko, N., Nohara, K., Yamaguchi, T., Mitsuyama, M., & Sakai, T. (2020). Influence of olfactory function on appetite and nutritional status in the elderly requiring nursing care. *The Journal of Nutrition, Health & Ageing, 24*(4), 398–403. https://doi.org/10.1007/s12603-020-1334-3

Avgerinou, C. (2020). Sarcopenia: Why it matters in general practice. *British Journal of General Practice, 70*(693), 200–201. https://doi.org/10.3399/bjgp20X709253

Bernstein, M., & Munoz, N. (2012). Position of the academy of nutrition and dietetics: Food and nutrition for older adults: Promoting health and wellness. *Journal of the Academy of Nutrition and Dietetics, 112*(8), 1255–1277. https://doi.org/10.1016/j.jand.2012.06.015

Buddeejeen, J., & Kengpol, A. (2018). *Criterion evaluation of accessible packaging design for ageing society*. 2018 2nd International Conference on Engineering Innovation (ICEI). https://doi.org/10.1109/ICEI18.2018.8448612

Chan, R., Leung, J., & Woo, J. (2015). Dietary patterns and risk of frailty in Chinese community-dwelling older people in Hong Kong: A prospective cohort study. *Nutrients, 7*(8), 7070–7084. https://doi.org/10.3390/nu7085326

Chan, R. S., Yu, B. W., Leung, J., Lee, J. S., Auyeung, T. W., Kwok, T., & Woo, J. (2018). How dietary patterns are related to inflammaging and mortality in community-dwelling older Chinese adults in Hong Kong—A prospective analysis. *The Journal of Nutrition, Health & Aging, 23*(2), 181–194. https://doi.org/10.1007/s12603-018-1143-0

Clegg, M. E., & Williams, E. A. (2018). Optimizing nutrition in older people. *Maturitas, 112*, 34–38. https://doi.org/10.1016/j.maturitas.2018.04.001

Dizon, F., Josephson, A., & Raju, D. (2021). Pathways to better nutrition in South Asia: Evidence on the effects of food and agricultural interventions. *Global Food Security, 28*, 100467. https://doi.org/10.1016/j.gfs.2020.100467

Esquivel, M. K. (2017). Nutritional assessment and intervention to prevent and treat malnutrition for fall risk reduction in elderly populations. *American Journal of Lifestyle Medicine, 12*(2), 107–112. https://doi.org/10.1177/1559827617742847

Febrian, F. & Ollivia, S. (2020). The risk analysis of malnutrition by tooth loss among elderly. *Denta: Jurnal Kedokteran Gigi, 14*(1), 51–57.

Food and Health Bureau. (2018, October 31). Key Functions and Features of DHC. Retrieved January 14, 2022, from https://www.dhc.gov.hk/en/key_functions_and_features.html

Gayer, J., & Smith, G. (2015). Micronutrient fortification of food in Southeast Asia: Recommendations from an expert workshop. *Nutrients, 7*(1), 646–658. https://doi.org/10.3390/nu7010646

Ghimire, S., Baral, B. K., Karmacharya, I., Callahan, K., & Mishra, S. R. (2018). Life satisfaction among elderly patients in Nepal: Associations with nutritional and mental well-being. *Health and Quality of Life Outcomes, 16*(1), 118. https://doi.org/10.1186/s12955-018-0947-2

Goss, A. M., Gower, B., Soleymani, T., Stewart, M., Pendergrass, M., Lockhart, M., Krantz, O., Dowla, S., Bush, N., Garr Barry, V., & Fontaine, K. R. (2020). Effects of weight loss during a very low carbohydrate diet on specific adipose tissue depots and insulin sensitivity in older adults with obesity: A randomized clinical trial. *Nutrition & Metabolism, 17*(164). https://doi.org/10.1186/s12986-020-00481-9

Huang, F., Wang, Z., Zhang, J., Du, W., Su, C., Jiang, H., et al. (2018). Dietary calcium intake and food sources among Chinese adults in CNTCS. *PLoS ONE, 13*(10), e0205045. https://doi.org/10.1371/journal.pone.0205045

Kalache, A., de Hoogh, A. I., Howlett, S. E., Kennedy, B., Eggersdorfer, M., Marsman, D. S., Shao, A., & Griffiths, J. C. (2019). Nutrition interventions for healthy ageing across the lifespan: A conference report. *European Journal of Nutrition, 58*, 1–11. https://doi.org/10.1007/s00394-019-02027-z

Katakam, N., & Durgaraju, S. (2020). Prevalence of vitamin B12 deficiency in elderly population with dementia. *International Journal of Health and Clinical Research, 3*(12), 110–114.

Lam, W., Loo, B., & Mahendran, R. (2020). Neighbourhood environment and depressive symptoms among the elderly in Hong Kong and Singapore. *International Journal of Health Geographics, 19*, 48. https://doi.org/10.1186/s12942-020-00238-w

Lips, P. (2019). Vitamin D Nutrition in the Elderly; Problems and Recommendations. In A. W. Norman, R. Bouillon & M. Thomasset (Eds.), *Vitamin D* (pp. 757–764). De Gruyter. https://doi.org/10.1515/9783110850345-258

Liu, Z., Zhao, L., Man, Q., Wang, J., Zhao, W., & Zhang, J. (2019). Dietary micronutrients intake status among Chinese elderly people living at home: Data from CNNHS 2010–2012. *Nutrients, 11*(8), 1787. https://doi.org/10.3390/nu11081787

Maggini, S., Pierre, A., & Calder, P. (2018). Immune function and micronutrient requirements change over the life course. *Nutrients, 10*(10), 1531. https://doi.org/10.3390/nu10101531

Malazonia, M., Anuashvili, A., Vashakmadze, N., & Corpas, E. (2021). Assessment of nutritional status in the elderly, causes and management of malnutrition in the elderly. *Endocrinology of Aging, 651–687*. https://doi.org/10.1016/B978-0-12-819667-0.00020-2

Mannar, M., & Hurrell, R. F. (2018). *Food fortification in a globalized world* (1st ed.). Academic Press.

Marsman, D., Belsky, D. W., Gregori, D., Johnson, M. A., Low Dog, T., Meydani, S., Pigat, S., Sadana, R., Shao, A., & Griffiths, J. C. (2018). Healthy ageing: The natural consequences of good nutrition-a conference report. *European Journal of Nutrition, 57*, 15–34. https://doi.org/10.1007/s00394-018-1723-0

Mensink, G., Fletcher, R., Gurinovic, M., Huybrechts, I., Lafay, L., Serra-Majem, L., Szponar, L., Tetens, I., Verkaik-Kloosterman, J., Baka, A., & Stephen, A. M. (2013). Mapping low intake of micronutrients across Europe. *British Journal of Nutrition, 110*(4), 755–773. https://doi.org/10.1017/S000711451200565X

Morais, C., Oliveira, B., Afonso, C., Lumbers, M., Raats, M., & de Almeida, M. D. V. (2013). Nutritional risk of European elderly. *European Journal of Clinical Nutrition, 67*, 1215–1219. https://doi.org/10.1038/ejcn.2013.175

Na, W., Kim, J., Chung, B. H., Jang, D. J., & Sohn, C. (2020). Relationship between diet quality and sarcopenia in elderly Koreans: 2008–2011 Korea national health and nutrition examination survey. *Nutrition Research and Practice, 14*(4), 352. https://doi.org/10.4162/nrp.2020.14.4.352

Ong, S., Woo, J., Parikh, P., Chan, R., Sun, J., Chan, Y. M., Wee, S.-L., Nghiem, N. T., Thang, P., Setiati, S., Huang, Y.-C., Wahlqvist, M. L., Bos, R., & de Groot, L. C. (2019). Addressing nutritional requirements of ageing consumers in Asia—Recommendations from an expert workshop. *Asia Pacific Journal of Clinical Nutrition, 28*(2), 204–213. https://doi.org/10.6133/apjcn.201906_28(2).0001

Rahi, B., Daou, T., Gereige, N., Issa, Y., Moawad, Y., & Zgheib, K. (2020). Effects of polypharmacy on appetite and malnutrition risk among institutionalized lebanese older adults—Preliminary results. *Current Developments in Nutrition, 4*(2), 69. https://doi.org/10.1093/cdn/nzaa040_069

Reid, I. R., & Bolland, M. J. (2020). Calcium and/or Vitamin D supplementation for the prevention of fragility fractures: Who needs it? *Nutrients, 12*(4), 1011. https://doi.org/10.3390/nu12041011

Remelli, F., Vitali, A., Zurlo, A., & Volpato, S. (2019). Vitamin D deficiency and sarcopenia in older persons. *Nutrients, 11*(12), 2861. https://doi.org/10.3390/nu11122861

Robinson, S. M. (2017). Improving nutrition to support healthy ageing: What are the opportunities for intervention? *Proceedings of the Nutrition Society, 77*(3), 257–264. https://doi.org/10.1017/s0029665117004037

Szilagyi, A., Walker, C., & Thomas, M. G. (2019). Lactose intolerance and other related food sensitivities. In M. Paques, & C. Lindner (Eds.), *Lactose: Evolutionary role, health effects, and applications* (pp. 113–153). Academic Press. https://doi.org/10.1016/B978-0-12-811720-0.00003-9

Watson, R. R. (2017). *Nutrition and functional foods for healthy aging* (1st ed.). Academic Press.

Whitelock, E., & Ensaff, H. (2018). On your own: Older adults' food choice and dietary habits. *Nutrients, 10*(4), 413. https://doi.org/10.3390/nu10040413

Wimalawansa, S. J., Razzaque, M. S., & Al-Daghri, N. M. (2018). Calcium and vitamin D in human health: Hype or real? *The Journal of Steroid Biochemistry and Molecular Biology, 180*, 4–14. https://doi.org/10.1016/j.jsbmb.2017.12.009

Wong, M. M. H., So, W. K. W., Choi, K. C., Cheung, R., Chan, H. Y. L., Sit, J. W. H., Ho, B., Li, F., Lee, T. Y., & Chair, S. Y. (2019). Malnutrition risks and their associated factors among home-living older Chinese adults in Hong Kong: Hidden problems in an affluent Chinese community. *BMC Geriatrics, 19*, 138. https://doi.org/10.1186/s12877-019-1148-5

Wong, K. & Yeung, M. (2019). *Population aging trend of Hong Kong*. https://www.hkeconomy.gov.hk/en/pdf/el/el-2019-02.pdf

Woo, J. (2017). Designing fit for Purpose Health and Social Services for ageing populations. *International Journal of Environmental Research and Public Health, 14*(5), 457. https://doi.org/10.3390/ijerph14050457

Yu, R., Tong, C., Ho, F., & Woo, J. (2020). Effects of a multicomponent frailty prevention program in prefrail community-dwelling older persons: A randomized controlled trial. *Journal of the American Medical Directors Association, 21*(2). https://doi.org/10.1016/j.jamda.2019.08.024

Zhao, F., He, L., Zhao, L., Guo, Q., Yu, D., Ju, L., & Fang, H. (2021). The status of dietary energy and nutrients intakes among Chinese elderly aged 80 and above: Data from the CACDNS 2015. *Nutrients, 13*(5), 1622. https://doi.org/10.3390/nu13051622

Zik, C. (2019). Late life vitamin B12 deficiency. *Clinics in Geriatric Medicine, 35*(3), 319–325. https://doi.org/10.1016/j.cger.2019.03.004

Chapter 17
Healthy Ageing and Regular Exercise

Ben Yuk Fai Fong, Yumi Y. T. Chan, Bryan P. C. Chiu, and Karly Oi-wan Chan

Abstract Ageing is an unprecedented international public health challenge. Studies show physically active older adults demonstrate individual benefits in terms of physical, cognitive function, intrinsic capacity, mobility and lower incidence of musculoskeletal pain, risk of falls and fractures, depression and quality of life and compression of disability. Older adults with physically inactive lifestyles are found to be associated with illnesses, increased risk of premature all-cause mortality, and the respective conditions include metabolic dysfunction, cardiovascular diseases, some types of cancer and sarcopenia. In response to ageing health problems, there are substantial studies to support the prevailing rationale of "Exercise is Medicine". An increasing number of studies are emerging to support and advocate regular exercise participation being a cost-effective, accessible, low and close to zero entrance requirement of health intervention, and most importantly exercise is non-invasive in nature. This chapter takes an initiative to examine the potential benefits of regular exercise for healthy ageing, and further investigate how personal, environmental, social and policy factors will shape the active and healthy ageing development. Effective behavioural change interventions in physical activity will be proposed to promote and facilitate healthy and sustainable ageing with dignity.

Keywords Physical activity · Physical inactivity · Active ageing · Healthy ageing · Environment · Social isolation · Social connectivity · Behavioural change

B. Y. F. Fong (✉) · K. O. Chan
College of Professional and Continuing Education, The Hong Kong Polytechnic University, Hong Kong, China
e-mail: byffong@gmail.com

K. O. Chan
e-mail: karly.chan@cpce-polyu.edu.hk

Y. Y. T. Chan · B. P. C. Chiu
Hong Kong College of Community Health Practitioners, Hong Kong, China

V. T. S. Law and B. Y. F. Fong (eds.), *Ageing with Dignity in Hong Kong and Asia*, Quality of Life in Asia 16, https://doi.org/10.1007/978-981-19-3061-4_17

17.1 Introduction

Physical activity refers to the movements of body generated by skeletal muscles, and generally describes activities that result in significant energy expenditure during leisure, work, exercise or travel. Studies have found that 30 to 60 min of daily moderate-intensity physical activity, which includes walking, moping the floor, doing the laundry, etc., per day is good for health. Regular physical activities can reduce the risk of colon cancer, lung cancer and heart diseases (Abou Elmagd, 2016). Exercise refers to the systematic and planned body movement produced by skeletal muscles. The Community Sports Committee of the Sports Commission had found that 32.5% of Hong Kong older adults did not carry out regular exercises (Sports Commission, 2012). The reasons included insufficient spare time, no interest, bad weather, tiredness and laziness. In addition, some older adults had misunderstandings about exercising. For instance, they have concern if their physical conditions can allow regular exercise (Kamerow, 2015).

There are studies on the benefits of regular exercise to the older adults. However, there is only a few studies on the solutions to encourage more older adults to exercise regularly (Langhammer et al., 2018; Reiner et al., 2013). This article is going to examine the potential benefits of regular exercise for healthy ageing. It will also investigate how personal, environmental and policy factors will shape the active and healthy ageing culture development. Effective behavioural change interventions in physical activity to promote and facilitate healthy ageing with dignity in a more humanistic way will be proposed.

17.2 Prevalence of Physical Activity of Older Adult

The increasing ageing population in the world has raised concerns about the physical conditions of the older adults. Studies have suggested that regular physical activity has a beneficial effect on health of the older adults (Bodeker et al., 2020). Physical activity guidelines for the older adults recommend multimodal programmes, including balance training, weight or resistance training, endurance training and flexibility exercises. It has been recommended the older adults should reach 150 min per week for moderate-to-vigorous exercise, not less than 30 min per day for 5 days or more each week. People who have met these conditions can be defined as physically active (Zhu et al., 2016). However, many older adults may not attain such level of physical activity because of bodily conditions, disabilities, psychological influence (fear of falls) and living environment. The authors would suggest walking for older adults who do not or cannot exercise as recommended since some exercise is better than none. A daily walk of around 10,000 steps should do the trick and be adopted as a routine. Getting out the house is beneficial to the older adults not only physically but also psychosocially as well.

Table 17.1 Proportion of physically active older adults among Asian countries/regions

Countries/Regions	Proportion of physically active elderly (%)
China	25.3–47.4
Hong Kong	36.5
India	27.1–41.6
Malaysia	19.0
South Korea	21.5
Taiwan	57.4
Thailand	58.7

The Community Sports Committee of the Sports Commission had found that the proportion of Hong Kong older adults who performed physical activity was 36.5% (Sports Commission, 2012). In China, the proportion of older adults who performed regular physical activity for 150 min of moderate or vigorous physical activities per week ranged from 25.30% to 47.44% (Sun et al., 2013). The ageing population is over 10% of the total in India, and Cramm and Lee (2014) have found 27 to 41.6% of their older people being physically active. In Thailand, 58.7% of the older adults were considered physically active (Ethisan et al., 2017). 57.4% of older adults in Taiwan had been carrying out exercise regularly (Chang et al., 2016). In 2015, 21.5% of older adults in South Korea were found to have conducted 5 times or more physical activities per week (Kim et al., 2018). Lastly, a cross-sectional study has demonstrated that only 19% of older adults in Malaysia had participated in exercise (Justine et al., 2013). The figures show that there is some room for improvement to increase the participation in physical activity by the older adults in all the Asian countries mentioned (Table 17.1). There ought to be more efforts to encourage them to carry out exercise regularly with the aim to reduce the risk of communicable diseases and improve the overall health and wellness (Abou Elmagd, 2016).

There are some inducements pushing the older adults to perform regular physical activity. A review had indicated that about 60% of participants responded that the immediate reason for starting physical activities was to maintain and improve health. About 20% of participants thought physical activity was a good use of leisure time (Kim et al., 2018). Other reasons included weight control, stress relief, self-satisfaction, personal relationship, personal pleasure, self-realisation and social gathering (Taylor, 2014). Nevertheless, there are also certain barriers pulling the older adults back from the activity. The most common reasons, or excuses, were ageing, lack of time or physical strength (Kamerow, 2015).

There are different types of physical activities suitable, and affordable, for the older adults. The Physical Fitness Test for the Community has shown that the top three favourite physical activities for Hong Kong older adults are walking (51.4%), hiking (21.3%) and Tai Chi (18.3%) (Sports Commission, 2012). A scoping review had also shown that walking was the most common physical activity among 43.8 to 63.4% of Taiwanese older adults. Other common activities included hiking, swimming, stretching, jogging, dancing, etc. (Kadariya et al., 2019). Malaysian older adults enjoyed mostly walking and gardening (Kaur et al., 2015). Walking, housework, stretching exercises, cycling at a regular pace, etc., are considered as light to moderate level of physical activity, while jogging, running, cycling, swimming or going to a gymnasium or health centre, etc., are vigorous activities for the older adults.

17.3 Health Impact of Physical Inactivity of Older Adults

Physical inactivity in the older adults is a significant public and social problem in the modern world (Hu et al., 2020). In fact, being physically inactive could lead to numerous negative impacts in the older adults. Such adverse effects can be embodied in various aspects, including the physical states, mental status and cognitive function as well as the intrinsic capacity (Langhammer et al., 2018). Older adults, with or without chronic conditions or disabilities, should do varied multicomponent physical activity that emphasises functional balance and strength training at moderate or greater intensity, on most days a week, to enhance functional capacity and to prevent falls.

With the deterioration of the health status, various adverse consequences may take place. In terms of physical states, sarcopenia is one of the most crucial issues to be considered. According to Chen, Woo, et al. (2020), sarcopenia is interpreted as an age-associated reduction in muscle mass, muscle strength, as well as poor physical performance. It is, however, a complex condition and the sarcopenic process is initiated by multi-factorial mechanisms induced by ageing, physical inactivity or a less active lifestyle (Montero-Fernández & Serra-Rexach, 2013). It is commonly known that older adults are prone to falls because of degenerative changes in the bones and muscle and subnormal coordination and balance of the body. Indeed, the outcome of falls can be severe, leading to morbidity and disability. Falls are a leading cause of death (Victoria State Government, 2017). The consequent restriction of mobility from being home-bound, wheelchair-bound or even bed-bound is detrimental to the unfortunate older adults, families and carers. Apart from sarcopenia and the risk of falls, inadequate physical activity can also bring negative impacts to the skeletal system, particularly the risk of traumatic, and possible spontaneous fractures, resulting in perceived poor health and loss of confidence (Duray & Genç, 2017). Falls result in a substantial economic and social burden for people, the families, community health services and the government, particularly with the increaseing ageing population globally. The costs associated with falls will escalate (Sherrington et al., 2017).

Physical inactivity can also influence the mental status or wellness. Dementia and depression are two of the common consequences of living a rather inactive lifestyle, especially after retirement. The association for dementia or Alzheimer's disease has not found to be strong but the excess risk is particularly observed in those with cardiometabolic disease, meaning not physically fit (Kivimäki et al., 2019). This is understandable as ageing would have led to the deterioration of cognitive functions among the older adults. It was found that people who did not do physical exercise, particularly common during the pandemic had higher scores of stress, anxiety and depression (Silva et al., 2020). Conversely, depressive symptomatology may be a barrier to physical activity and not related to chronic conditions like cardiovascular diseases (Achttien et al., 2019). It was noted that up to half of the older adults may have anxiety symptoms which are particularly common in those with chronic diseases. Anxiety often presents as physical symptoms such as insomnia, behavioural, sensory, urinary, cardiovascular and gastrointestinal disorders in the older adults. Negative consequences of anxiety are significant, with increased health needs and mortality, as well as affecting the quality of life (Kazeminia et al., 2020).

17.4 Potential Benefits of Regular Exercise for Healthy Ageing

Essential regular exercise is good for the heart and lungs, the muscles and the mind. Positive benefits are observed in cardiorespiratory fitness, muscle endurance and power, body vitality, morale and emotion and performance at work and daily activities. The gains are potentially greater in the older adults. Regular exercise programme should be included in all community older adults care programmes (Kazeminia et al., 2020).

17.4.1 Mortality

More physical activity had been shown to increase longevity substantially in middle aged and older adults, irrespective of risk factors such as medical history, diet quality, blood pressure, lipids and body mass index. The potential population health impact would result if efforts in public health focused on the maintenance of physical activity levels after midlife. It was suggested the benefits was related to the reduction of death from cardiovascular diseases from physical activity (Mok et al., 2019). There was some evidence that jogging or running, swimming and recreational football had health benefits (Oja et al., 2017). Effective population-level health-enhancing sport programmes with the aim to achieve a big number of participants should be promoted in the community to reduce the all-cause and cause specific mortality (Lai et al., 2020; Zhao et al., 2020). The association is strong when the physical activity guideline is met by the participants.

17.4.2 Fall and Fracture Prevention

Physical activity and sports are well recognised as the simple, cheap and readily available therapeutic activities for the older adults. Different parts of the muscle and skeletal system to interact with each other to allow the joints to perform desired ranges of motions with flexibility, thus helping to avoid accidents and injuries. Inactivity results in the loss of strength and flexibility of the joints and shorter connective tissues. Exercise should be an important and integral agenda of everyone's daily activities (Kazeminia et al., 2020). Most falls arise from more than one factor and are related to biological, physiological and social risk factors. Maintenance of physical activity helps to prevent falls by improving health-related fitness such as muscular strength, endurance, coordination, balance and flexibility of the body (Duray & Genç, 2017; Soares et al., 2018). On the other hand, resistance exercises and weight-bearing exercises were effective for prevention of fractures, and osteoporosis among community-dwelling older population. The effectiveness of exercise interventions on fracture prevention has more significant effect on women (Bolam et al., 2013; Wong et al., 2020).

17.4.3 Anxiety and Depression

Regular exercise, in the form of moderate-to-vigorous physical activity, helps to control anxiety and improves general health significantly, both subjectively and objectively (Hu et al., 2020). Sport and exercise have biological effects on the neurotransmitters and stress hormones and muscle tension, with anti-anxiety results and physical fitness. Psychologically, more activity levels and positive conditional reinforcements from regular exercise will distract the attention from threatening stimuli and anxiety, and allow individuals enhanced self-esteem, self-empowerment and physical competence. Regular physical activities are complementary treatment ("Exercise is Medicine") to medications in the management of anxiety (Kazeminia et al., 2020; Schuch et al., 2018). Schuch et al. (2018) cited that physical activity could protect against the occurrence of depression among different ages and geographical locations. Even light activity and reduced sedentary behaviour would help people with depression. Yoga, with breath control, bodily postures and meditation, had been found to alleviate anxiety, and Tai Chi, a Chinese martial art, worked for older adults on medical therapy for anxiety (Hu et al., 2020).

Using exercise as treatment for anxiety or depression should be recommended by health professionals such as family doctors, psychiatrists, advanced practice nurses, psychologists, counsellors, family therapists, community health practitioners, etc., because people may have lower cardiorespiratory fitness from lower physical activity related to mental wellness, or comorbid physical conditions such as diabetes, hypertension and heart diseases, that are common in the older adults. Thus, communication with sufferers and their carers is important, more so in the anticipation of potential mental health emergencies like suicidal ideation (Chad, 2019).

17.4.4 Dementia and Alzheimer's Disease

A review had found physical activity beneficial to Alzheimer's disease, all-cause dementia, and cognitive decline as a modifiable risk factor. Moderate physical activity would reduce the risk of all-cause dementia and associated unexpected hospitalisation (Guure et al., 2017). Passive finger exercises could help to improve urinary control, defecation function, the gait and activities of daily living (ADL) in older adults with dementia (Chen, Chen, et al., 2020). There were fewer cases of falls, pneumonia and urinary tract infection. Suitable exercise methods for the older adults included fast walking, running, swimming, Tai Chi, dance, fitness classes, etc., to maintain their independence muscle strength and flexibility, agility and dynamic balance and endurance fitness. However, there is often inadequate opportunities for physical activity in institutions (Sampaio et al., 2021) although exercise programmes are useful in distress management of caregivers of the people institutionalised for dementia.

17.4.5 Factors Shaping Active and Healthy Ageing

In 2020, the World Health Organisation (WHO) launched the Decade of Healthy Ageing 2021–2030 in response to increasing ageing populations in the world. In shaping the active and healthy ageing culture, hence the longevity of the older adults, there are positive personal factors such as sex, age, ethnicity, culture, education, strength, motivation, exercise history, self-efficacy, financial situation and social supportive and networking. The health and activity participation of the older adults can be significantly determined by a combination of both personal and environmental characteristics (Annear et al., 2014).

The environment generally means both physical (natural and built) and social situations. For older adults, their health and physical activity are influenced by environmental and residential conditions related to elements of built, natural and social settings. Environmental influences include natural surroundings and scenery, availability of public spaces and fitness facilities (playgrounds and walking trails), climate, road traffic, street lighting, age-appropriate community services and facilities, pedestrian-friendly conditions, level of urbanism, population density, cultural and spiritual traditions, socio-economic development, affluent areas, social network participation, recreational venues, responsible residents, trustworthy neighbourhood, community functions, social support, pollution, etc. However, environmental attributes, like poverty, high areas, inappropriate infrastructure, antisocial behaviour, crime, environmental degradation, heavy traffic, can form barriers to active engagement with life (Annear et al., 2014).

Although low socio-economic status appears to be a negative factor, but it indeed requires the individual to be physically active through working and moving around mainly by walking or public transport for obvious financial reasons. Social, cultural, civic, spiritual and economic endeavours are concerned with active ageing. They include living in an urban city, close access to services, nice local environment, feeling attached to the neighbourhood, home security and available social networks. Conversely, fear of violence in the neighbourhood, social disconnection, strange environments, air pollution, the presence of rubbish and chaotic and noisy traffic are considered as barriers. Aspects of the social environment also play a role, including social networks, social capital, community literacy, incidental social interactions, levels of social participation, frequency of social contacts, etc. Disability, functional decline, morbidity and mortality of the older adults are associated with the social environment. Moreover, a combination of personal and environmental influences is observed on the health and activity participation of the older adults (Annear et al., 2014).

17.5 Behavioural Change Interventions in Physical Activity for Healthy Ageing

Old adults are understandably the inactive age group. They spend most time sitting in the home, parks and pubs. Although increasing physical activity has found to be beneficial to health and well-being, changing an inactive lifestyle is a real challenging endeavour for most people, more so for the older adults (Taylor et al., 2021). Many strategies have been proposed to increase physical activity in the community to improve the health and social outcomes, such as doing exercise during leisure time in small quantities, education about the benefits of exercise, using activity trackers as an enjoyable workout to get to develop self-regulation, forming an exercise habit with the aids of internet and smartphone apps, increasing accessibility to sport facilities and purpose-built environments, etc. (Hu et al., 2020).

Physical activity is widely recognised as important for supporting healthy ageing. Structured exercise, including strength, balance and resistance training, as well as physical recreation, has been found to benefit the older adults in view of chronic comorbidity. Physical activity interventions for older adults requires active societies, active environments and active people, to slow the decline in functional ability, and to maintain physical and mental intrinsic capacity, all related to well-being and quality of life. Hence, physical activity is a key enabler of work, social contribution, autonomy and dignity as well as health in the older adults. "Active Societies, Active Environments, Active People, and Active Systems" are policy objectives to address the issues, and research gaps have been noted in the areas of societies, environments and systems, rather than people. Behaviour change techniques (BCTs) are acknowledged by academics and practitioners as useful tools of intervention in facilitating autonomy support, instructions for exercise behaviour and credible information about physical activities (Taylor et al., 2021).

Practically, making an informed choice is essential in changing the behaviour or habit. In addition, health literacy in terms of understanding of the health consequences, setting the goals, social and family support, coping mechanism, financial resources are determinants in the behavioural adoption of physical activity in the older adults. In programme implementation, face-to-face delivery has been considered the most important. This is more so during the global pandemic when most educational activities are either suspended or organised online, with older adults being affected seriously. Their daily life is "shutdown" or much reduced, including routine physical activity. Other important factors of exercise programme implementation are learning materials, cost, availability of time, level of activity, cognitive capacities and individualised approach. It is suggested that interventions to augment participation of older adults in physical activity should incorporate BCTs in the processes and allow for the preferences of the older adults to support their habitual engagement in different settings. Furthermore, key motivational factors include attitudes, social norms, self-efficacy and behavioural control and intention, which are constructs in the theory of planned behaviour (Arnautovska et al., 2018).

Ideally, habit formation is regarded as the best intervention as an activity is repeated consistently and the automatic behaviour occurs without the "conscious" movements by the older adults. BCTs, such as prompting rehearsal of the behavioural change or substitution, restructuring the environment by introducing cues for the desired behaviour, can facilitate automatic engagement in behaviour and help the older adults in carrying out daily physical activity whether at home or community facilities. However, the issue of confidence is also important in interventions by BCTs that will enhance self-efficacy beliefs, leading to behavioural changes (Arnautovska et al., 2018).

Lastly, a supportive social environment to promote the engagement in more physical activity is necessary. Engaging in regular exercise with a friend or group of peers of similar physical capacities and forming a community buddy system are significant factors. In fact, "having fun" is also applicable to older adults, who, in the Chinese saying, are "just like children". So, making group physical activities enjoyable is welcome by the older adults. However, the social interaction should be gauged to appropriate capacities of each individual to maximise the health, social and cognitive benefits from physical activity. Therefore, interventions should be designed for different levels and tailored activities to the preferences and capacities of individuals (Arnautovska et al., 2018).

In Victoria, Australia, their local government conducted the 2016 Victorian Active Ageing Partnership (VAAP) Physical Activity Audit and Gap Analysis to identify existing physical activity programmes and the associated gaps in their area. The VAAP self-assessment tool helped people to find out good practice and encourage the older adults to participate in physical activity. VicHealth, the health promotion foundation established by the Victorian state parliament in 1987, has conducted studies on attitudes and barriers to physical activity with the aim to explore what would motivate Victorians to change their behaviours (Victoria State Government, 2017). Social interaction is the main facilitator to walking for travel or leisure in older adults. The desire for social interaction may motivate seniors to form or join a walking group. This may be particularly true of women, who will often feel safer walking in groups. As people age and become more conscious of maintaining their health, they may also become more receptive to programmes that promote the health benefits of walking (Victoria State Government, 2017).

In Singapore, a community embedded peer-led programme, involving the local government, national departments, non-profit organisations, private sector, academia and the community, to redesign health with a life course approach, and to promote healthy ageing, was introduced to improve cognition, physical function and frailty status, reduce social isolation and improve perceived health through planning national and subnational programmes on age-friendly cities and communities to foster the abilities of the older adults. The objectives included ageing in place, increase in physical activity, reduction of loneliness and maintenance of functional and cognitive capability and these are a public health priority (Merchant et al., 2021).

They started the Healthy Ageing Promotion Programme for You (HAPPY) programme in 2017 to engage older adults with prefrailty, frailty or cognitive impairment in exercise led by health coaches or trained volunteers in the community. They aimed to improve the function, cognition and decrease social isolation among these older adults. Actually, many robust older adults also participated in the exercises of the programme embed with multi-sectoral collaboration. The programme was recognised to conform to the ageing and health policy framework for healthy ageing with accessible, person-centred, and integrated care and primary health services and the goal of functional ability and age-friendly environment, associated with lifelong learning and autonomy of the older adults (Merchant et al., 2021).

In Hong Kong, the Department of Health had established Elderly Health Services in 1998 to enhance primary health care to older adults living in the community (Department of Health, 2022). It includes 18 elderly health centres and 18 visiting health teams to encourage healthy living such as promotion of healthy diet, mental health and physical activity and strengthen family support. Clinic service and outreach service are provided. Older adults enrolled at the Elderly Health Centres have regular examinations. The data collected from daily service operations are used for monitoring the health status of older adults and research purposes (Schooling et al., 2014). The Elderly Health Service Cohort was then set up since 1998. Such a cohort with large sample size and long duration of follow-up have established a solid basis for longitudinal studies of older adults to track health, functional status, health services utilisation and the effects of other lifestyle and mental health factors.

Within the community setting, healthy ageing initiatives and ageing with dignity are possible. Commitment from multiple sectors and stakeholders with joint accountability is essential. Community for active and healthy ageing should entail integrated social and health care with the commitments to improve personal health and wellness, autonomy, safe homes and public environment, social connectivity, lifelong learning opportunities, financial security and ultimately achieving “productive ageing” with dignity. In practice, the WHO Integrated Care for Older People, ICOPE handbook Guidance and Rapid Geriatric Assessment, which are examples of person-centred assessment and management pathway, can be adopted by countries and regions in the world to introduce them in primary care and community health practice. These tools are instruments to prevent and enable early detection of age-related conditions (Merchant et al., 2021).

17.6 Conclusion

"Exercise is Medicine" is particularly important for older adults that regular exercise reduces all-cause mortality, reduces the incidence of falls and fall-related injuries, prevents sarcopenia, reduces feelings of anxiety and depression and risk of dementia. Considering the less satisfactory proportion of active older adults among Asian cities, the pressing question is how to effectively promote this cost-effective, accessible health intervention to all older adults. Environmental conditions including built, natural and social settings show predominant effects on older adult health and activity participation. Enhancing good habit formation through BCTs, facilitating social interaction and promoting fun physical activity programmes are the fundamental directions of programme design. With the person-centred strategies and commitment from multiple sectors including governments, community health centres, as well as university/research centres, ageing with dignity is possible.

References

Abou Elmagd, M. (2016). Benefits, need and importance of daily exercise. *International Journal of Physical Education, Sports and Health, 3*(5), 22–27.

Achttien, R., van Lieshout, J., Wensing, M., van der Sanden, M. N., & Staal, J. B. (2019). Symptoms of depression are associated with physical inactivity but not modified by gender or the presence of a cardiovascular disease; a cross-sectional study. *BMC Cardiovascular Disorders, 19*, 95. https://doi.org/10.1186/s12872-019-1065-8

Annear, M., Keeling, S., Wilkinson, T., Cushman, G., Gidlow, B., & Hopkins, H. (2014). Environmental influences on healthy and active ageing: A systematic review. *Ageing and Society, 34*(4), 590–622. https://doi.org/10.1017/S0144686X1200116X

Arnautovska, U., O'Callaghan, F., & Hamilton, K. (2018). Behaviour change techniques to facilitate physical activity in older adults: What and how. *Ageing and Society, 38*(12), 2590–2616. https://doi.org/10.1017/S0144686X17001027

Bodeker, G., Pundit, M., Quising, P., & Tian, S. (2020). *Ageing and wellness in Asia*. https://www.adb.org/sites/default/files/institutional-document/633886/adou2020bp-ageing-wellness-asia.pdf

Bolam, K. A., van Uffelen, J. G., & Taaffe, D. R. (2013). The effect of physical exercise on bone density in middle-aged and older men: A systematic review. *Osteoporosis International, 24*(11), 2749–2762. https://doi.org/10.1007/s00198-013-2346-1

Chad, R. (2019). Exercise for persons with depression and/or anxiety disorders. *Acsm's Health & Fitness Journal, 23*(2), 44–46. https://doi.org/10.1249/FIT.0000000000000463

Chang, S.-H., Chien, N.-H., & Chen, M.-C. (2016). Regular exercise and depressive symptoms in community-dwelling elders in northern Taiwan. *Journal of Nursing Research, 24*(4), 329–336. https://doi.org/10.1097/jnr.0000000000000117

Chen, K. H., Chen, H. H., Li, L., Lin, H. C., Chen, C. L., & Chen, N. C. (2020). The impact of exercise on patients with dementia: A 2-year follow-up. *Medicine, 99*(23), e20597. https://doi.org/10.1097/MD.0000000000020597

Chen, L. K., Woo, J., Assantachai, P., Auyeung, T. W., Chou, M. Y., Iijima, K., Jang, H. C., Kang, L., Kim, M., Kim, S., Kojima, T., Kuzuya, M., Lee, J. S. W., Lee, S. Y., Lee, W.-J., Lee, Y., Liang, C.-K., Lim, J.-Y., … Arai, H. (2020). Asian working group for Sarcopenia: 2019 consensus update on sarcopenia diagnosis and treatment. *Journal of the American Medical Directors Association, 21*(3), 300–307. https://doi.org/10.1016/j.jamda.2019.12.012

Cramm, J. M., & Lee, J. (2014). Smoking, physical activity and healthy aging in India. *BMC Public Health, 14*, 526. https://doi.org/10.1186/1471-2458-14-526

Duray, M., & Genç, A. (2017). The relationship between physical fitness and falling risk and fear of falling in community-dwelling elderly people with different physical activity levels. *Turkish Journal of Medical Sciences, 47*, 455–462. https://doi.org/10.3906/sag-1511-101

Department of Health. (2022) Elderly Health Service- Main Services. The Government of the Hong Kong Special Administrative Region. https://www.elderly.gov.hk/english/about_us/main_services.html

Ethisan, P., Somrongthong, R., Ahmed, J., Kumar, R., & Chapman, R. S. (2017). Factors related to physical activity among the elderly population in rural Thailand. *Journal of Primary Care & Community Health, 8*(2), 71–76. https://doi.org/10.1177/2150131916675899

Guure, C. B., Ibrahim, N. A., Adam, M. B., & Said, S. M. (2017). Impact of physical activity on cognitive decline, dementia, and its subtypes: Meta-analysis of prospective studies. *BioMed Research International, 2017*, 9016924. https://doi.org/10.1155/2017/9016924

Hu, S., Tucker, L., Wu, C., & Yang, L. (2020). Beneficial effects of exercise on depression and anxiety during the Covid-19 pandemic: A narrative review. *Frontiers in Psychiatry, 11*, 587557. https://doi.org/10.3389/fpsyt.2020.587557

Justine, M., Azizan, A., Hassan, V., Salleh, Z., & Manaf, H. (2013). Barriers to participation in physical activity and exercise among middle-aged and elderly individuals. *Singapore Medical Journal, 54*(10), 581–586. https://doi.org/10.11622/smedj.2013203

Kadariya, S., Gautam, R., & Aro, A. R. (2019). Physical activity, mental health, and wellbeing among older adults in South and Southeast Asia: A scoping review. *BioMed Research International, 2019*, 6752182. https://doi.org/10.1155/2019/6752182

Kamerow, D. (2015). Why don't people exercise, even a little? *BMJ, 350*, h3024. https://doi.org/10.1136/bmj.h3024

Kaur, J., Kaur, G., Ho, B. K., Yao, W. K., Salleh, M., & Lim, K. H. (2015). Predictors of physical inactivity among elderly Malaysians: Recommendations for policy planning. *Asia Pacific Journal of Public Health, 27*(3), 314–322. https://doi.org/10.1177/1010539513517257

Kazeminia, M., Salari, N., Vaisi-Raygani, A., Jalali, R., Abdi, A., Mohammadi, M., Daneshkhah, A., Hosseinian-Far, M., & Shohaimi. (2020). The effect of exercise on anxiety in the elderly worldwide: A systematic review and meta-analysis. *Health and Quality of Life Outcomes, 18*, 363. https://doi.org/10.1186/s12955-020-01609-4

Kim, M., Parl, S., Kim, H., Yi, E., & Jeon, S. (2018). Trend of daily sports participation in Korean aged population and sports policy: A review of research on public daily sports participation. *Iranian Journal of Public Health, 47*(Suppl 1), 9–18.

Kivimäki, M., et al. (2019). Physical inactivity, cardiometabolic disease, and risk of dementia: An individual-participant meta-analysis. *BMJ, 365*, l1495. https://doi.org/10.1136/bmj.l1495

Lai, Y.-J., Yen, Y.-F., Chen, L.-J., Ku, P.-W., Chen, C.-C., & Lin, Y.-K. (2020). Association of exercise with all-cause mortality in older Taipei residents. *Age and Ageing, 49*(3), 382–388. https://doi.org/10.1093/ageing/afz172

Langhammer, B., Bergland, A., & Rydwik, E. (2018). The importance of physical activity exercise among older people. *BioMed Research International, 2018*, 7856823. https://doi.org/10.1155/2018/7856823

Merchant, R. A., Tsoi, C. T., Tan, W. M., Lau, W., Sandrasageran, S., & Ara, H. (2021). Community-based peer-led intervention for healthy ageing and evaluation of the 'HAPPY' program. *The Journal of Nutrition, Health & Aging, 25*, 520–527. https://doi.org/10.1007/s12603-021-1606-6

Mok, A., Khaw, K.-T., Luben, R., Wareham, N., & Brage, S. (2019). Physical activity trajectories and mortality: Population based cohort study. *BMJ, 365*, l2323. https://doi.org/10.1136/bmj.l2323

Montero-Fernández, N., & Serra-Rexach, J. (2013). Role of exercise on sarcopenia in the elderly. *European Journal of Physical and Rehabilitation Medicine, 49*(1), 131–143.

Oja, P., Kelly, P., Pedisic, Z., Titze, S., Bauman, A., Foster, C., Hamer, M., Hillsdon, M., & Stamatakis, E. (2017). Associations of specific types of sports and exercise with all-cause and cardiovascular-disease mortality: A cohort study of 80 306 British adults. *British Journal of Sports Medicine, 51*, 812–817. https://doi.org/10.1136/

Reiner, M., Niermann, C., Jekauc, D., & Woll, A. (2013). Long-term health benefits of physical activity–a systematic review of longitudinal studies. *BMC Public Health, 13*, 813. https://doi.org/10.1186/1471-2458-13-813

Sampaio, A., Marques-Aleixo, I., Seabra, A., Mota, J., & Carvalho, J. (2021). Physical exercise for individuals with dementia: Potential benefits perceived by formal caregivers. *BMC Geriatrics, 21*, 6. https://doi.org/10.1186/s12877-020-01938-5

Schooling, C., Chan, W., Leung, S., Lam, T., Lee, S., Shen, C., et al. (2014). Cohort profile: Hong Kong department of health elderly health service cohort. *International Journal of Epidemiology, 45*(1), 64–72. https://doi.org/10.1093/ije/dyu227

Schuch, F. B., Vancampfort, D., Firth, J., Rosenbaum, S., Ward, P. B., Silva, E. S., Hallgren, M., Ponce De Leon, A., Dunn, A. L., & Deslandes, A. C. (2018). Physical activity and incident depression: A meta-analysis of prospective cohort studies. *American Journal of Psychiatry, 175*(7), 631–648. https://doi.org/10.1176/appi.ajp.2018.17111194

Silva, L. R. B., Seguro, C. S., de Oliveira, C. G. A., Santos, P. O. S., de Oliveira, J. C. M., de Souza Filho, L. F. M., de Paula Júnior, C. A., Gentil, P., & Rebelo, A. C. S. (2020). Physical inactivity is associated with increased levels of anxiety, depression, and stress in brazilians during the COVID-19 pandemic: A cross-sectional study. *Frontiers in Psychiatry, 11*, 565291. https://doi.org/10.3389/fpsyt.2020.565291

Soares, W. J., Lopes, A. D., Nogueira, E., Candido, V., de Moraes, S. A., & Perracini, M. R. (2018). Physical activity level and risk of falling in community-dwelling older adults: Systematic review and meta-analysis. *Journal of Aging and Physical Activity, 27*(1), 34–43. https://doi.org/10.1123/japa.2017-0413

Sports Commission. (2012). *Healthy exercise for all campaign—Physical fitness test for the community*. https://www.lcsd.gov.hk/en/healthy/physical_fitness_test/common/physical_fitness_test/download/SummaryReport_en.pdf

Sherrington, C., Michaleff, Z. A., Fairhall, N., Paul, S. S., Tiedemann, A., Whitney, J., Cumming, R. G., Herbert, R. D., Close, J. C. T., & Lord, S. R. (2017). Exercise to prevent falls in older adults: An updated systematic review and meta-analysis. *British Journal of Sports Medicine, 51*(24), 1750–1758. https://doi.org/10.1136/bjsports-2016-096547

Sun, F., Norman, I. J., & While, A. E. (2013). Physical activity in older people: A systematic review. *BMC Public Health, 13*, 449. https://doi.org/10.1186/1471-2458-13-449

Taylor, D. (2014). Physical activity is medicine for older adults. *Postgraduate Medical Journal, 90*(1059), 26–32. https://doi.org/10.1136/postgradmedj-2012-131366

Taylor, J., Walsh, S., Kwok, W., Pinheiro, M. B., de Oliveira, J. S., Hassett, L., Bauman, A., Bull, F., Tiedemann, A., & Sherrington, C. (2021). A scoping review of physical activity interventions for older adults. *International Journal of Behavioral Nutrition and Physical Activity, 18*, 82. https://doi.org/10.1186/s12966-021-01140-9

Victoria State Government. (2017). *Active & healthy ageing local government action guide*. https://www2.health.vic.gov.au/-/media/health/files/collections/policies-and-guidelines/a/active-and-healthy-ageing-local-govt-action-guide---pdf.pdf

Wong, R. M. Y., Chong, K. C., Law, S. W., Ho, W. T., Li, J., Chui, C. S., Chow, S. K. H., & Cheung, W. H. (2020). The effectiveness of exercises on fall and fracture prevention amongst community elderlies: A systematic review and meta-analysis. *Journal of Orthopaedic Translation, 24*, 58–65. https://doi.org/10.1016/j.jot.2020.05.007

Zhao, M., Veeranki, S. P., Magnussen, C. G., & Xi, B. (2020). Recommended physical activity and all cause and cause specific mortality in US adults: Prospective cohort study. *BMJ, 370*, m2031. https://doi.org/10.1136/bmj.m2031

Zhu, W., Chi, A., & Sun, Y. (2016). Physical activity among older Chinese adults living in urban and rural areas: A review. *Journal of Sport and Health Science, 5*(3), 281–286. https://doi.org/10.1016/j.jshs.2016.07.004

Chapter 18
Osteosarcopenia and Fragility Fracture: A Community Perspective

Leon Wai Li, Wing Tung Ho, and Sin Yee Lau

Abstract Osteosarcopenia is a syndrome with co-existence of osteoporosis and sarcopenia. Osteoporosis is a disease in which the microarchitecture and quality of bone is reduced. Globally, 1 in 3 women and 1 in 5 men aged 50 years and above are at risk of osteoporotic fracture. In fact, the lifetime fracture risk in osteoporosis patients reaches up to 40% and mortality of osteoporotic hip fractures is 33% at 1 year. Hospital expenditures for osteoporotic fractures are hence a major socioeconomic burden. Sarcopenia is a common geriatric syndrome, in which there is progressive loss of lean body mass and function. In normal ageing, muscle mass decreases at a rate of 1% annually after the age of 40 years. More importantly, a high prevalence of sarcopenia in patients with fragility fractures has been reported recently, reaching 95% in males and 64% in females. The disease affects patient balance, gait and muscle strength resulting in falls and fractures. Therefore, the treatment of both osteoporosis and sarcopenia is essential to prevent morbidity and mortality in the elderly. Primary prevention, early diagnosis and treatment of these diseases are found to be extremely important in reducing diseases-related falls and subsequence fractures, mortality rate, healthcare costs as well as poor physical function and quality of life.

Keywords Ageing · Bone · Elderly · Falls · Fractures · Frailty · Muscle · Osteosarcopenia · Osteoporosis · Sarcopenia · Holistic care

18.1 Introduction

Osteosarcopenia is a syndrome with overlap in the pathophysiology of low bone density including osteopenia and osteoporosis and sarcopenia. The World Health

L. W. Li (✉) · W. T. Ho
Hong Kong College of Community Health Practitioners, Hong Kong, China
e-mail: leonwai9413@gmail.com

S. Y. Lau
Hong Kong Children's Hospital, Hospital Authority, Hong Kong, China

V. T. S. Law and B. Y. F. Fong (eds.), *Ageing with Dignity in Hong Kong and Asia*, Quality of Life in Asia 16, https://doi.org/10.1007/978-981-19-3061-4_18

Organisation (WHO) has established a quantified definition of osteopenia and osteoporosis with T-scores of bone mineral density (BMD) ranging from –1 to –2.5, respectively (World Health Organisation, 2007). For sarcopenia, The European Working Group on Sarcopenia in Older People (EWGSOP) defines this syndrome to be characterised with progressive loss of muscle mass, strength and function. These syndromes could lead to adverse health outcomes such as physical incapacity, declined quality of life and increased mortality rate (Cruz-Jentoft et al., 2010). Although there is a lack of standard criteria to define clinical diagnosis of osteosarcopenia, there are increasing knowledge on interpreting this unique syndrome as the association between musculoskeletal system and age-related metabolic alterations (Hassan & Duque, 2017; Hirschfeld et al., 2017; Kirk, Al Saedi, et al., 2019).

Osteosarcopenia has created a major global health problem among the older adults. Global ageing population is expected to be increased by more than 20% from 841 million in 2013 to more than 2 billion by 2050 (Greco et al., 2019). 1 in 3 women and 1 in 5 men aged 50 years or above are at risk of osteoporotic fractures (Hernlund et al., 2013). Studies have shown that patients with osteoporosis have a significantly higher risk of fractures by 40%, with the annual mortality due to osteoporotic hip fracture increases by 20—30% (Barnsley et al., 2021; Klop et al., 2014). A cross-sectional study has further reported that sarcopenia patients are at higher risk to develop into osteosarcopenia, with around 20% and 60% in 60–64 years and 75 years or above age group, respectively, as compared to older adults without sarcopenia (Fahimfar et al., 2019). Complications of osteosarcopenia including falls, fracture frailty, loss of independence, depression and hospitalisation could therefore increase the burden on healthcare systems (Kirk, Zanker, et al., 2020).

The objectives of this chapter are to increase the awareness of primary prevention, early diagnosis and treatment of osteosarcopenia in the older population through examining its mechanism, epidemiology and consequences, and provide recommendations for the development of a holistic care model for osteosarcopenia elderlies.

18.2 Epidemiology

The prevalence of osteosarcopenia in different countries varies because of the diverse populations and different methods or criterion applied in the diagnosis and screening of this syndrome such as examination of BMD, muscle mass and function. Nonetheless, by reviewing the consensus definition and diagnostic criteria for sarcopenia as developed by the EWGSOP and different established studies, the trend and general population affected by osteosarcopenia can still be projected (Kirk, Al Saedi, et al., 2019; Paintin et al., 2018).

In Germany, 28% of the community-dwelling elderly were characterised with osteosarcopenic symptoms (Drey et al., 2015). In Italy, 29% of the older adults aged $\geq$ 50 who are living in community settings are affected by sarcopenia, and of those, 33% are staying in long-term care facilities (Cruz-Jentoft et al., 2010). In

United Kingdom, 10% of the osteosarcopenic patients are acute hospitalised geriatric patients (Cruz-Jentoft et al., 2010; Nielsen et al., 2018).

Studies related to the prevalence of osteosarcopenia have also been conducted in Australia. Results have shown that there are approximately 40% of older population suffering from osteosarcopenia (Huo et al., 2015; Scott et al., 2018; Suriyaarachchi et al., 2018). Whereas in United States, 31% of individuals who participated in Louisiana Healthy Ageing Study had been indicated with adverse functional consequences of osteosarcopenia (Poggiogalle et al., 2019).

Back in Asia, the prevalence of osteosarcopenia in community-dwelling elderlies ranged from 4.7 to 14% in Japan and China, respectively (Kirk, Al Saedi, et al., 2019; Yoshimura et al., 2018). In Korea, a retrospective observational study had reported that more than 20% of their subjects with hip fracture were diagnosed with osteosarcopenia (Yoo et al, 2018).

18.3 Mechanism and Consequences of Osteosarcopenia and Fragility Fracture

18.3.1 Mechanism

Osteosarcopenia is a multifactorial musculoskeletal disorder associated with the pathophysiology of osteoporosis and sarcopenia (Hirschfeld et al., 2017; Saeki et al., 2020). Apart from the mechanical, genetic and lifestyle factors, which are established interrelated conditions that can exacerbate the development of osteosarcopenia (Paintin et al., 2018), a complex biochemical mechanism that is involved in the "Bone-muscle crosstalk" also brings a significant effect in the pathogenesis of osteosarcopenia (Girgis et al., 2014). The intricate paracrine and endocrine mechanisms, which are involved in muscle atrophy and bone homeostasis, are essentially governing the interacting system of "Bone-muscle crosstalk" through the secretion of myokines, osteokines and adipokines from their specific precursor cell (myocytes, osteocytes and adipocytes) and maintaining cellular communication in between (Girgis et al., 2014; Kirk, Miller, et al., 2020). To maintain the bone density, and muscle and associated tissue (e.g. tendons, ligaments) strength, weight bearing or gravitational loading activities are essential to avoid atrophy, because such mechanical stimuli can facilitate protein metabolism in muscle and collagen synthesis in bone matrix (Dolan & Sale, 2018).

Genetic traits (e.g. vitamin D receptor, collagen 1 alpha 1, myocyte enhancer factor-2 (MEF2C), etc.) that determine the Peak Bone Mass (PBM) and muscle development in early life also have significant association to the risk of developing osteosarcopenia in late life (Estrada et al., 2012; Gordon et al., 2017; Kirk, Miller, et al., 2020). These polymorphisms of the genes can affect molecular interaction and vary cellular mechanisms, causing an imbalance in protein and bone matrix turnover (Bikle et al., 2015; Karasik & Kiel, 2010).

With the effects of the aforementioned factors, occurrence of osteosarcopenia will increase with ageing. The musculoskeletal system is the major reservoir for calcium and glucose to regulate bone mineral density (BMD) and muscle mass and strength. Progressive decline of such metabolic conditions when people reaching their advanced age will result in higher sensitivity to utilise dietary protein and vitamin D degradation that can lead to establishment of impaired neuromuscular functioning, decreased muscle bone mass and joint catabolism (Bhat et al., 2013; Kirk, Al Saedi, et al., 2019). Without sufficient nutrients, the bone-forming (osteoblasts) and bone-resorbing (osteoclasts) cells cannot reach equilibrium for bone turnover. At the same time, in the presence of reduction in physical activity and immunological changes among elderly, hormonal imbalances will be likely to occur, characterised by low growth hormone (e.g. testosterone, oestrogen) and insulin-like growth factor 1 (IGF-1). These biological events can deteriorate bone remodelling and muscle protein turnover, and thus the likelihood to further develop osteosarcopenia will be increased (Kirk, Zanker, et al., 2020).

18.3.2 Consequences

With the localised and systemic factors affecting age-related muscle and bone loss, Zanker and Duque (2018) have demonstrated that muscle bone anabolism and catabolism among ageing persons have strong tendency to accumulate intramuscular and bone marrow fat, and this could stimulate secretion of adipokines and trigger the apoptosis of myocytes and osteocytes. Such phenomenon can deteriorate muscle regeneration and impair bone structures for replacement due to fat infiltration to muscle and bone marrow. It further creates a Lipoprotein lipase (LPL)-mediated lipotoxic environment to the surrounded connective tissue (Tamilarasan et al., 2012) which can cause inflammation in tissues already affected by age-associated osteosarcopenia (Al Saedi et al., 2019; Hassan & Duque, 2017).

Substantial negative outcomes, including mobility, disability and mortality, can be brought by osteosarcopenia. For mobility problems, since people affected by osteosarcopenia are characterised with atrophied skeletal muscles, the loss of strength can affect chair rising time, sit-to-stand power or other physical limitations that can affect patients' quality of life (Inoue et al., 2021). With reduced outdoor activities and social interactions, a psychological impact such as depression will also be more likely to develop (Park et al., 2021).

Evidence has shown that frailty (i.e. multisystem physical impairment) can lead to higher vulnerability to emotional or psychological events and conditions in elderly with osteosarcopenia, and subsequently increase the risk of falls and fractures (Salech et al., 2021; Yoshimura et al., 2018), especially for patients with chronic diseases including hypertension, dementia and chronic liver disease (Barnsley et al., 2021; Chen et al., 2019; Saeki et al., 2020). A study conducted among community-dwelling older adults (mean age > 60 years) revealed that osteosarcopenic participants had higher frequency of falls and hip fractures and associated with significant higher mortality risk in comparing to those without sarcopenia or osteopenia (Balogun et al., 2019).

Besides, the socioeconomic impact that could be caused by osteosarcopenia must not be overlooked. In Europe, it had cost over €30 billion for treating fragility fractures and was estimated to surge by 25% in 2025 (Hernlund et al., 2013). This medical condition also creates substantial economic burden on individuals and the public. For instance, in China, a rapid rise in hospital costs associated with osteoporotic fractures had increased 60% from 2008 to 2010 (i.e. from nearly ¥16,700 to ¥26,700 for each patients) (Yang et al., 2015), while more than 60% of hospital costs had been spent on treating patients with osteoporotic hip fracture due to prolonged hospitalisation (Luo & Xu, 2005).

18.4 Holistic Model for Prevention, Early Diagnosis and Treatment of Osteosarcopenia

With growing concerns on treating osteoporosis and sarcopenia synchronously and more prospective therapeutic approaches and knowledge shared among clinical practices, pathophysiological mechanisms in the interaction between muscle and bone dysfunction has drawn more attention of study (Kirk, Miller, et al., 2020). The provision of care to patients with osteosarcopenia is no longer limited to pharmacologic treatments, but also advanced in holistic care approaches which consider patients as whole persons through caring of their physical, psychological, emotional and environmental conditions. Holistic care contains wide aspects of treatment that emphasise on reassuring patients' self-care abilities, spirituality, self-esteem and dignity and liveliness (Thompson et al., 2008).

In clinical settings, a holistic care approach needs to be applied in prevention programmes, early diagnosis and therapeutic treatments while addressing patients' total needs at the same time (McEvoy & Duffy, 2008; Fig. 18.1).

18.4.1 Prevention

18.4.1.1 Healthy lifestyle

Smoking and alcohol consumption have potential negative impacts on muscle and bone health. A meta-analysis has established that elderly smokers experienced higher risk of osteoporotic fracture and hip fracture (Kanis et al., 2004). Abate et al. (2013) have also revealed that bone metabolism will be interfered by chemical components produced from cigarette smoking which have induced skeletal muscle damage and tendon rupture. Another meta-analysis had further identified that people who had ceased smoking for more than 10 years had lower chance of developing hip fracture

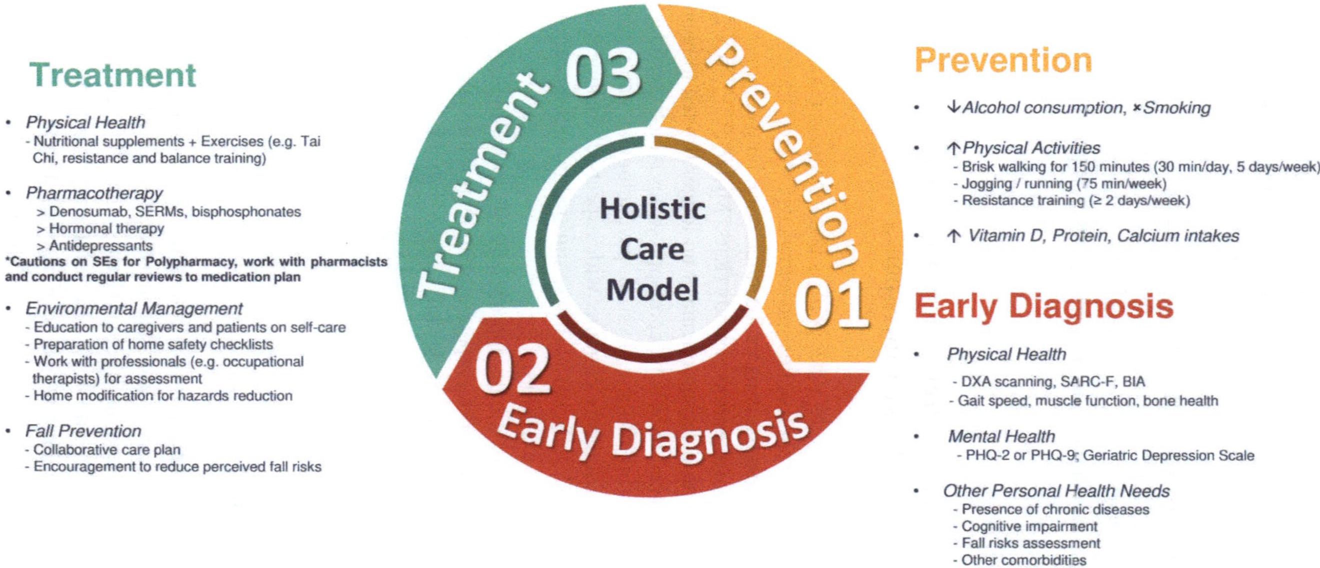

Fig. 18.1 Holistic care model for prevention, early diagnosis and treatment of osteosarcopenia

(Shen et al., 2015). Hence, potential beneficial effects on skeletal muscle structure and function brought by smoking cessation have also been demonstrated (Ajime et al., 2020). Alcohol consumption among ageing people, especially heavy drinkers, have also been well documented with greater risk from attaining osteoporotic fracture, loss of bone density and skeletal myopathies due to alcohol-mediated deficiencies in nutrients metabolism (Berg et al., 2008; Steiner & Lang, 2015).

18.4.1.2 Physical Activity

Avoidance of sedative lifestyle is also regarded as first-line prevention choice for osteosarcopenia (Hassan & Duque, 2017). Resistance exercises have been documented with positive effects in mitigating age-related muscle and bone density loss and reducing fracture risk in older adults (Daly et al., 2019; Kemmler et al., 2013). If exercise programmes with multiple categories, such as combining resistance exercise with balance and functional exercises (e.g. Tai Chi, dance or walking programmes), can be established in long-term care to elderly, the risk of falls can be reduced by nearly 30% (Sherrington et al., 2019; Silva et al., 2013).

With a series of physical activities, the resistant exercises can provide a whole-body vibration (WBV) process to bone and muscle and contribute to constant locomotion and bone-muscle remodelling (Fatima et al., 2019). Moderate to vigorous intensity aerobic activities among older adults, such as brisk walking for 150 min (30 min a day, 5 days a week), and jogging / running (75 min every week), along with resistance training on all major muscle groups ($\geq$ 2 days/week), have been recommended by Centres for Disease Control and Prevention (2021). In addition, to have regular resistant exercises (3 times/week) over 12—24 weeks, the rate of muscle loss can be reduced among obese elderly and this provides extra benefit in lowering the risk of developing hypertension caused by osteosarcopenia associated obesity (Chen et al., 2019; Sardeli et al., 2018).

18.4.1.3 Dietary Nutrients Intake

Dietary protein intake has been proved to be an important nutrient source of the bone and muscle matrix and involved in musculoskeletal functioning through adapting roles in calcium absorption and hormonal controls (Rizzoli et al., 2014). Dietary protein intake in elderly (aged > 65 years) is recommended at least 1–1.2 g/kg daily (i.e. 25–30 g of protein in each meal) (Fatima et al., 2019; Yoo et al., 2020). If combined with continuous intake of protein supplements (6–30 g/day) for over 6–12 months, and together with adequate resistance exercises, the muscle strength could also be improved in elderly (Koutsofta et al., 2018).

Calcium is another essential micronutrient for the elderly to avoid osteosarcopenia. As an important mineral of bone, it is also suggested as an important role in muscle function (Endo, 2009). Dietary calcium and calcium supplements intake by elderly can contribute to their increases of BMD so as to reduce risks of falls and fractures (Fatima et al., 2019). The National Institute of Health (NIH) (2018) and the guideline established by Institute of Medicine (2011) recommend an adequate intake of calcium to be 1,000—1,300 mg/day in the diet for better bone health, and if dietary calcium is insufficient to meet the recommended level, additional calcium supplement ($\leq$ 500 mg/day) should be taken with food for better absorption. However, it should be taken with caution not to supplement high doses of calcium over 2,000 mg daily as evidence has shown that high dosage of calcium intakes can potentially increase cardiovascular side-effects among older adults (Tankeu et al., 2017).

Vitamin D also acts as an important nutrient for elderly and is vital for the formation of hormone calcitriol which facilitates calcium absorption from the diet and store in the skeleton for bone formation (NIH, 2018). With insufficient vitamin D, the bone and muscle mass will decline, worsened by weakened bioavailability of vitamin D when ageing. Subsequently the risk of getting osteosarcopenia will be higher. The ideal vitamin D daily intake for the elderly is 800 IU (20 μg) from a diet that can be derived from supplements or foods (e.g. oily fish, red meats, egg yolk, liver, fortified milk and cereal). Moreover, daily vitamin D intake should not exceed 4,000 IU/day or Vitamin D toxicity can occur, leading to adverse effects of hypercalcemia, bone pain and formation of calcium stones in the kidney (De Rui et al., 2019; Institute of Medicine, 2011; Meehan & Penckofer, 2014).

18.4.2 Early Diagnosis

18.4.2.1 Muscle Function and Bone Health

Dual-energy X-ray Absorptiometry (DEXA) scanning is used to measure BMD for diagnosis of osteoporosis. If T-score (i.e. standard deviation of mean BMD) is below the mean reference value of a healthy population, say, by 1.0 and 2.5 standard deviations, the examinees will be considered to be at higher risk of osteoporotic fractures (Karasik & Kiel, 2010). Among the elderly, the BMD will tend to be lower as compared to the general population due to co-occurrence of other complications, such as degenerative spine disease, vertebral collapse and disc disease (Barnsley et al., 2021). In addition, an alternative diagnostic tool for the elderly who are too weak or inconvenient to move or have no access to DEXA facility, the European Working Group on Sarcopenia in Older People (EWGSOP) has suggested the application of bioelectrical impedance analysis (BIA) for measurements of appendicular skeletal muscle mass, whole fat mass and water (Cruz-Jentoft et al., 2010; Fujimoto et al., 2018).

To diagnose for muscle functions and presence of sarcopenia, the Strength, Assistance with walking, Rising from a chair, Climbing stairs, and Falls (SARC-F) questionnaire has been developed for quick analysis of the condition. The five components in the questionnaire can assess the perceived muscle strength, needs for assistance with walking, difficulty to transfer from a chair or a bed, difficulty to climb stairs and frequency of falls of an individual. Questions are scored from 0 to 2 points for each component depending on the answers. If the overall scores are ≥ 4, an individual will probably have a condition of sarcopenia and weak grip strength (Malmstrom & Morley, 2013). By referring to the consensus report published by Asian Working Group for Sarcopenia (AWGS), muscle mass measured smaller than 7.0 kg/m2 for men and 5.4 kg/m2 for women; grip strength lower than 26 kg for men and 18 kg for women, and gait speed equal or fewer than 0.8 m/s will be considered to have sarcopenia. These reference values have been widely used in Asia (Chen et al., 2014).

18.4.2.2 Fall Risk Assessment

According to the clinical practice guideline on prevention of falls in elderly by the American Geriatrics Society/British Geriatrics Society, annual screening for fall risk can contribute to better follow-up exercises and better health outcomes of patients (The American Geriatrics Society, 2011). The application of Fall Risk Questionnaire (FRQ) can offer a timely and effective self-assessment screening tool to assess the fall risk of an individual by answering a 12-item questionnaire about fall risk factors, abnormal sensations and self-perceived fall risks. A total score equal or higher than 4 is indicative of higher risk of falling (Rubenstein et al., 2011).

National Centre for Injury Prevention and Control and the Centres for Disease Control and Prevention have also suggested a series of assessment methods to help in identifying, understanding and reducing the fall risk factors. They include (i) Mobility test on gait speed, sit and stand in a chair; (ii) Leg length and endurance test by assessing number of sets from sitting, crossing arms, standing up in a chair by the patient within 30s; and (iii) Balance test by assigning different standing positions from easy to hard degree of difficulty to the patients and ask them to hold each position for 10s (Eckstrom et al., 2021). The gait, muscle strength and underlying fall risks can be identified, and together with other measurement tools, such as hand-held dynamometry and DXA, the level of physical functions of the patients can be examined more accurately (Cruz-Jentoft et al., 2010). In addition, low body mass index (BMI) has also been demonstrated to have higher risk from developing osteosarcopenia and its progression (Okamura et al., 2020).

18.4.2.3 Depression

To find out symptoms of depression among elderly, the Patient Health Questionnaire (PHQ-2 or PHQ-9) asks about nine key symptoms of depression, e.g. lack of interest in most of activities, sense of hopelessness, frequent sleepiness, loss of appetite, etc. They are commonly used in primary care (Kroenke et al., 2003).

Korea has also developed a Korean version of the Geriatric Depression Scale (GDS-KR) and adapted it in the clinical setting to evaluate the major and minor depression disorders in the elderly. This questionnaire has been proved to have high validity and reliability on diagnosing psychiatric health (Bae & Cho, 2004; Kim et al., 2008).

18.4.2.4 Identification of Comorbidities

Extra care is required for the elderly with neurologic conditions (e.g. dementia, Parkinson's disease) and chronic diseases. An elderly with cognitive problems and osteosarcopenia will have significantly higher fall risks (Allan et al., 2009). Screening tools like Mini-Cog and Montreal Cognitive Assessment (MoCA) can be used to identify cognitive impairment (Eckstrom et al., 2021).

Chronic diseases, such as diabetes and hypertension, will increase the likelihood of developing cardiac complications that are associated with greater deterioration on patients' quality of life which is also affected by osteosarcopenia (Chen et al., 2019; Fahimfar et al, 2019).

18.4.3 Quality Improvement of Treatment Programmes

Use of the standardised quality improvement approach in treatment programme implementation can facilitate the establishment of patient-centred initiative throughout the treatment and support for better follow-up and care coordination (Eckstrom et al., 2021). Under this approach, a continual improvement of the programme should be pursued to achieve patient satisfaction. The Institute for Healthcare Improvement has proposed the Plan-Do-Study-Act (PDSA) cycles as a framework to achieve the initiatives. This framework advocates the monitoring plan to determine patient satisfaction and learning from feedbacks can help healthcare providers to plan for long-term care programmes with sustainability and reliability, while ensuring patients' compliance to the treatment programme (Langley et al, 2009).

To maintain a long-term programme sustainability and a successful programme at the clinical level, the Centres for Disease Control and Prevention has published a coordinated care plan to emphasise for identifying and tracking programme outcomes by setting up quantifiable targets. The strategies include regular scheduled training sessions for clinic team members to ensure they can perform proper screening exercise and are able to identify and implement suitable interventions for the modifiable risk factors (e.g. fall prevention in elderly). Programme coordinators are assigned to evaluate the programme process and assure the correct process by following Plan-Do-Study-Act (PDSA) cycles. Programme impact is demonstrated and new quality metric, e.g. annual outcome measures on rate of hospitalisation due to fall-related injuries for pre- and post-programme comparison, will be set up. Clinic leadership will be updated by evaluating annual outcomes and identifying quality improvement opportunities, for example, the use of Merit-Based Incentive Payment System (MIPS) established by the United States Centres for Medicare and Medicaid Services that encouraged clinicians to earn payment adjustment by implementing high quality and efficient practice in preventive activities to the patients and continuously submitting data to designated information system (Eckstrom et al., 2021; U.S Centres for Medicare & Medicaid Services, n.d.).

18.4.4 Nutritional Intakes and Exercises

Adequate nutrient intake with optimal exercise interventions should be adopted to maximise the treatment outcomes to improve muscle functions and maintain bone mass (Kirk, Mooney, et al., 2019). Nutritional supplementation includes vitamin D (at least 1,000 IU/day), calcium (600 mg per day), protein (($\geq$ 1.2 g/kg/day), creatine (3–5 g/day) and multicomponent exercise interventions comprise Tai Chi, resistance and balance training (e.g. leg press, shoulder press, Sit to Stand etc.) and flexibility exercises, etc. The combination of optimal nutritional intakes and physical activities has been well documented in the improvement of muscle strength, gait speed, functional capacity and fracture risks in the elderly (Daly et al., 2019; Kemmler et al., 2013; Saeki et al., 2020; Silva et al., 2013; Stanghelle et al., 2020).

18.4.5 Pharmacotherapy

Currently, there are lack of specific pharmacological agents that are targeted to treat sarcopenia but a wide range of pharmacotherapy has been developed for treating osteoporosis specifically (Paintin et al., 2018; Hassan & Duque, 2017). Nevertheless, with growing research on bone-muscle crosstalk, medications that are typically regarded to treat osteoporosis alone have been established to have beneficial effects in restoring muscle mass and strength as well. For example, Denosumab (receptor activator of nuclear factor kappa B (RANKL) inhibitor) that can break osteoclastic action by blocking the specific receptor to activate osteoclastogenesis, promotes the increases of BMD, mitigates muscle alterations and maintain glucose uptakes in skeletal muscles (Bonnet et al., 2020). Other major treatment agents for osteoporosis, such as Bisphosphonates (e.g. Alendronate, Risedronate, Zoledronate), selective oestrogen receptor modulators (SERMs) (e.g. raloxifene, anadarine), recombinant follistatin and teriparatide are recommended by the Clinical Guidelines Committee of the American College of Physicians (Qaseem et al., 2017).

Studies have also shown the potential benefits of hormonal therapies in treating osteosarcopenia. Testosterone replacement therapy has been demonstrated to have positive effects on BMD and muscle strength through the promotion of bone mineralisation and protein synthesis (Fatima et al., 2019). Other new therapies targeting the central signalling pathway to regulate bone and muscle, including recombinant growth hormone (GH) and GH secretagogues, are found to increase lean body mass and lumbar BMD (Girgis et al., 2014). Anti-myostatin therapies have been tested for its efficacy to improve functional capacity in people aged more than 75 years with increasing muscle strength and gait speed (Becker et al., 2015). Despite the potential promises, these therapies should be used with caution for their associated androgenic side effects, like joint and muscle pain, oedema, hyperglycaemia and potential concerns of cardiovascular events and even prostate cancer in men (Liu et al., 2007).

18.4.6 Cautions of Polypharmacy

Caregivers and patients should also be aware of the side effects of the medications, especially those that can affect the central nervous system, including antidepressants and anti-Parkinson medicines. The use of multiple psychoactive medicines has been shown to increase fall risks among elderly (Pratt et al., 2014). Therefore, medical treatments provided to elderly patients should be formulated and screened by the pharmacists. Optimisation of the medication plan should also be reviewed regularly with the aims to advise on tapering plans (i.e. reduce dosage of certain medications) and seek possible alternatives according to The American Geriatrics Society's Updated Beers Criteria which list out the potentially inappropriate medication use in older adults (Eckstrom et al., 2021; The American Geriatrics Society, 2019). Individualised medical therapy is crucial to avoid potential harmful side effects in the elderly because of the age-related changes of pharmacodynamics and pharmacokinetics caused by declining functions of organs in the body (Aymanns et al., 2010).

18.4.7 Evaluation of Home Hazards and Effective Communication

A safe living environment can assure independent living arrangements for the elderly. The removal of hazards can be achieved by preparation of home safety checklists by occupational therapists, home inspectors or other personnel with proper training in home safety assessment. With proper home modification for hazards reduction, the risk of injury, fall risks and falls related mortality can be effectively avoided (Pynoos et al., 2010). Fall prevention tips at home includes i) awareness of the environmental hazard; ii) choosing suitable and appropriate shoes and clothing; iii) performing self-care and household chores safely; iv) staying alert when going out such as avoid rushing and always having a free hand for emergencies; and v) using social resources such as housework services and family care services wisely (Elderly Health Service, 2020). Interventions include installation of handrails in the bathroom, removal of throw rugs, improved indoor lightning, etc. (Blanchet & Edwards, 2018; Eckstrom et al., 2021).

In addition to the modifications on the physical environment, psychological factors should also be assessed when studying the risk of falling. An elderly who has falling experience will have higher susceptibility to future fall than non-fallers, and they are associated with more attentional focus on controlling body movement deliberately. Such ruminations about previous falls can result in lower balance confidence, walking efficiency and gait stability in elderly with falling experience (Mak et al., 2019). Hence, a comprehensive care plan that can be easily implemented by healthcare team, patient, and family with effective communication for recommending interventions, analysing outcomes, understanding patient's perceived fall risks and encouraging objective fall risk management are essentials to assist patient behavioural change actively and continuously (Eckstrom et al., 2021).

18.5 Conclusion

Osteoporosis and sarcopenia are often being treated separately in the past. Recently, the new concept of osteosarcopenia is rapidly evolving and this is a very novel concept to tackle the knowledge gap between osteoporosis and sarcopenia. Instead of treating osteoporosis and sarcopenia alone and separately, the prevention and treatment of osteosarcopenia, by adopting the holistic care model mentioned in this chapter will be making an important role and impact in solving a cross-disciplinary problem from the bone and the muscle fields. Further studies should focus on minimising the knowledge gap between osteoporosis and sarcopenia, as well as the investigation methods or models to prevent or treat osteosarcopenia.

By adopting a holistic care model in caring elderly with osteosarcopenia, the health services and care programme targeting the elderly can focus on both physical and psychological sides whereas the approach should be evidence-based, supportive and sustainable. The continuous evaluation of programmes or interventions can ensure the measures are being more individualised to fit the varying emotions of the elderly while environmental alternations are also important to make the elderly live independently and safely. With the minimisation of their depression due to declining mobility, loss of self-care capability and weakened cognitive ability, the dignity and autonomy of patients can be preserved by showing more care and developing collaborative care plan with them (Lothian, 2001; Tranvåg et al., 2014).

References

Abate, M., Vanni, D., Pantalone, A., & Salini, V. (2013). Cigarette smoking and musculoskeletal disorders. *Muscle, Ligaments and Tendons Journal*, *3*(2). https://doi.org/10.11138/mltj/2013.3.2.063

Ajime, T. T., Serré, J., Wüst, R. C. I., Messa, G. A. M., Poffé, C., Swaminathan, A., Maes, K., Janssens, W., Troosters, T., Degens, H., & Gayan-Ramirez, G. (2020). Two weeks of smoking cessation reverse cigarette smoke-induced skeletal muscle atrophy and mitochondrial dysfunction in mice. *Nicotine & Tobacco Research, 23*(1), 143–151. https://doi.org/10.1093/ntr/ntaa016

Al Saedi, A., Hassan, E. B., & Duque, G. (2019). The diagnostic role of fat in osteosarcopenia. *Journal of Laboratory and Precision Medicine, 4*, 7. https://doi.org/10.21037/jlpm.2019.02.01

Allan, L. M., Ballard, C. G., Rowan, E. N., & Kenny, R. A. (2009). Incidence and prediction of falls in dementia: A prospective study in older people. *PLoS ONE, 4*(5), e5521. https://doi.org/10.1371/journal.pone.0005521

Aymanns, C., Keller, F., Maus, S., Hartmann, B., & Czock, D. (2010). Review on pharmacokinetics and pharmacodynamics and the ageing kidney. *Clinical Journal of the American Society of Nephrology, 5*(2), 314–327. https://doi.org/10.2215/cjn.03960609

Bae, J. N., & Cho, M. J. (2004). Development of the Korean version of the geriatric depression scale and its short form among elderly psychiatric patients. *Journal of Psychosomatic Research, 57*(3), 297–305. https://doi.org/10.1016/j.jpsychores.2004.01.004

Balogun, S., Winzenberg, T., Wills, K., Scott, D., Callisaya, M., Cicuttini, F., Jones, G., & Aitken, D. (2019). Prospective associations of osteosarcopenia and osteodynapenia with incident fracture and mortality over 10 years in community-dwelling older adults. *Archives of Gerontology and Geriatrics, 82*, 67–73. https://doi.org/10.1016/j.archger.2019.01.015

Barnsley, J., Buckland, G., Chan, P. E., Ong, A., Ramos, A. S., Baxter, M., Laskou, F., Dennison, E. M., Cooper, C., & Patel, H. P. (2021). Pathophysiology and treatment of osteoporosis: Challenges for clinical practice in older people. *Ageing Clinical and Experimental Research, 33*(4), 759–773. https://doi.org/10.1007/s40520-021-01817-y

Becker, C., Lord, S. R., Studenski, S. A., Warden, S. J., Fielding, R. A., Recknor, C. P., Hochberg, M. C., Ferrari, S. L., Blain, H., Binder, E. F., Rolland, Y., Poiraudeau, S., Benson, C. T., Myers, S. L., Hu, L., Ahmad, Q. I., Pacuch, K. R., Gomez, E. V., & Benichou, O. (2015). Myostatin antibody (LY2495655) in older weak fallers: A proof-of-concept, randomised, phase 2 trial. *The Lancet Diabetes & Endocrinology, 3*(12), 948–957. https://doi.org/10.1016/s2213-8587(15)00298-3

Berg, K. M., Kunins, H. V., Jackson, J. L., Nahvi, S., Chaudhry, A., Harris, K. A., Malik, R., & Arnsten, J. H. (2008). Association between alcohol consumption and both osteoporotic fracture and bone density. *The American Journal of Medicine, 121*(5), 406–418. https://doi.org/10.1016/j.amjmed.2007.12.012

Bhat, M., Kalam, R., Qadri, S. S., Madabushi, S., & Ismail, A. (2013). Vitamin D deficiency-induced muscle wasting occurs through the ubiquitin proteasome pathway and is partially corrected by calcium in male rats. *Endocrinology, 154*(11), 4018–4029. https://doi.org/10.1210/en.2013-1369

Bikle, D. D., Tahimic, C., Chang, W., Wang, Y., Philippou, A., & Barton, E. R. (2015). Role of IGF-I signaling in muscle bone interactions. *Bone, 80*, 79–88. https://doi.org/10.1016/j.bone.2015.04.036

Blanchet, R., & Edwards, N. (2018). A need to improve the assessment of environmental hazards for falls on stairs and in bathrooms: Results of a scoping review. *BMC Geriatrics, 18*(1). https://doi.org/10.1186/s12877-018-0958-1

Bonnet, N., Bourgoin, L., Biver, E., Douni, E., & Ferrari, S. (2020). RANKL inhibition improves muscle strength and insulin sensitivity and restores bone mass. *Journal of Clinical Investigation, 130*(6), 3329. https://doi.org/10.1172/jci138278

Centers for Disease Control and Prevention. (2021, February 11). *How much physical activity do older adults need?*. Centers for Disease Control and Prevention (CDC). https://www.cdc.gov/physicalactivity/basics/older_adults/index.htm

Chen, L. K., Liu, L. K., Woo, J., Assantachai, P., Auyeung, T. W., Bahyah, K. S., Chou, M. Y., Chen, L. Y., Hsu, P. S., Krairit, O., Lee, J. S., Lee, W. J., Lee, Y., Liang, C. K., Limpawattana, P., Lin, C. S., Peng, L. N., Satake, S., Suzuki, T., . . . Arai, H. (2014). Sarcopenia in Asia: Consensus report of the Asian working group for sarcopenia. *Journal of the American Medical Directors Association, 15*(2), 95–101. https://doi.org/10.1016/j.jamda.2013.11.025

Chen, X., Kong, C., Yu, H., Gong, J., Lan, L., Zhou, L., Gong, J., Liu, P., Xu, L., & Deng, Q. (2019). Association between osteosarcopenic obesity and hypertension among four minority populations in China: A cross-sectional study. *British Medical Journal Open, 9*(7), e026818. https://doi.org/10.1136/bmjopen-2018-026818

Cruz-Jentoft, A. J., Baeyens, J. P., Bauer, J. M., Boirie, Y., Cederholm, T., Landi, F., Martin, F. C., Michel, J. P., Rolland, Y., Schneider, S. M., Topinkova, E., Vandewoude, M., & Zamboni, M. (2010). Sarcopenia: European consensus on definition and diagnosis: Report of the European working group on sarcopenia in older people. *Age and Ageing, 39*(4), 412–423. https://doi.org/10.1093/ageing/afq034

Daly, R. M., Gianoudis, J., Kersh, M. E., Bailey, C. A., Ebeling, P. R., Krug, R., Nowson, C. A., Hill, K., & Sanders, K. M. (2019). Effects of a 12-Month supervised, community-based, multimodal exercise program followed by a 6-month research-to-practice transition on bone mineral density, trabecular microarchitecture, and physical function in older adults: A randomized controlled trial. *Journal of Bone and Mineral Research, 35*(3), 419–429. https://doi.org/10.1002/jbmr.3865

De Rui, M., Inelmen, E. M., Pigozzo, S., Trevisan, C., Manzato, E., & Sergi, G. (2019). Dietary strategies for mitigating osteosarcopenia in older adults: A narrative review. *Ageing Clinical and Experimental Research, 31*(7), 897–903. https://doi.org/10.1007/s40520-019-01130-9

Dolan, E., & Sale, C. (2018). Protein and bone health across the lifespan. *Proceedings of the Nutrition Society, 78*(1), 45–55. https://doi.org/10.1017/s0029665118001180

Drey, M., Sieber, C. C., Bertsch, T., Bauer, J. M., & Schmidmaier, R. (2015). Osteosarcopenia is more than sarcopenia and osteopenia alone. *Ageing Clinical and Experimental Research, 28*(5), 895–899. https://doi.org/10.1007/s40520-015-0494-1

Eckstrom, E., Parker, E. M., Shakya, I., & Lee, R. (2021). *Coordinated care plan to prevent older adult falls* (11th ed.). National Center for Injury Prevention and Control, Centers for Disease Control and Prevention. https://www.cdc.gov/steadi/pdf/Steadi-Coordinated-Care-Plan.pdf

Elderly Health Service. (2020) *Fall prevention.* https://www.elderly.gov.hk/english/healthy_ageing/home_safety/falls.html

Endo, M. (2009). Calcium-induced calcium release in skeletal muscle. *Physiological Reviews, 89*(4), 1153–1176. https://doi.org/10.1152/physrev.00040.2008

Estrada, K., Styrkarsdottir, U., Evangelou, E., Hsu, Y. H., Duncan, E. L., Ntzani, E. E., Oei, L., Albagha, O. M. E., Amin, N., Kemp, J. P., Koller, D. L., Li, G., Liu, C. T., Minster, R. L., Moayyeri, A., Vandenput, L., Willner, D., Xiao, S. M., Yerges-Armstrong, L. M., . . . Rivadeneira, F. (2012). Genome-wide meta-analysis identifies 56 bone mineral density loci and reveals 14 loci associated with risk of fracture. *Nature Genetics, 44*(5), 491–501. https://doi.org/10.1038/ng.2249

Fahimfar, N., Zahedi Tajrishi, F., Gharibzadeh, S., Shafiee, G., Tanha, K., Heshmat, R., Nabipour, I., Raeisi, A., Jalili, A., Larijani, B., & Ostovar, A. (2019). Prevalence of osteosarcopenia and its association with cardiovascular risk factors in Iranian older people: Bushehr Elderly Health (BEH) Program. *Calcified Tissue International, 106*(4), 364–370. https://doi.org/10.1007/s00223-019-00646-6

Fatima, M., Brennan-Olsen, S. L., & Duque, G. (2019). Therapeutic approaches to osteosarcopenia: Insights for the clinician. *Therapeutic Advances in Musculoskeletal Disease, 11*, 1–15. https://doi.org/10.1177/1759720x19867009

Fujimoto, K., Inage, K., Eguchi, Y., Orita, S., Suzuki, M., Kubota, G., Sainoh, T., Sato, J., Shiga, Y., Abe, K., Kanamoto, H., Inoue, M., Kinoshita, H., Norimoto, M., Umimura, T., Koda, M., Furuya, T., Akazawa, T., Toyoguchi, T., . . . Ohtori, S. (2018). Use of bioelectrical impedance analysis for the measurement of appendicular skeletal muscle mass/whole fat mass and its relevance in assessing osteoporosis among patients with low back pain: A comparative analysis using dual X-ray absorptiometry. *Asian Spine Journal, 12*(5), 839–845. https://doi.org/10.31616/asj.2018.12.5.839

Girgis, C. M., Mokbel, N., & DiGirolamo, D. J. (2014). Therapies for musculoskeletal disease: Can we treat two birds with one stone? *Current Osteoporosis Reports, 12*(2), 142–153. https://doi.org/10.1007/s11914-014-0204-5

Gordon, C. M., Zemel, B. S., Wren, T. A., Leonard, M. B., Bachrach, L. K., Rauch, F., Gilsanz, V., Rosen, C. J., & Winer, K. K. (2017). The determinants of peak bone mass. *The Journal of Pediatrics, 180*, 261–269. https://doi.org/10.1016/j.jpeds.2016.09.056

Greco, E. A., Pietschmann, P., & Migliaccio, S. (2019). Osteoporosis and sarcopenia increase frailty syndrome in the elderly. *Frontiers in Endocrinology, 10*(255). https://doi.org/10.3389/fendo.2019.00255

Hassan, E. B., & Duque, G. (2017). Osteosarcopenia: A new geriatric syndrome. *Australian Family Physician, 46*(11), 849–853. https://www.racgp.org.au/download/Documents/AFP/2017/November/AFP-2017-11-Clinical-Osteosarcopenia.pdf

Hernlund, E., Svedbom, A., Ivergård, M., Compston, J., Cooper, C., Stenmark, J., McCloskey, E. V., Jönsson, B., & Kanis, J. A. (2013). Osteoporosis in the European Union: Medical management, epidemiology and economic burden. *Archives of Osteoporosis, 8*(1–2). https://doi.org/10.1007/s11657-013-0136-1

Hirschfeld, H. P., Kinsella, R., & Duque, G. (2017). Osteosarcopenia: Where bone, muscle, and fat collide. *Osteoporosis International, 28*(10), 2781–2790. https://doi.org/10.1007/s00198-017-4151-8

Huo, Y. R., Suriyaarachchi, P., Gomez, F., Curcio, C. L., Boersma, D., Muir, S. W., Montero-Odasso, M., Gunawardene, P., Demontiero, O., & Duque, G. (2015). Phenotype of osteosarcopenia in older individuals with a history of falling. *Journal of the American Medical Directors Association, 16*(4), 290–295. https://doi.org/10.1016/j.jamda.2014.10.018

Inoue, T., Maeda, K., Nagano, A., Shimizu, A., Ueshima, J., Murotani, K., Sato, K., Hotta, K., Morishita, S., & Tsubaki, A. (2021). Related factors and clinical outcomes of osteosarcopenia: A narrative review. *Nutrients, 13*(2), 291. https://doi.org/10.3390/nu13020291

Institute of Medicine. (2011). *Dietary reference intakes for calcium and vitamin D*. The National Academies Press. https://doi.org/10.17226/13050

Kanis, J. A., Johnell, O., Oden, A., Johansson, H., De Laet, C., Eisman, J. A., Fujiwara, S., Kroger, H., McCloskey, E. V., Mellstrom, D., Melton, L. J., Pols, H., Reeve, J., Silman, A., & Tenenhouse, A. (2004). Smoking and fracture risk: A meta-analysis. *Osteoporosis International, 16*(2), 155–162. https://doi.org/10.1007/s00198-004-1640-3

Karasik, D., & Kiel, D. P. (2010). Evidence for pleiotropic factors in genetics of the musculoskeletal system. *Bone, 46*(5), 1226–1237. https://doi.org/10.1016/j.bone.2010.01.382

Kemmler, W., Häberle, L., & von Stengel, S. (2013). Effects of exercise on fracture reduction in older adults. *Osteoporosis International, 24*(7), 1937–1950. https://doi.org/10.1007/s00198-012-2248-7

Kim, J. Y., Park, J. H., Lee, J. J., Huh, Y., Lee, S. B., Han, S. K., Choi, S. W., Lee, D. Y., Kim, K. W., & Woo, J. I. (2008). Standardization of the Korean version of the geriatric depression scale: Reliability, validity, and factor structure. *Psychiatry Investigation, 5*(4), 232–238. https://doi.org/10.4306/pi.2008.5.4.232

Kirk, B., Al Saedi, A., & Duque, G. (2019). Osteosarcopenia: A case of geroscience. *AGEING MEDICINE, 2*(3), 147–156. https://doi.org/10.1002/agm2.12080

Kirk, B., Miller, S., Zanker, J., & Duque, G. (2020). A clinical guide to the pathophysiology, diagnosis and treatment of osteosarcopenia. *Maturitas, 140*, 27–33. https://doi.org/10.1016/j.maturitas.2020.05.012

Kirk, B., Mooney, K., Amirabdollahian, F., & Khaiyat, O. (2019b). Exercise and dietary-protein as a countermeasure to skeletal muscle weakness: Liverpool Hope University—Sarcopenia ageing trial (LHU-SAT). *Frontiers in Physiology, 10*. https://doi.org/10.3389/fphys.2019.00445

Kirk, B., Zanker, J., & Duque, G. (2020). Osteosarcopenia: Epidemiology, diagnosis, and treatment—facts and numbers. *Journal of Cachexia, Sarcopenia and Muscle, 11*(3), 609–618. https://doi.org/10.1002/jcsm.12567

Klop, C., Welsing, P. M., Cooper, C., Harvey, N. C., Elders, P. J., Bijlsma, J. W., Leufkens, H. G., & de Vries, F. (2014). Mortality in British hip fracture patients, 2000–2010: A population-based retrospective cohort study. *Bone, 66*, 171–177. https://doi.org/10.1016/j.bone.2014.06.011

Koutsofta, I., Mamais, I., & Chrysostomou, S. (2018). The effect of protein diets in postmenopausal women with osteoporosis: Systematic review of randomized controlled trials. *Journal of Women & Ageing, 31*(2), 117–139. https://doi.org/10.1080/08952841.2018.1418822

Kroenke, K., Spitzer, R. L., & Williams, J. B. W. (2003). The patient health questionnaire-2: Validity of a two-item depression screener. *Medical Care, 41*(11), 1284–1292. https://doi.org/10.1097/01.mlr.0000093487.78664.3c

Langley, G. J., Moen, R. D., Nolan, K. M., Nolan, T. W., Norman, C. L., & Provost, L. P. (2009). *The Improvement Guide: A Practical Approach to Enhancing Organizational Performance* (2nd ed.). Jossey-Bass. http://www.ihi.org/resources/Pages/Publications/ImprovementGuidePracticalApproachEnhancingOrganizationalPerformance.aspx

Liu, H., Bravata, D. M., Olkin, I., Nayak, S., Roberts, B., Garber, A. M., & Hoffman, A. R. (2007). Systematic review: The safety and efficacy of growth hormone in the healthy elderly. *Annals of Internal Medicine, 146*(2), 104. https://doi.org/10.7326/0003-4819-146-2-200701160-00005

Lothian, K. (2001). Care of older people: Maintaining the dignity and autonomy of older people in the healthcare setting. *BMJ, 322*(7287), 668–670. https://doi.org/10.1136/bmj.322.7287.668

Luo, L. Z., & Xu, L. (2005). Study on direct economic-burden and its risk factors of osteoporotic hip fracture. *Chinese Journal of Epidemiology, 26*(9), 669–672. http://rs.yiigle.com/CN112338200509/591774.htm

Mak, T. C. T., Young, W. R., Lam, W. K., Tse, A. C. Y., & Wong, T. W. L. (2019). The role of attentional focus on walking efficiency among older fallers and non-fallers. *Age and Ageing, 48*(6), 811–816. https://doi.org/10.1093/ageing/afz113

Malmstrom, T. K., & Morley, J. E. (2013). SARC-F: A simple questionnaire to rapidly diagnose sarcopenia. *Journal of the American Medical Directors Association, 14*(8), 531–532. https://doi.org/10.1016/j.jamda.2013.05.018

McEvoy, L., & Duffy, A. (2008). Holistic practice – A concept analysis. *Nurse Education in Practice, 8*(6), 412–419. https://doi.org/10.1016/j.nepr.2008.02.002

Meehan, M., & Penckofer, S. (2014). The role of vitamin D in the ageing adult. *Journal of Ageing and Gerontology, 2*(2), 60–71. https://doi.org/10.12974/2309-6128.2014.02.02.1

Nielsen, B. R., Abdulla, J., Andersen, H. E., Schwarz, P., & Suetta, C. (2018). Sarcopenia and osteoporosis in older people: A systematic review and meta-analysis. *European Geriatric Medicine, 9*(4), 419–434. https://doi.org/10.1007/s41999-018-0079-6

Okamura, H., Ishikawa, K., Kudo, Y., Matsuoka, A., Maruyama, H., Emori, H., Yamamura, R., Hayakawa, C., Tani, S., Tsuchiya, K., Shirahata, T., Toyone, T., Nagai, T., & Inagaki, K. (2020). Risk factors predicting osteosarcopenia in postmenopausal women with osteoporosis: A retrospective study. *PLoS ONE, 15*(8), e0237454. https://doi.org/10.1371/journal.pone.0237454

Paintin, J., Cooper, C., & Dennison, E. (2018). Osteosarcopenia. *British Journal of Hospital Medicine, 79*(5), 253–258. https://doi.org/10.12968/hmed.2018.79.5.253

Park, K. S., Lee, G. Y., Seo, Y. M., Seo, S. H., & Yoo, J. I. (2021). Disability, frailty and depression in the community-dwelling older adults with osteosarcopenia. *BMC Geriatrics, 21*(1). https://doi.org/10.1186/s12877-021-02022-2

Poggiogalle, E., Cherry, K. E., Su, L. J., Kim, S., Myers, L., Welsh, D. A., Jazwinski, S. M., & Ravussin, E. (2019). Body composition, IGF1 status, and physical functionality in Nonagenarians: Implications for osteosarcopenia. *Journal of the American Medical Directors Association, 20*(1), 70–75. https://doi.org/10.1016/j.jamda.2018.07.007

Pratt, N. L., Ramsay, E. N., Kalisch Ellett, L. M., Nguyen, T. A., Barratt, J. D., & Roughead, E. E. (2014). Association between use of multiple psychoactive medicines and hospitalization for falls: Retrospective analysis of a large healthcare claim database. *Drug Safety, 37*(7), 529–535. https://doi.org/10.1007/s40264-014-0179-2

Pynoos, J., Steinman, B. A., & Nguyen, A. Q. (2010). Environmental assessment and modification as fall-prevention strategies for older adults. *Clinics in Geriatric Medicine, 26*(4), 633–644. https://doi.org/10.1016/j.cger.2010.07.001

Qaseem, A., Forciea, M. A., McLean, R. M., & Denberg, T. D. (2017). Treatment of low bone density or osteoporosis to prevent fractures in men and women: A clinical practice guideline update from the American college of physicians. *Annals of Internal Medicine, 166*(11), 818. https://doi.org/10.7326/m15-1361

Rizzoli, R., Stevenson, J. C., Bauer, J. M., van Loon, L. J., Walrand, S., Kanis, J. A., Cooper, C., Brandi, M. L., Diez-Perez, A., & Reginster, J. Y. (2014). The role of dietary protein and vitamin D in maintaining musculoskeletal health in postmenopausal women: A consensus statement from the European Society for Clinical and Economic Aspects of Osteoporosis and Osteoarthritis (ESCEO). *Maturitas, 79*(1), 122–132. https://doi.org/10.1016/j.maturitas.2014.07.005

Rubenstein, L. Z., Vivrette, R., Harker, J. O., Stevens, J. A., & Kramer, B. J. (2011). Validating an evidence-based, self-rated fall risk questionnaire (FRQ) for older adults. *Journal of Safety Research, 42*(6), 493–499. https://doi.org/10.1016/j.jsr.2011.08.006

Saeki, C., Kanai, T., Nakano, M., Oikawa, T., Torisu, Y., Abo, M., Saruta, M., & Tsubota, A. (2020). Relationship between osteosarcopenia and frailty in patients with chronic liver disease. *Journal of Clinical Medicine, 9*(8), 2381. https://doi.org/10.3390/jcm9082381

Salech, F., Marquez, C., Lera, L., Angel, B., Saguez, R., & Albala, C. (2021). Osteosarcopenia predicts falls, fractures, and mortality in Chilean community-dwelling older adults. *Journal of the American Medical Directors Association, 22*(4), 853–858. https://doi.org/10.1016/j.jamda.2020.07.032

Sardeli, A., Komatsu, T., Mori, M., Gáspari, A., & Chacon-Mikahil, M. (2018). Resistance training prevents muscle loss induced by caloric restriction in obese elderly individuals: A systematic review and meta-analysis. *Nutrients, 10*(4), 423. https://doi.org/10.3390/nu10040423

Scott, D., Seibel, M., Cumming, R., Naganathan, V., Blyth, F., Le Couteur, D. G., Handelsman, D. J., Waite, L. M., & Hirani, V. (2018). Does combined osteopenia/osteoporosis and sarcopenia confer greater risk of falls and fracture than either condition alone in older men? The concord health and ageing in men project. *The Journals of Gerontology: Series A, 74*(6), 827–834. https://doi.org/10.1093/gerona/gly162

Shen, G. S., Li, Y., Zhao, G., Zhou, H. B., Xie, Z. G., Xu, W., Chen, H. N., Dong, Q. R., & Xu, Y. J. (2015). Cigarette smoking and risk of hip fracture in women: A meta-analysis of prospective cohort studies. *Injury, 46*(7), 1333–1340. https://doi.org/10.1016/j.injury.2015.04.008

Sherrington, C., Fairhall, N. J., Wallbank, G. K., Tiedemann, A., Michaleff, Z. A., Howard, K., Clemson, L., Hopewell, S., & Lamb, S. E. (2019). Exercise for preventing falls in older people living in the community. *Cochrane Database of Systematic Reviews, 1*(1). https://doi.org/10.1002/14651858.cd012424.pub2

Silva, R. B., Eslick, G. D., & Duque, G. (2013). Exercise for falls and fracture prevention in long term care facilities: A systematic review and meta-analysis. *Journal of the American Medical Directors Association, 14*(9), 685–689. https://doi.org/10.1016/j.jamda.2013.05.015

Stanghelle, B., Bentzen, H., Giangregorio, L., Pripp, A., Skelton, D., & Bergland, A. (2020). Effects of a resistance and balance exercise programme on physical fitness, health-related quality of life and fear of falling in older women with osteoporosis and vertebral fracture: A randomized controlled trial. *Osteoporosis International, 31*(6), 1069–1078. https://doi.org/10.1007/s00198-019-05256-4

Steiner, J. L., & Lang, C. H. (2015). Dysregulation of skeletal muscle protein metabolism by alcohol. *American Journal of Physiology-Endocrinology and Metabolism, 308*(9), E699–E712. https://doi.org/10.1152/ajpendo.00006.2015

Suriyaarachchi, P., Gomez, F., Curcio, C. L., Boersma, D., Murthy, L., Grill, V., & Duque, G. (2018). High parathyroid hormone levels are associated with osteosarcopenia in older individuals with a history of falling. *Maturitas, 113*, 21–25. https://doi.org/10.1016/j.maturitas.2018.04.006

Tamilarasan, K. P., Temmel, H., Das, S. K., Al Zoughbi, W., Schauer, S., Vesely, P. W., & Hoefler, G. (2012). Skeletal muscle damage and impaired regeneration due to LPL-mediated lipotoxicity. *Cell Death & Disease, 3*(7), e354. https://doi.org/10.1038/cddis.2012.91

Tankeu, A. T., Agbor, V. N., & Noubiap, J. J. (2017). Calcium supplementation and cardiovascular risk: A rising concern. *The Journal of Clinical Hypertension, 19*(6), 640–646. https://doi.org/10.1111/jch.13010

The American Geriatrics Society. (2011). Summary of the updated American geriatrics society/British geriatrics dociety clinical practice guideline for prevention of falls in older persons.

Journal of the American Geriatrics Society, 59(1), 148–157. https://doi.org/10.1111/j.1532-5415.2010.03234.x

The American Geriatrics Society. (2019). American geriatrics society 2019 updated AGS beers criteria® for potentially inappropriate medication use in older adults. *Journal of the American Geriatrics Society, 67*(4), 674–694. https://doi.org/10.1111/jgs.15767

The National Institutes of Health (NIH). (2018, October). *Calcium and Vitamin D: Important at Every Age*. NIH Osteoporosis and Related Bone Diseases—National Resource Center. https://www.bones.nih.gov/health-info/bone/bone-health/nutrition/calcium-and-vitamin-d-important-every-age

Thompson, E. A., Quinn, T., Paterson, C., Cooke, H., McQuigan, D., & Butters, G. (2008). Outcome measures for holistic, complex interventions within the palliative care setting. *Complementary Therapies in Clinical Practice, 14*(1), 25–32. https://doi.org/10.1016/j.ctcp.2007.10.001

Tranvåg, O., Petersen, K. A., & Nåden, D. (2014). Relational interactions preserving dignity experience. *Nursing Ethics, 22*(5), 577–593. https://doi.org/10.1177/0969733014549882

U.S Centers for Medicare & Medicaid Services. (n.d.). *Merit-based incentive payment system—Participation options overview*. Quality Payment Program. https://qpp.cms.gov/mips/overview

World Health Organization. (2007). *WHO scientific group on the assessment of osteoporosis at primary health care level*. WHO Press, World Health Organization. https://www.who.int/chp/topics/Osteoporosis.pdf

Yang, Y., Du, F., Ye, W., Chen, Y., Li, J., Zhang, J., Nicely, H., & Burge, R. (2015). Inpatient cost of treating osteoporotic fractures in mainland China: A descriptive analysis. *ClinicoEconomics and Outcomes Research, 2015*(7), 205–212. https://doi.org/10.2147/ceor.s77175

Yoo, J. I., Kim, H., Ha, Y. C., Kwon, H. B., & Koo, K. H. (2018). Osteosarcopenia in patients with hip fracture is related with high mortality. *Journal of Korean Medical Science, 33*(4). https://doi.org/10.3346/jkms.2018.33.e27

Yoo, J. I., Lee, K. H., Choi, Y., Lee, J., & Park, Y. G. (2020). Poor dietary protein intake in elderly population with sarcopenia and osteosarcopenia: A nationwide population-based study. *Journal of Bone Metabolism, 27*(4), 301–310. https://doi.org/10.11005/jbm.2020.27.4.301

Yoshimura, N., Muraki, S., Oka, H., Iidaka, T., Kodama, R., Horii, C., Kawaguchi, H., Nakamura, K., Akune, T., & Tanaka, S. (2018). Do sarcopenia and/or osteoporosis increase the risk of frailty? A 4-year observation of the second and third ROAD study surveys. *Osteoporosis International, 29*(10), 2181–2190. https://doi.org/10.1007/s00198-018-4596-4

Zanker, J., & Duque, G. (2018). Osteoporosis in older persons: Old and new players. *Journal of the American Geriatrics Society, 67*(4), 831–840. https://doi.org/10.1111/jgs.15716

Chapter 19
Chemical Pollution and Healthy Ageing: The Prominent Need for a Cleaner Environment

Wang-Kin Chiu and Ben Yuk Fai Fong

Abstract Chemical contaminants in our living environment are the basic contributing factors of air, water and food pollution, which pose a serious threat to the human health. This is a particular concern for the elderly population. In fact, a growing body of epidemiologic evidence supports the association between certain environmental pollutants and age-related diseases. There are various sources of pollutants in air and the adverse effects of different pollutants to the elderly cannot be neglected. For an instance, exposure to fine particulate matter ($PM_{2.5}$) has been suggested to play a role in the development of dementia, with which its global prevalence among the elderly has been extensively reported. Besides air pollution, water and food quality, a health concern that may be easily overlooked, is actually an influential factor to the success of healthy ageing. The elderly is prone to the serious effects from contaminants in drinking water and food due to the higher risk of suffering from chronic diseases, as well as weakened immune systems and functions of liver and kidney. Recently, there has been growing concern worldwide regarding health problems resulting from exposure to heavy metals, such as lead, mercury and cadmium. For example, there is report supporting the association of high levels of heavy metals and prevalence of dyslipidemia in the elderly population. In this chapter, the various issues of chemical pollution and the adverse effects to the health of the elderly will be discussed. Research findings of related investigations will also be reviewed and summarised. The important implications and recommendations on research, policy and education will be further identified to give insights towards a cleaner environment which is indispensable for the success of healthy ageing.

Keywords Chemical pollution · Healthy ageing · Sustainable development · Sustainable chemistry · Environmental sustainability

W.-K. Chiu (✉) · B. Y. F. Fong
College of Professional and Continuing Education, The Hong Kong Polytechnic University, Hong Kong, China
e-mail: oscar.chiu@cpce-polyu.edu.hk

V. T. S. Law and B. Y. F. Fong (eds.), *Ageing with Dignity in Hong Kong and Asia*, Quality of Life in Asia 16, https://doi.org/10.1007/978-981-19-3061-4_19

19.1 Introduction

Chemicals can be found everywhere with indispensable applications in our daily life. However, the presence of chemicals in a certain place with concentration higher than the safety level results in chemical contamination, which poses serious adverse health effects. Various sources can release different types of chemical contaminants to the environment, causing hazardous effects which include air, water and food pollution (Rather et al., 2017). In fact, the extensive use of chemicals is just like a double-edged sword. Different chemicals find their broad daily applications. On the other hand, the widespread use of chemicals has been a critical issue of environmental concern. For example, advanced techniques in synthetic chemistry are emerging as promising tools deployed for drug design and development. However, growing concern has also evolved due to the presence of pharmaceutical residues in effluents from drug manufacturing factories at some regions. The chemicals are finally released to the aquatic environment causing reported detection of substantial amount of groundwater pollutants (Fick et al., 2009; Larsson et al., 2007).

The deteriorating environmental quality resulted from the increasing chemical pollution is of particular concern to elderly health due to the higher susceptibility of this population group (Simoni et al., 2015). The growing ageing population also adds to the prominent importance of a sustainable environment (Fong et al., 2021). In this chapter, the various issues of chemical pollution and the adverse effects on the elderly health will be discussed. Research findings in the context of Asian studies will also be reviewed and summarised. The important implications and recommendations behind will be further identified to give insights towards a clean sustainable environment which is indispensable for the success of healthy ageing.

19.2 Air Pollution

The advancement of modern technology has been seen as the main culprit of air pollution. Notably, starting from the mid-nineteenth century, a substantial increase of pollutants, including sulphur dioxide (SO_2), nitrogen oxides (NO_x) and particulate matter (PM_x), has been observed which was accompanied with the significant increase in the extensive consumption of coal since the first industrial revolution (Han et al., 2020). Various sources could release chemical contaminants to the environment causing air pollution and bad impacts to human health (Brusseau & Artiola, 2019). Atmospheric pollutants could be originated from naturally induced processes such as an accidental forest fire caused by lightning. Apart from natural pollutants, the term "primary pollutants" is used to describe the majority of air pollutants which are chemicals released into the atmosphere from various types of human activities. Notable examples include volatile hydrocarbons and carbon monoxide from the incomplete combustion of fossil fuels, as well as $PM_{2.5}$ (particulate matter with an aerodynamic diameter equal to or less than 2.5 μm), NO_x and SO_2 from the burning of fuels. A $PM_{2.5}$ measurement study of organic and black carbon concentrations at an urban traffic site in Bangladesh, a densely populated country in South Asia, revealed that the pollutant sources could be from traffic emissions and the burning of coal and biomass (Begum et al., 2012).

Besides, primary pollutants are generated due to the intrinsic inefficiency of an industrial process. Moreover, chemicals released from human activities such as extraction of raw materials and manufacturing of products can further react under the condition of sufficient energy. As a result, secondary pollutants including ozone (O_3) and other reactive compounds are produced which may also have adverse health effects (Mabahwi et al., 2014). Notably, a significant source of air pollutants come from the burning of biomass and the adverse effects on health due to the biomass burning-induced smoke haze should not be overlooked. In Southeast Asia, the biomass burning-induced smoke haze with elevated PM levels is a common phenomenon. A recent review by Adam et al. (2020) also indicated that substantial amounts of PM (in different sizes and chemical compositions) were released by vegetation, peatland and forest fires in various Southeast Asia regions. This caused elevating levels of air pollutants in regions not only restricted to those within the proximity of sources of biomass burning, but also in areas with dense population further away from the sources. The frequent occurrence of biomass burning-induced smoke haze in Southeast Asia and transboundary effects due to strong winds have led to decreased air quality across several Southeast countries. For example, Fujii et al. (2015) have studied the effects of Indonesian peatland fires and analysed the annual variations in the concentrations of $PM_{2.5}$ in Malaysia, which focused on various organic substances released from sources of biomass burning. Recently, Phairuang et al. (2017) investigated the effects of forest fires and burning of crop residues on the air quality across several provinces in Thailand and reported the association of increased PM concentrations with the agricultural activities and forest fires. Meanwhile, polycyclic aromatic hydrocarbons (PAHs), a remarkable category of persistent organic compounds found in PM, have been the specific focus of many research studies investigating their physio-chemical properties due to the potent carcinogenic nature of the chemicals (Pongpiachan, 2016).

Major sources of $PM_{2.5}$-bound PAHs include vehicle emissions, industrial flue gas, tobacco smoking, household activities such as heating and cooking, in addition to biomass burning (Zhang et al., 2021). In 2016, Han et al. conducted a personal exposure assessment to PM-bound PAHs in a retirement community of Tianjin, a mega city in Northern China. The study revealed the association of inhalation exposure to elevated levels of particulate PAHs with a higher cancer risk among the elderly. In addition, a recent study has examined the relationship between exposure to PAHs and functional dependence, which is also an important factor affecting quality of life among the elderly (Chen et al., 2019). The study reported findings which supported high association of exposure to PAHs with an increased risk of total disability in an elderly population although the underlying pathophysiological mechanisms leading to possible cognitive and functional impairment are subject to further research investigations.

While there have been calls for urgent actions to mitigate the deterioration of air quality in Asia as a result of the evolving industrialisation and urbanisation in the past decades, there have been limited studies on the long-term effects of air pollution on mortality in Asia (Wong et al., 2015). The study by Wong et al. (2015) is one of the remarkable examples which studied the effects of long-term $PM_{2.5}$ exposure and mortality among the elderly in Hong Kong. The statistical analysis of data recruited from a cohort of 66,820 elderly participants (aged 65 or above) in this satellite-based investigation revealed a high association between individual long-term exposure to $PM_{2.5}$ and mortality in the elderly population for all natural and cardiovascular causes. Furthermore, another study harnessing the use of land use regression models for estimating air pollutant concentrations, which served as an extension of the prior analysis, also supported a significant association of cardiovascular mortality among the same elderly cohort in Hong Kong with long-term exposure to $PM_{2.5}$ (Yang et al., 2018). Considering the adverse effects of air pollution on human health, it is important that studies investigating the health effects resulting from either long-term exposure or short-term exposure should also be emphasised. For elderly people, they are more susceptible to the detrimental effects of air pollution and such effects can be lethal even for a short-term exposure to air pollutants because of comorbidity (Simoni et al., 2015) and pathological ageing (Bentayeb et al., 2012).

Findings from various time-series studies have suggested the positive association between short-term exposure to air pollutants and the adverse effects on human health (Bhaskaran et al., 2013). In addition, significant results from epidemiological studies have supported the association with increased respiratory morbidity among the elderly population (Bentayeb et al., 2012). Meanwhile, it is noteworthy that psychological well-being is also important to healthy ageing. The relationship between exposure to air pollution and the mental health of elderly people has attracted considerable attention in health research during the recent decades in view of the prevalence of mental disorders such as cognitive impairment and depression in the later stage of life (Pun et al., 2017). In 2015, Tian et al. had reported an analytical study on the effect of air pollution on mental health among the elderly in China. The results suggested significant influence of air pollution (air pollution degree being measured by SO_2 emission) on the elderly mental health. Furthermore, a recent study by Tang et al. (2020), focusing on the elderly Chinese residents in Ningbo, has reported findings supporting the positive association between short-term exposure to air pollution and sleep disorder, a common symptom among the elderly which has frequent co-occurrence with other neurological and mental disorders. More recently, a cohort study recruiting elderly participants from the same city reported evidence suggesting the association between exposure to $PM_{2.5}$ and increased incidence of Parkinson's disease (Yu et al., 2021). The research study has also indicated the importance of a green environment for reduction in the risk of Parkinson's disease. Notably, the literature findings also support that exposure to solvents or pesticides may increase the risk of developing Parkinson's disease (Pezzoli & Cereda, 2013).

19.3 Water and Food Pollution

A healthy environment is not just merely referring to the presence of clean air. Serious considerations should also be put on water and food. Chemical contaminations of water and food can lead to severe health effects with the elderly having a high susceptibility to the adverse impact. Heavy metals, such as lead, mercury and cadmium, have potent toxicity even at trace amounts and heavy metal pollution is considered a probable environmental factor contributing to dyslipidemia, which is a prevalent disease of having abnormal blood lipid levels. Dyslipidemia is also a critical risk factor for the onset of cardiovascular diseases (Ghandehari et al., 2008), and its continually increasing prevalence in different countries, including those in the Asia Pacific region (Lin et al., 2018), has aroused worldwide concern especially considering its association with cardiovascular diseases and the growing worldwide ageing population. One of the major causes of the dramatic increase of heavy metal contamination is the continued sewage discharge and industrial effluents resulted from the rapid growth of industrialisation. The impacts of heavy metal contamination on food safety and emerging issues related to food security have been extensively documented (Lu et al., 2015; Rai et al., 2019).

Contaminations of water and food by heavy metals continue to pose serious threats to public health. This gives rise to growing concern in regions where wastewater is reused for agricultural irrigation due to limited availability of freshwater (Jan et al., 2015; Rattan et al., 2005). In the past decades, various studies have suggested the association between cardiovascular morbidity and exposure to lead in drinking water or irrigation water (Bjørklund et al., 2018). Recently, Zhu et al. (2021) have evaluated the correlation between blood metal levels and dyslipidemia. The study recruited participants from the elderly community in a city in China. The findings have suggested the association of lead exposure with increased risk of dyslipidemia. Moreover, the study by Asgary et al. (2017) presented findings on the observation of elevated serum levels of lead, cadmium and mercury among the elderly patients with coronary artery disease.

In addition to heavy metal pollution, chemical contaminations of food can also be caused by plastic pollution. There is growing concern towards the deteriorating situation caused by the environmental pollution with microplastic particles. Reported examples include contamination of table salts, drinking water, sediment and air (Prata et al., 2020). In their study, Lee et al. (2019) reported that microplastics were found in 94% of salt products. Polyethylene terephthalate (PETE), polypropene (PP) and polyethene (PE) were among those identified as the major examples of polymer particles found in the tested samples. Although further research is required for investigating the effects of human exposure to microplastics, increasing pollution of the environment by microplastics is attracting significant attentions with current evidence of findings suggesting the possible health impacts including inflammatory lesions, toxicity resulted from oxidative stress, disruption of immune functions and neurodegenerative diseases (Prata et al., 2020).

19.4 Implications and Recommendations on Research, Policy and Education

The worldwide elderly population continues to grow and a healthy environment is essential for healthy ageing (Chiu & Fong, 2021; Fong et al., 2021). Chemical pollution poses serious threat to a sustainable environment. This severely affects healthy ageing in view of the prevalence of chronic diseases and higher susceptibility of the elderly to the adverse health effects caused by pollution (Simoni et al., 2015). Considering that various sources can give rise to chemical pollution of the environment, different intervention measures should be taken for remediating actions. One of the main focuses is to address the alarming situation of worsening environmental quality caused by air pollution. In view of the significant findings from various epidemiological studies which suggested the associations of exposures to air pollution with increased risks of cancers, cardiovascular and respiratory diseases, there have been calls for urgent need to identify and implement efficient mitigation strategies for the reduced emission of hazardous chemicals (Sofia et al., 2020). Further planning of policy on chemical management and regulatory system, with special attention to vulnerable population groups including the elderly and children, is necessary to include promotional programmes for both sustainable chemistry and the circular economy as strategic measures to enhance the efficient use of chemicals and reduce the adverse impacts of hazardous chemicals on public health and environmental quality (Matus, 2021). Specific guidelines and pathways to healthy urban living have been discussed including the advocation of smart city and car-free city (Nieuwenhuijsen & Khreis, 2016; Sofia et al., 2020).

In Hong Kong, there are various environment initiatives put forth under the major area of "Smart Environment" in the second edition of Hong Kong Smart City Blueprint (2020). Remarkable examples include implementation of decarbonisation technologies to reduce carbon intensity by a target of 65–70% by 2030 in comparison with the 2005 level, gradual phase down of power generation by burning of coals and scaled-up application of renewable energy. As for the development of a green and smart community, important components such as green building design and provision of electric-car charging facilities are required for new land sale sites. Furthermore, with regards to pollution monitoring, examples include the adoption of remote sensing devices for monitoring air pollution and unmanned vessels for monitoring water quality, respectively. Meanwhile, concerted efforts are required from the scientific community. Further research investigations are needed for applying green chemistry and sustainable chemistry technologies in the transformation of the chemical industry (Matus, 2021). At the same time, sustainable chemistry, a relatively new development of applied sciences, is expected to play an important role in moving the society towards a sustainable future and achieving the Sustainable Development Goals (SDGs) globally (Barra & González, 2018). More investigations are needed for the development of chemical knowledge and incorporating sustainable chemistry into the extraction, synthetic, disposing and recycling processes. Incorporation of the principles of sustainability in the design, production and application of chemicals and chemical products is critical to the development of a sustainable environment. Establishing green solvents for industrial processes and reaction chemistry has been an important research agenda in recent years (Byrne et al., 2016). Emerging issues on the development and use of green solvents are worth investigating considering the harmful effects of certain chemicals on human health. A recent research study conducted in China revealed that the use of dimethylformamide (DMF), a common solvent for chemical synthesis and being exposed to a large population in the country, poses significantly higher health risks to the elderly residents living in the regions around the synthetic plants (Hu et al., 2020). The findings of the study suggested the association of DMF exposure with a higher risk of kidney and liver dysfunction for the elderly people residing around synthetic leather factories.

In addition to the development of green solvents in replacement of solvents which have harmful health effects, there have been extensive discussions on the reduction in the use of pesticides since pesticide poisoning has long been a critical issue in public health (Cha et al., 2014). In the past decades, various studies have reported the association of exposure to pesticides with cognitive impairment and dementia, which heavily affects an elder's quality of life (Aloizou et al., 2020). Also, the study by Cha et al. (2014) found that both the mortality rate due to pesticide poisoning and incidence rate of pesticide poisoning were higher among the elderly, and higher rates were also observed in rural than in urban areas of South Korea. While further efforts are needed to prevent pesticide self-poisonings, agricultural activities such as organic farming with minimised use of synthetic fertilisers or pesticides are worth investigations in view of the importance of a sustainable environment (Chiu & Fong, 2021).

Furthermore, due to the rapid growth of industrial development and worldwide population, investigations to address issues related to global sustainability will continue to be a major research agenda in the coming future. For example, development of materials and technologies for the removal of contaminants such as heavy metals from water have attracted significant attention in recent years, with zeolites finding promising applications due to its excellent adsorption and ion-exchange properties. It is further suggested that more research studies are needed on the practicability of large-scale industrial removal of heavy metals by zeolites. In addition, recent studies on zeolites have reported the high potential in areas of renewable energy and mitigation of air pollution, which are important towards environmental sustainability (Li et al., 2017).

Meanwhile, it is noteworthy that plastic pollution remains a serious global threat to public health and the environment despite being the research focus of numerous studies. It is estimated that in the near future, large quantities of plastic will continue to accumulate in the environment and extraordinary efforts are required in major areas of strategies including reduction of plastic wastes, waste management and environmental recovery (Borrelle et al., 2020). While more education campaigns are expected to enhance the reduction of plastic pollution, more efforts in research study of sustainable materials, policy and legislation to reduce the use of plastic bags and microbeads are also urgently required. Furthermore, incorporation of behavioural sciences into the design of effective policy interventions for mitigation actions has been suggested and further research on design of interventions to reduce consumption of plastics at population level is highly desired (Jia et al., 2019).

To achieve a sustainable environment, education plays a crucial role. On the grounds that many examples of PAHs have been identified as potent carcinogens, it is recommended that public education should be enhanced to raise awareness on the sources of emission and health effects of PAH exposure (Abdel-Shafy & Mansour, 2016). While there are emerging research investigations on the advancement of green and sustainable chemistry, including new molecular and material design, innovation of synthetic and catalytic processes, aiming to contribute to the achievement of the SDGs, it is equally important that educational reform in chemistry to be adopted which incorporates inter-disciplinary approaches as informed by systems thinking (Mahaffy et al., 2019; Matlin et al., 2015). As a central science, the education and practice of chemistry in the context of sustainability will play pivotal contributions to a sustainable future. To address chemical pollution of the environment, one of the major global sustainability challenges, concerted efforts from various stakeholders, including governments, academia, healthcare professionals, the industry, chemists and engineers, are needed for realisation of practical and sustainable solutions.

19.5 Conclusion

In summary, chemical contamination, including air, water and food pollution, is a serious threat to global sustainability. This article has reviewed various studies in Asia regions reporting findings about the adverse effects of chemical pollution on the elderly health. Implications and recommendations on research, policy interventions and education are further discussed. Contributions that chemical science can provide to achieve a sustainable future require close collaborations across different disciplines for identifying solutions to global sustainability challenges.

References

Abdel-Shafy, H. I., & Mansour, M. S. (2016). A review on polycyclic aromatic hydrocarbons: Source, environmental impact, effect on human health and remediation. *Egyptian Journal of Petroleum, 25*(1), 107–123. https://doi.org/10.1016/j.ejpe.2015.03.011

Adam, M. G., Tran, P. T., Bolan, N., & Balasubramanian, R. (2020). Biomass burning-derived airborne particulate matter in Southeast Asia: A critical review. *Journal of Hazardous Materials, 407*, 124760. https://doi.org/10.1016/j.jhazmat.2020.124760

Aloizou, A. M., Siokas, V., Vogiatzi, C., Peristeri, E., Docea, A. O., Petrakis, D., Provatas, A., Folia, V., Chalkia, C., Vinceti, M., & Wilks, M. (2020). Pesticides, cognitive functions and dementia: A review. *Toxicology Letters, 326*, 31–51. https://doi.org/10.1016/j.toxlet.2020.03.005

Asgary, S., Movahedian, A., Keshvari, M., Taleghani, M., Sahebkar, A., & Sarrafzadegan, N. (2017). Serum levels of lead, mercury and cadmium in relation to coronary artery disease in the elderly: A cross-sectional study. *Chemosphere, 180*, 540–544. https://doi.org/10.1016/j.chemosphere.2017.03.069

Barra, R., & González, P. (2018). Sustainable chemistry challenges from a developing country perspective: Education, plastic pollution, and beyond. *Current Opinion in Green and Sustainable Chemistry, 9*, 40–44. https://doi.org/10.1016/j.cogsc.2017.12.001

Begum, B. A., Hossain, A., Nahar, N., Markwitz, A., & Hopke, P. K. (2012). Organic and black carbon in PM2. 5 at an urban site at Dhaka, Bangladesh. *Aerosol and Air Quality Research, 12*(6), 1062–1072. https://doi.org/10.4209/aaqr.2012.05.0138

Bentayeb, M., Simoni, M., Baiz, N., Norback, D., Baldacci, S., Maio, S., Viegi, G., Annesi-Maesano, I., & Geriatric Study in Europe on Health Effects of Air Quality in Nursing Homes (GERIE) Group. (2012). Adverse respiratory effects of outdoor air pollution in the elderly. *The International Journal of Tuberculosis and Lung Disease, 16*(9), 1149–1161. https://doi.org/10.3978/j.issn.2072-1439.2014.12.10

Bhaskaran, K., Gasparrini, A., Hajat, S., Smeeth, L., & Armstrong, B. (2013). Time series regression studies in environmental epidemiology. *International Journal of Epidemiology, 42*(4), 1187–1195. https://doi.org/10.1093/ije/dyt092

Bjørklund, G., Dadar, M., Chirumbolo, S., & Aaseth, J. (2018). High content of lead is associated with the softness of drinking water and raised cardiovascular morbidity: A review. *Biological Trace Element Research, 186*(2), 384–394. https://doi.org/10.1007/s12011-018-1336-8

Borrelle, S. B., Ringma, J., Law, K. L., Monnahan, C. C., Lebreton, L., McGivern, A., Murphy, E., Jambeck, J., Leonard, G. H., Hilleary, M. A., Eriksen, M., Possingham, H. P., De Frond, H., Gerber, L. R., Polidoro, B., Tahir, A., Bernard, M., Mallos, N., Barnes, M., & Rochman, C. M. (2020). Predicted growth in plastic waste exceeds efforts to mitigate plastic pollution. *Science, 369*(6510), 1515–1518. https://doi.org/10.1126/science.aba3656

Brusseau, M. L., & Artiola, J. F. (2019). Chemical contaminants. In M. L. Brusseau, I. L. Pepper & C. P. Gerba (Eds.), *Environmental and pollution science* (3rd ed., pp. 175–190). Academic Press. https://doi.org/10.1016/B978-0-12-814719-1.00012-4

Byrne, F. P., Jin, S., Paggiola, G., Petchey, T. H., Clark, J. H., Farmer, T. J., Hunt, A. J., Robert McElroy, C., & Sherwood, J. (2016). Tools and techniques for solvent selection: Green solvent selection guides. *Sustainable Chemical Processes, 4*, 7. https://doi.org/10.1186/s40508-016-0051-z

Cha, E. S., Khang, Y. H., & Lee, W. J. (2014). Mortality from and incidence of pesticide poisoning in South Korea: Findings from national death and health utilization data between 2006 and 2010. *PLoS ONE, 9*(4), e95299. https://doi.org/10.1371/journal.pone.0095299

Chen, Y. Y., Kao, T. W., Wang, C. C., Chen, Y. J., Wu, C. J., Lai, C. H., & Chen, W. L. (2019). Exposure to polycyclic aromatic hydrocarbons and risk of disability among an elderly population. *Environmental Science and Pollution Research, 26*(11), 10719–10726. https://doi.org/10.1007/s11356-019-04498-3

Chiu, W. K., & Fong, B. Y. F. (2021). Green Diet and Public Health. In B. Y. F. Fong, & M. C. S. Wong (Eds.), *Routledge Handbook of Public Health and the Community.* Singapore: Routledge. https://www.routledge.com/The-Routledge-Handbook-of-Public-Health-and-the-Community/Fong-Wong/p/book/9780367634193

Fong, B. Y., Chiu, W. K., Chan, W. F., & Lam, T. Y. (2021). A review study of a green diet and healthy ageing. *International Journal of Environmental Research and Public Health, 18*(15), 8024. https://doi.org/10.3390/ijerph18158024

Fick, J., Söderström, H., Lindberg, R. H., Phan, C., Tysklind, M., & Larsson, D. J. (2009). Contamination of surface, ground, and drinking water from pharmaceutical production. *Environmental Toxicology and Chemistry, 28*(12), 2522–2527. https://doi.org/10.1897/09-073.1

Fujii, Y., Tohno, S., Amil, N., Latif, M. T., Oda, M., Matsumoto, J., & Mizohata, A. (2015). Annual variations of carbonaceous PM 2.5 in Malaysia: Influence by Indonesian peatland fires. *Atmospheric Chemistry and Physics, 15*(23), 13319–13329. https://doi.org/10.5194/acp-15-13319-2015

Ghandehari, H., Kamal-Bahl, S., & Wong, N. D. (2008). Prevalence and extent of dyslipidemia and recommended lipid levels in US adults with and without cardiovascular comorbidities: The

National Health and Nutrition Examination Survey 2003–2004. *American Heart Journal, 156*(1), 112–119. https://doi.org/10.1016/j.ahj.2008.03.005

Han, B., Liu, Y., You, Y., Xu, J., Zhou, J., Zhang, J., Niu, C., Zhang, N., He, F., Ding, X., & Bai, Z. (2016). Assessing the inhalation cancer risk of particulate matter bound polycyclic aromatic hydrocarbons (PAHs) for the elderly in a retirement community of a mega city in North China. *Environmental Science and Pollution Research, 23*(20), 20194–20204. https://doi.org/10.1007/s11356-016-7209-9

Han, L., Zhou, W., Li, W., & Qian, Y. (2020). China's complex urban air pollution: An improved understanding with ground operational measurements. *Integrated Environmental Assessment and Management, 16*(3), 306–313. https://doi.org/10.1002/ieam.4254

Hong Kong Smart City Blueprint. (2020). *Smart environment*. Innovation and Technology Bureau, HKSAR. https://www.smartcity.gov.hk/environment.html

Hu, Z. Y., Chang, J., Guo, F. F., Deng, H. Y., Pan, G. T., Li, B. Y., & Zhang, Z. L. (2020). The effects of dimethylformamide exposure on liver and kidney function in the elderly population: A cross-sectional study. *Medicine, 99*(27). https://doi.org/10.1097/md.0000000000020749

Jan, A. T., Azam, M., Siddiqui, K., Ali, A., Choi, I., & Haq, Q. M. (2015). Heavy metals and human health: Mechanistic insight into toxicity and counter defense system of antioxidants. *International Journal of Molecular Sciences, 16*(12), 29592–29630. https://doi.org/10.3390/ijms161226183

Jia, L., Evans, S., & van der Linden, S. (2019). Motivating actions to mitigate plastic pollution. *Nature Communications, 10*(4582), 1–3. https://doi.org/10.1038/s41467-019-12666-9

Larsson, D. J., de Pedro, C., & Paxeus, N. (2007). Effluent from drug manufactures contains extremely high levels of pharmaceuticals. *Journal of Hazardous Materials, 148*(3), 751–755. https://doi.org/10.1016/j.jhazmat.2007.07.008

Lee, H., Kunz, A., Shim, W. J., & Walther, B. A. (2019). Microplastic contamination of table salts from Taiwan, including a global review. *Scientific Reports, 9*, 10145. https://doi.org/10.1038/s41598-019-46417-z

Li, Y., Li, L., & Yu, J. (2017). Applications of zeolites in sustainable chemistry. *Chem, 3*(6), 928–949. https://doi.org/10.1016/j.chempr.2017.10.009

Lin, C. F., Chang, Y. H., Chien, S. C., Lin, Y. H., & Yeh, H. Y. (2018). Epidemiology of dyslipidemia in the Asia Pacific region. *International Journal of Gerontology, 12*(1), 2–6. https://doi.org/10.1016/j.ijge.2018.02.010

Lu, Y., Song, S., Wang, R., Liu, Z., Meng, J., Sweetman, A. J., Jenkins, A., Ferrier, R. C., Li, H., Luo, W., & Wang, T. (2015). Impacts of soil and water pollution on food safety and health risks in China. *Environment International, 77*, 5–15. https://doi.org/10.1016/j.envint.2014.12.010

Mabahwi, N. A. B., Leh, O. L. H., & Omar, D. (2014). Human health and wellbeing: Human health effect of air pollution. *Procedia-Social and Behavioral Sciences, 153*, 221–229. https://doi.org/10.1016/j.sbspro.2014.10.056

Mahaffy, P. G., Matlin, S. A., Whalen, J. M., & Holme, T. A. (2019). Integrating the molecular basis of sustainability into general chemistry through systems thinking. *Journal of Chemical Education, 96*(12), 2730–2741. https://doi.org/10.1021/acs.jchemed.9b00390

Matlin, S. A., Mehta, G., Hopf, H., & Krief, A. (2015). The role of chemistry in inventing a sustainable future. *Nature Chemistry, 7*(12), 941–943. https://doi.org/10.1038/nchem.2389

Matus, K. (2021). Factoring in public policy and perception. In T. Clark & A. Pasternak (Eds.), *How to commercialize chemical technologies for a sustainable future* (pp. 103–118). John Wiley & Sons Ltd. https://doi.org/10.1002/9781119604860.ch6

Nieuwenhuijsen, M. J., & Khreis, H. (2016). Car free cities: Pathway to healthy urban living. *Environment International, 94*, 251–262. https://doi.org/10.1016/j.envint.2016.05.032

Pezzoli, G., & Cereda, E. (2013). Exposure to pesticides or solvents and risk of Parkinson disease. *Neurology, 80*(22), 2035–2041. https://doi.org/10.1212/wnl.0b013e318294b3c8

Phairuang, W., Hata, M., & Furuuchi, M. (2017). Influence of agricultural activities, forest fires and agro-industries on air quality in Thailand. *Journal of Environmental Sciences, 52*, 85–97. https://doi.org/10.1016/j.jes.2016.02.007

Pongpiachan, S. (2016). Incremental lifetime cancer risk of PM2. 5 bound polycyclic aromatic hydrocarbons (PAHs) before and after the wildland fire episode. *Aerosol and Air Quality Research, 16*(11), 2907–2919. https://doi.org/10.4209/aaqr.2015.01.0011

Prata, J. C., da Costa, J. P., Lopes, I., Duarte, A. C., & Rocha-Santos, T. (2020). Environmental exposure to microplastics: An overview on possible human health effects. *Science of the Total Environment, 702*, 134455. https://doi.org/10.1016/j.scitotenv.2019.134455

Pun, V. C., Manjourides, J., & Suh, H. (2017). Association of ambient air pollution with depressive and anxiety symptoms in older adults: Results from the NSHAP study. *Environmental Health Perspectives, 125*(3), 342–348. https://doi.org/10.1289/EHP494

Rai, P. K., Lee, S. S., Zhang, M., Tsang, Y. F., & Kim, K. H. (2019). Heavy metals in food crops: Health risks, fate, mechanisms, and management. *Environment International, 125*, 365–385. https://doi.org/10.1016/j.envint.2019.01.067

Rather, I. A., Koh, W. Y., Paek, W. K., & Lim, J. (2017). The sources of chemical contaminants in food and their health implications. *Frontiers in Pharmacology, 8*, 830. https://doi.org/10.3389/fphar.2017.00830

Rattan, R. K., Datta, S. P., Chhonkar, P. K., Suribabu, K., & Singh, A. K. (2005). Long-term impact of irrigation with sewage effluents on heavy metal content in soils, crops and groundwater—A case study. *Agriculture, Ecosystems & Environment, 109*(3–4), 310–322. https://doi.org/10.1016/j.agee.2005.02.025

Simoni, M., Baldacci, S., Maio, S., Cerrai, S., Sarno, G., & Viegi, G. (2015). Adverse effects of outdoor pollution in the elderly. *Journal of Thoracic Disease, 7*(1), 34. https://doi.org/10.3978/j.issn.2072-1439.2014.12.10

Sofia, D., Gioiella, F., Lotrecchiano, N., & Giuliano, A. (2020). Mitigation strategies for reducing air pollution. *Environmental Science and Pollution Research, 27*(16), 19226–19235. https://doi.org/10.1007/s11356-020-08647-x

Tang, M., Li, D., Liew, Z., Wei, F., Wang, J., Jin, M., Chen, K., & Ritz, B. (2020). The association of short-term effects of air pollution and sleep disorders among elderly residents in China. *Science of The Total Environment, 708*, 134846. https://doi.org/10.1016/j.scitotenv.2019.134846

Tian, T., Chen, Y., Zhu, J., & Liu, P. (2015). Effect of air pollution and rural-urban difference on mental health of the elderly in China. *Iranian Journal of Public Health, 44*(8), 1084–1094. https://www.ncbi.nlm.nih.gov/pmc/articles/PMC4645728/

Wong, C. M., Lai, H. K., Tsang, H., Thach, T. Q., Thomas, G. N., Lam, K. B. H., Chan, K. P., Yang, L., Lau, A. K., Ayres, J. G. & Lam, T. H. (2015). Satellite-based estimates of long-term exposure to fine particles and association with mortality in elderly Hong Kong residents. *Environmental Health Perspectives, 123*(11), 1167–1172. https://doi.org/10.1289/ehp.1408264

Yang, Y., Tang, R., Qiu, H., Lai, P. C., Wong, P., Thach, T. Q., Allen, R., Brauer, M., Tian, L., & Barratt, B. (2018). Long term exposure to air pollution and mortality in an elderly cohort in Hong Kong. *Environment International, 117*, 99–106. https://doi.org/10.1016/j.envint.2018.04.034

Yu, Z., Wei, F., Zhang, X., Wu, M., Lin, H., Shui, L., Jin, M., Wang, J., Tang, M., & Chen, K. (2021). Air pollution, surrounding green, road proximity and Parkinson's disease: A prospective cohort study. *Environmental Research, 197*, 111170. https://doi.org/10.1016/j.envres.2021.111170

Zhang, X., Yang, L., Zhang, H., Xing, W., Wang, Y., Bai, P., Zhang, L., Hayakawa, K., Toriba, A., Wei, Y., & Tang, N. (2021). Assessing approaches of human inhalation exposure to polycyclic aromatic hydrocarbons: A review. *International Journal of Environmental Research and Public Health, 18*(6), 3124. https://doi.org/10.3390/ijerph18063124

Zhu, X., Fan, Y., Sheng, J., Gu, L., Tao, Q., Huang, R., Liu, K., Yang, L., Chen, G., Cao, H., Li, K., Tao, F., & Wang, S. (2021). Association between blood heavy metal concentrations and dyslipidemia in the elderly. *Biological Trace Element Research, 199*(4), 1280–1290. https://doi.org/10.1007/s12011-020-02270-0

Chapter 20
Pet Ownership and Social Wellness of Elderly

Andrea Chu and Ben Yuk Fai Fong

Abstract Elderlies are facing with problems not only limited to chronic diseases and functional disabilities, but also loneliness and feeling of isolation, and even rejection. For some older adults, especially those who have disabilities, their spouse and children are unable to take care of them. They may have to live in residential care homes for the elderly for the rest of their lives. This makes the elderly very unhappy and becoming more and more pessimistic. They may treat themselves as a burden to the family and society as they continue to age and degenerate. Pet ownership is known to help in promoting health and increasing the quality of life of older adults by calming the elderly, combating loneliness, providing companionship and unconditional love, encouraging mobility, providing a sense of purpose and making the elderly hosts feel safe. This review will discuss the physical and psychosocial benefits, as well as the potential harms and dangers of owning pets. Owning a pet is not only costly, but there is increased risk of fall injuries, risk of developing allergies and asthma, and risk of acquiring zoonotic diseases. Furthermore, losing a pet may cause huge emotional and psychological burden to the elderly. Collaborating service animals with community elderly services increases the physical and psychosocial health as well as the dignity of the older adults and their families.

Keywords Pet ownership · Service animals · Elderly · Quality of life

20.1 Introduction

Animals have different roles in the society. During the First and Second World Wars, dogs were professionally trained as messengers, ambulance dogs and war dogs (Cummins, 2003). Pets also play an important role in acting as a companion

A. Chu
School of Professional Education and Executive Development, The Hong Kong Polytechnic University, Hong Kong, China

B. Y. F. Fong (✉)
College of Professional and Continuing Education, The Hong Kong Polytechnic University, Hong Kong, China
e-mail: byffong@gmail.com

V. T. S. Law and B. Y. F. Fong (eds.), *Ageing with Dignity in Hong Kong and Asia*, Quality of Life in Asia 16, https://doi.org/10.1007/978-981-19-3061-4_20

animal in households, while providing health benefits to their owners not only physically but also emotionally. Some animal breeds are specifically trained to serve the community as service animals, including emotional support animals, guide dogs, dementia assistance dogs and more. The abilities of trained animals also benefit the elderly enormously.

Animals have been owned by people for service uses other than just as companion animals since wartime in the 1910s. For example, during the Great War, dogs were trained as messengers to deliver messages, as rescue dogs to search for and aid injured soldiers, and as guide dogs to help in the rehabilitation and as a guardian and companion of the blind veterans after the war (Frankel, 2014; Haller, 2011).

Pet ownership is common in Hong Kong as in many societies. Pet owners share the same household and environment with their animals, and this may be beneficial or bad to one's health. There is increasing interest in digging deeper into the association between pet ownership and human health than just claiming that 'pets are good to human'. There is increasing evidence that pet ownership does have an effect on the physical and psychosocial health of the elderly, maintaining mobility, reducing loneliness, avoiding depression by acting as an emotional supporter and also an ice breaker to help the owner make new friends. The chapter aims to explore the benefits and risks of pet ownership and how it is related to the health and dignity of the elderly.

20.2 Pet Population and Patterns

Pets were found in over 241,900 households in Hong Kong in 2018. 5.7% of them were keeping dogs and 4.0% of them were keeping cats. Among them, 67.6% were keeping one dog only, and 59.2% were keeping one cat only at the same time. Pet ownership was common in the comparatively richer families. Among household with HK$40,000 or above monthly household income, 44.3% were keeping dogs and 44.8% were keeping cats (Census and Statistics Department, 2019).

In the United Kingdom (UK), 17 million, equivalent to 59% of the households, owned a pet in 2021. The most commonly owned animals included dogs owned by 12.5 million or 33% of the households and cats owned by 12.2 million or 27% of the households. Other animals owned by people in UK include rabbits, fowls, birds, insects, etc. (Pet Food Manufacturers' Association, 2021).

In the United States (US), pet ownership is also common. Dogs and cats are the most commonly owned companion animal. There are totally 77 million of dogs and 58 million cats owned by 38.4 and 25.4% of all households, respectively. Birds and horses are also commonly owned by 2.8 and 0.7% of the households in the United States (American Veterinary Medical Association, 2020).

20.2.1 Service and Emotional Support by Animals

Animals do not just act as pets but can also contribute to the community as service animals. Friendly and calm pets can take examinations to become approved service pets. The Hong Kong Therapy Dog Association (HKTDA) is a charitable organisation established in 2014, with the aim to provide therapy to people in need through therapy dog services. There are different forms of interventions to assist them in overcoming stress and difficulties. HKTDA provides trainings and assessments to potential dogs. Dogs are registered as dog ambassadors or therapy dogs when they passed specific assessments and requirements. HKTDA runs visitation programmes to hospitals and hospice homes for the elderly etc. as entertainment, distractions from pain and things for people to look forward to (Hong Kong Therapy Dog Association [HKTDA], 2021).

20.2.2 Guide Dogs

The origin of guide dogs could be traced back to the First World War. The brutal World War created a lot of injuries. The advancement in the military increased the use of new weapons, such as flash grenades and sound bomb, causing a significant number of blind soldiers and veterans whom despite having lost their eyesight, were young and physically healthy. The blind veterans were left isolated and visually impaired. In 1916, the German state implemented the professional training of guide dogs for war veterans as a rehabilitation service, aiming to support the disabled veterans to recover as a self-efficient, independent taxpayer and to prevent the economy from exhaustion. The use of guide dogs has become an inspiration as people start to realise that dogs can act more than just domestic pets, but also a companion and the eyes of the blind (Baár, 2015).

When thinking about the visually impaired, guide dogs often come in mind. The Hong Kong Guide Dog Association (HKGDA) was established in January 2011 with the aim to ensure that people with disabilities can live independently and with dignity through the right choice of service dogs. HKGDA provides professional training to guide dogs and support and care to the visually impaired persons with respect (Hong Kong Guide Dog Association [HKGDA], 2021). Guide dogs are capable in providing not only assistance like guidance and safety while going out, but also unconditional love and companionship to the visually impaired people. According to HKGDA, guide dogs are trained to lead a person safely around obstacles, to have good manners in public places, avoiding distractions and most importantly, they are trained not to obey any unsafe commands given by the trainer or owner (HKGDA, 2019). These skills help in supporting the daily needs of the visually impaired to live their life independently and confidently.

The Hong Kong Jockey Club (HKJC) Charities Trust donated over HKD $9 billion to HKGDA in 2017 to establish the Jockey Club Education and Training Centre in

Kwun Tong (The Hong Kong Jockey Club [HKJC], 2019). The centre aimed at training guide dogs and service dogs for animal-assisted therapies for children with special needs. The centre also enhanced public knowledge on guide dogs as well as promotion of social inclusion through public education (HKJC, 2019).

20.2.3 Dementia Assistance Dogs

Apart from serving people with impaired vision and emotional problems, dogs can also help people with dementia. In Scotland, people diagnosed with early stage dementia can apply for a dementia assistance dog from the Dementia Dog Project. Like guide dogs, dementia assistance dogs are trained to help in daily routines, including waking up, taking medications and more. This makes demented elderly feel more confident and independent living with dementia and relieves the workload of caregivers (Dementia Dog Project, 2019).

20.2.4 Hearing Dogs

Deaf people are often forgotten by the society as they look just the same as people with normal hearing. Although they could handle daily routines and can be independent, they may feel isolated and stressed as they are different from normal people in their silent world. In the United Kingdom, hearing dogs are trained to assist deaf people by alerting them to important sounds like doorbells and fire alarms. Having a hearing dog helps the owner in avoiding accidents (Hearing Dogs for Deaf People, 2011).

20.2.5 Seizure-Alert Dogs and Seizure-Response Dogs

Seizure-alert dogs are dogs that have innate ability to detect oncoming seizures. They alert the caretaker or owner's family in the same household that a seizure is going to happen, so that the owner can be well-prepared. Seizure-response dogs are dogs that are trained to identify seizures and respond to it immediately. They are trained to warn caregivers by having long eye contact and barking, depending on how the dog is trained. They also assist the owner with epilepsy, preventing the owner from getting injured by leaning on the floor next to the patient to prevent falls during a seizure. They can also bring medications and activate alerting devices. Patients with epilepsy tends to avoid socialising for fear that they would have a seizure in public, and the seizure alert dogs give these patients the assistance and confidence needed (Canine Partners for Life, 2020a; Epilepsy Foundation of America, 2019).

20.2.6 Ambulance Dogs

Ambulance dogs, also known as Red Cross dogs or rescue dogs, were originated during war periods and used by the military. During the Franco-Prussian War in 1870 and the First World War, the German military trained dogs for difficult and dangerous missions. Rescue is one of the function military trained dogs do for the injured soldiers during the war. Militaries employ ambulance dogs to substitute motorised ambulances, thus allocate them accordingly to each military to help armies in stationary wars and trenches. In 1890, ambulance dogs were trained to carry at his collar first-aid kit, bandages and supplies in a pocket. They located overlooked or injured soldiers in the battlefield and aided them in bandaging by pulling stretchers. The use of ambulance dog in European armies were common in 1912 (Frankel, 2014; Haller, 2011). During the Great War in 1914, Germany had at least 6,000 military dogs, primarily functioned as messengers and ambulance dogs. Only the ambulance dogs alone saved at least 4,000 injured German soldiers (Cummins, 2003).

20.3 Costs of Pet Ownership

20.3.1 Cost to Community

To facilitate and support pet ownership, the society has developed some facilities, guidelines and laws for pet owners. According to the Leisure and Cultural Services Department (2011), there are dog parks provided in 45 venues and sites in Hong Kong, including11, 11 and 23 dog parks in Hong Kong, Kowloon and New Territories, respectively. The size of the parks varies from 96 square metres in Tai Hang to 107,000 square metres in The Peak. The ancillary varies from basic dog latrines and benches, to dog excreta collection bins, pet play equipment and hand-washing facilities (Leisure & Cultural Services Department, 2019).

There are several animal laws in Hong Kong. Among all, Prevention of Cruelty to Animals Ordinance, Cap 169, is the most important law that safeguards the welfare of animals. Under this ordinance, not only companion animals, but food and laboratory animals are also protected from being abused, neglected, inappropriately transported and used for fighting, or unnecessary suffering during import. Offenders will be fined a maximum of HKD $200,000 and imprisoned for up to 3 years (SPCA, 2019).

20.3.2 Cost to Pet Owners

Owning a pet is a serious financial commitment, especially when considering some pets may have long life span. Owners can adopt pets in different organisations such as the Society for the Prevention of Cruelty to Animals (SPCA) or Hong Kong Dog Rescue. In SPCA, the acquiring cost varies from HK$700 for a domestic cat to up to HK$1,500 for a pure-breed or crossbreed dog. An additional HK$1,000 desexing deposit must be paid before adoption (SPCA, 2019). The acquiring cost is just the beginning. Regular expenses for dogs include food, heartworm prevention, flea control and vaccination. All dogs must be licensed by the Law and have rabies vaccination every 3 years. Regular expenses for cats include food, annual vaccination, flea control, litter box and cat litter. Pets, especially dogs, may need dental care a few times in their lifetime to ensure good oral health. In addition, cost for equipment like food bowls, nail cutters, collars and leashes, shampoo, toys etc. are mostly optional.

The long-term cost depends on the type of pet owned. Smaller breeds require less food compared to the larger breeds, and breeds with shorter hair requires less grooming. Some types of pets are prone to having diseases. Breeds with protruding eyeballs like pugs are prone to having eye injuries and disorders and flat face breeds such as himalayans and bulldogs are prone to having breathing problems. Smaller breeds like chihuahua are prone to having patellar luxation. These breeds require special care and may require long-term medical care, medicines and supplements.

20.4 Special Pet Owners and Conditions

Pet ownership is beneficial to people who are functionally or psychosocially unwell. Here are some examples.

20.4.1 Elderlies

Elderly may suffer from diseases such as Alzheimer's disease, arthritis and heart disease as they age. However, according to the Centre for Suicide Research and Prevention (2019), suicide rate among elderlies has always been a lot higher than the other age groups. In spite the fact that there had been a decreasing trend in Hong Kong from over 20% in 2008 to less than 15% in 2016, it is still a problem that service animals and companion animals can help.

Well olds are elderly who are independent and capable of taking care of themselves. As people retires, they may have more free time for their hobbies and other activities including looking after kids as well as pets. Keeping pets is beneficial to their physical and mental wellness particularly after retirement.

Home-bound elderly refers to a person that requires considerable and taxing effort leaving home, and that infrequent absences from home for a short duration or to receive medical treatment are acceptable (U.S. Department of Health and Human Services, 2001). For these older adults who may need wheelchairs to help them to move around, mobility assistance dogs can provide assistance from closing a door to helping the physically challenged moving in and out of public transport (Canine Partners for Life, 2020b).

Bed-bound older adults are usually disabled from post-stroke or dementia conditions. They are dependent, lack of physical activities and lack of motivation in daily activities. Most of them needs intensive care and support, usually in elderly homes and facilities. They may feel lonely and may have the feelings of being a burden to their partner and family. Service animals may provide comfort and happiness by just accompanying the patient in the bedside and as a facilitation of communication. Companion animals may even help in facilitating grief in the family that is going through bereavement (Geisler, 2004).

20.4.2 Depression and Anxiety

Major depression is characterised by at least five of the diagnostic symptoms of which at least one of the symptoms is either an overwhelming feeling of sadness or a loss of interest and pleasure in most usual activities. It can be caused by experiencing stressful events such as losing a loved one or going through hard times. Anxiety is different from depression, but they experience similar symptoms including nervousness, irritability and problems sleeping and concentrating (Anxiety & Depression Association in America, 2018).

20.4.3 Visual Impairment

The National Federation of the Blind defines blindness as having 20/200 or less central visual acuity in the better eye with the best possible correction (The National Federation of the Blind, 2019). There were 174,800 people or 2.4% of the population have seeing difficulties in 2014 in Hong Kong (Census and Statistics Department, 2014). Losing the vision does cause inconvenience, ranging from navigating new environments to being perceived as disabled or even being discriminated. Visually impaired people rely very much on memory and frequency of walking in one path, thus owning a trained guide dog benefits them in avoiding obstacles when travelling to new areas.

20.5 Benefits of Owning Pets

20.5.1 *Reducing Chance of Having Chronic Diseases*

Earlier research and studies on how owning pets affect the owners in chronic diseases suggested that pet ownership lowers the blood pressure, particularly when an individual was dealing with stress (Allen et al., 2003; Cole et al., 2007). The study of heart failure patients conducted by Cole et al. (2007) reflected that the group with visits by a volunteer and a therapy dog had a greater improvement in blood pressure and anxiety. In a more recent research conducted by Chowdhury et al. (2017) on the relationship between pet ownership and the survival in elderly treated for hypertension, among 4,039 participants aged between 65 and 84 years old treated with hypertension and responded to the pet-ownership questionnaire, 86% of them owned at least one pet during their life time whereas the other 14% have never owned a pet. Follow ups were conducted and the survival information of participants were analysed over a median of 10.9 years. Results suggested that any type of pet ownership was associated with less all-cause or cardiovascular mortality compared to non-pet owners. Another research on a population in Nanjing, China, points out that owning pets, especially dogs, has a protective effect on coronary artery disease patients and that the associated risks of hypertension and hyperlipidaemia are decreased, with correlation to the duration and early age of pet keeping (Xie et al., 2017).

20.5.2 *Encouraging Physical Activity and Maintaining Mobility*

Inadequate physical activity is common in Hong Kong resulting from the sedentary habit of people. According to the Population Health Survey conducted by the Department of Health (2020), every one out of two Hong Kong people aged 15 to 84 is either overweight or obese. The survey also shows that there is an increase in proportion of older adults by age group who did not meet the WHO recommendation of physical activity level. Physical inactivity may lead to frailty in elderly and chronic illnesses such as heart diseases, hypertension cerebrovascular diseases, diabetes mellitus and obesity (Department of Health, 2006; McPhee, et al., 2016). The sedentary behaviour of older adults, especially aged 85 or above, is common, with 30.5% of them spending more than 600 minutes sitting or reclining a day.

Companion animals can help owners to increase mobility. Visually impaired owners can rely on guide dogs to travel from one place to another at the same time avoid any obstacles. They can also gain confidence, companionship, independence, socialising and security by owning and living with a guide dog (Whitmarsh, 2009). A study conducted by Andreassen et al. (2013) assessed the relationship between how attached the owner was with their dogs and time of walking their dogs, and the results showed that the more time spent walking their dogs, the more attached they were with their dogs.

Another example is the responsibility for owners to walk their dogs. Yabroff et al. (2008) have found that dog owners are more likely to walk for leisure than non-pet owners, showing that there is a moderate association between owning a dog and having higher level of physical activity. The habit of going out for a walk regularly helps improve the overall health and lose weight (State of Victoria, 2020).

20.5.3 Pain Management

Few studies have reported the effect of animal-assisted therapies in reducing pain in patients. In a study conducted by Engelman (2013), 19 in-patients and out-patients were referred for animal-assisted interventions for a one-year with Lizzy, the therapy dog. The palliative care patients were reported to feel pleased and there was reduction in pain and discomfort, and their quality of life was improved. In another study conducted by Marcus et al. (2012), 235 patients from a pain clinic were divided into the experimental and control groups. Surveys were taken before and after sitting in the waiting room. The experimental group had interactions with a therapy dog during waiting and reported improvements in pain when compared to the control group. Although therapy dogs may not have the same pain management effect to everyone, it is in a fact a good therapy, particularly when there are no side effects as in many medical treatments.

20.5.4 Acting as Emotional Support

Pets improve people's mood and health. Pets provide unconditional love to their owners, relieving loneliness, which tends to go together with depression (Doheny, 2012). Pet therapy improves depressive symptoms by 50% and cognitive functions in elderly patients with different mental illnesses in care facilities (Moretti et al., 2011). Furthermore, having a companion animal, especially those with stronger human-animal bond may aid owners in reducing loneliness and stress brought from life transitions and life events like retirement and loss of a loved one (Banks & Banks, 2002; Suthers-McCabe, Summer 2001).

In a study conducted by Moretti et al. (2011), 21 elderly patients with dementia were recruited from a nursing home in northern Italy for a 6-weeks pet visitation. The pet group ($n = 10$) were allowed to interact with the pet, while the control group ($n = 11$) were only allowed to watch the therapy dogs without directly interacting with them. A significant reduction in depression symptoms and cognitive functions was recorded and have improvements in the participants' perceived quality of life in both the pet group and the control group.

In a study conducted by Moreira et al. (2016), the response of patients was evaluated before and after assisted therapies with dogs. It was concluded that the service dog helped reducing the anxiety level of patients, making them happier and more relaxed during waiting as well as during the assisted therapy. Assisted therapies do not only benefit patients but also make it easier for health professionals to do their job.

20.5.5 Acting as Social Support

'Humans are inherently social' and the need and importance of social interactions are relatively neglected (Young, 2008). Older adults may become lonely and are socially isolated (National Institute on Aging, 2019). The presence of a pet or a service animal acts as a social 'lubricant' and is proved to facilitate interactions and reduce and overcome social isolation.

Companion animals help in facilitating social interactions. Wood et al. (2015) reported that pets facilitate their owners in building friendship to acquiring social support, and the feeling of being involved makes elderly feel less lonely and socially isolated. The friends they made through their pets could provide different forms of support, no matter emotional or practical support to the pet owner when needed (Wood et al., 2015).

A study conducted by Richeson (2003) reported how animal-assisted therapy (AAT) benefits elderly with dementia in nursing homes. The one-hour intervention was conducted from Mondays to Fridays for three weeks during the change of nurse shifts. The results suggest that AAT intervention do not only keep participants alert and responsive, but it also helps in lowering agitated behaviours as well as increasing social interactions in elderly with dementia. The AAT intervention also helps everyone including nursing staff to be engaged and involved prior and during the intervention.

20.5.6 Combating Loneliness

Few studies have reported the effect of AAT in combating loneliness in older adults. Vrbanac et al. (2013) reported the effect of dog companionship three times a week for 90 minutes in a six-months period on 21 elderlies. The results showed that participants felt less lonely after the AAT intervention. There was no difference between non-pet owners and prior pet owners in the influence of AAT intervention. Participants who used to live in solitary and have minimum communication with other participants started sharing stories to other participants during the AAT programme. The findings suggested that spending time with animals helped in combating loneliness.

20.6 Potential Harms and Dangers of Owning Pets

20.6.1 Risk of Falls

Falls are a common and major cause of injuries in elderlies. In Hong Kong, 1 out of 4 community dwelling elderlies experienced from a fall, while 75% of them had injuries including fractures and head injuries (Department of Health, 2018). When the elderly and companion animals share the same environment, the risk of older adults tripping over by their pets increases, as the elderly may have limited mobility and hearing impairments.

A study on pet-related fractures has concluded that pets, most likely cats and dogs, constitute environmental hazard in fall-related injuries among the elderly (Kurrle et al., 2004). Chasing the pet is another common cause of pet-related falls. When an indoor pet accidentally gets outdoor, the owner may chase the pet before it gets hurt. Owners usually put the pet's safety in the priority. This increases the risks of fall in owners, especially older adults who have less mobility. Pet equipment including dishes, beds and toys may also pose a risk to pet owners (Rehder, 2016).

20.6.2 Risk of Zoonoses

Zoonotic diseases may be transmitted from animals to humans, especially the immunocompromised including pregnant women, elderly, patients with immunological diseases and patients who needs immunosuppressive treatments. One of the greatest concern is methicillin-resistant *Staphylococcus aureus* (MRSA), though it is rare. Over 200 zoonotic diseases can be transmitted to human beings when pets are used as companion animals in elderly nursing homes (Guay, 2001). However, there is limited knowledge, information and awareness of the zoonotic risks from household pets (Stull et al., 2012).

Bites are one of transmission path of zoonotic diseases. Many people have been bitten by pets once and most of them did not seek medical help from doctors. A study has shown that cats (51.6%), followed by dogs (42.2%) are involved in pet-related injuries, when people are playing with the pet (59.4%), cleaning the pets (9.4%) or training the pets (7.8%) (Chan et al., 2017). Animal bites and scratches are one way of transmitting zoonotic diseases, as there are many pathogens in the saliva of pets especially in cats (Guay, 2001).

Elderly is especially vulnerable to dog bite injuries. As elderly may have impaired eyesight, and degenerative diseases leading to slower response. Older adults may be slow to react to the dog's change in behaviour and get injured more easily (Pfortmueller et al., 2013). They are also susceptible to infection due to weaker immunity. According to Wilson et al. (2016), a 70-year old Caucasian woman was treated for a severe sepsis caused by *Capnocytophaga canimorsus*, a bacterium found in the cavities of dogs and cats, without having any scratches or bites but just licks from her dog. If small bites or scratches are left untreated with the correct antibiotics, it may increase the victim's risk of getting secondary infections which could be serious (Pfortmueller et al., 2013).

20.6.3 Bereavement when Losing a Pet

Most pet owners treat their pets as a part of the family. Pets are especially valuable to the elderly. The loss of a pet may indicate and remind elderly owners of their own mortality (Testoni et al., 2017). Not accepting the fact that their valued pet is dead may cause serious mental distress to the owner, thus affecting the physical and mental wellness of elderly. The experience and feeling of grief in the loss of a pet is similar to the loss of a significant human. The owner has significant levels of negative emotions like anger and despair. Mood improvements take place earlier in owners who have acquired a new pet than those who do not (Gerwolls & Labott, 2015).

McNicholas et al. (2005) have mentioned in their review paper that 'the death of a pet may cause great distress to owners, especially when the pet has associations with a deceased spouse or former lifestyle'. It does not only mean losing a pet, but it also means losing a companion. The lifestyle may never be the same, and the owner has to face the reality in order to get back to the right track. Unfortunately, the bereaved owner may not receive enough sympathy or support (Morales, 1997). The inadequate support given by family and society may weaken their determination in overcoming the obstacle, and thus isolating the bereaved owner from the society. Therefore, it is important to address the potential issues elderly may have in the bereavement of losing a pet and to provide assistance and support by social workers and veterinary professionals.

20.7 Conclusion

Owning a companion animal brings the owners health benefits, both physically and psychosocially, by having intimate companionship and unconditional love. Pets can help reducing chronic diseases, increasing mobility and are always there when a person is facing with hardship or life events which are difficult to get over with. However, pets age like humans and the elderly may not be able to afford the cost for owning pets as they need more financial support and care as they grow old. The elderly may have difficulties in taking care of them. For example, an elderly with arthritis may have trouble in cleaning sand box for cats or walking dogs. Companion animals may also increase the risk of fall injuries for owners. This may be traumatic and may have serious consequences for elderly who are vulnerable to falls. In addition, elderly may unintentionally or accidently harm the pet, for example, stepping on the pet's tail or losing the pet when the door was left open.

Although it is proved that companion animals bring positive health effects to older adults by providing companionship to reducing pain, it is not always feasible to collaborate service animals and elderly care facilities, and it is even less practical for elderly care facilities to own animals due to the prohibition of animals from these facilities. Moreover, a risk–benefit analysis is necessary before bringing animals into a healthcare facility (D'Arcy, 2011). It is necessary to assess the suitability of animal interventions especially when some of the patients are afraid of or are allergic to animals. In addition, staff of nursing facility and pet therapy programmes need to pay attention not only to the therapy dogs but also the patients, as not all of them have experience interacting an animal and may accidently hurt the therapy animal (Bowder, 2009).

The older adults face different problems ranging from physical illness like degenerative diseases to mental distress including feeling lonely and being a burden. By researching on the benefits of pet ownership, the elderly can benefit from pets not only in aiding their illness, but providing them love and companionship, thus making hardships become much easier for them. Future research can investigate about how animal-assisted therapy could become the mainstream in assisting elderly patients, especially in Hong Kong.

References

Allen, K., Shykoff, B. E., & Izzo, J. L. (2003). Pet ownership, but not ACE inhibitor therapy, blunts home blood pressure responses to mental stress. *Hypertension, 38*(4), 815–820. https://doi.org/10.1161/hyp.38.4.815

American Veterinary Medical Association. (2020). *U.S. pet ownership statistics*. https://www.avma.org/resources-tools/reports-statistics/us-pet-ownership-statistics

Andreassen, G., Stenvold, L. C., & Rudmin, F. W. (2013). "My dog is my best friend": Health benefits of emotional attachment to a pet dog. *Psychology & Society, 5*(2), 6–23. http://www.psychologyandsociety.org/__assets/__original/2013/04/2.pdf

Anxiety and Depression Association in America. (2018). *Understanding the Facts: Depression*. https://adaa.org/understanding-anxiety/depression

Baár, M. (2015). Prosthesis for the body and for the soul: The origins of guide dog provision for blind veterans in interwar Germany. *First World War Studies, 6*(1), 81–98. https://doi.org/10.1080/19475020.2015.1047890

Banks, M. R., & Banks, W. A. (2002). The effects of animal-assisted therapy on loneliness in an elderly populations in long-term care facilities. *The Journals of Gerontology, 57*(7), M428–M432. https://doi.org/10.1093/Gerona/57.7.M428

Bowder, L. M. (2009). Paws and relax: One hospice's pet therapy journey. *Home Healthcare Nurse: the Journal for the Home Care and Hospice Professional, 27*(7), 443–448. https://doi.org/10.1097/01.nhh.0000358280.84670.68

Canine Partners for Life. (2020a). *Seizure alert dogs*. https://k94life.org/seizure-alert/

Canine Partners for Life. (2020b). *Mobility assistance dogs*. https://k94life.org/mobility-assistance-dogs/

Census and Statistics Department. (2014). *Special topics report no. 62*. https://www.statistics.gov.hk/pub/B11301622014XXXXB0100.pdf

Census and Statistics Department. (2019). *Thematic household survey report No.66*. https://www.statistics.gov.hk/pub/B11302662019XXXXB0100.pdf

Centre for Suicide Research and Prevention. (2019). *Number of suicides rates in Hong Kong, 1997–2017.* https://csrp.hku.hk/wp-content/uploads/2018/09/2018WSPD_slide.pdf

Chan, Y. Y., Gao, Y., Li, L., & Lee, P. Y. (2017). Injuries caused by pets in Asian urban households: A cross-sectional telephone survey. *British Medical Journal Open, 7*(1), e012813. https://doi.org/10.1136/bmjopen-2016-012813

Chowdhury, E. K., Nelson, M. R., Jennings, G. L. R., Wing, L. M. H., & Reid, C. M. (2017). Pet ownership and survival in the elderly hypertensive population. *Journal of Hypertension, 35*(4), 769–775. https://doi.org/10.1097/HJH.0000000000001214

Cole, K. M., Gawlinski, A., Steers, N., & Kotlerman, J. (2007). Animal-assisted therapy in patients hospitalized with heart failure. *American Journal of Critical Care, 16*(6), 575–585. https://doi.org/10.4037/ajcc2007.16.6.575

Cummins, B. D. (2003). *Colonel richardson's airedales: The making of the British war dog school, 1990–1918.* Destselig.

D'Arcy, Y. (2011). "Paws" to provide comfort, relieve pain. *Nursing2011, 41*(4), 67–68. https://doi.org/10.1097/01.NURSE.0000395305.83786.93

Dementia Dog Project. (2019). *Dogs at home and dogs in the community.* http://dementiadog.org/how-we-help-2/#DogsHome

Department of Health. (2006). *Fact sheet on physical activity.* https://www.dh.gov.hk/english/useful/useful_dykt/useful_dykt_exercise.html

Department of Health. (2018). *Fall prevention.* https://www.elderly.gov.hk/english/books/files/fall_prevention/Fall_Prevention_booklet.pdf

Department of Health. (2020). *Report of health behaviour survey 2018/19.* https://www.chp.gov.hk/files/pdf/report_of_health_behaviour_survey_2018_en.pdf

Doheny, K. (2012). *Pets for depression and health.* http://www.wellnessinitiatives.org/wp-content/uploads/2017/11/Pets-Reduce-Depression.pdf

Engelman, S. R. (2013). Palliative care and the use of animal-assisted therapies. *OMEGA—Journal of Death and Dying, 67*(1–2), 63–67. https://doi.org/10.2190/OM.67.1-2.g

Epilepsy Foundation of America. (2019). *Seizure dogs.* https://www.epilepsy.com/learn/seizure-first-aid-and-safety/seizure-dogs

Frankel, R. (2014). *War dogs: Tales of canine heroism, history, and love.* Palgrave Macmillan.

Geisler, A. M. (2004). Companion animals in palliative care: Stories from the bedside. *American Journal of Hospice and Palliative Medicine, 21*(4), 285–288. https://doi.org/10.1177/104990910402100411

Gerwolls, M. K., & Labott, S. M. (2015). Adjustment to the death of a companion animal. *Anthrozoös, 7*(3), 172–187. https://doi.org/10.2752/089279394787001826

Guay, D. R. P. (2001). Pet-assisted therapy in the nursing home setting: Potential for zoonosis. *American Journal of Infection Control, 29*(3), 178–186. https://doi.org/10.1067/mic.2001.115873

Haller, J. S. (2011). *Battlefield medicine: A history of the military ambulance from the Napoleonic Wars through World War I: With a new preface.* Southern Illinois University Press.

Hearing Dogs for Deaf People. (2011). *Helping deaf people.* https://www.hearingdogs.org.uk/helping-deaf-people/

Hong Kong Guide Dogs Association. (2021). *About us.* https://www.guidedogs.org.hk/about-us/

Hong Kong Therapy Dog Association. (2021). *About us.* http://www.hktda.org/About

Kurrle, S. E., Day, R., & Cameron, I. D. (2004). The perils of pet ownership: A. *Medical Journal of Australia, 181*(11), 682–683. https://sci-hub.se/10.5694/j.1326-5377.2004.tb06060.x

Leisure and Cultural Services Department. (2011). *The 23 LCSD leisure venue/sites that are provided with pet gardens.* https://gia.info.gov.hk/general/201105/04/P201105040141_0141_78391.pdf

Leisure and Cultural Services Department. (2019). *List of facilities & venues—Dog garden/pet garden.* https://www.lcsd.gov.hk/clpss/en/webApp/Facility/District.do?ftid=47

Marcus, D. A., Berstein, C. D., Constantin, J. M., Kunkel, F. A., Breuer, P., & Hanlon, R. B. (2012). Animal-assisted therapy at an outpatient pain management clinic. *Pain Management, 13*(1), 45–57. https://doi.org/10.1111/j.1526-4637.2011.01294.x

McNicholas, J., Gilbey, A., Rennie, A., Ahmedzai, S., Dono, J., & Ormerod, E. (2005). Pet ownership and human health: A brief review of evidence and issues. *BMJ, 331*(7527), 1252–1254. https://doi.org/10.1136/bmj.331.7527.1252

McPhee, J. S., French, D. P., Jackson, D., Nazroo, J., Pendleton, N., & Degens, H. (2016). Physical activity in older age: Perspectives for healthy ageing and frailty. *Biogerontology, 17*, 567–580. https://doi.org/10.1007/s10522-016-9641-0

Morales, P. C. (1997). Grieving in silence: The loss of companion animals in modern society. *Journal of Personal and Interpersonal Loss, 2*(3), 243–254. https://doi.org/10.1080/10811449708414419

Moreira, R. L., Gubert, F. A., Sabino, L. M., Benevides, J. L., Tomé, M. A., Martins, M. C., & Brito, M. A. (2016). Assisted therapy with dogs in pediatric oncology: Relatives' and nurses' perceptions. *Brazilian Journal of Nursing, 69*(6), 1188–1194. https://doi.org/10.1590/0034-7167-2016-0243

Moretti, F., De Ronchi, D., Bernabei, V., Marchetti, L., Ferrari, B., Forlani, C., Negretti, F., Sacchetti, C., & Atti, A. R. (2011). Pet therapy in elderly patients with mental illness. *Psychogeriatrics, 11*(2), 125–129. https://doi.org/10.1111/j.1479-8301.2010.00329.x

National Institute on Aging. (2019). *Social isolation, loneliness in older people poses health risks.* https://www.nia.nih.gov/news/social-isolation-loneliness-older-people-pose-health-risks

Pet Food Manufacturers' Association. (2021). *Pet population 2019.* https://www.pfma.org.uk/pet-population-2021

Pfortmueller, C. A., Efeoglou, A., Furrer, H., & Exadaktylos, A. K. (2013). Dog bite injuries: Primary and secondary emergency department presentations—A retrospective cohort study. *The Scientific World Journal, 2013*, 393176. https://doi.org/10.1155/2013/393176

Rehder, J. (2016, February 2). *Pets and the elderly—What are the risks?*. The Davis Community. https://www.thedaviscommunity.org/2016/02/02/pets-elderly-risks/

Richeson, N. E. (2003). Effects on animal-assisted therapy on agitated behaviours and social interactions of older adults with dementia. *American Journal of Alzheimer's Disease & Other Dementias, 18*(6), 353–358. https://doi.org/10.1177/153331750301800610

Society for the Prevention of Cruelty to Animals (SPCA). (2019). *Adoption process.* https://www.spca.org.hk/en/services/animals-for-adoption/adoption-process

State of Victoria. (2020). *Walking for good health.* https://www.betterhealth.vic.gov.au/health/healthyliving/walking-for-good-health

Stull, J. W., Peregrine, A. S., Sargeant, J. M., & Weese, J. S. (2012). Household knowledge, attitudes and practices related to pet contact and associated zoonoses in Ontario, Canada. *BMC Public Health, 12*(553). https://doi.org/10.1186/1471-2458-12-553.

Suthers-McCabe, H. M. (Summer, 2001). Take one pet and call me in the morning. *Generations: Journal of the American Society on Aging, 25*(2), 93–95. http://www.jstor.org/stable/44877613

Testoni, I., De Cataldo, L., Ronconi, L., & Zamperini, A. (2017). Pet loss and representations of death, attachment, depression, and euthanasia. *Anthrozoös, 30*(1), 135–148. https://doi.org/10.1080/08927936.2017.1270599

The Hong Kong Guide Dog Association. (2019). *Guide dog.* https://www.guidedogs.org.hk/services/

The Hong Kong Jockey Club. (2019). *Jockey Club supports establishment of education and guide dog training centre to promote social inclusion.* https://corporate.hkjc.com/corporate/corporate-news/english/2018-10/news_2018100601400.aspx

The National Federation of the Blind. (2019). *Blindness statistics.* https://nfb.org/resources/blindness-statistics

U.S. Department of Health and Human Services (2001). *Clarifying the definition of homebound and medical necessity using OASIS data: Final report.* https://aspe.hhs.gov/execsum/clarifying-definition-homebound-and-medical-necessity-using-oasis-data-final-report

Vrbanac, Z., Zečević, I., Ljubić, M., Belić, M., Stanin, D., Bottegaro, N. B., Jurkić, G., Škrlin, B., Bedrica, L., & Žubčić, D. (2013). Animal assisted therapy and perception of loneliness in geriatric nursing home residents. *Collegium Antropologicum, 37*(3), 973–976. https://pubmed.ncbi.nlm.nih.gov/24308245/

Whitmarsh, L. (2009). The benefits of guide dog ownership. *Visual Impairment Research, 7*(1), 27–42. https://doi.org/10.1080/13882350590956439

Wilson, J. P., Kafetz, K., & Fink, D. (2016). Lick of death: Capnocytophaga canimorsusis an important cause of sepsis in the elderly. *BMJ Case Reports, 2016*,. https://doi.org/10.1136/bcr-2016-215450

Wood, L., Martin, K., Christian, H., Nathan, A., Lauritsen, C., Houghton, S., Kawachi, I., & McCune, S. (2015). *The pet factor—Companion animals as a conduit for getting to know people, friendship formation and social support*. https://doi.org/10.1371/journal.pone.0122085

Xie, Z. Y., Zhao, D., Chen, B. R., Wang, Y. N., Ma, Y., Shi, H. J., Yang, Y., Wang, Z. M., & Wang, L. S. (2017). Association between pet ownership and coronary artery disease in a Chinese population. *Medicine, 96*(13), e6466. https://doi.org/10.1097/MD.0000000000006466

Yabroff, K. R., Troiano, R. P., & Berrigan, D. (2008). Walking the dog: Is pet ownership associated with physical activity in California? *Journal of Physical Activity and Health, 5*, 216–228. https://doi.org/10.1097/10.1123/jpah.5.2.216

Young, S. (2008). The neurobiology of human social behaviour: An important but neglected topic. *Journal of Psychiatry & Neuroscience, 33*(5), 391–392. https://pubmed.ncbi.nlm.nih.gov/18787656/

Part III
Capacity Building for Ageing with Dignity

Chapter 21
Building Living Capacity for Senior Citizens in Asia

Catherine K. Y. Kwong and Ben Yuk Fai Fong

Abstract Hong Kong has the increasing ageing population with the longest life expectancy in the world. The older adults are seeking good quality of life from their living conditions. Elderly housing with supportive facilities and care is one of the essential components to achieve an advanced living condition. In Hong Kong, different types of elderly accommodations are provided by the Hong Kong Housing Authority, the Hong Kong Housing Society and the Social and Welfare Department. Elderly Village is an ordinary accommodation for retired seniors in many countries, where it shares a similar concept of the Senior Citizen Residences Scheme and Joyous Living Scheme launched by the Hong Kong Housing Society. Based on the local and foreign experience, it has figured out the opportunities and barriers of providing elderly housing to allow them to live with comfort and dignity. This chapter describes accommodations for elderlies in Hong Kong and the barriers of implementation. Examples of elderly residence from Singapore, Korea and Australia are presented.

Keywords Ageing in place · Elderly villages

21.1 Introduction

Senior citizens, like everybody in the society, pursue better living conditions and good quality of life. These are the principles in ageing in place, which should be enjoyed by all older adults because they have contributed to the community all life. However, there are inadequate subsidised places for independent elderly living, particularly for those from the low income group and those who need assisted services or home care services. A concept in building livable homes for joyous seniors is being

C. K. Y. Kwong
Hong Kong College of Community Health Practitioners, Hong Kong, China

B. Y. F. Fong (✉)
College of Professional and Continuing Education, The Hong Kong Polytechnic University, Kowloon, Hong Kong, China
e-mail: byffong@gmail.com

V. T. S. Law and B. Y. F. Fong (eds.), *Ageing with Dignity in Hong Kong and Asia*, Quality of Life in Asia 16, https://doi.org/10.1007/978-981-19-3061-4_21

examined in this chapter. Elderly villages, also known as retirement villages, provide comprehensive supports of housing, healthcare and community services. They have been successfully implemented in countries Australia, the United Kingdom (UK), Singapore, Japan and South Korea.

21.2 Accommodations for Hong Kong Elderly

In Hong Kong, China, the population aged 65 or above is estimated to reach 2.28 million by 2034 and will further grow up to 2.58 million by 2064, being equal to 1 in 3 in the population (Research Office, 2015). Moreover, 0.36 million of elders, or 30.9% of the aged population, lived under poverty in 2018. These poor elders mainly resided in elderly households without any pre-intervention income and the majority of them lived alone (Census and Statistics Department, 2019). The growing poor senior population not only will increase the burden on healthcare expenses, but also on the supply of residential and long-term care services, especially in subsidised residential care homes for the elderly (RCHE). Subsidised elderly accommodations are provided in the public sector by the Hong Kong Housing Authority, a government department, and Hong Kong Housing Society (HKHS), a statutory body, while housing in the private sector is non-subsidised. HKHS provides elderly housings and services to the low, middle and higher income groups, such as the Ageing-in-Place (AIP) scheme, Senior Citizen Residences Scheme (SEN) and the quality elderly housing project at Tanner Hill on Hong Kong Island (Wong, 2018). For those who need institutional care services, the Social Welfare Department (SWD) of the government provides funded residential care homes, e.g. nursing homes, care and attention homes for the elderly, and homes and hostels for the aged (Wong, 2016).

It is unfortunate that the many older adults on the central waiting list for subsidised RCHE have died before getting a place. As of 30 June 2021, there were a total of 36,531 applicants being waitlisted for various types of subsidised residential care services (RCS) for the elderly in the Central Waiting List for subsidised long-term care services. As of 31 March 2020, 39,655 older adults were on the waiting list, but only 29,088 subsidised places were available in both Care and Attention Homes for the elderly and nursing homes (SWD, 2021a). At the meantime, the overall waiting time for different types of sponsored RCS for the elderly is 21 months, where the longest waiting time for a place in subvented or contract homes is 41 months (SWD, 2021b). The appalling situation does not appear to change.

21.2.1 Housing for Senior Citizens

The government provides housing for the healthy and well elderly who are capable of living independently. Housing for Senior Citizens (HSC) was launched by the

Hong Kong Housing Authority for singleton elderly applicants (Hong Kong Housing Authority, 2021). Specifically designed facilities for elderly are provided in such housing, including emergency alarm system, rocker-type light switches, non-slip floor tiles and handrails in corridors. There are common areas like solarium, activity rooms, shared kitchen and dining area. However, there was a high vacancy rate of HSC in the 90s because applicants would prefer self-contained flats. Hence, production of HSC was ceased in 2000. Currently, HKHA has no provision of specific public housing rental flats merely for the residence of elderly applicants. For those elderly applicants who prefer hostel type of accommodation with communal facilities and warden service, they might opt to be rehoused to HSC Type 2 and Type 3 design units.

21.2.2 Ageing-in-Place Scheme

The Hong Kong Housing Society initiated the Ageing-in-Place (AIP) Scheme since 2012, mainly targeted at the low income group (HKHS, 2020a). An integrated concept consisting of home safety, health and wellness support and social support was implemented in 20 HKHS rental estates. In the AIP Scheme, there are screening and promotion of home safety by estate-based ambassadors. Home modifications such as installing handrails, lifting up sockets, removing curbs and provision of shower chairs are conducted after home environment assessments by occupational therapists from the HKHS. Regular health checkup, rehabilitation services, chronic diseases management, fall prevention exercises and mental wellness training programmes are included in the scheme to achieve the wellness and autonomy of the elderly. Social activities are also organised to promote happy ageing and prevent cognitive decline (HKHS, 2020a; Wong, 2018). A longitudinal study conducted by the University of Hong Kong has proved the sustainable effect of the AIP Scheme in terms of reduction of the utilisation of institutional care and the accident and emergency services, positive outcomes in preventing fall, encouragement active-ageing participation and improvement of mental wellness and cognition (HKHS, 2017a).

21.2.3 Senior Citizen Residences Scheme

The Senior Citizen Residences Scheme (SEN) had been initiated by HKHS since 1999. Two pilot projects were completed and they were Jolly Place located in Tseung Kwan O by 2003 and Cheerful Court sited in Ngau Tau Kok by 2004 (HKHS, 2020c). The residents, middle-class elders, are provided with a comprehensive one-stop housing, entailing medical care, recreation and social supporting services. There are 576 residential units of studio and 1-bedroom flats under a long lease contract arrangement (HKHS, 2020c). There are built-in home safety installations including non-slip homogenous tiles, handrails in shower area, fire system and emergency support facilities such as smoke detectors, fire signal lights, emergency lighting, sprinklers, hands free door phone, emergency nurse call system and two-way opening door etc. Club facilities like restaurant, gymnasium, swimming pool and library are available to improve the psychosocial wellbeing and quality of life (Wong, 2018). In addition, Jolly Place Care Home and Cheerful Court Care Home in the scheme function as residential care homes to provide holistic care to the elderly through a multi-disciplinary professional team which consists of registered nurses, geriatricians, psychogeriatricians, social workers, physiotherapists and occupational therapists (HKHS, 2017b). In addition, a polyclinic and a rehabilitation centre are built to enhance the physical wellness of the residents.

21.2.4 The Joyous Living Scheme

The Tanner Hill project in North Point, on Hong Kong Island, is the first non-subsidised elderly housing scheme under the Joyous Living Platform of HKHS. It was completed in 2015 as a one-stop quality living initiative of ageing in place which targeted at the more financially affordable clientele aged 60 or above. It is near North Point Mass Transit Railway (MTR) Station and accessible to different public transports such as the buses, trams and ferries. There are also community facilities in the neighbourhood within walking distance, including shopping malls, restaurants, municipal parks and a public library (HKHS, 2019; Wong, 2016).

588 units are provided in the 3 residential towers, with unit size from 344 sq. ft. to 1,231 sq. ft. All units are designed with elder-friendly characteristics and technologies which aim to provide a convenient and safe setting. There are widened and kerbless entrances, waist level power sockets, two-way light switching system, adjustable cabinets in open kitchen, bathroom designated for wheelchair users, visual and audio fire alarm, two-level security viewers, health data collection and monitoring system, and no-motion response detection senor with emergency call response services, etc. (HKHS, 2020d; Wong, 2018). These smart systems are integrated to record the health conditions of residents and monitor the household safety. The senior friendly design is also found in lifts, installed with handrails and seats and big and clear lift buttons with braille signs, as well as sufficient space for manoeuvring wheelchairs (HKHS, 2019). The Joyous Hub and Resident Club provides facilities to encourage an active and happy lifestyle for the residents and community members. There are a gymnasium, an indoor heated swimming pool, a library, a mini-theatre and a child playroom etc.

The Tanner Hill project also offers professional care and comprehensive support services to look after the functional, mental, spiritual and social health of the tenants by Hong Kong Baptist University Chinese Medicine Specialty Clinic (North Point), HKSH Healthcare Family Medicine and Primary Care Centre (Tanner Hill) and Senior Citizen Wellness Centre (HKHS, 2019). Domestic services such as handyman service, housekeeping service and companion service are also available (Wong, 2016). In addition, the RCHE in Tanner Hill provides a one-stop quality services of 24-h nursing and personalised care, while the day and training centre offers cognitive training for residents with severe disabilities or dementia, and the rehabilitation centre offers tailor-made rehabilitation programmes by physiotherapists and occupational therapists (HKHS, 2020b).

21.2.5 Dependent Older Adults

For older adults who are incapable of self-care at home, the Social and Welfare Department provides residential care homes for elderly citizens aged 65 or above. They are Homes for the Aged, Care and Attention Homes and Nursing Homes. Homes for the Aged offer a limited range of assistance in daily cleaning activities, for seniors with no or mild impairment, who are not capable of living independently, but no nursing care is available (SWD, 2018b). For older adults who suffer from deteriorating physical or psychological health and with moderate impairment, Care and Attention Homes for Elderly would offer limited nursing care, therapeutic exercises and personal care services to improve their body functioning (SWD, 2018a). Nursing Homes are catered for bed-bound elderlies with severe physical or mental impairment and disabilities (SWD, 2018c). Care and Attention Homes and nursing homes are suitable for either home-bound or bed-bound elders who are incapable of living alone. They can receive proper daily living services, counselling service, nursing care and social and recreational activities attended by professional staff.

21.2.6 Poor Living Environment

The living environment of some elderly people is rather poor, especially those who live in private subdivided flats (Hui et al, 2014). The poor living conditions often result not only in higher cost of repair and maintenance, but also risk to personal safety. On the other hand, the quality of living in RCHEs varies in terms of living spacing and services in the homes (Research Office, 2015). It is thus desirable to provide sufficient living environment for the elderly with optimal settings in residential building, medical care services and spacious areas. Another issue of public concern is the hygiene in the RCHEs, which are in confined settings and residents are sharing dining and bathing facilities. The prevalence of infection among residents of RCHs was about 2.7%. A local study has found that the transmission of infection would be potentially fostered by close contact (Choy et al., 2016). Worse still, elderly care homes became a potential disaster during the COVID-19 pandemic, due to insufficient ventilation and cramped spaces, and the older people are generally lack the physical strength to fight the infection (Mohana, 2022).

21.3 Senior Housing in Asia–Pacific Economies

21.3.1 Singapore

Kampung Admiralty located in Woodlands town is the first public housing innovation for senior Singapore citizens aged 55 and above (Civil Service College, 2019). It was launched in 2014 with integration of residential buildings, healthcare, leisure and commercial facilities for the senior citizens and residents of all ages under one roof. The one-stop hub aims to achieve healthy ageing-in-place with good living quality, active living in communities and healthy lives through the communal spaces designed with innovative and sustainable features.

Within the kampung (village), a total of 104 studio apartments are provided in two 11-storey residential blocks. Every unit is supported with elderly friendly settings and fittings, such as anti-slip and moisture-resistant flooring, grab bars, a ramp at the entrance of the unit, bigger switches and retractable clothes drying rack etc., to ensure a secure, comfortable and convenient environment for senior residents (Centre for Liveable Cities, 2019). Moreover, a huge and fully sheltered community plaza of $1000m^2$ is used for social activities like large-scale sports and fitness activities, educational events, performances, festivities and more, encouraging active living and social interactions. The Active Ageing Hub provides care services and activities for vicinal seniors to enjoy active ageing, and it is co-located with the childcare centre and the community park so as to enhance the intergenerational bonding. The Admiralty Medical Centre inside the kampung is a one-stop centre providing comprehensive medical services by specialists from nearby hospitals. Diabetes centre, integrated pharmacy, day surgery, endoscopies and rehabilitation services are the in-situ facilities and disease management services offered in order to maintain aged wellness and facilitate health education. In addition, the kampung supplies basic living needs and a holistic living community for the third age by including many shops, supermarket, bank, hawker centre and community garden inside.

21.3.2 South Korea

Shinnae Medical Housing (SMH) in Shinnae-dong, Seoul is a public rental housing opened in 2015 for the disadvantaged elderly with medical needs (Centre for Liveable Cities, 2019). It is an integrative housing project combining the public rental residential facilities with public healthcare and medical services, which are sponsored by the Seoul Metropolitan Government. SMH is a medical-based housing for eligible residents in Seoul who are older than 65 with a chronic disease or use of a wheelchair. SMH provides 222 households, while 10 of the housing units are allocated to Seoul Medical Center staff who are responsible for emergency situations.

Both interior and exterior facilities in the SMH are barrier-free, designed for ease access by wheelchairs and mobile beds. There are handrails on the walls and grab bars, and emergency alarms installed in the bathroom and living room. The life rhythm checking system installed in each unit is a motion detector to check the use of facilities in the unit for the SMH superintendent to monitor personal conditions of the residents so as to safeguard elderlies living alone. The emergency alarms inside the unit and emergency-bell necklace provided to residents are supported with a 'two-way safety system'. The alarm is connected to the office of the superintendent, and referred to the 119 emergency service and Seoul Medical Centre emergency room when necessary.

The Seoul Medical Centre in the SMH provides both healthcare treatment and community health services, e.g. free health consultation twice a month, healthcare checking equipment like blood pressure gauge, a diabetograph and emergency boxes, as well as the emergency hotline service. In addition, community facilities including fitness centres, restaurants, hobby centre, guesthouse and rooftop garden are provided to support the physical and emotional health of residents, promote neighbourhood communication and enhance community spirit.

21.3.3 Australia

Retirement villages in Australia are a widely accepted concept which aims to promote independent living and enhance the quality of life of elder adults (Xia et al., 2015). Keperra Sanctuary located in a suburban area in Brisbane is a private retirement village with decades of history. There are 254 homes in the village with the unit format of 1 to 3 bedrooms per home. Most of the units in the village have an age-friendly design. There are no entrance stairs and this is convenient for those who have mobility difficulties. Keperra Sanctuary provides an enjoyable living environment with various facilities and services in the communal area such as the solar heated swimming pool, bowling green, clubhouse, library, dance floor, salon, pet services and village shuttle bus etc. A community centre is located at the central of the village so that all units can access easily. Besides, the village provides 31 emergency assembly points as the safe locations for emergency evacuation.

When residents become incapable of living independently or in need for the higher-level aged care service, the Aged Care Centre in the village provides care accommodation in the forms of single or double rooms for 49 residents (Xia et al., 2015). The care services include on-site aged care, visiting medical practitioners, visiting podiatrists and visiting acupuncturists. Keperra Sanctuary is a good example of connecting an elderly village with the local community with the objective of sustainability for active ageing. On the other hand, the fee structure is complicated and the costs of living are varied among different elderly villages. Thus a usual three-tiered model is used for financial payment. The first is a lump-sum payment paid as the entry contribution, then ongoing costs are the daily running costs of retirement village, and the last is deferred management fee when resale, moving out or passing away (Hu et al., 2017).

21.4 Elderly Villages for the Future

There are different forms of housing for senior citizens. Elderly villages are a community-based living style in a planned area where accommodation and supportive services are provided for the elderly who voluntarily want to live there in either long-term or temporarily (Retirement Living Council, 2013). The accommodation generally caters for people aged 55 or above and mainly retired from full-time employment.

Most villages are single-storey or low-rise houses occupying spacious landscapes, providing multi-unit complexes equipped with medical and recreational facilities to offer a range of health and entertainment services, with purposes to maintain physical, mental and social wellness to residents. The village environments are conducive to achieving the basic needs of the elderly in providing independence, security and supports in their homes, encouraging social participation in order to minimise the feeling of loneliness and isolation and promoting social belonging, connectivity and integration (Yeung et al, 2017). For example, services by visiting doctors and allied healthcare professionals will support the long-term health of residents. Community halls are places for social communication during workshops, special programmes and trainings. Since elderly villages share the similar concept as SEN projects and quality retirement living established by the HKHS in Hong Kong, the experience of Jolly Place, Cheerful Court and Tanner Hill is significant for the infrastructure of elderly villages in the future. Several local studies are conducted on the satisfaction of the residential citizens in the three elderly housings. Chan and Cheung (2008) found that about 84% of respondents who lived in Jolly Place and Cheerful Court had a positive feedback on the living environment and were satisfied with the residential locations and neighbourhood facilities, e.g. hospital, supermarket, wet market and department stores etc. Both studies by Chan and Cheung (2008) and Ma (2013) noted that most respondents (70%) from Jolly Place and Cheerful Court were very gratified with various kinds of elderly facilities provided in the housing estates. On the other hand, a study on the Tanner Hill project by Wong et al. (2012) found that respondents had positive comments on the facilities in Tanner Hill and the public facilities in North Point as their daily needs could be sufficiently fulfilled. They were also satisfied with the medical facilities, healthcare services and sport facilities supplied in the Tanner Hill for maintaining good physical health.

There are cultural differences in the concept of elderly housing between the Asian and Western societies. First is the different design in the housing structure. Singapore and South Korea use one-hub vertical buildings with multiple floor levels, while apartments or houses with one level are constructed in Australia, where it may be due to the larger availability of land. Second, the multi-functional facilities provided are specific to the local target groups of resident customers. Keperra Sanctuary in Australia focuses more on recreational facilities, while Kampung Admiralty in Singapore emphasises the intergenerational community and Shinnae Medical Housing in South Korea mainly provides medical services to their residents. Differences in selection of location and external supporting facilities are observed. Keperra Sanctuary is situated in the Australian suburban district. Kampung Admiralty, Shinnae Medical Housing and Tanner Hill are close to the urban area where the residents have easy access to public facilities and are thus readily connected and involved in the society. Nonetheless, residents at Keperra Sanctuary can escape from the busy city life and enjoy the natural scenery and environment.

In Hong Kong, changes of the traditional Chinese cultures are apparent because of a long history of high level of influence of Western cultures, which bring changes to the society in terms of living style and housing approaches. Children are traditionally responsible in living together with their parents and taking care of them, as well as providing financial supports whether they have married or not. In contrast, Western cultures entail ideas like separation, segregation, small household size and individualism, and Hong Kong people have adopted the philosophy of individualism (Wong, 2018). From the latest census report, the number of domestic household size of 1–2 persons was greatly increased, but the number of larger family that consists of 5–6 persons was shrinking consistently (Census & Statistic Department, 2020).

21.5 Barriers in Implementing Elderly Residence

21.5.1 Affordability

The entry contribution and living costs in the Australian retirement villages are the main concern for prospective residents (Hu et al., 2017). Even though they have made a comprehensive planning on financial decision, money is still the main concern in some groups such as persons who do not own a house. The housing affordability may create an issue of limiting the financial management abilities and resources in their retirement. Thus, some villages provide a financial package with a lower entry contribution yet a higher deferred management fee to suit different types of clients (Hu et al., 2017).

On the contrary, the SEN scheme in Hong Kong has launched with a minimum requirement of financial ability of applicants. The total asset of singleton should be at least HK$3.26 million and the combined total asset of doubleton is not less than HK$4.89 million. The entry contribution for a studio of Jolly Place and Cheerful Court ranges from approximately HK$770 thousand to HK$1.23 million, while for a 1-bedroom it ranges from HK$1.14 million to HK$ 1.90 million. Regarding to the quality living project, the entry contribution and operation cost are expected to be much higher. The high rental cost in Tanner Hill has been expressed by the elderly, since most senior adults are unable to pay the monthly rental of about HK$15,000 to $24,000 (Wong et al., 2012). Furthermore, there are additional costs of the management fee and other activities or services. The hidden cost would create uncertainty to the potential clients and may thus deter their wish to apply for the residence.

21.5.2 Low Intention of Moving Home

A local Hong Kong study found that an overwhelming percentage (89%) of elderly respondents tended to live in the community for ageing and continue to receive community care, while about 75% of them preferred ageing in place even when their physical conditions are getting worse (HKHS, 2018). There is a higher chance of physical disability among elderly people. Hui et al. (2014) noted about 69% of the elderlies interviewed had no intention to move within the following five years because of their physical disability. The lowered moving ability would bring difficulties for them in adapting to a new living environment. Therefore, the older adults considered ageing in place as their optimal preference and they had no or low incentive to consider housing relocation (Hui et al., 2014). Moreover, many older adults had stayed in the accommodation, and the same district and community, for many years. In Hui's et al. study (2014), more than 40% of the elderlies had lived in the current home for more than 20 years, where they were already familiar with the surroundings. They had also developed their social network in the nearby communities and a strong sense of social belonging. Their friends and social connections would be lost if they moved to a new community.

21.5.3 Traditional Values

As a society dominated with Chinese culture, Hong Kong people consider housing as an important possession to support family unity and maintain stability, particularly older adults who have offsprings (Wong, 2018). Elderly people want to secure the future living of their children so they would bequest their living homes to the children after they pass away. Either of the SEN scheme and Tanner Hill projects are run by the rental concept, the elderly has no property rights of the units. This explains why places in SEN scheme and Tanner Hill are not attractive to the older residents. The ideology of traditional value cannot be changed easily. They may feel less secure without the right of property because they could not pass the assets to their offspring (Wong et al., 2012).

21.5.4 Lack of Policy Support

Lack of governmental support is a common issue in planning appropriate housing for older people. In Australia, retirement village is not a prior industry to receive direct governmental support in the land use planning policies. The village developers have to invest more to prepare a superior living environment, and sufficient care and services. It would raise the living cost in the villages, while the majority of residents are financially unaffordable from the limited pension (Hu et al., 2017).

In Hong Kong, lack of government policy support in land allocation and land premium concession has not encouraged the development of retirement housing in the society (Wong, 2018). Even after the completion of two pilot projects in 2003, the government had not advocated or initiated further development of similar elderly housing, particularly for the middle class (Wong et al., 2012). The ageing population and longer life expectancy have created great increase in the needs of elderly housing units, but insufficient supply of SEN and quality living housing has led to a longer waiting time for the elder applicants. Lack of long-term care planning is observed in the elderly policy (Wong et al., 2012).

21.6 The Way Forward

The Hong Kong government should promulgate comprehensive policies on elderly residence and long-term care to allow the older population to live more comfortably and safely with dignity. Elderly housing must be provided in a holistic consideration and humanistic manner to assure quality of life for the elderly in the last leg of life. Alternative options of elderly housing for different classes should be planned. There ought to be increased financial assistance and improved facilities (Wong et al., 2012). The elderly housing scheme should include all districts to give incentive to elderlies to move to elderly homes within the same district. Furthermore, with the success of the SEN Scheme, the government should reserve land for the HKHS and make ageing in place a routine practice (Dashun Policy Research Centre, 2015; Ma, 2013).

Hong Kong Housing Society has made a great contribution to elderly housing with quality living. The high satisfaction of residents under SEN Scheme and Tanner Hill is noted by some studies (Chan & Cheung, 2008; Ma, 2013; Wong et al., 2012). HKHS should consider extending the Scheme to all districts and building relevant elderly housing for seniors of different income levels, providing more housing options for elderlies who are not eligible to apply for public estates or financial subsidies (Ma, 2013). HKHS may also consider providing SEN-like housing units with the special elder-friendly fittings and basic care facilities but not the extra and additional services. This can help to meet the demand of seniors with different affordability levels. On the other hand, the high-entry contribution brings stress to potential clients. Thus, using Australian's experience on retirement village as a reference, HKHS can consider lowering the entry contribution or letting the elderly residents to pay by instalments, in order to decrease the sudden financial burden.

There are several types of elderly housings provided in Hong Kong, but not including elderly villages in the current options. This new model of elderly housing is designated to provide residential, medical, recreational and social supports for elder adults to attain active ageing community. The SEN Scheme and Tanner Hill projects share a similar concept of elderly village. However, some factors like high living costs, low moving incentive and lack of related policy are the barriers.

References

Census and Statistics Department. (2019). *Hong Kong poverty situation report 2018.* https://www.statistics.gov.hk/pub/B9XX0005E2018AN18E0100.pdf

Census and Statistic Department. (2020). *Table E032: Domestic households by household size and monthly household income (excluding foreign domestic helpers) (Table 9.4A in quarterly report on general household survey).* https://www.censtatd.gov.hk/hkstat/sub/sp150.jsp?productCode=D5250036

Centre for Liveable Cities. (2019). *Age-friendly cities: Lessons from Seoul and Singapore.* https://www.clc.gov.sg/research-publications/publications/books/view/age-friendly-cities-lessons-from-seoul-and-singapore

Chan, C. M. A., & Cheung, K. W. K. (2008). *An evaluation study on the elderly housing initiative in Hong Kong* (APIAS Working Paper Series No. 14). http://commons.ln.edu.hk/apiaswp/15/

Choy, C. S. M., Chen, H., Yau, C. S. W., Hsu, E. K., Chik, N. Y. & Wong, A. T. Y. (2016). Prevalence of infections among residents of Residential Care Homes for the Elderly in Hong Kong. *Hong Kong Medical Journal, 22*, 347–355. https://doi.org/10.12809/hkmj164865

Civil Service College. (2019). *Kampung admiralty: Building for all ages.* https://www.csc.gov.sg/articles/kampung-admiralty-building-for-all-ages

Dashun Policy Research Centre. (2015). *Age-friendly housing policies.* http://www.dashun.org.hk/en/research_details.php?id=7

Hong Kong Housing Authority. (2021). *Types of senior housing.* https://www.housingauthority.gov.hk/en/public-housing/meeting-special-needs/senior-citizens/types-of-senior-housing/index.html

Hong Kong Housing Society. (2017a). *Housing society today. Building age-friendly community and promoting ageing in place. Issue no. 77.* https://www.hkhs.com/home/upload/pdf/hst_77_HST_77_Eng.pdf

Hong Kong Housing Society. (2017b). *Jolly place care home (Residential care home for the elderly).* https://www.hkhs.com/sen_20040903/eng/jolly_place/fs/tko_care.htm

Hong Kong Housing Society. (2018). *Ageing in Place: Joyful elderly home (in Chinese).* https://www.hkhs.com/home/upload/pdf/AIP_Booklet_resize_20190121100054.pdf

Hong Kong Housing Society. (2019). *Building livable homes for joyous senior living.* https://www.hkhs.com/home/pdf/TTH_eBook/en/78/index.html#zoom=z

Hong Kong Housing Society. (2020a). *Ageing-in-place scheme.* https://www.hkhs.com/en/our-business/elderly-housing/ageing-in-place

Hong Kong Housing Society. (2020b). *Joyous circle skilled care service.* https://www.tth-joyouscircle.hkhs.com/en/home/rche/rche_environment_facilities/index.html

Hong Kong Housing Society. (2020c). *Senior citizen residences scheme.* https://www.hkhs.com/en/our-business/elderly-housing/senior-citizen

Hong Kong Housing Society. (2020d). *Senior-friendly features.* https://www.thetannerhill.hkhs.com/en/design/senior_friendly_features/index.html

Hu, X., Xia, B., Skitmore, M., Buys, L., & Zuo, J. (2017). Retirement villages in Australia: A literature review. *Pacific Rim Property Research Journal, 23*(1), 101–122. https://doi.org/10.1080/14445921.2017.1298949

Hui, E. C. M., Wong, F. K. W., Chung, K. W., & Lau, K. Y. (2014). Housing affordability, preferences and expectations of elderly with government intervention. *Habitat International, 43*, 11–21. https://doi.org/10.1016/j.habitatint.2014.01.010

Ma, H. K. J. (2013). *Housing for the elders in Hong Kong: Arrangement of housing policy to cater for the special needs of the elders* [Master dissertation, The University of Hong Kong]. https://hub.hku.hk/bitstream/10722/194935/1/FullText.pdf

Mohana, D. (2022). COVID-19 and the elderlies: How safe are Hong Kong's care homes? *Frontiers in Public Health*, 10. https://doi.org/10.3389/fpubh.2022.883472

Research Office. (2015). *Challenges of population ageing. Hong Kong Special Administrative Region.* https://www.legco.gov.hk/research-publications/english/1516rb01-challenges-of-population-ageing-20151215-e.pdf

Retirement Living Council. (2013). *Retirement living council fact sheet retirement villages and residential aged care facilities compared*. Property Council of Australia. http://www.retirementliving.org.au/wp-content/uploads/2013/12/Nursing-Homes.pdf

Social Welfare Department. (2018a). *Care and attention homes for elderly.* https://www.swd.gov.hk/storage/asset/section/628/en/C&A_Home_Leaflet.pdf

Social Welfare Department. (2018b). *Home for the aged.* https://www.swd.gov.hk/en/index/site_pubsvc/page_elderly/sub_residentia/

Social Welfare Department. (2018c). *Nursing homes.* https://www.swd.gov.hk/storage/asset/section/630/en/NH_Leaflet.pdf

Social Welfare Department. (2021a). *Overview of residential care services for the elderly.* https://www.swd.gov.hk/en/index/site_pubsvc/page_elderly/sub_residentia/id_overviewon/

Social Welfare Department. (2021b). *Statistics on 'Waiting list for subsidised residential care services for the elderly', 'Waiting time for residential care services' and 'Turn for placement offer for cases applying for residential care services'.* https://www.swd.gov.hk/storage/asset/section/632/en/LTC_statistics_HP-Eng(202003).pdf

Wong, F., Hui, E., Chung, K. W., Li, T., & Lui, E. (2012). *Housing for the elderly in Hong Kong—Affordability and preferences.* https://www.hkis.org.hk/ufiles/Elderly-FinalReport.pdf

Wong, K. L. (2016, December 9). *The Hong Kong institute of engineers engineering forum—Quality retirement Living in Hong Kong* [Seminar presentation]. Engineering forum seminar on "Engineering Hong Kong housing supply—Challenges, changes, continuity", Hong Kong. http://www.engineeringforum.hk/publications/2016-12-09/4_Quality%20Retirement%20Living%20in%20Hong%20Kong.pdf

Wong, K. L. (2018, November 2). *Quality housing for an ageing community* [Conference presentation]. HKHS International Housing Conference, Hong Kong. https://www.hkhs.com/home/pdf/hkhsconference2018/Keynote_Wong_Kit_Loong.pdf

Xia, B., Zuo, J., Skitmore, M., Chen, Q., & Rarasati, A. (2015). Sustainable retirement village for older people: A case study in Brisbane, Australia. *International Journal of Strategic Property Management, 19*(2), 149–158. https://doi.org/10.3846/1648715x.2015.1029564

Yeung, P., Good, G., O'Donoghue, K., Spence, S., & Ros, B. (2017). What matters most to people in retirement villages and their transition to residential aged care. *Aotearoa New Zealand Social Work, 29*(4), 84–96. https://doi.org/10.11157/anzswj-vol29iss4id419.

Chapter 22
Healthy Ageing and Lifelong Learning in Hong Kong

Hilary H. L. Yee, Ben Yuk Fai Fong, Tommy K. C. Ng, and Vincent Tin Sing Law

Abstract By 2030, the older population is expected to outnumber children under the age of 10 and now ageing population remains a fundamental and major worldwide challenge for the more developed economies. It has been nearly 20 years since the World Health Organization (WHO) developed the active ageing and healthy ageing policy frameworks that aim to optimise 'opportunities for health, participation and security in order to enhance quality of life as people age'. It has aroused the attention of policymakers to adopt relevant action plans to promote active ageing. Lifelong learning is one of the ways to facilitate older adults to stay engaged, healthy and secure in the society and has been proved to help to maintain quality of life in the physical, mental and social health aspects. In the physical aspects, some studies have shown that many elders are distracted from their chronic conditions by taking part in various activities, which might have resulted in the delay of physical deterioration. In addition, wider benefits of lifelong learning have been found in the mental and social context. Several studies have combined these two as psychological well-being in lifelong learning. The opportunity to further engage in education allows older adults to develop new skills and confidence which in turn helps them to stay connected with the community and enhance community well-being. The benefits of lifelong education among older adults can help them to achieve healthy ageing and to age with dignity. This chapter lists out the advantages of lifelong education to older adults and the current education policy for older learners in Hong Kong. Taking a group of senior citizens who studied a diploma as an example, new insights are drawn and limitations and future opportunities are evaluated.

H. H. L. Yee
The Hong Kong Polytechnic University, Kowloon, Hong Kong, China
e-mail: hiulam.yee@polyu.edu.hk

B. Y. F. Fong · T. K. C. Ng (✉) · V. T. S. Law
School of Professional Education and Executive Development, College of Professional and Continuing Education, The Hong Kong Polytechnic University, Kowloon, Hong Kong, China
e-mail: tommy.ng@cpce-polyu.edu.hk

V. T. S. Law
e-mail: vincent.law@cpce-polyu.edu.hk

V. T. S. Law and B. Y. F. Fong (eds.), *Ageing with Dignity in Hong Kong and Asia*, Quality of Life in Asia 16, https://doi.org/10.1007/978-981-19-3061-4_22

Keywords Older learner · Lifelong learning · Quality of life · Healthy ageing · Education policy

22.1 Introduction

Ageing is a universal and natural biological process that happens to everyone. Ageing population due to long lifespan has become a worldwide trend and issue. While having longer life expectancy, most older adults develop chronic diseases or disabilities associated with ageing. Although getting old is inevitable, people can still enjoy life as long as healthy ageing can be experienced. Defined by World Health Organization (WHO), healthy ageing is about creating environments and opportunities for people to be able to continue doing what they value through 'a process of developing and maintaining the functional ability that enable well-being in older age' (World Health Organization [WHO], 2020). It is impossible to be completely free of diseases but achieving healthy ageing in the community can provide optimal opportunities and environments for people to age well and enjoy quality life.

Engaging in lifelong learning is a process to stimulate and empower older learners to acquire 'new' knowledge, skills and values, which then enable them to cope with challenges and adapt to changes later in life (Laal & Salamati, 2012; Thang et al., 2019). WHO acknowledges lifelong learning in the active ageing framework in 2002 as an important factor that helps participation, health and security in late adulthood (WHO, 2002). Evidence from studies has shown lifelong learning is still considered as a multidimensional activity that benefits individual's psychological and social well-being, and enhances life satisfaction (Narushima et al., 2018a, 2018b; Oliver et al., 2017; Thang et al., 2019; Yamashita et al., 2017). Learning allows older adult to keep up with technology like computer and internet-related developments, as well as socio-economic resources in retirement (González-Palau et al., 2014; Limone et al., 2018; Talmage et al., 2016).

While there is a range of definitions of what is meant by 'lifelong learning' in literatures, it generally includes any learning activities over the lifespan and can be classified into formal and informal learning (Yamashita et al., 2017). More opportunities have been given to older learners to participate in degree-levels courses at higher educational institutions. Higher education plays a role in facilitating adult and continuing education and provides older people chances to acquire educational qualifications. Some people prefer informal and leisure pursuit of learning that focuses more on self-learning to gain new skills and knowledge through the context of daily lives (Thang et al., 2019). On the whole, both formal and informal learning are important forms of learning engagements which encourage older adults to continue to participate in various contexts of personal growth and social development beyond academic and work qualifications (Thang et al., 2019). Thus lifelong education is one of the ways to achieve healthy ageing and has been receiving more attention around the world.

22.2 Lifelong Education and Healthy Ageing

The Active Ageing Framework endorsed by the WHO advocates physical, mental and social health as equally important elements in quality of life and therefore has influenced ageing policies around the world. WHO acclaimed a strong relationship between activity and opportunities for healthy living and emphasised the need to create opportunities for older people to age actively (Formosa, 2019). The Active Ageing Framework in 2002 acknowledged lifelong learning as an important factor that facilitates active ageing. WHO then added lifelong learning in 2015 as the fourth pillar that supported active ageing, along with the other three pillars, namely participation, health and security. Since 2015, active ageing was replaced by 'healthy ageing', extending to 'maintaining functional ability that enables well-being in older age' (WHO, 2021). Given the context of population ageing, increasing number of studies and literature have investigated the effects of lifelong learning among older adults and found positive links between learning and better well-being and health (Narushima et al., 2018b).

Early studies focused on how lifelong learning assisted older people to adapt the transformation to old age such as declining physical health, reducing income and changing social roles and civic obligations. Formosa (2018) identified the benefits of lifelong learning including empowering older people with the advocacy skills to counteract social and financial changes arising from ageing. The learning needs among old people can be addressed in a variety of contexts through formal and informal modes, such as formal classrooms, self-directed learning, volunteering and intergenerational learning. These needs can be related to employment, health and wellness, personal interests and development, leisure and travel, technology literacy like computer usage and so on (Merriam & Kee, 2014). There are numerous benefits of engaging in lifelong learning (Formosa, 2018; Laal & Salamati, 2012):

- To enrich self-fulfilment, self-esteem, self-satisfaction through adapting to ageing transition such as degenerations in physical strength and health, changes in social and civic obligations, retirement and reduced income
- To make new friends and establish valuable social networking and social solidarity
- To increase wisdom and understanding on previous success and failures
- To open up the mind by exchanging ideas and viewpoints among older learners and younger peers
- To adapt to changes in the society especially technological innovations including computer and internet-related developments
- To improve opportunities to either remain in or re-enter the labour market

A growing number of research has found well-being and health are positively linked with lifelong education among adult learners. It was stated by Field (2009) that 'adult learning makes a small but significant, measurable positive contribution to well-being', and 'adult education is effective in enhancing the well-being, helping to develop social competencies, extending social networks, and promoting shared norms and tolerance of others'. Vulnerable older adults with poorer health conditions, socio-economic status and social support benefit most from lifelong learning as it mitigates the effects of risk conditions and restores the psychological reserves including well-being, motivation in participation and coping capacity (Narushima et al., 2013).

It is found that education and learning activities have the most influences on older adult's physical and psychological well-being, thus impacting their quality of life (Escuder-Mollon et al., 2014; Thang et al., 2019). Despite having various chronic diseases, elderly participants still enjoy activities at health centres, suggesting that engagement in social and/or physical activities may help the elderly to focus on wellness than illness, and even delay further physical deterioration (Lassen, 2015). Psychological well-being is measured by evaluation of various aspects of an individual's life, including concerns about general health, life satisfaction, depressive moods, anxiety and stress, autonomy and personal growth. A cross-sectional survey with 699 older learners enrolled in community-based continuing education programmes demonstrated that the longer they participated in the programmes, the better their psychological well-being was reported, regardless of the types of programmes (Narushima et al., 2013). They also showed positive healthy lifestyles such as non-smoking and regular exercise. Lifelong learning also helps to stimulate mind activities by increase processing speed and creativity thinking among older learners, ultimately preventing cognition decline and decreasing the probability to develop dementia by 12% (Basu, 2013; Boulton-Lewis, 2010).

In a study, post-work participants found that their learning in retirement had kept their mind active by gaining new knowledge (Withnall, 2009). Furthermore, a longitudinal study showed that participation in informal and non-credit type learning had been especially beneficial in maintaining psychological well-being of older adults, while formal learning and training did not have such effects (Jenkins & Mostafa, 2013). It was suggested that publicly funded and non-credit programmes often offered diverse general-interest subjects and locations that were easy to access, making it easier for older adults with physical and mental health condition to continue to pursue their personal interests (Narushima et al., 2013, 2018b). After adjusting for life satisfaction determinants such as demographic factors, educational attainment and income, it was found that participation in additional lifelong learning activities, including self-learning activities such as reading was associated with greater life satisfaction (Yamashita et al., 2017).

Socially engaged individuals with good personal networking are at lower risk of physical health problems and psychological distress than those who are isolated and being social withdrawn (Minagawa & Saito, 2015). Being more active in the community and social group facilitates emotional and material supports, thus fostering a sense of purpose and belonging to the community. Learning from and communicating with teachers and classmates can promote social health by building and enlarging the social circle, developing connections and a stronger sense of identity in the community (Narushima et al., 2018b). Such social participation of learning helps to develop larger personal network and is important among older adults because it has a substantial positive effect on social trust and life satisfaction (Tomini et al., 2016).

After all, engaging in lifelong learning programmes is not only 'a process of acquiring knowledge, skills and dispositions throughout one's life to achieve well-being', but also well-being for the community (Laal & Salamati, 2012; Merriam & Kee, 2014). Communities benefit from having all segments of their citizens staying healthy, actively engaging and contributing to community resources (Merriam & Kee, 2014). Older adults contribute to community well-being in substantive ways through civic engagement, social connectivity, volunteering, service-learning and intergenerational activities. Service-learning projects involving different age groups of people facilitate intergenerational harmony in the community by deconstructing stereotypes between the younger and older generations. In terms of promoting social and educational inputs, young students can benefit from their academic and professional learning, while the elderly can gain by having social interaction and feelings of successful ageing (Ruiz-Montero et al., 2020). Lifelong learning among the elderly contributes to both human and social capitals as they become more knowledgeable and more socially engaged, thus enhancing personal and community well-being (Merriam & Kee, 2014).

22.3 Lifelong Education in Hong Kong

22.3.1 Elder Academy (EA)

Lifelong education opportunities have been provided to older adults in Hong Kong, mostly informal learning, that addresses the leisure and practical needs, organised in community elderly centres (Formosa, 2019). Common courses include computer lessons, Tai Chi, dancing and painting. The diversity of learning becomes wider after the establishment of Elder Academy Scheme in 2007. It promotes intergenerational learning with young students and older adults. Partnering with non-governmental organisations and local volunteer organisations, primary, secondary and post-secondary institutions are encouraged to register as members of EA and offer both formal and informal programmes and courses for older persons to pursue studies or participate in learning activities.

There are around 180 EAs in total and they comply with objectives (1) to encourage older persons to acquire new knowledge and learn new skills to keep pace with the society (2) to offer a platform for older persons to share knowledge, demonstrate creativity, serve the community and contribute to the society, (3) to enhance sense of achievement and self-confidence through learning in order to maintain physical health and mental well-being, (4) to optimise the existing resources of schools for running elder learning programmes after school hours, (5) to promote intergenerational harmony between young students and elders, (6) to strengthen civic education among younger students, and (7) to promote collaboration between different stakeholders and strengthen ties between schools and local community services (Elder

Academy, 2020). As some older adults have not had the chance to study in universities, EAs in City University of Hong Kong, The Education University of Hong Kong, Hong Kong Shue Yan University and The Open University of Hong Kong have provided places in selected undergraduate courses for the elderly to attend as auditing students. It does not involve any assessment nor earn credits for a degree award.

22.3.2 University of 3rd Age Network (U3A)

U3A, originated in France, aims to provide opportunities for later-life learning, and has later been promoted in many other places around the world. Co-founded by Hong Kong Electric Centenary Trust (HK Electric) and Hong Kong Council of Social Service (HKCSS), U3A is promoted in Hong Kong to encourage lifelong learning and volunteerism among retirees. The principle of U3A is 'learning for pleasure', and therefore U3A advocates interest-based and self-initiated learning for the elderly. 48 learning centres are established for elders, providing more than 70,000 learning opportunities (Formosa, 2019). U3A has also organised 'Outstanding Third Age Citizens Awards' every two years to recognise outstanding students, teachers and centres. U3A has found that elders enrolled in this network demonstrate more socially and mentally active, better organisational and teaching skills and confidence of expressing one's views. Despite the COVID-19 pandemic since 2020, U3A has continued to conduct online training programmes and successfully trained 130 retirees to be green ambassadors to promote green messages and low-carbon lifestyle (HK Electric Investments, 2020).

22.3.3 A Case of Older Learners in Achieving Formal Qualification—Diploma in Active Ageing

A study showed that older age and being retired reduced the probability of formal learning, but not informal learning (Jenkins & Mostafa, 2013). This may be because older people prefer comparatively flexible, leisure and personalised, but less structured methods of education (Halliday-Wynes & Beddie, 2009; Tam et al., 2017). Engaging in formal learning usually undergoes testing or accreditation process which is more 'threatening' to the elderly. Therefore, informal learning remains more popular among older adults. There are very limited formal qualifications and degree-level of programmes that are specifically designed for older learners.

The Diploma in Active Ageing (DAA), designed for students over 50 years old and organised by the School of Professional Education and Executive Development (SPEED) of The Hong Kong Polytechnic University (PolyU) is an example of a university diploma award for older adults. DAA is a formal academic programme and aims to equip students with the required transferable skills and knowledge for enhancement of the daily living activities. Students are preferably required to have secondary 6 or equivalent level of qualification to enrol in the programme. There are 10 compulsory subjects covering a wide range of areas, categorised into three areas, namely (i) overview of ageing-related knowledge, (ii) holistic health wellness and (iii) finance and re-employment, including nutrition and physical fitness, brain health, traditional Chinese medicine, finance and investment planning, life review, psychology, etc. Unlike informal courses, DAA has a structured learning approach with assessments to test the knowledge of the students and learning outcomes of the subjects. Students who have successfully completed 30 credits with satisfactory results will be awarded the DAA while those who have only completed 9 credits will be awarded a Certificate in Active Ageing.

Students enrolled in the 2019–2020 academic year demonstrated a cheerful attitude towards life and good understanding of subject contents. Reflected from their individual assessments in the subject 'Brain health and dementia care', students had gained deeper understanding on how to prevent and handle dementia. Some of them shared their experiences in taking care of their own parents who suffered from dementia. Although feeling a bit worried about the symptoms of dementia in affecting memory, thinking and social abilities, they realised that remaining active in daily living was important to maintain autonomy in older people. They realised that sickness and ageing were unavoidable but keeping a healthy lifestyle and holding an optimistic vision would allow them to enjoy later life happily.

Students also demonstrated active learning attitudes and the majority of them participated in research activities conducted by the Centre for Ageing and Healthcare Management Research (CAHMR), PolyU SPEED. 20 DAA students aged between 50 and 73 participated in a study about the impact of lifelong learning conducted by the Centre. In both the questionnaire and focus group discussion, participants agreed that they experienced positive changes in psychological and social health, including thinking more positively, feeling less fatigue, meeting more new friends and expressing more with classmates. Some of them commented that most older adults, especially those who had retired, preferred informal learning as they liked flexible timetable and considered the tuition fees for academic programmes expensive. They remained neutral on the promotion of lifelong education as the public generally knew little about formal education programmes. Participants also reflected that financial subsidies by the government for continuing education and training were insufficient in Hong Kong. There was a big 'loophole' in the eligible age being limited from between 18 and 70 for subsidy reimbursement. Elders beyond 70 of age were not covered by the scheme when life expectancy of both men, at 82, and women, at 87, in Hong Kong topped the world.

In another study conducted by CAHMR on the same DAA cohort, 20 students volunteered to participate in focus groups to share their opinions and views about the use of technological devices in online learning. During the COVID-19 pandemic, education has changed dramatically with online learning via digital platforms. Although older adults were more digitally connected in recent years, they were generally less experienced in technology than younger generations. Nonetheless, majority of the 20 participants, with a mean age of 63.5 years, showed positive attitudes towards online learning. Some of them admitted that they had once refused to learn by the new way as they had not experienced online learning before. They later realised that it was not as difficult as what they had expected, and they even overcame the challenges such as memorising the correct buttons and dealing with technical issues. However, they commented that such learning modality had affected their interactions with classmates and the benefits in social connectivity. Although they still preferred face-to-face learning, they regarded online learning as convenient. Some of them felt confident in handling new technology in future.

The studies of DAA students provided new insights into lifelong learning in Hong Kong. Informal learning like interest classes was indeed popular among older adults but there would also be a potential market in formal higher education for this age group. Students emphasised that meeting new friends who shared similar learning attitudes and working together in group projects were very rewarding. This suggests that formal education is effective in enhancing social interaction as learners need to work towards the same goals that lead to an academic qualification, which is not offered in the usual interest classes. DAA students had also demonstrated that older adults were willing to learn new things including technology skills. Although they were 'forced' to engage in online learning due to the COVID-19 pandemic, they managed well and learned fast in handling online platforms. DAA students received technical and social supports from the Information Technology Unit of the university and lecturers. They built up their confidence in the new learning modality. They might be slow in adopting new skills but adequate support and training were indispensable in motivating and supporting them to use technology for online learning. From the experience of this group, online learning should have significant potential for growth and should be promoted to older adults, not limited to informal or formal learning.

22.4 Future Opportunities

The population of the world is ageing quickly, and the pace of population ageing in Hong Kong is projected to be doubled from 1.27 million to 2.44 million from 2018 to 2038 (Wong & Yeung, 2019). Research has shown lifelong education among older adults will bring positive health benefits and facilitates healthy ageing. Promotion of lifelong education among older adults also contributes to community well-being through volunteering and intergenerational activities. Therefore, enhancing learning opportunities for older adults is important for them to maintaining active and engaged lifestyle, preserving community well-being and ultimately achieving healthy ageing. As some older people may no longer have the purpose in life anchored to employment, most of their learning is naturally through informal means (Merriam & Kee, 2014). Learning activities organised in health community centres and NGOs are popular informal platforms for older adults to participate in lifelong education. The Hong Kong government endorses the WHO's framework on healthy ageing and addresses the important of maximising learning opportunities for older adults. In response to the demand of older adult's learning, the establishment of EA network, U3A and CEF are examples of providing more opportunities and incentives for older adults in engaging continuous learning.

Results about physical dimension and leisure activities suggest that helping older adults to maintain participation in formal or informal leisure pursuits are important implications for promoting well-being and enhancing satisfaction in later life (Ra et al., 2013). The case of the DAA students brings out different insights into and important messages regarding learning opportunities for older learners in Hong Kong, including the exploration of formal education. Old age should no longer be regarded as having lower learning abilities. The positive learning attitudes and passions from DAA students reflect that similar courses are appropriate alternatives for older learners to be engaged in lifelong learning. Universities have adequate and fruitful resources such as library, computer laboratories and technical support to fully address the challenges and barriers faced by older adults, who are eager to adopt new technology when clear instructions and supports are available. The creation of appropriate and supportive learning environment is matters that affect the initiatives of lifelong learning in older adults.

The current lifelong learning policies for older adults are not without criticisms. Institutions that offer programmes and courses tend to target at maintaining competitiveness and meeting what is immediately needed in the market, in a sense practical economic values are mostly concerned. There is also criticism that learning providers for older adults only promote community-based forms of learning rather than learning activities that can help to improve quality of life and achieve healthy ageing (Tam, 2012). Financial support is another issue especially important to older adults as not many of them can afford the extra money on inessential items or activities. There is a big loophole in the application criteria of CEF that only individuals aged from 18 to 70 are eligible applicants. The amount of CEF is not sufficient for those who aim to obtain higher education qualifications as the amount of subsidy could only cover one to two modules of a degree course. The scope of registered courses of CEF has yet to include Massive Open Online Courses (MOOCs). MOOCs provide more flexible programmes for learners to access online course materials and video lectures at their own learning pace, bringing benefits on promoting information technology to older learners and overcoming mobility difficulties. MOOCs should also be of particular relevance to older learners to stay responsive to changes of technology and digital literacy.

The limitations inhibit older adults to achieve healthy ageing through lifelong education. To increase lifelong education participation rate and encourage education provision among older adults, the existing policies and lifelong education programmes must be restructured and revamped. Research has to be conducted to review and evaluate current effectiveness, adequacy and financial arrangement of lifelong education and related policy from the perspectives of older learners and education institutions. Future opportunities for lifelong education among older adults may include more higher education qualifications, online learning programmes and integrational activities to help them to achieve healthy ageing.

Acknowledgements The work described in this paper was partially supported by a grant from the Research Grants Council of the Hong Kong Special Administrative Region, China (Project Reference No.: UGC/IDS24/18). *The authors wish to thank students of the Diploma in Active Ageing for the participation and contribution to the studies cited in this chapter.

References

Basu, R. (2013). Education and dementia risk: Results from the aging demographics and memory study. *Research on Aging, 35*(1), 7–31. https://doi.org/10.1177/0164027511434086

Boulton-Lewis, G. M. (2010). Education and learning for the elderly: Why, how, what. *Educational Gerontology, 36*(3), 213–228. https://doi.org/10.1080/03601270903182877

Elder Academy. (2020). *About elder academy.* https://www.elderacademy.org.hk/en/aboutea/index.html

Escuder-Mollon, P., Esteller-Curto, R., Ochoa, L., & Bardus, M. (2014). Impact on senior learners' quality of life through lifelong learning. *Procedia-Social and Behavioral Sciences, 131*, 510–516. https://doi.org/10.1016/j.sbspro.2014.04.157

Field, J. (2009). Good for your soul? Adult learning and mental well-being. *International Journal of Lifelong Education, 28*(2), 175–191. https://doi.org/10.1080/02601370902757034

Formosa, M. (2018). National policies for healthy aging in Malta: Achievements and limitations. *Healthy Aging Research, 7*(1). https://doi.org/10.12715/har.2018.7.3

Formosa, M. (2019). The university of the third age and active ageing. *European and Asian-Pacific Perspectives. Cham: Springer.* https://doi.org/10.1007/978-3-030-21515-6

González-Palau, F., Franco, M., Bamidis, P., Losada, R., Parra, E., Papageorgiou, S. G., & Vivas, A. B. (2014). The effects of a computer-based cognitive and physical training program in a healthy and mildly cognitive impaired aging sample. *Aging & Mental Health, 18*(7), 838–846. https://doi.org/10.1080/13607863.2014.899972

Halliday-Wynes, S., & Beddie, F. (2009). *Informal learning. At a glance.* National Centre for Vocational Education Research.

HK Electric Investments. (2020). *Sustainability report 2020.* https://www.hkelectric.com/en/CorporateSocialResponsibility/CorporateSocialResponsibility_CDD/Documents/SR2020E.pdf

Jenkins, A., & Mostafa, T. (2013). *Learning and well-being trajectories among older adults in England.* Working paper series. https://discovery.ucl.ac.uk/id/eprint/10018762/

Laal, M., & Salamati, P. (2012). Lifelong learning; why do we need it? *Procedia-Social and Behavioral Sciences, 31*, 399–403. https://doi.org/10.1016/j.sbspro.2011.12.073

Lassen, A. J. (2015). Keeping disease at arm's length-how older Danish people distance disease through active ageing. *Ageing and Society, 35*(7), 1364. https://doi.org/10.1017/S0144686X14000245

Limone, P., Monacis, L., Ceglie, F., Sinatra, M., & de Palo, V. (2018). Enhancing e-learning in old age. *Australian Journal of Adult Learning, 58*(1), 88–109.

Merriam, S. B., & Kee, Y. (2014). Promoting community well-being: The case for lifelong learning for older adults. *Adult Education Quarterly, 64*(2), 128–144. https://doi.org/10.1177/0741713613513633

Minagawa, Y., & Saito, Y. (2015). Active social participation and mortality risk among older people in Japan: Results from a nationally representative sample. *Research on Aging, 37*(5), 481–499. https://doi.org/10.1177/0164027514545238

Narushima, M., Liu, J., & Diestelkamp, N. (2013). The association between lifelong learning and psychological well-being among older adults: Implications for interdisciplinary health promotion in an aging society. *Activities, Adaptation & Aging, 37*(3), 239–250. https://doi.org/10.1080/01924788.2013.816834

Narushima, M., Liu, J., & Diestelkamp, N. (2018a). I learn, therefore I am: A phenomenological analysis of meanings of lifelong learning for vulnerable older adults. *The Gerontologist, 58*(4), 696–705. https://doi.org/10.1093/geront/gnx044

Narushima, M., Liu, J., & Diestelkamp, N. (2018b). Lifelong learning in active ageing discourse: Its conserving effect on well-being, health and vulnerability. *Ageing & Society, 38*(4), 651–675. https://doi.org/10.1017/S0144686X16001136

Oliver, A., Tomás, J. M., & Montoro-Rodriguez, J. (2017). Dispositional hope and life satisfaction among older adults attending lifelong learning programs. *Archives of Gerontology and Geriatrics, 72*, 80–85. https://doi.org/10.1016/j.archger.2017.05.008

Ra, J., An, S., & Rhee, K. J. (2013). The relationship between psychosocial effects and life satisfaction of the Korean elderly: Moderating and mediating effects of leisure activity. *Journal of Arts and Humanities, 2*(11), 21–35. https://doi.org/10.18533/journal.v2i11.229

Ruiz-Montero, P. J., Chiva-Bartoll, O., Salvador-García, C., & González-García, C. (2020). Learning with older adults through intergenerational service learning in physical education teacher education. *Sustainability, 12*(3), 1127. https://doi.org/10.3390/su12031127

Talmage, C. A., Mark, R., Slowey, M., & Knopf, R. C. (2016). Age Friendly Universities and engagement with older adults: Moving from principles to practice. *International Journal of Lifelong Education, 35*(5), 537–554. https://doi.org/10.1080/02601370.2016.1224040

Tam, M. (2012). Lifelong learning for elders in Hong Kong: Policy and practice. *International Journal of Lifelong Education, 31*(2), 157–170. https://doi.org/10.1080/02601370.2012.663805

Tam, M., Boulton-Lewis, G., Buys, L., & Chui, E. (2017). Similarities and differences in views of ageing and learning in Hong Kong and Australia. *Educational Gerontology, 43*(8), 393–403. https://doi.org/10.1080/03601277.2017.1309634

Thang, L. L., Lim, E., & Tan, S. L. S. (2019). Lifelong learning and productive aging among the baby-boomers in Singapore. *Social Science & Medicine, 229*, 41–49. https://doi.org/10.1016/j.socscimed.2018.08.021

Tomini, F., Tomini, S. M., & Groot, W. (2016). Understanding the value of social networks in life satisfaction of elderly people: A comparative study of 16 European countries using SHARE data. *BMC Geriatrics, 16*(1), 1–12. https://doi.org/10.1186/s12877-016-0362-7

Withnall, A. (2009). *Improving learning in later life*. Routledge.

Wong, K., & Yeung, M. (2019). Population ageing trend of Hong Kong. *Hong Kong: Office of the government economist—Economic letter 2019/02*. https://www.hkeconomy.gov.hk/en/pdf/el/el-2019-02.pdf

World Health Organization. (2002). *Active ageing: A policy framework* (No. WHO/NMH/NPH/02.8). World Health Organization.

World Health Organization. (2020). *Ageing: Healthy ageing and functional ability*. https://www.who.int/westernpacific/news/q-a-detail/ageing-healthy-ageing-and-functional-ability

World Health Organization. (2021). *Ageing: Healthy ageing and functional ability*. https://www.who.int/westernpacific/news/q-a-detail/ageing-healthy-ageing-and-functional-ability

Yamashita, T., López, E. B., Stevens, J., & Keene, J. R. (2017). Types of learning activities and life satisfaction among older adults in urban community-based lifelong learning programs. *Activities, Adaptation & Aging, 41*(3), 239–257. https://doi.org/10.1080/01924788.2017.1310583

Chapter 23
Roles and Training of Community Health Practitioners in Elderly Care

Sean Hon Yin Hui and Ellen Ku

Abstract Primary healthcare covers a wide range of high-quality preventive care services to the public. With the phenomenon of the ageing population, expenditure spent on healthcare activities is increasing. By improving the primary care structure, the heavy medical burden is expected to be eased to a considerable extent. Therefore, there should be an increasing number of healthcare practitioners providing community-based healthcare to the public as community health practitioners (CHP) and community health coaches (CHC) in Hong Kong. Community health practitioners are trained with the roles in monitoring health behaviours, supporting health promotion activities and strengthening community actions and capabilities to get rid of health risks, thus helping to reduce the prevalence of chronic diseases, monitor disease progression, improve quality of life as well as reduce the workload of other healthcare professionals to tackle insufficient manpower in primary care. Community health coaches take up a critical role to reinforce citizens with health knowledge to assist them in self-monitoring of health or disease progression and to promote and encourage positive doctor-patient cooperation and healthy behaviours. This chapter presents the development of comprehensive medical services to enhance the continuity of medical services as well as to optimise preventive care to cope with the burden caused by major diseases, ageing population and patients with chronic diseases and explores the continuous development training of community health practitioners and community health coaches by discussing their roles and training guidelines for elderly care in the provision of holistic and humanistic approaches with the aim of ageing with dignity for the older adults.

Keywords Community health practitioners · Patient empowerment programme · Bodenheimer model · Starfield 4 pillars · Team-based care · Teamlet model

S. H. Y. Hui (✉)
Hong Kong College of Community Health Practitioners, Hong Kong, China
e-mail: seanhui1997@gmail.com

E. Ku
Caritas Institute of Higher Education, Hong Kong, China
e-mail: eku9229@gmail.com

V. T. S. Law and B. Y. F. Fong (eds.), *Ageing with Dignity in Hong Kong and Asia*, Quality of Life in Asia 16, https://doi.org/10.1007/978-981-19-3061-4_23

23.1 Introduction

Primary healthcare covers a wide range of high-quality preventive care services to the public. With the phenomenon of the ageing population, expenditure spent on healthcare activities is increasing. By improving the primary care structure, the heavy medical burden is expected to be eased to a considerable extent. Therefore, there is an increasing number of healthcare practitioners providing community-based healthcare to the public as Community Health Practitioners (CHP) and Community Health Coaches (CHC). Community health practitioners are trained with the roles of monitoring health behaviours, supporting health promotion activities and strengthening community actions and capabilities to get rid of health risks, helping to reduce the prevalence of chronic diseases, monitor disease progression, improve quality of life as well as reduce the workload of other healthcare professionals to tackle insufficient manpower in primary care. Community health coaches take up a critical role to reinforce citizens with health knowledge to assist them in self-monitoring of health or disease progression and to promote and encourage positive doctor-patient cooperation and healthy behaviours. The objectives of this chapter are: (i) to develop comprehensive health services that cooperate across professional teams and sectors to enhance the continuity of health services as well as to optimise preventive care to cope with the burden caused by major diseases, ageing population and patients with chronic diseases and (ii) to promote continuous development training of community health practitioners and community health coaches by discussing their roles and training guidelines for elderly care in the provision of holistic and humanistic approaches with the aim of ageing with dignity for the older adults.

23.1.1 Non-Communicable Disease of the Elderly

Non-Communicable Diseases (NCDs) are an umbrella term that covers several non-infectious diseases including cardiovascular diseases, cancers, diabetes and chronic respiratory disease (World Health Organization, 2021). The risk factors of NCDs include high blood pressure, high cholesterol, high blood glucose, smoking, alcohol consumption, inactive physical lifestyle, unhealthy diet, stress and occupation (Bonita et al., 2003; Uddin et al., 2020).

Across the globe, 70% of deaths are attributed to NCDs while the prevalence of NCDs in China is more than 65% in the population of elderly aged more than 65 (Gong et al., 2018). The Chinese population is currently facing a sharp increase in the prevalence of NCDs and the World Health Organization figure out that 8,600,000 deaths, which represents more than 85% of the total death of the Chinese population, are attributed to NCDs. In Hong Kong, there are about 36,000 deaths, of which about 77% of total deaths are due to NCDs (Chang et al., 2020). With the advancing age, the risk and severity of diseases disability and death increases. The increased morbidity and mortality are usually related to NCDs, for which cardiovascular diseases, cancers, diabetes and chronic respiratory disease account for more than four-fifths of the death due to NCDs (Nethan et al., 2017).

23.1.2 The Burden Brought to the Elderly and Caregivers

Health conditions are affected by several factors that are not limited to mental conditions, physical well-being nor social functioning (Litvak et al., 1987). Moreover, burdens can also be found in the perspectives of medications and treatment. Medications are usually prescribed for the long-term management of chronic diseases to prevent or delay of adverse outcomes and complications. Treatment guidelines focus on individual chronic diseases and there is a lack of structured strategies to manage the elderlies, especially when most of them suffer from multiple NCDs. Patients have to follow complex instructions of the medications for several NCDs for the rest of their lives and thus the burdens to them and caregivers are apparent. The burdens are greatly related and affected by family support, duration of medicine, disease control and drug therapy adherence (Zidan et al., 2018). Some caregivers may be responsible for the costs of the treatments and management plan, and this will become a financial burden on them as well. To take care of the patients, caregivers have to pay attention to the illness-related characteristics, personal dispositions and resources. These are the primary stressors to the caregivers (Möller-Leimkühler & Wiesheu, 2011).

23.1.3 Ageing Population and Healthcare Facilities in Hong Kong

Hong Kong is an ageing society. Older adults, aged 65 or above, increasingly occupied from 17% in 2016 to 37% in 2066 while people who were aged under 65 would decrease from 83% in 2016 to 63% in 2066 (Woo et al., 2020). The general household survey conducted during October 2011 to January 2012 showed that about three-forth of the elderly, aged more or equal to 65, suffered from chronic health conditions, especially hypertension, diabetes mellitus, heart diseases, cancer and stroke (Centre for Health Protection, 2015). With such a highly and constantly increasing of the ageing population, and the fact that the elderly is highly reliant on the healthcare services provided by the public sector, it is expected that there will be an even longer queuing in public healthcare services (Lam, 2017). Together with the early onset of chronic illnesses, the Hospital Authority has estimated that there will be a constant increase in the demand for healthcare services of lifestyle-related diseases. Apart from healthcare services of chronic diseases, the needs for medical treatment from the elderly are compounded to four times than the others. Hong Kong will need 8,000 more beds in the coming 20 years to meet the expected growth in the ageing population which equals six comprehensive hospitals with the size of Queen Mary Hospital, teaching hospital of The University of Hong Kong (Lo et al., 2014, pp. 1–14).

23.1.4 Importance of Preventive Care in Alleviation of Burdens

Chronic diseases are characterised by their slow process of disease stages which are long lasting. They do not only affect the living quality of individuals and their care givers, but also escalate the healthcare costs and bring limitations to affordability of healthcare services and facilities. These problems can be alleviated by preventive care measures by identifying behavioural habits, which include lacking physical activities, uncontrolled dietary intake, smoking and alcohol drinking. Although it is widely agreed that it is not easy to do, but by promoting positive behavioural changes, chronic diseases can be prevented (Raghupathi & Raghupathi, 2017).

In the clinical aspect, preventive care measures can bring positive outcomes with better clinical status. In Hong Kong, the Hospital Authority has launched the large population-based Patient Empowerment Programme (PEP) for diabetes patients. Patient empowerment refers to a process enabling patients to make a greater and better decision on their health. PEP curriculum includes lifestyle behavioural changes, disease-specific knowledge and skills education. According to an observational matched cohort study, it show that patients with PEP participation had better outcomes in clinical aspects such as improved HbA1c level, LDL-C level and reduced visits to general outpatient clinics than those without PEP participation (Wong et al., 2014). The improvements in laboratory results could bring secondary prevention to the development of complications in diabetes patients and prevent further lowering, or even improving, the standard of living.

It has also been shown that with efficient investment in healthcare programmes, opportunities are seemingly equal for prevention and treatment with full ranged cost-effectiveness in accordance to the literature reviewed (Cohen et al., 2008). A recent cost-effectiveness analysis was performed from a societal perspective with the adoption of the patient-level simulation model. It showed that PEP could be highly cost-effective as a supplementary intervention to patients with diabetes from societal perspectives (Ferrario et al., 2016). From the health system perspective, programmes that help reduce long-term complications are cost-effective (Brownson et al., 2009). Moreover, the queuing time would also be reduced as there will be fewer patients who need care or treatment for complications. Putting all these into a nutshell, preventive care can help to alleviate the burden brought by the ageing population in clinical aspects which helps reducing complications and also in societal and health system aspects that promoting cost-effectiveness in healthcare expenditure and queuing burden. The improvement outcomes from the holistic and humanistic approaches have significant impacts on the elderly in their health and its long-term management, amounting dignity care.

23.2 Community Health

Community health refers to the health of the whole population and to emphasise what the population is suffering by discovering the root cause of problems from not only the aspects of the individuals, but also the family, community and the environment, and to use the community resources to solve the problems while aiming to strive for the balance between physical, emotional, social, spiritual and intellectual health (Solomon Ibama & Dennis, 2016). For community health services, it takes an essential part in the primary healthcare constitution. There is an association between client's satisfaction, quality of life and health outcomes (Ha et al., 2019). Community health services also build bridges between health services and community, even when some groups that are difficult to be accessible, such as the ethnic minorities or the underprivileged. Those from low socioeconomic status or low and middle-income backgrounds are more prone to have higher morbidity and mortality relating to NCDs. Through community health services, the risk factors are expected to be alleviated through improving the accessibility of community health services, which can help to solve concerns about mutual accountability between healthcare providers and patients, poor medication adherence, care plan misunderstanding, language and cultural barrier, lack of lifestyle modification and care plan, and lack of supporting means in the community for the elderly and care providers.

23.3 Community Health Practitioners and Their Roles in Elderly Care in Community Health Services

Community Health Practitioners (CHP) are healthcare providers who work in community settings, including outreach healthcare services or other healthcare which is not hosted by conventional healthcare professionals like doctors, nurses and allied health professionals (Fong, 2020). As CHPs work in the community and performs outreach activities such as home visits, they function as the first contact point of healthcare while mutual trust is usually developed here to start the healthcare delivery by the CHPs. The primary mission of a CHP is to prevent problems from occurring or re-occurring through a patient educational programme, healthcare service administration and research (Solomon Ibama & Dennis, 2016).

The roles of CHPs are well described in the ten building blocks of high performing primary care which is also called the Bodenheimer model (Bodenheimer et al., 2014). Bodenheimer model is composed of (Barbara) Starfield 4 pillars, elements of the Joint Principles and Patient-Centered Medical Home (PCMH) recognition standards, and other core components. The 4 pillars of primary care practice represent the first-contact care, continuity of care, comprehensive care and coordination of care. Although the Starfield 4 pillars together with the Joint Principles describe the important functions of primary care, there is no practical and specific guideline to carry out the operation of these functions. Therefore, 10 building blocks are presented as guidance to carry out high performance primary care. There are four foundation building blocks that almost every practice will be first established, which are engaged leadership, data-driven improvement, empanelment and team-based care. After fulfilling these four foundation blocks, higher building blocks can be achieved which are the patient-team partnership, population management, continuity of care, prompt access to care, comprehensiveness and care coordination while the highest level is about the template of the future. The following is the description of the 10 building blocks:

1. Engaged leadership

   It is expected that there is a leader who fully engages in the changing process into high performing practices at all levels of the organisation. Apart from healthcare providers, patients can also take up the leadership role to set improvement priorities.
2. Data-driven improvement

   In this building block, a data system is employed to keep tacking and analysing the data in clinical, operational and patient experience aspects. Performance and improvements are evaluated and will be discussed regularly.
3. Empanelment

   Empanelment represents that a primary health clinician and a healthcare team are linked to a patient to provide foundational constant monitoring to the patient which is quintessential for ideal primary care and the basis of block 5, patient-team partnership, and block 7, continuity. Apart from these, empanelment allows the healthcare provider to adjust the workload for each care team and clinician as work overload may cause hamper on block 8, prompt access to care.
4. Team-based care

   There is a problem that patient cannot identify any healthcare providers who have thorough understanding of the patient's situation that may decrease the mutual accountability between patients and healthcare providers. To solve this problem, a team consistently made up of a regular clinician and his assistant should be formed that they share the work and responsibility on an everyday basis.
5. Patient-team partnership

   In this building block, patients are motivated to take part in the decision-making process, including evidence base and medical judgments to respect their personal goals.
6. Population management

   Three population-based functions share the care of the needs of patients and the design of team roles of healthcare providers include panel management, health coaching and complex care management. For panel management, which usually includes a healthcare assistant or nurses, to identify if a patient should do the routine checking. They also check for the health status of each patient to identify the care gaps. For health coaching, it focuses on assisting patients in changing their lifestyle behaviours by providing education on knowledge and skills and guiding the patient to engage in the action plan. For complex care management, it addresses the medical and psychosocial problems together. Both health coaching and complex care management require more time and thus it is suggested to give the healthcare providers a protracted time to ensure the ideal service delivery.

7. Continuity of care

   Continuity of care requires the effect of block 3, empanelment, that patients are partnered with the primary healthcare team. It is associated with improved preventive and chronic care, decreased expenditure and a better experience. Continuity of health services is a concept that providing patients with seamless services through the integration, coordination and sharing of information between multidisciplinary healthcare providers, and have to be evaluated with the experience from the perspective of patients and healthcare providers (Gulliford et al., 2006). The continuity of health services is made up of three main components which are relational continuity, management continuity and informational continuity (Haggerty et al., 2003). Informational continuity is about bridging separate healthcare events by patient's information to ensure that care is responsive to patient's needs. Management continuity emphasises on the service delivery quality of service management that services should be provided in a complementary and timely manner. Relational continuity is expecting not only from past to current care but also the future care to ensure the needed service is provided to patients.

8. Prompt access to care

   Access is always related to patient satisfaction which is greatly affected by waiting time. Access can be improved sustainably when block 3, empanelment, and block 4, team-based care can be successfully fulfilled. However, prompt access can harm the continuity of care when patients want prompt access to a provider when he or she is not the partnered healthcare provider.

9. Comprehensiveness and care coordination

   Comprehensiveness and care coordination are two of the Starfield 4 pillars. Comprehensiveness refers to the ability to offer what patient needs while care coordination refers to the ability of primary care providers to arrange services that they cannot provide to patients by referral. However, physicians are usually too busy to manage the coordination of services and thus a care coordinator should be engaged.

10. Template of the future

   The ultimate block is the template of the future. It is expected that there will be fewer in-patient visits while there will be more e-visits (telehealth) and telephone visits. It is noted that the full implementation of the template of the future requires payment reform that does not promote in-person clinical visits but also e-visits. It would be more cost-effective if non-essential emergency department and hospital costs for their patients can be reduced.

With these roles, it is expected that CHPs can improve the inaccessibility of service delivery in high performance primary care, especially when they look for ethnic minorities or those who are excluded from healthcare services by different barriers, such as language, the cultural or economic situation in health systems.

23.4 Community Health Coach and Their Roles in Elderly Care in Community Health Services

Currently, community health coach (CHC) is not clearly defined in the healthcare system and there is no established definition on it. They serve with a health education approach that emphasises lifestyle behaviour changes to bring out chronic disease self-management whereas its effect is proved (Dye et al., 2018). The major duty of a CHC is to help patients learning the knowledge, techniques, tools and confidence enabling patients to actively participate in their care and therefore attaining their self-identified goals (Bennett et al., 2010). CHC can perform in the following two models, which are the teamlet model and the hospital-to-home model.

In San Francisco General Hospital's Family Health Center, they used the teamlet model and the model included a clinician and a health coach (Ngo et al., 2010). They explain that the larger the team is, the more time and effort are spent and wasted on communicating among team members and more risk of fumbled handoffs. In a large team, it is resource consuming and it requires time for a single message to spread. It needs healthcare providers to hold a meeting to share the risk of human error and some non-relative healthcare providers have to waste the time to listen. Resources are consumed and wasted.

On the other hand, the hospital-to-home model is also a model for engaging community health coaches. From being discharged from the hospital, many elderlies eventually return to the hospital due to complications and confusion or the inability for their caregivers in care management. They especially require health coaches to assist patients to schedule the follow-up clinical visits, explain to patients the rationale for the instructions and requirements given by healthcare professionals, identify whether patients agree to treatment plans, provide patients support on behavioural modification, to assist patients in drug understanding and adherence, and be a support, a portal as well as a point of access and a cultural bridge (Bennett et al., 2010).

A study was conducted for diabetes care among Chinese patients using the Bodenheimer teamlet model (Ivey et al., 2013). The whole intervention was as follows. First, health coaches would conduct a pre-visit meeting that they would perform the routine assessment, medication reconciliation, patient agenda arrangement for consultation and data collection. The health coaches would enter the data into the chronic disease management database and generate a summary report for the physician to analyse during the physician visit. During the visit, the physician would explain the summary report to the patient. A health coach would not show up in this process, but the physician would share the findings with the health coaches and discuss the care plan during their meeting. After the consultation, health coaches would perform the post-visit meeting to make sure that patients were clear about the care plan and to emphasise the important parts to them. The agreed behavioural or self-care goals would be recorded on the Self-Management Action Plan Form. A copy would be given to the patients. Finally, health coaches would help patients to schedule the next follow-up appointments, perform navigations on referral systems and clerical work on ordered tests of patients. A week after each consultation, health coaches would dial into patients for self-management support and queries answering by themselves or by liaising with physicians. Two weeks after, patients also would be referred to attend health education for their conditions. Comparing to the original Bodenheimer model, they hired five health coaches to work with four physicians instead of two coaches for one physician. All health coaches, dietitians and most of the physicians are ethnically and linguistically matched to patients.

Hong Kong is an international metropolitan where groups of ethnic minorities are living with the Chinese. There are people from Pakistan, Indian, the Philippines, Indonesian, etc. These ethnic minorities always encounter the problem of the lack of translating resources for them to understand their health concerns. Services are provided with the forms of translated reading materials or translation services during consultations. However, if they encounter problems during lifestyle behaviour modification, it is difficult to seek aid. If health coaches are matched with ethnicity and linguistically, problems can be solved while mutual accountability can also be improved. This model of community care with the engagement of and services by health coaches is worth thinking about by the policymakers across the nations.

23.5 Continuing Professional Development and Training for CHP and CHC

Continuing professional development (CPD) is a self-driven lifelong learning process to maintain and enhance the standards of providers in knowledge, skills, altitude and behaviour development. In addition, management, team building, professionalism, interpersonal communication, technology, teaching and accountability should also be enhanced in CPD (Filipe et al., 2014).

CHC should be well trained to enable them to promote adherence to health activities by the clients, to educate the clients in self-management approaches to manage their health more effectively (Dye et al., 2018; Hartzler et al., 2018). Moreover, in the development of a successful teamlet model, CHPs and CHCs should be familiar with the availability and access of the community resources. They can act as a portal to help their clients locate and connect to such resources, thus improving optimal accessibility to the healthcare services in the community.

In self-management, CHCs should be well equipped with the skills to teach and encourage their clients to monitor their body health status, such as their body weights, blood glucose readings, blood pressure or heartbeat rate. CHCs need to show the clients how the equipment, like the blood glucose metre and blood pressure monitor, works. CHCs should also help their clients to maintain a health status log to trace their health outcomes and seek medical advice if symptoms appear or get worsened.

To facilitate their clients to bring out continuous and effective behaviour changing processes, CHCs should assist their patients to have self-motivation to bring out lifestyle behavioural changes. CHCs should also teach their clients to build up their tailor-made plan for behavioural changes and to reward themselves when they meet the goals. CHCs should also develop skills in preventing their clients from retake risk factors and return to the related behaviours to ensure the changes are more permanent.

Success of team formation is crucial among the CHPs and CHCs (Babiker et al., 2014). First of all, the team, patients and their supporting persons should share a common and unambiguous goal. The functions, responsibilities and accountability should be clearly described to each team member to maximise efficiency while mutual trust and respect are developed. Thirdly, the team should keep on improving their communication skills and provide an accessible communication platform for team members to use in all settings. Fourthly, the outcomes and processes should be measurable. Records of them should be agreed and upon implemented for tracking and improvements for future strategies. The last and fifth principle is that there should be a leader in the team to guide and coordinate the activities for other team members.

The Hong Kong Jockey Club, in conjunction with major non-government organisations (NGOs), and in research partnership with the Hong Kong Institute of Asia–Pacific Studies of The Chinese University of Hong Kong, sponsored the two-year Professional Traineeship Programme designed for first time jobseekers in 2020 for 400 degree and subdegree graduates in four disciplines including healthcare (PROcruit, n. d.). The trainees were given an intensive training and orientation course before they were posted to facilities managed by the NGOs to work as full-time Community Care Practitoners, Wellness Planners and Health Coaches. They delivered care and services in the community to promote self-management, health literacy, health awareness, holistic health practice, community psychosocial wellness, health maintenance, training of carers, etc. to older adults. The project aimed to develop these young upcoming professionals in the respective areas of work and to recommend to the government and the healthcare sector the practical professional and career pathways in the future.

23.6 Conclusion

Ageing population is a globally concerning issue that may bring problems from the perspectives of economics and health resources. To deal with the problems, community health services are a cost-effective approach to help slowing the onset of non-communicable diseases and their complications. In adherence to the Bodenheimer model's ten building blocks of high performing primary care, CHPs should strive for achieving higher blocks. By forming patient-CHC-CHP partnerships, the continuity of care can be improved while mutual trust can be developed among them, and therefore behaviour changing plan can be more effective. CHPs and CHCs should understand their roles and keep improving themselves to maintain and improve the community health service delivery while educational and communication skills are the most important. In the ideal situation, the partnership should be formed in well planning and even linguistically and culturally matching to their clients. Besides, there are different minorities and people from underprivileged backgrounds. Therefore, health coaches should learn more on how to connect the community resources to help those in need or whom are excluded from healthcare services by different barriers, such as language, the cultural or economic situation. CHPs should remember the common goals in promoting health activities to the community and aiming to bring health behavioural changes to strive for the balance between physical health, mental health, social health and spiritual health. With a good balance on different aspects of health, chronic diseases and complications can be delayed or prevented. Thus, by the promotion of community health services, CHPs not only maintain and extend the life of the elderlies, but also maintain and improve the quality of life of the older adults and their caregivers. It would be an ideal situation for the government to promote health coaching and education in the community and to invite the public to be health coaches to mitigate the challenges brought by the ageing population.

References

Babiker, A., Husseini, M. E., Nemri, A. A., Frayh, A. A., Juryyan, N. A., Faki, M. O., Assiri, A., Saadi, M. A., Shaikh, F., & Zamil, F. A. (2014). Health care professional development: Working as a team to improve patient care. *Sudanese Journal of Paediatrics, 14*(2), 9–16. https://www.ncbi.nlm.nih.gov/pmc/articles/PMC4949805/

Bennett, H. D., Coleman, E. A., Parry, C., Bodenheimer, T., & Chen, E. H. (2010). Health coaching for patients with chronic illness. *Family Practice Management, 17*(5), 24–29. http://www.aafp.org/fpm/20100900/p24

Bodenheimer, T., Ghorob, A., Willard-Grace, R., & Grumbach, K. (2014). The 10 building blocks of high-performing primary care. *The Annals of Family Medicine, 12*(2), 166–171. https://doi.org/10.1370/afm.1616

Bonita, R., Winkelmann, R., Douglas, K. A., & De Courten, M. (2003). The WHO stepwise approach to surveillance (Steps) of non-communicable disease risk factors. In D.V. McQueen, & P. Puska (Eds.), *Global behavioral risk factor surveillance* (pp. 9–22). Springer. https://doi.org/10.1007/978-1-4615-0071-1_3

Brownson, C. A., Hoerger, T. J., Fisher, E. B., & Kilpatrick, K. E. (2009). Cost-effectiveness of diabetes self-management programs in community primary care settings. *The Diabetes Educator, 35*(5), 761–769. https://doi.org/10.1177/0145721709340931

Centre for Health Protection. (2015, February). *Ageing well and optimal golden years. Centre for Health Protection.* https://www.chp.gov.hk/files/pdf/ncd_watch_feb2015.pdf

Chang, A., Schulz, P. J., & Wenghin Cheong, A. (2020). Online newspaper framing of non-communicable diseases: Comparison of Mainland China, Taiwan, Hong Kong and Macao. *International Journal of Environmental Research and Public Health, 17*(15), 5593. https://doi.org/10.3390/ijerph17155593

Cohen, J. T., Neumann, P. J., & Weinstein, M. C. (2008). Does preventive care save money? Health economics and the presidential candidates. *New England Journal of Medicine, 358*(7), 661–663. https://doi.org/10.1056/nejmp0708558

Dye, C., Willoughby, D., Aybar-Damali, B., Grady, C., Oran, R., & Knudson, A. (2018). Improving chronic disease self-management by older home health patients through community health coaching. *International Journal of Environmental Research and Public Health, 15*(4). https://doi.org/10.3390/ijerph15040660

Ferrario, M. G., Lizán, L., Montagnoli, R., & Ramírez de Arellano, A. (2016). Liraglutide vs. sitagliptin add-on to metformin treatment for type 2 diabetes mellitus: Short-term cost-per-controlled patient in Italy. *Primary Care Diabetes, 10*(3), 220–226. https://doi.org/10.1016/j.pcd.2015.10.002

Filipe, H., Golnik, K., Silva, E., & Stulting, A. (2014). Continuing professional development: Best practices. *Middle East African Journal of Ophthalmology, 21*(2), 134. https://doi.org/10.4103/0974-9233.129760

Fong, B.Y. F. (2020). *Health and the community*. https://hklaureateforum.org/en/science-in-the-community/185-health-and-the-community

Gong, J. B., Yu, X. W., Yi, X. R., Wang, C. H., & Tuo, X. P. (2018). Epidemiology of chronic noncommunicable diseases and evaluation of life quality in elderly. *Aging Medicine, 1*(1), 64–66. https://doi.org/10.1002/agm2.12009

Gulliford, M., Naithani, S., & Morgan, M. (2006). What is 'continuity of care'? *Journal of Health Services Research & Policy, 11*(4), 248–250. https://doi.org/10.1258/135581906778476490

Ha, N. T., Harris, M., Preen, D., Robinson, S., & Moorin, R. (2019). A time-duration measure of continuity of care to optimise utilisation of primary health care: A threshold effects approach among people with diabetes. *BMC Health Services Research, 19*(1). https://doi.org/10.1186/s12913-019-4099-9

Haggerty, J. L., Reid, R. J., Freeman, J. K., Starfield, B. F., Adair, C. E., & McKendry, R. (2003). Continuity of care: A multidisciplinary review. *BMJ, 327*(7425), 1219–1221. https://doi.org/10.1136/bmj.327.7425.1219

Hartzler, A. L., Tuzzio, L., Hsu, C., & Wagner, E. H. (2018). Roles and functions of community health workers in primary care. *The Annals of Family Medicine, 16*(3), 240–245. https://doi.org/10.1370/afm.2208

Ivey, S. L., Tseng, W., Kurtovich, E., Lui, B., Weir, R. C., Liu, J., Song, H., Wang, M., & Hubbard, A. (2013). Evaluating a culturally competent health coach intervention for Chinese American patients with diabetes. *Diabetes Spectrum, 25*(2). https://doi.org/10.2337/diaspect.25.2.93

Lam, H. Y. (2017). *Strategies of Hong Kong's healthcare system in aging population* [Paper presentation]. The Asian Conference on Aging & Gerontology 2017, Kobe, Japan. https://papers.iafor.org/submission36030/

Litvak, J., Ruiz, L., Restrepo, H. E., & McAlister, A. (1987). The growing noncommunicable disease burden, a challenge for the countries of americas. *PAHO Bulletin, 21*(2), 156–171.

Lo, S. H., Fong, K. W., Yuen, P. P., Lo, M. K., Kwong, K. K., & Lo, W. H. (Eds.). (2014). Public Administration and Policy. *An Asia-Pacific Journal, 17*(1), 1–14.

Möller-Leimkühler, A. M., & Wiesheu, A. (2011). Caregiver burden in chronic mental illness: The role of patient and caregiver characteristics. *European Archives of Psychiatry and Clinical Neuroscience, 262*(2), 157–166. https://doi.org/10.1007/s00406-011-0215-5

Nethan, S., Sinha, D., & Mehrotra, R. (2017). Non communicable disease risk factors and their trends in India. *Asian Pacific Journal of Cancer Prevention, 18*(7), 2005–2010. https://doi.org/10.22034/APJCP.2017.18.7.2005

Ngo, V., Hammer, H., & Bodenheimer. (2010). Health coaching in the Teamlet model: A case study. *Journal of General Internal Medicine, 25*(12), 1375–1378. https://doi.org/10.1007/s11606-010-1508-5

PROcruit. (n. d.). *Programme Overview*. https://www.procruitc.hk/en/aboutus

Raghupathi, V., & Raghupathi, W. (2017). Preventive healthcare: A neural network analysis of behavioral habits and chronic diseases. *Healthcare, 5*(1), 8. https://doi.org/10.3390/healthcare5010008

Solomon Ibama, A., & Dennis, P. (2016). Role of community health practitioners in national development: The Nigeria situation. *International Journal of Clinical Medicine, 7*(7), 511–518. https://doi.org/10.4236/ijcm.2016.77056

Uddin, R., Lee, E., Khan, S. R., Tremblay, M. S., & Khan, A. (2020). Clustering of lifestyle risk factors for non-communicable diseases in 304,779 adolescents from 89 countries: A global perspective. *Preventive Medicine, 131*, 105955. https://doi.org/10.1016/j.ypmed.2019.105955

Wong, C. K., Wong, W. C., Lam, C. L., Wan, Y. F., Wong, W. H., Chung, K. L., Dai, D., Tsui, E. L., & Fong, D. Y. (2014). Effects of patient empowerment programme (PEP) on clinical outcomes and health service utilization in type 2 diabetes mellitus in primary care: An observational matched cohort study. *PLoS ONE, 9*(5), e95328. https://doi.org/10.1371/journal.pone.0095328

Woo, J., Leung, D., Yu, R., Lee, R., & Wong, H. (2020). Factors affecting trends in societal indicators of ageing well in Hong Kong: Policies, politics and pandemics. *The Journal of Nutrition, Health & Aging, 25*(3), 325–329. https://doi.org/10.1007/s12603-020-1488-z

World Health Organization. (2021, April 13). *Non communicable diseases.* https://www.who.int/news-room/fact-sheets/detail/noncommunicable-diseases

Zidan, A., Awisu, A., El-Hajj, M. S., Al-Abdulla, S. A., Figueroa, D. C., & Kheir, N. (2018). Medication-related burden among patients with chronic disease conditions: Perspectives of patients attending non-communicable disease clinics in a primary healthcare setting in Qatar. *Pharmacy, 6*(3), 85. https://doi.org/10.3390/pharmacy6030085

Raghupathi, V., & Raghupathi, W. (2017). Preventive healthcare: A neural network analysis of behavioral habits and chronic diseases. *Healthcare*, 5(1), 8. https://doi.org/10.3390/healthcare5010008

[illegible]

[illegible]

[illegible]

[illegible]

[illegible]

Chapter 24
Ageing with Dignity Through Service-Learning—Hong Kong Experience

Ben Yuk Fai Fong, Tommy K. C. Ng, Hilary H. L. Yee, and Billie S. M. Chow

Abstract Service-learning is offered at universities with the aim to provide students an experiential learning pedagogy that integrates meaningful community service with academic study and reflections to enrich students' learning experience. The learning process will not only enhance students' sense of civic responsibility and engagement, but also benefit the community at large. It is learning through engagement in services by incorporating academic learning, service experience and reflection in learning, and demonstrating positive outcomes on personal development, including improved skills in critical thinking, problem solving, communication, enhanced sense of social responsibility and a deeper understanding of learning concept in the community. Service-learning in a health promotion subject will develop students' ability to apply principles and concepts of health behaviour from the classroom into a community setting, in which the collaboration with non-government organisations provides students the opportunity to engage in meaningful community service to the recipients, under the guidance of teachers and site staff. Students are expected to reflect critically on academic contents and civic engagement during service-learning. The most important objective of the health promotion subject is to instil in students a strong sense of empathy, social responsibility and professionalism. Results have indicated that students have learned different skills and overcome most of the challenges when communicating with the older adults. Through serving the elderly, students learn on how to promote health with dignity in a community setting through the application

B. Y. F. Fong · T. K. C. Ng (✉) · B. S. M. Chow
School of Professional Education and Executive Development, College of Professional and Continuing Education, The Hong Kong Polytechnic University, Kowloon, Hong Kong, China
e-mail: tommy.ng@cpce-polyu.edu.hk

B. Y. F. Fong
e-mail: byffong@gmail.com

B. S. M. Chow
e-mail: billie.chow@cpce-polyu.edu.hk

H. H. L. Yee
The Hong Kong Polytechnic University, Kowloon, Hong Kong, China
e-mail: hiulam.yee@polyu.edu.hk

V. T. S. Law and B. Y. F. Fong (eds.), *Ageing with Dignity in Hong Kong and Asia*, Quality of Life in Asia 16, https://doi.org/10.1007/978-981-19-3061-4_24

of principles and concepts of health behaviour to motivate older adults to adopt a healthy lifestyle and self-management of chronic conditions.

Keywords Service-learning · Social responsibility · Professionalism · Empathy

24.1 Introduction

Service-learning is the combination of academic learning and community service. It provides an opportunity for students to apply what they have learnt in the classroom to practical situation. This learning pedagogy integrates meaningful community service with academic study and reflections to enrich students' learning experience. Although service-learning is similar to volunteerism and internship, the emphasis of these learning approaches is completely different. In internship, service providers can obtain specific career-oriented skills and work experiences and, so the service providers will be the main beneficiary. In volunteerism, the primary concern is to provide service to the recipients at the volunteer's own free will. The main beneficiary is service recipients. In contrast, service providers and recipients will both have the benefits under service-learning, which focuses more on enhancing providers' theoretical knowledge in the community service experience (Salam et al., 2019; Sandaran, 2012). Service providers can have more reflection, preparation and active participation in the services, while recipients gain services from the providers.

Service-learning incorporates with four Rs, namely respect, reciprocity, relevance and reflection (Butin, 2010). Students should always respect the situation of service recipients no matter what the circumstances and outlook are. For reciprocity, mutual benefits to students and community will be gained from service-learning. Learning knowledge and insights from others, influenced by the participants and generating something new together are the reciprocity of service-learning (Asghar & Rowe, 2017). The relevance of academic learning between the community services is essential since students can get more involved in the community and the relevant engagement and participation of the community service. In addition, reflection is the necessary element of service-learning for students to make connections between theory learnt and service provided.

Service-learning integrates learning, reflection and community services but the adoption of service-learning in secondary and tertiary education is not common in Hong Kong. Several challenges may hesitate the implementation of service-learning in education. Time and resources allocation are among the main challenges of service-learning. Lecturers may consider that there is limited time to teach students while the course content remains the same (Speck, 2001). Since the teaching schedule to equip students with the requisite knowledge and skills for community service is tight, teachers need more time and resources to facilitate students' learning. Teachers may need to put greater effort to develop and adjust assessment measurement, and address experience difficulty among students (Stefaniak, 2015). Time constraints imposed by the academic semester is one of the key challenges in the implementation of service-learning. From the students' perspective, more time are needed to prepare the service content, compared with traditional learning (Whitley et al., 2017). Therefore, additional time is needed for both teachers and students to prepare for service-learning.

24.2 Service-Learning in Hong Kong

To promote social capital and interpersonal relationship, volunteering is commonly discussed instead of service-learning in Hong Kong. Since 1998, the Social Welfare Department (SWD) had launched a programme 'Volunteer Movement' to build up a caring community, utilising community resources to enhance the sense of social belonging and promoting volunteer service in a systematic and more effective manner in Hong Kong (Ma, 2018; Volunteer Movement, 2020). With the emphasis on volunteerism, the education system has adopted service-learning as an extracurricular activity and non-credit-bearing subject in higher education. The Chinese University of Hong Kong was the first university to adopt service-learning in Hong Kong since 1995 (Ma, 2018). In 2006, Lingnan University set up the first Office of Service-learning (Ma & Chan, 2013). Three different modes of service-learning were set up at Lingnan University, including community-based service-learning activities (non-credit-bearing courses), partially integrated course mode and fully integrated course mode (credit-bearing courses). 21% of students studying in Lingnan University joined service-learning programmes in 2012, and this was a 9% increase compared with the figures in 2007, showing that Lingnan University was offering more service-learning opportunities to the students (Ma & Chan, 2013). Apart from Lingnan University, other universities in Hong Kong, such as the Hong Kong Polytechnic University (PolyU), The University of Hong Kong, The Chinese University of Hong Kong and Education University of Hong Kong, set up units to promote and coordinate service-learning for undergraduate students.

Service-learning subjects become credit-bearing subject and a graduation requirement for undergraduate students in many universities. At The Hong Kong Polytechnic University, a 3-credit-bearing subject on service-learning has been compulsory for students of the 4-year university programme in order to be qualified for graduation since 2012 (Chan et al., 2019; Service-Learning & Leadership Office, 2020). All faculties and academic departments at PolyU can design service-learning subjects. The service-learning opportunity allows students to apply their multidisciplinary knowledge in different areas, levels and recipients, with services such as designing and developing assistive devices to handicapped students to use computers, designing a financial literacy package for youth in low-income families and constructing the assistive devices for the elderly and disabled (Service-Learning & Leadership Office, 2021). In the following section, the development of and experience in conducting intergenerational service-learning subjects at the School of Professional Education and Executive Development (SPEED) will be discussed.

24.3 School of Professional Education and Executive Development

The School of Professional Education and Executive Development offers self-financed undergraduate top-up degree programmes in the two-year full-time and four-year part-time modes. With the support from PolyU, SPEED had developed the first service-learning subject, which was age-related, for students since the 2016/2017 academic year (College of Professional & Continuing Education, 2018). In 2019, PolyU SPEED offered another intergenerational service-learning subject for students in the Bachelor of Science (Honours) in Applied Sciences (Health Studies) programme.

24.3.1 'Using Human-Centred Design to Work with the Elderly: A Memoir Project'

The first service-learning subject in SPEED was 'Using Human-Centered Design to Work with the Elderly: A Memoir Project', and it was running smoothly over the past semesters. This service-learning subject involved students and elderlies. The objectives of this subject consisted of raising students' awareness of the needs of the elderly, bringing satisfaction to the elderly by recapturing their lifetime stories and enhancing students' problem solving and communication skills. As students needed to design and produce a memoir book for the elderly in order to recapture their past experience and achievement, students were required to attend lectures to learn the basic knowledge and skills in design. Students had 40 h of contact with the older adults, who were recruited by the service partner (Sai Kung District Community Centre or Salvation Army), to build the trust relationship, collect information about recipient's lifetime story and produce the memoir book together with the elderly. Two reflective journals and an in-class discussion were conducted during and after the service-learning. Through this intergenerational experience, students did not only apply what they had learned and improved the communication skills with the elderly, but also understood the responsibility and role to provide care and concern to the older adults (Chan, 2020). During the review of recipient's life, students needed to communicate and listen well with the elderly to gather the most important and impressive stories. At the same time, the elderly could recall their memories, share their past experiences and express their feelings to the students through close communication. This subject had allowed students to step out of the campus and be engaged in the community.

24.3.2 *'Practices in Health Promotion'*

Another intergenerational service-learning subject developed at SPEED was 'Practices in Health Promotion', which was a compulsory subject for students studying in the Bachelor of Science in Applied Sciences (Health Studies) programme. This subject was introduced in 2019/2020, and it aimed to equip students with the knowledge of health promotion in different settings, and instil a strong sense of empathy, social responsibility and professionalism in students. It had been held for two consecutive years and the total number of students enrolled was 76. The taught part of this subject consisted of three three-hour weekly classroom contacts to discuss the concepts, knowledge and strategies of health promotion before students made direct contact with the target older adults and their caregivers.

Four groups of students in each year were sent to visit and provide services to the elderly assigned by the four community or neighbourhood centres for senior citizens operated by the service partner, Sik Sik Yuen, one of the largest local non-government organisations (NGOs) in Hong Kong. Students needed to promote health either through home visits or organising centre activities under the supervision of site supervisors. Students in one of the four groups paired up to serve mildly demented older adults under the Dementia Community Support Scheme, jointly launched by SWD and the Hospital Authority, and the other groups were arranged to serve older adults with chronic diseases. Home visits and centre activities helped to build relationships between students and the elderly. At the same time, general health knowledge, including nutrition, physical exercise and mental wellness, could be introduced to the older adults and their carers. Each visit and activity lasted for four hours every week for a total of ten weeks. The needs of the elderly were assessed by the students in order to determine the delivery of health topics, such as management of hypertension and diabetes, teaching of sitting Tai Chi, introduction and practice of mindfulness, etc. Site supervisors and centres staff provided suggestions to the students after each visit and activity as part of the learning process and to enhance the outcomes of the service delivery. Students submitted two reflective journals during and after the services in order to stimulate their reflection on the service-learning experience and personal gains from this community project.

For the groups conducting home visits, students communicated and discussed with the elderly for at least 45 min per visit. At the beginning of the field services, students encountered difficulties in communication with the elderly because they were not familiar with each other. Some older adults were conservative and not too willing to share with the students. However, the relationship was built, and the elderly became more open to talk with the students. Home visits allowed the students to know not only the health background of the elderlies but also their family and living environment. Most of the recruited older adults lived in the public housing alone or with their partner, and so the home visits were an eye-opening experience for the students. Furthermore, home safety issue and food storage were also directly assessed by the students on site.

Compared to home visits, the groups organising centre activities had a different approach. Students organised health talks on topics such as drug management, pain management and prevention of chronic diseases, and they also conducted exercise sessions at the centres. They demonstrated their skills and leadership in organising activities, in both of the individual-based and group-based approaches to achieve the core aims of health promotion.

The two reflective journals by each student showed positive learning outcomes, including communicating effectively with the elderly, reflecting the civic roles and social responsibilities, demonstrating empathy and organising health promotion activities. In addition, the intergenerational service-learning was an unforgettable learning experience because they could apply what they had learned from the classes in the real life situation (Fung & Fong, 2020; Yee et al., 2020). The services had also benefited the older adults as they received up-to-date health knowledge from the students and shared their precious life experience with the younger generation. This intergenerational service-learning subject is recognised by all teachers, students and centre staff to be a 'win–win' project for the students and the elderly, as well as Sik Sik Yuen and PolyU SPEED.

24.4 Effects of Service-Learning on Ageing

The worldwide life expectancy is increasing due to improved living conditions, advanced medical care and effective disease prevention programmes. However, ageing population and low fertility rate will result in increased spending on health-care and social services, decline in manpower and negative impact on economic growth (Howdon & Rice, 2018; Nagarajan et al., 2016). Government policy is the key factor to ease the impacts of ageing population and avoid deficiency in caring, because looking after older adults is a long-term and sustainability issue worldwide. To enhance the participation in healthcare and serving the elderly by the youth, education plays an important and pivotal role in offering students a practical chance to be better acquainted and connected with the elderly. As such, the effects of service-learning on students, as service providers, and older adults, as service recipients, will be reviewed in the following sections.

24.4.1 Students as Service Providers

Learning is the major and core component in service-learning and students are expected to gain knowledge and understanding regarding the learning outcomes and course contents through the participation in service-learning. Before the start of the services, students acquire relevant knowledge and skills in the classroom. This helps them to understand how to meet the needs of the recipients and allows students to prepare for the application of what they have learnt from the university to meet the needs of the older adults in the community (Tam, 2014). Intergenerational service-learning does not only result in the better understanding of ageing by the students but also their practical and direct learning from the elderly (Andreoletti & Howard, 2018; Tam, 2014). To nursing students participating in service-learning, they can learn about community health nursing skills and apply them through the real life experience with older adults (Gipson et al., 2020). Furthermore, their overall knowledge of ageing and understanding of mental health needs among older adults are significantly increased (Leung et al., 2012). In a study, students studying sport science thought intergenerational service-learning had facilitated their development of planning exercise programmes for older people (Ruiz-Montero et al., 2020). It showed that service-learning could provide practical experience for these students to apply the knowledge they have learnt to the elderly and achieved the learning objectives of the courses. Likewise, the experience shared by elderly can inspire and enlighten the students on issues of daily living, home environment, mental wellness, etc. that are not readily found in books.

Furthermore, communication skills with the elderly can be strengthened via service-learning. Young people may not have the chance to live or connect with older adults. The intergenerational service-learning provides an opportunity for students to contact directly with the elderly. The students are able to serve and communicate with them. Using eye contacts, talking louder and showing empathy are the skills learnt by the students in service-learning (Gipson et al., 2020; Yee et al., 2020). Although students may encounter difficulties in communicating with the elderly at the beginning of their encounter, their communication skills are improved and thus the challenges to interact with the elderly can be minimised. Service-learning give a great opportunity to students to actually apply the skills learned from formal lessons.

In addition, students are given the chance outside the campus to examine some social issues regarding ageing population in the community. Reflection is one of the components of service-learning, and it helps students to have a thorough thought on what they have encountered in the project. Students develop the awareness of social issues and civic responsibility (Mey et al., 2018). Through providing services to the elderly, students can clearly apprehend the situations of the elderly in the community, such as their loneliness, their living environment and decline in physiological functions. Likewise, students will reflect what they can do for the recipients and they may participate more in community services. Sense of social responsibility, community engagement and respect for others can be built and enhanced (Heo et al., 2014; Shek et al., 2019). Generally, adolescents are found to have misconceptions regarding older adults, possibly because of the lack of knowledge about ageing (Cherry et al., 2016). Such insufficiency is negatively correlated to the ageist attitudes and behaviours, including negative stereotypes and discrimination against the elderly. After the participation in intergenerational service-learning project, there is a significant decrease in the level of ageism among students (Santini et al., 2018; Yoelin, 2021). Their attitude towards the elderly would be shifted to positive (Andreoletti & Howard, 2018; Kalisch et al., 2013). Although some students have perceived older adults being difficult to communicate and lacking of interest in the outside world but they have found that older people are enjoyable to talk with and are really interesting people.

Through service-learning, students will have a positive youth development, which focuses on enhancing their strengths and establishing their potential for positive and healthy development, particularly in terms of psychosocial and mental health (Chung & McBride, 2015; Taylor et al., 2017). The positive youth development framework consists of five elements, including competence, confidence, connection, character and caring. Furthermore, by increasing the development in positive relationships, supports and environmental enhancement, young people can develop personal competencies, confidence and social skills. Therefore, service-learning enables students to consolidate their academic knowledge, interpersonal skills and problem solving ability. Likewise, students also develop fuller understanding of and empathy to the elderly (Roodin et al., 2013). These skills are essential for their future career development. Moreover, students can strive positive bonding with their classmates and teachers, and the recipients from the field experience, from which they also know the community organisations and their services to better prepare for their career options.

24.4.2 Older Adults as Service Recipients

Meeting the needs of older adults is vital for achieving a successful and meaningful service-learning course. Students will try to assess and understand the needs of the elderly and provide appropriate and suitable services to them. Multidisciplinary and multi-prone activities are conducted to entertain the different needs of the elderly. For example, students in engineering design and anthropology courses were required to understand the difficulties of livings among older adults, and thus custom-designed artefacts that aimed to resolve their problems were designed (Lynch et al., 2014). One of the artefacts was a cutting board that assisted the elderly with visual impairments to cook independently. Such engineered products could improve the quality of life of older adults. Similarly, reduction of risk of fall and improvement of living environment of older adults can be attained as a result of service-learning programmes (Hegeman et al., 2010). This is important for the elderly because the falls may lead to severe injuries or even death.

Psychological needs of elderly can be met and even improved through numerous communications and interactions in service-learning. Older adults are at higher risk of suffering from loneliness and social isolation, leading to anxiety, depression, cardiovascular disease, diminished sleep quality and even premature mortality (Domènech-Abella et al., 2019; Holt-Lunstad et al., 2015; Valtorta et al., 2018). Through intergenerational service-learning, they can feel connected to the community which contributes to their physical and emotional health, particularly for those living alone (Teater, 2016). They can also share past life experiences and express their recent feelings with students (Underwood & Dorfman, 2006). During the communication, the elderly can learn about the latest world development from the younger generation, such as understanding the use of technology. The service-learning encounters help to enhance emotional wellness of the elderly, deal with the stressful situation and build the bonding between the elderly and students (Segrist, 2004; Underwood & Dorfman, 2006). A study has found that the scores of depressive symptoms of the elderly were reduced after attending the programme (Hernandez & Gonzalez, 2008). Therefore, service-learning has a positive impact on the psychological health and social wellness of the participating elderly.

Intergenerational service-learning is often designed to meet the needs and improve the physical and psychological health of the elderly. To achieve ageing with dignity, supportive networks is one of the perceptions on supports to dignity among older adults (Black & Dobbs, 2014). Intergenerational service-learning can provide not only tangible supports but also intangible ones. Tangible supports include physical support. Family recognition and social supports are intangible supports. Through the participation in service-learning, elderly can broaden their social network. They share their own experiences and exchange different ideas with the students (Au Underwood & Dorfman, 2006; Yeung et al., 2019). Moreover, they also establish a relationship with the students (Tam, 2012). The older adults can expand their social life by meeting the students regularly. Participation in social encounters and recognition by others are core components for older adult to develop a true sense of dignity (Clancy et al., 2020). Sharing experiences with the students allows elderly to feel that they are valuable and being respected in the society. Generally speaking, intergenerational service-learning programmes can help to promote ageing with dignity. All schools and universities should take on this initiative in the education of the next generation for the wellness of the older adults.

24.4.3 Community Organisations

To arrange and organise service-learning, tertiary institutions need to communicate and partner with local community organisations, depending on the nature of the programme. Intergenerational service-learning involves older adults, and so the tertiary institutions have to work in close collaboration and partnership with community organisations that provide elderly care and services. This partnership can facilitate the knowledge and information exchange, improve service delivery and inject new impetus to community services (Roodin et al., 2013). Students' idea and creativity may bring new insights into the community organisations in addressing some social and health issues in the local community. Furthermore, service-learning provides an opportunity for students to be involved in community services, and the experience can bring inspiration for them to consider their future career in elderly care. Career direction is one of the students' expectation and gain from the participation in service-learning, which facilitates students to develop skills and interest for future careers because they get a better understanding of the types of works available in the community (McClam et al., 2008; Mitchell & Rost-Banik, 2019). Therefore, intergenerational service-learning provides an opportunity for students to know and understand the nature, operations and development of community elderly services.

Intergenerational service-learning can stimulate civic engagement, which aims to meet the needs of all those involved and improve the community. Both the students and older adults are the beneficiaries. Students can put what they learn into practice, such as promoting health to the elderly. Apart from practical learning, some intangible skills can be improved and beneficial to their future career pathway and life. The active participation in community services allows students to have better reflections on community involvement. For the older adults, they continue to be more involved in the community after the participation in the intergenerational service-learning because they can communicate and interact more with the community. Their contribution can strengthen their bonding to the community with an objective of ageing with dignity.

24.5 The Path Forward

Service-learning is adopted in the government funded universities in Hong Kong, and it is one of the graduation requirements for students in some universities. However, service-learning is not commonly found in self-financing tertiary institutions because it needs more time and resources to prepare and organise these subjects. Hence, to promote service-learning in self-financing tertiary institutions, financial and manpower supports are the main constraints. Moreover, intergenerational service-learning can be adopted in different programmes. In the short term, students and older adults can gain knowledge, obtain valuable experience and learn how to communicate between generations. The needs of the elderly, including both physical and mental wellness, can be met through the intergenerational service-learning. In the long run, promoting the awareness of social issues and civic responsibility of the students are important to the entire society. Likewise, service-learning provides an opportunity for students to explore the elderly care services and prepare them for future career development. To conclude, developing intergenerational service-learning in tertiary institutions is beneficial to students, older adults and the community, and facilitates the promotion of ageing with dignity in the society.

Acknowledgements The work described in this chapter was partially supported by a grant from the Research Grants Council of the Hong Kong Special Administrative Region, China (Project Reference No.: UGC/IDS24/18).

References

Andreoletti, C., & Howard, J. L. (2018). Bridging the generation gap: Intergenerational service-learning benefits young and old. *Gerontology & Geriatrics Education, 39*(1), 46–60. https://doi.org/10.1080/02701960.2016.1152266

Asghar, M., & Rowe, N. (2017). Reciprocity and critical reflection as the key to social justice in service learning: A case study. *Innovations in Education and Teaching International, 54*(2), 117–125. https://doi.org/10.1080/14703297.2016.1273788

Au Yeung, S. N. C., Lam, L. K., & Fong, J. J. (2019). How service-learning promotes intergenerational harmony: Case study of a service-learning project in a science course. *Metropolitan Universities, 30*(3), 20–35. https://doi.org/10.18060/23194

Black, K., & Dobbs, D. (2014). Community-dwelling older adults' perceptions of dignity: Core meanings, challenges, supports and opportunities. *Ageing & Society, 34*(8), 1292–1313. https://doi.org/10.1017/S0144686X13000020

Butin, D. (2010). Service-learning in theory and practice: The future of community engagement in higher education. *Springer*. https://doi.org/10.1057/9780230106154

Chan, P. (2020). Providing elderly care through Service-Learning: A case study and proposal to generate subject ideas in an effective manner. *Paper presented at the CPCE Health Conference 2020, Hong Kong*. http://healthconf2020.cpce-polyu.edu.hk/doc/F2.2020-01-13PatrickSharesServiceLearning.pdf

Chan, S. C., Ngai, G., & Shek, D. T. (2019). Service-learning as a mandatory credit-bearing subject at The Hong Kong Polytechnic University. *International Journal of Child and Adolescent Health, 12*(1), 19–32.

Cherry, K. E., Brigman, S., Lyon, B. A., Blanchard, B., Walker, E. J., & Smitherman, E. A. (2016). Self-reported ageism across the lifespan: Role of aging knowledge. *The International Journal of Aging and Human Development, 83*(4), 366–380. https://doi.org/10.1177/0091415016657562

Chung, S., & McBride, A. M. (2015). Social and emotional learning in middle school curricula: A service learning model based on positive youth development. *Children and Youth Services Review, 53*, 192–200. https://doi.org/10.1016/j.childyouth.2015.04.008

Clancy, A., Simonsen, N., Lind, J., Liveng, A., & Johannessen, A. (2020). The meaning of dignity for older adults: A meta-synthesis. *Nursing Ethics, 1–17*,. https://doi.org/10.1177/0969733020928134

College of Professional and Continuing Education. (2018). *Connecting SPEED Students and the Elderly through a Service-Learning Subject*. https://www.cpce-polyu.edu.hk/f/newsletter/1735/5401/CPCE_connect_2018_10th_03_P3-4.pdf

Domènech-Abella, J., Mundó, J., Haro, J. M., & Rubio-Valera, M. (2019). Anxiety, depression, loneliness and social network in the elderly: Longitudinal associations from The Irish longitudinal study on ageing (TILDA). *Journal of Affective Disorders, 246*, 82–88. https://doi.org/10.1016/j.jad.2018.12.043

Fung, R. C. H., & Fong, B. Y. F. (2020). Treasure in elderly care learning: A service-learning experience at a neghborhood centre in Hong Kong. *Asia Pacific Journal of Health Management, 15*(2), 5–10. https://doi.org/10.24083/apjhm.v15i2.405

Gipson, C. S., Delello, J. A., & McWhorter, R. R. (2020). Engaging nursing students and older adults through service-learning. *Working with Older People, 25*(1), 84–93. https://doi.org/10.1108/WWOP-10-2020-0053

Hegeman, C. R., Roodin, P., Gilliland, K. A., & Ó'Flathabháin, K. B. (2010). Intergenerational service learning: Linking three generations: Concept, history, and outcome assessment. *Gerontology & Geriatrics Education, 31*(1), 37–54. https://doi.org/10.1080/02701960903584418

Heo, J., King, C., Lee, J. W., Kim, H. M., & Ni, C. (2014). Learning from healthy older adults: An analysis of undergraduate students' reflective essays. *The Asia-Pacific Education Researcher, 23*(3), 537–545. https://doi.org/10.1007/s40299-013-0128-3

Hernandez, C. R., & Gonzalez, M. Z. (2008). Effects of intergenerational interaction on aging. *Educational Gerontology, 34*(4), 292–305. https://doi.org/10.1080/03601270701883908

Holt-Lunstad, J., Smith, T. B., Baker, M., Harris, T., & Stephenson, D. (2015). Loneliness and social isolation as risk factors for mortality: A meta-analytic review. *Perspectives on Psychological Science, 10*(2), 227–237. https://doi.org/10.1177/1745691614568352

Howdon, D., & Rice, N. (2018). Health care expenditures, age, proximity to death and morbidity: Implications for an ageing population. *Journal of Health Economics, 57*, 60–74. https://doi.org/10.1016/j.jhealeco.2017.11.001

Kalisch, H. R., Coughlin, D. R., Ballard, S. M., & Lamson, A. (2013). Old age is a part of living: Student reflections on intergenerational service-learning. *Gerontology & Geriatrics Education, 34*(1), 99–113. https://doi.org/10.1080/02701960.2012.753440

Leung, A. Y. M., Chan, S. S. C., Kwan, C. W., Cheung, M. K. T., Leung, S. S. K., & Fong, D. Y. T. (2012). Service learning in medical and nursing training: A randomized controlled trial. *Advances in Health Sciences Education, 17*(4), 529–545. https://doi.org/10.1007/s10459-011-9329-9

Lynch, C., Stein, L. A., Grimshaw, S., Doyle, E., Camberg, L., & Ben-Ur, E. (2014, October). The impacts of service learning on students and community members: Lessons from design projects for older adults. In *2014 IEEE frontiers in education conference (FIE) proceedings* (pp. 1–9). https://doi.org/10.1109/FIE.2014.7044320

Ma, C. (2018). Service-learning development in higher education in Hong Kong. In Lim, T. W. & Kong, T. Y. (Eds.) *Studying Hong Kong: 20 years of political, economic and social developments* (pp. 43–61). World Scientific Publishing. https://doi.org/10.1142/9789813223554_0004

Ma, C. H. K., & Chan, A. C. M. (2013). A Hong Kong university first: Establishing service-learning as an academic credit-bearing subject. *Gateways: International Journal of Community Research and Engagement, 6,* 178–198. https://doi.org/10.5130/ijcre.v6i1.3286

McClam, T., Diambra, J. F., Burton, B., Fuss, A., & Fudge, D. L. (2008). An analysis of a service-learning project: Students' expectations, concerns, and reflections. *Journal of Experiential Education, 30*(3), 236–249. https://doi.org/10.1177/105382590703000304

Mey, M., Werner, A., & de Villiers, B. (2018). Student experiences of service learning through a community outreach project. *Development in Practice, 28*(6), 764–774. https://doi.org/10.1080/09614524.2018.1473340

Mitchell, T. D., & Rost-Banik, C. (2019). How Sustained Service-Learning Experiences Inform Career Pathways. *Michigan Journal of Community Service Learning, 25*(1), 18–29. https://doi.org/10.3998/mjcsloa.3239521.0025.102

Nagarajan, N. R., Teixeira, A. A., & Silva, S. T. (2016). The impact of an ageing population on economic growth: An exploratory review of the main mechanisms. *Análise Social, 51*(218), 4–35.

Roodin, P., Brown, L. H., & Shedlock, D. (2013). Intergenerational service-learning: A review of recent literature and directions for the future. *Gerontology & Geriatrics Education, 34*(1), 3–25. https://doi.org/10.1080/02701960.2012.755624

Ruiz-Montero, P. J., Chiva-Bartoll, O., Salvador-García, C., & González-García, C. (2020). Learning with older adults through intergenerational service learning in physical education teacher education. *Sustainability, 12*(3), 1127. https://doi.org/10.3390/su12031127

Salam, M., Iskandar, D. N. A., Ibrahim, D. H. A., & Farooq, M. S. (2019). Service learning in higher education: A systematic literature review. *Asia Pacific Education Review, 20*(4), 573–593. https://doi.org/10.1007/s12564-019-09580-6

Sandaran, S. C. (2012). Service learning: Transforming students, communities and universities. *Procedia-Social and Behavioral Sciences, 66*, 380–390. https://doi.org/10.1016/j.sbspro.2012.11.281

Santini, S., Tombolesi, V., Baschiera, B., & Lamura, G. (2018). Intergenerational programs involving adolescents, institutionalized elderly, and older volunteers: Results from a pilot research-action in Italy. *BioMed Research International, 2018*,. https://doi.org/10.1155/2018/4360305

Segrist, K. (2004). Assessing impact of service-learning project on older, isolated adults in rural America. *Journal of Intergenerational Relationships, 2*(2), 51–66. https://doi.org/10.1300/J194v03n01_11

Service-Learning and Leadership Office. (2020). *Service-learning handbook*. https://www.polyu.edu.hk/osl/student/Student%20SL%20Handbook_Aug%202020.pdf

Service-Learning and Leadership Office. (2021). *Service-learning subjects on offer*. https://www.polyu.edu.hk/osl/index.php?option=com_content&view=article&id=141&Itemid=114#s1_2021

Shek, D. T. L., Ma, C. M. S., & Yang, Z. (2019). Transformation and development of university students through service-learning: A corporate-community-university partnership initiative in Hong Kong (Project WeCan). *Applied Research in Quality of Life, 15*, 1375–1393. https://doi.org/10.1007/s11482-019-09738-9

Speck, B. W. (2001). Why service-learning? *New Directions for Higher Education, 2001*(114), 3–13. https://doi.org/10.1002/he.8

Stefaniak, J. E. (2015). The implementation of service-learning in graduate instructional design coursework. *Journal of Computing in Higher Education, 27*(1), 2–9. https://doi.org/10.1007/s12528-015-9092-7

Tam, M. (2012). *Intergenerational learning through service with the elderly*. The Third Conference of the ESREA Network on Education and Learning of Older Adults.

Tam, M. (2014). Intergenerational service learning between the old and young: What, why and how. *Educational Gerontology, 40*(6), 401–413. https://doi.org/10.1080/03601277.2013.822201

Taylor, R. D., Oberle, E., Durlak, J. A., & Weissberg, R. P. (2017). Promoting positive youth development through school-based social and emotional learning interventions: A meta-analysis of follow-up effects. *Child Development, 88*(4), 1156–1171. https://doi.org/10.1111/cdev.12864

Teater, B. (2016). Intergenerational programs to promote active aging: The experiences and perspectives of older adults. *Activities, Adaptation & Aging, 40*(1), 1–19. https://doi.org/10.1080/01924788.2016.1127041

Underwood, H. L., & Dorfman, L. T. (2006). A view from the other side: Elders' reactions to intergenerational service-learning. *Journal of Intergenerational Relationships, 4*(2), 43–60. https://doi.org/10.1300/J194v04n02_04

Valtorta, N. K., Kanaan, M., Gilbody, S., & Hanratty, B. (2018). Loneliness, social isolation and risk of cardiovascular disease in the English longitudinal study of ageing. *European Journal of Preventive Cardiology, 25*(13), 1387–1396. https://doi.org/10.1177/2047487318792696

Volunteer Movement. (2020). *Background*. https://volunteermovement.hk/en/about-volunteer-movement

Whitley, M. A., Farrell, K., Maisonet, C., & Hoffer, A. (2017). Reflections on service-learning: Student experiences in a sport-based youth development course. *Journal of Physical Education, Recreation & Dance, 88*(7), 23–29. https://doi.org/10.1080/07303084.2017.1340202

Yee, H. H. L., Fong, B. Y. F., Ng, T. K. C., & Chow, B. S. M. (2020). Community ageing with health and dignity through a service-learning initiative. *Asia Pacific Journal of Health Management, 15*(2), 11–17. https://doi.org/10.24083/apjhm.v15i2.399

Yoelin, A. B. (2021). Intergenerational service learning within an aging course and its impact on undergraduate students' attitudes about aging. *Journal of Intergenerational Relationships, 1–16*,. https://doi.org/10.1080/15350770.2021.1881019

Chapter 25
Social Enterprises in Elderly Care

Vincent Tin Sing Law

Abstract Ageing population is a universal phenomenon which needs the combined efforts of the public, private and third sectors to tackle. Social enterprises are non-profit-making organisations which provide goods and services with a social mission to benefit the community. Social enterprises have been developing and provide a suitable model for the sustainable delivery of some public services, including health care. While social enterprises also strike to make a profit, profits will be reinvested to substantiate their social mission and to create positive social change. Hence, social enterprise is defined as a business with social objectives whose surplus is reinvested in the business or in the community, rather than maximising profit for shareholders and owners. Up to now, there are limited research on the impacts of social enterprises on the health and well-being of older people. Based on examples in Hong Kong, this chapter discusses the nature of social enterprises, their roles in the care and community services for older adults, and give recommendations on further enhancing the roles of social enterprises in the care for older adults.

Keywords Social enterprises · Care for older adults · Ageing with dignity · Community health workers

25.1 Introduction

From the public health perspectives, both the private and third sector can deploy public health interventions to tackle social determinants of health (Macaulay, Mazzei, et al., 2018; Suchowerska et al., 2020). For years, Macaulay (2016) views the third sector organisations have been filling the gap between the public and private sector regarding provision of social and health services. Social enterprises (SEs) are important providers of public services (Garnett et al., 2018), including services for the older adults. SEs have been rapidly growing and have become a global economic phenomenon (Leung et al., 2019), and their concept has been making significant

V. T. S. Law (✉)
School of Professional Education and Executive Development, College of Professional and Continuing Education, The Hong Kong Polytechnic University, Hong Kong, China
e-mail: vincent.law@cpce-polyu.edu.hk

V. T. S. Law and B. Y. F. Fong (eds.), *Ageing with Dignity in Hong Kong and Asia*, Quality of Life in Asia 16, https://doi.org/10.1007/978-981-19-3061-4_25

breakthroughs in Europe, the USA, Latin America and Eastern Asia (Defourny & Nyssens, 2008). However, SE is a contested concept (Teasdale, 2012), and there is no unified definition (Chan et al., 2011; Galera & Borzaga, 2009; Leung et al., 2019). One of the characteristics of SEs is the utilisation of business strategies which aims at improving social, economic and environmental well-being together with maximising social impact (Leung et al., 2019). SEs are expected to balance dual while competing objectives, i.e. create social value and achieve financial sustainability (Battilana et al., 2014; Galera & Borzaga, 2009). There is a continuum of SEs due to the variations in social and economic objectives (Stevens et al., 2015). With a clear and specific social mission, SEs can assist NGOs to achieve their social goals (Leung et al., 2019).

Due to change in demographic structure, the problem of accommodating the ageing society has received a lot of attention (Sakulkijkarn, 2020). Individual health outcomes are linked with socio-economic contexts. Researching older people is complicated since chronological age does not necessarily reflect the variation in individual ageing processes (Kotter-Grühn et al., 2016). Older people need more care since they are commonly regarded as a noticeable risk group for social isolation (Kelly et al., 2019b) due to the loss of friends and family members, reduced mobility, as well as poor physical health (Gardiner et al., 2018). Besides, older people residing in rural locations have higher chance of suffering from social isolation as compared to their counterparts in urban areas (Kelly et al., 2019b).

Ageing population is a universal phenomenon, and every government is endeavour to explore public policy to cope with it. Among various policies in the care for older adults, the establishment and utilisation of SEs is considered a viable solution. Well-being is located in the opportunities provided by society for social integration and participation (Baumgartner & Burns, 2013) which SEs play a vital role (Gordon et al., 2018). Governments are faced with the challenge of developing a just and fair caring system for older adults that is high quality, cost-effective, offers individual choices on care and its delivery and provides enriched quality of life (Jones, 2009). It is desirable to see SEs to serve as a business model of choice in caring for the older adults in order to deliver personalised, innovative and cost-effective care (Jones, 2009).

25.2 Dignity of Older Persons Who Need Care

Ageing is an unavoidable process for everyone since it is related to various molecular and cellular damages at the biological level (Steves et al., 2012). However, ageing brings changes to the physical body and associated functioning, affects self-efficacy of individuals and influences self-perceptions of ageing of the older persons (Tovel et al., 2019). The ageing older adults also face social and psychological situations. Weiss and Freund (2012) found that there are wide societal perceptions that the older people are incompetent with a lower social status. Older persons also face societal stigma and feel negative about the ageing process which lowers their social status and capability (Hatzenbuehler et al., 2013; Weiss & Freund, 2012). Besides, the older adults are also being stereotyped as resistant to change (Cuddy et al., 2005). Older persons become vulnerable to the negative self-perceptions as 'old' and thus reinforcing their negativity towards ageing (Shenkin et al., 2014). Older adults living in the rural areas cannot receive comprehensive long-term care service and thus face problems during ageing (Wang et al., 2021).

While dignity is important to the older adults (Woolhead et al., 2004), there is little consensus on how dignity can be achieved (Jacobson, 2007). To help the older adults to age with dignity, handling of health and social situations is not undignified for the older adults (Woolhead et al., 2004). In addition, services providers tend to view the elderly as a homogenous group and ignore individual variation in abilities and physical functioning (Henderson et al., 2019). Ultimately, the mental well-being of the older adults can be improved if they feel being valued and appreciated by others (Woolhead et al., 2004), including their caregivers and service providers. SEs provide care for the older adults and partly uphold dignity of the older adults via its designated services and social support.

25.3 Social Enterprises

25.3.1 Definitions of Social Enterprises

Social enterprise (SE) is a disputed concept (Teasdale, 2012), and there is no unified definition of a SE (Chan et al., 2011; Galera & Borzaga, 2009; Leung et al., 2019). Different people view the concept of SE differently since the concept evolves in accordance with specific environment (Defourny & Kim, 2011). Generally speaking, SEs involve an activity carried out by particular organisations (Galera & Borzaga, 2009), and they are not-for-profit organisations which provide goods and services based on a social mission that is beneficial to the community (Defourny & Nyssens, 2008).

Definition of a SE can focus on the social objective, market needs, and solutions provided. SEs are typically hybrid organisations with a social mission (Leung et al., 2019). From the perspective of social objectives, the Department of Trade and Industry (2002) of the United Kingdom defined a SE as an enterprise with social objectives whose profits are primarily reinvested in the business or in the community. Government views SEs as providing a unique portfolio of public-orientated services with a flexible business focus (Hall et al., 2015).

From the perspective of market needs, McKague and Harrison (2019) defined SEs as organisations that have built models to fulfil basic human needs unmet by the existing public and private sectors. Based on a need and problem approach, Social Enterprise Alliance (2021) defined a SE as an organisation that addresses a basic unmet need or solve a social or environmental problem via a market-driven method. Garnett et al. (2018) defined SEs as ventures driven by social missions that use social innovation to solve social problems (Garnett et al., 2018).

25.3.2 Nature of Social Enterprises

SEs generally have dual aims of maximising financial objective and creating social value (Cornforth, 2014). In terms of profit, SEs do not aim at maximising profit for shareholders and owners but reinvest their profits to the business to advance their social mission (Galera & Borzaga, 2009; Jones, 2009; Leung et al., 2019). For example, SEs in the United States are non-profit organisations that generate revenue and exploit business opportunities (Kerlin, 2006) while their counterparts in Europe focus on fostering social value (Defourny & Nyssens, 2010). In terms of community connection, SEs are featured to have strong connection with the community and service users (Jones, 2009). SEs frequently act at the local level to alleviate the pressing social problems with the most vulnerable people in the society, including the older adults (Roy & Hackett, 2017).

Unlike their private counterparts, SEs are managed in an entrepreneurial manner while their managerial activities touch on general interests (Galera & Borzaga, 2009). SEs can use entrepreneurial spirit and market-oriented strategies to attain social objectives (Kerlin, 2013). SEs are more flexible (Caló et al., 2019; Kelly et al., 2019b) as compared with the private and public providers because they can form partnerships with various organisations (Henderson et al., 2019) which include local authorities, private businesses, other SEs, as well as other third sector organisations (Jones, 2009). SEs can provide tailor-made solutions and are more responsive and proactive as compared with their public and private counterparts (Garnett et al., 2018; Jones, 2009; Kelly et al., 2019b).

SEs are comparatively creative and provide niche responsiveness to changing demands (Garnett et al., 2018; Jones, 2009). In terms of scope of services, SEs can provide broader and more unique services as compare with government departments or units. While many SEs tend to heavily depend on funding from government or donation in the startup stage (Luke, 2016), with more innovative and holistic approaches, SEs can provide better service if they adopt a commercial approach when negotiating contracts and perform strategic business planning (Jones, 2009).

25.3.3 Benefits of Social Enterprises to Population

SEs play vital roles in the society since they can handle a variety of social, economic and environmental issues and touch on various economic facets (Defourny & Nyssens, 2008). However, the overarching goal of SEs is to solve social issues through business profits, but the role varies considerably with countries (Agarwal et al., 2018). Evaluation of the impact of social enterprises face challenges such as different actors in partnership may have different priorities in outcomes, limited comparable data on outcomes, as well as the benefits of engaging a SE may take longer time to observe (Macaulay, Mazzei, et al., 2018; Munoz et al., 2015).

In many countries, SEs have been gaining governmental recognition as a channel of offering public services to meet changing needs (Teasdale, 2012) because SEs give multiple benefits to the society. SEs lead to improved self-reliance and self-esteem by enhancing skills and employability (Roy et al., 2014), reduce stigmitisation of the marginalised groups (Roy et al., 2014) including the older adults, facilitate interactions families with communities, cultivate feelings of engagement, improve feeling of social support, and enhance sense of self-worth (Caló et al., 2019), absorb disconnected people via social reconnection (Caló et al., 2019), as well as casting positive impacts on social determinants of health at both individual and community levels (Gordon et al., 2018).

25.4 Social Enterprises, Health Outcomes and Care for Older Adults

There is relatively little empirical research concerning SEs in health (Borzaga & Fazzi, 2014; Roy et al., 2014) while only limited studies have used specific outcome measures related to health to gauze the health effects of SEs (Milton et al., 2015). Scholars have been attempting to close the gap in knowing how activities conducted by SEs impact on health and well-being. For example, Roy et al. (2014) found that activities led by SEs can contribute to overall health and well-being by promoting mental health, self-reliance and health behaviours. Besides, Farmer et al. (2016) depict an emergent concept that SEs can serve as 'spaces of well-being' and have growing role in public health (Garnett et al., 2018; Roy et al., 2014). Based on thematic qualitative analysis in the United Kingdom, Henderson et al. (2019) found the antecedences, namely downward social comparison and social identity, that impact SE activities on the health and well-being of informants aged over 50.

25.4.1 Well-Being at Individual/Community Level

SEs are related to health in terms of improving well-being of its clients at the individual or community level, improve the social determinants of health and improve the quality of health care services. First, at individual level, Caló et al. (2018), through a systematic review method, found that SEs may improve health outcomes particularly mental health and well-being of clients being served. Activities of the SEs can generate health and well-being benefits to the community (Kelly et al., 2019b) and reach many communities (Jones, 2009). Besides, assessment of the SEs led to a substantial improvement in well-being (Sakulkijkarn, 2020). In view of the various forms of SEs, the impacts of SEs on health and well-being vary and cast a need to understand how they enhance health of the population (Roy et al., 2014).

25.4.2 *Social Determinants of Health*

From a public administration perspective, government is the formulator and implementor of health care policy and it should understand and address various social determinants of health for societal benefits (Roy et al., 2017). Health-related SEs are normally managed so that improvement to the business and improvement to health outcomes come together (McKague & Harrison, 2019). SEs can leverage the concern in the broader and 'upstream' factors of health for innovative programmes for specific client groups such as mentally ill persons and the older adults (Garnett et al., 2018). SEs can enhance individual and community health by facilitating employment, developing social networks, improve social and environmental environments of the community, improve physical and mental health of citizens (Macaulay, Roy, et al., 2018), as well as help building up social capital and improve health behaviours (Roy et al., 2014). From a broader social perspective, as a peer support and knowledge exchange between co-workers, self-help among the elder offer good support (Sakulkijkarn, 2020).

25.4.3 *Quality of Health Services*

At the social or population level, citizens' involvement in SEs is itself a health intervention instead of a way of service provision (Garnett et al., 2018). Small-scale SEs can address upstream health improvement goals by responding to public health needs innovatively although they may not have the necessary skills or variety of services to win in tender competition (Garnett et al., 2018). SEs have become desired vehicles for delivering various public services particularly related to health (Agarwal et al., 2018) and social care (Roy et al., 2017). According to a UK case study (Garnett et al., 2018), SEs emerge as significant publicly funded providers of health improvement services. SEs can create new health care markets, catalyse new entrepreneurs, create new job opportunities and help customers at the bottom of society (Agarwal et al., 2018). Through standardisation of health care service, SEs can improve transparency and upgrade quality standards of health care services (Agarwal et al., 2018).

To facilitate positive health and well-being outcomes for the older adults (Kelly et al., 2019a), SEs need to organise their activities flexibly for the older adults to cater for the diverse and evolving cohorts (Perissinotto & Covinsky, 2014). SEs provide access to social care, improve social connectedness of target groups, reduce social isolation of marginalised older people (Henderson et al., 2019), as well as giving positive psychological outcomes associated with self-efficacy, self-stigma and confidence (Villotti et al., 2018).

25.5 Social Enterprises and Care for Older Adults in Hong Kong

In Hong Kong, the development of social enterprises has been closely related to the institutional changes, which have significantly affected the operational efficiency of SE programmes initiated by non-profitmaking organisations (NPOs) (Chan et al., 2011). The typical social mission of SEs in Hong Kong is to create employment and provides job-related training opportunities to the concerned target groups. Some SEs provide the community with services that cater for unmet social demands (Chan et al., 2011).

Social enterprises in Hong Kong get funding either from the government, non-profit organisations or the private sector. Among various funding schemes, the government-funding schemes for SEs aim at achieving specific social mission such as self-reliance of the socially disadvantaged via employment initiatives. The major government funding schemes are the *Enhancing Self-Reliance through District Partnership Programme* is funded by the Home Affairs Department of the government of the Hong Kong Special Administrative Region (HKSARG), the *Enhancing Employment of People with Disabilities through Small Enterprise* is funded by the Social Welfare Department of the HKSARG, and the *Social Innovation and Entrepreneurship Development Fund* is funded by the Innovation and Technology Bureau of the HKSAR government.

In Hong Kong, SEs which provide care for the older adults offer 24-h call service, one-stop advice on selecting elderly homes, improvement of accessibility of residences and promotion of active ageing as separately highlighted below.

25.5.1 24/7 Call Service

In Hong Kong, there are various SEs that offer niche care for the older adults. For example, the Senior Citizen Home Safety Association (SCHSA) was established in 1996 as a non-profit charitable organisation in Hong Kong (SCHSA, 2021). SCHSA provides Care-on-Call Service, a comprehensive 24/7 support service, which consists of emergency aid, integrated care, around-the-clock monitoring service, health management, active ageing services and day-to-day living support. Leveraging technology and innovation, the SCHSA provides people-centred services to the service users of older adults so that they can age in place with a quality life. The SCHSA also provides enrichment services to cope with the changes and needs of the older adults and their caregivers at different stages of life by initiatives such as organising digital innovation and technology workshops, to enrich the knowledge and skills of the older adults in technology, organising caregiver workshops and domestic helper caregivers workshops to provide in-place and considerate services, as well as online brain health training to cater for the needs of the older adults and carers.

25.5.2 *One-Stop Advises on Selecting Elderly Homes*

To fulfil its social responsibility of encouraging the older adults to live a joyful life when they get old, the LifeDB Limited in Hong Kong provides services in elderly home placement so as to help families to identify appropriate elderly home for their loved ones at an old age (LifeDB, 2021). With its strong social mission in mind and support by both private and NGO partners, the LifeDB provides comprehensive services on choosing elderly homes but does not charge any service fees.

25.5.3 *Improvement of Accessibility of Residences*

With a mission to assist the older adults and people with physical disabilities, Longevity Design House (LDH) in Hong Kong was a SE established in 2015. LDH helps the elderly, regardless of their financial background, to renovate their residences to improve home safety and accessibility. Other than renovation, LDH also offer additional services such as provision of temporary accommodation during home renovation, application for government older adults grants for eligible older adults, and even occupational therapist support. With social innovation in mind, LDH helps the older adults to age at home so as to support the grand goal of Hong Kong to become a smarter ageing city.

25.5.4 *Promotion of Active Ageing*

Operating under Upper Fusion Company Limited under the Hong Kong Council of Social Service (HKCSS), we60.com is a web portal for people approaching retirement age and beyond. This portal provides comprehensive information on how to build a healthy and quality later life especially for carers who care about older adults at home.

25.6 Recommendations

Based on qualitative analysis of interview data, Sakulkijkarn (2020) found that the critical factors that affect the role of SE for older adults include supportive environment, self-determining, rebuilding connections, and job enrichment. To strengthen the role of SEs in the care for older adults, the following recommendations were made.

25.6.1 Holistic Public Policy with Stakeholder Support

From the government perspective, public policy renders the entrepreneurial approaches more popular by supporting the setting up of SEs and community interest firms (HM Treasury, 2007). Woolhead et al. (2004) founded that policy documents are important in stressing the significance of dignity for older people. With a supportive SE policy environment (Steiner & Teasdale, 2017), the potential of SEs to deliver health care service provision in caring for the ageing population would be leveraged. Government should review its policy in long-term care (LTC) so as to assist businesses, including SEs, to offer economic incentives which serve the marginalised older adults or those residing in remote areas (Wang et al., 2021).

In improving the services of SEs to the elderly, government needs the support of both service providers and community organisations. Government should promote policy that community health promotion organisations can be transformed to SEs which generate income without government funding (Zasada, 2017). Besides, the public, private and third sectors should cooperate closely and develop partnerships in the welfare business (Wong & Tang, 2006). From the perspective of the service provider, SEs should use government subsidy effectively and simultaneously devise diversified business strategies to maximise resources utilisation (Wang et al., 2021) to meet ever-increasing needs of long-term care by the elderly.

25.6.2 Enhanced Social and Family Support

Although mixed outcomes may be generated when establishing supportive social groups regardless of age, gender or chronic health issues (Masi et al., 2011), the older adults need social support and gain their own social identity so that they can age with dignity. On one hand, the SEs should provide the older adults with supportive environments, facilitate the creation of self-help groups among the elderly and promote self-determination among the older adult clients (Sakulkijkarn, 2020). In addition, all older adults in SEs must be evaluated yearly as part of the service standard (Sakulkijkarn, 2020). Such individualised service treats each older person as a separate identity and the latter value their own dignity.

Since social identity is a beneficial factor which can improve health and well-being of older people (Gleibs et al., 2011; Haslam et al., 2014), family support is equally important for the older adults (Wang et al., 2021). Regarding the care of dependent elderly, training quality of practitioners working in long-term institutions for the older adults has been a concern (Trombeta et al., 2020). Both organisational training and individual training for SEs are vital to the success of delivering social and family support. SEs as institutions and their staff should be trained on the care for older adults to serve the their needs better (Sakulkijkarn, 2020).

25.6.3 *Improving Governance and Financial Sustainability of Social Enterprises*

Based on Hong Kong's experience, SEs in the care for older adults provide a wide range of services for the older adults. However, SEs also need to fulfil its financial objectives before they can substantiate their social missions. As depicted by Spear et al. (2007), SEs need suitable governance to thrive and be sustainable since sustainable SEs are the same to those profitmaking businesses in terms of adopting the best practices to serve clients (Leung et al., 2019). SEs need to establish an oversight or advisory committee to improve their business planning and financial management (Leung et al., 2019). SEs can deploy a problem-solving behaviour to structure and bundle resources (Bacq et al., 2015). In this regard, the government can subsidy the SEs in the care for older adults with suitable schemes while the private sector can subsidy the SEs from the perspectives of corporate social responsibility.

25.6.4 *Social Innovation in Care for Older Adults*

There is growing interest in social innovation (Ziegler, 2017). Social entrepreneurship has non-economic positioning and involves activists and visionary individuals, and it is perceived as a social innovation (Howaldt & Schwarz, 2016; Lisetchi & Brancu, 2014). Social entrepreneurs should employ more strategic thinking by developing the older adults to serve as a strategic partner in their company's mission (Sakulkijkarn, 2020). At the community level, community-based SEs can serve as a viable way for service innovation, cultural change and cultivation of social capital (Caló et al., 2019) whereas the older adults being cared of can serve as a social capital.

25.6.5 *Community Health Workers (CHWs) as Vital Workforce*

With the global trend has shifted back to community health workers (CHWs) programmes (Schneider et al., 2016), the potential of utilising CHWs to fill gaps in health coverage has been improving. CHWs help achieve the sustainable development goals (SDGs) to reach the remote and marginalised communities in developing countries (Schaaf et al., 2018). Based on regaining of interest in CHWs, NGOs and SEs are now interested in the deployment of CHWs in their services (McKague & Harrison, 2019). In this regard, SEs can expand its employment of CHWs to provide care for the older adults at the community level.

25.7 Conclusions

Ageing population is a universal phenomenon and every government needs to formulate public policy to cope with it. Seriously affected by various factors related to ageing, older adults are regarded as a risk group for social isolation, they need more care and individualised care. To help the older adults to age with dignity, services for the older adults should not simply adopt a one-size-fits-all approach and ignore the diversity of the older adults and individual capabilities. Well-being of the older adults partly rest on the provision of opportunities for social integration and participation by various sectors of the society whereas the third sector play a vital role.

SEs are not-for-profit organisations which provide goods and services with a social mission. Although SEs need to meet dual objectives of creating social value and achieving financial sustainability, they are considered suitable vehicles to improve well-being of the older adults in the economic, social and environmental perspectives. SEs can serve as a business model of caring the older adults by delivering individualised, cost-effective, and innovative care. SEs in elderly care can promote well-being of the older adults at both individual and community levels, address social determinants of health so as to uphold health of the older adults and help enhancing the quality of care services for them.

To further strengthen the role of SEs in the care for older adults, government should formulate and implement holistic public policy for older adult care with the support by SEs. At the service level, SEs should strike to enhance social and family support for the older adults, ideally with initiatives with social innovation. Finally, SEs can consider further utilise community health workers (CHWs) and a vital workforce for the care for older adults at the community level.

References

Agarwal, N., Chakrabarti, R., Brem, A., & Bocken, N. (2018). Market driving at Bottom of the Pyramid (BoP): An analysis of social enterprises from the healthcare sector. *Journal of Business Research, 86*, 234–244. https://doi.org/10.1016/j.jbusres.2017.07.001

Bacq, S., Ofstein, L. F., Kickul, J. R., & Gundry, L. K. (2015). Bricolage in Social Entrepreneurship: How creative resource mobilization fosters greater social impact. *The International Journal of Entrepreneurship and Innovation, 16*(4), 283–289. https://doi.org/10.5367/ijei.2015.0198

Battilana, J., Sengul, M., Pache, A., & Model, J. (2014). Harnessing productive tensions in hybrid organizations: The case of work integration social enterprises. *Academy of Management Journal, 58*(6), 1658–1685. https://doi.org/10.5465/amj.2013.0903

Baumgartner, J., & Burns, J. (2013). Measuring social inclusion—a key outcome in global mental health. *International Journal of Epidemiology, 43*(2), 354–364. https://doi.org/10.1093/ije/dyt224

Borzaga, C., & Fazzi, L. (2014). Civil society, third sector, and healthcare: The case of social cooperatives in Italy. *Social Science & Medicine, 123*, 234–241. https://doi.org/10.1016/j.socscimed.2014.10.001

Caló, F., & Roy, M. J., Donaldson, C., Teasdale, S., & Baglioni, S. (2019). Exploring the contribution of social enterprise to health and social care: A realist evaluation. *Social Science & Medicine, 222*(C), 154–161. https://doi.org/10.1016/j.socscimed.2019.01.007

Caló, F., Teasdale, S., Donaldson, C., Roy, M. J., & Baglioni, S. (2018). Collaborator or competitor: Assessing the evidence supporting the role of social enterprise in health and social care. *Public Management Review, 20*(12), 1790–1814. https://doi.org/10.1080/14719037.2017.1417467

Chan, K. T., Kuan, T. T., & Wang, S. T. (2011). Similarities and divergences: Comparison of social enterprises in Hong Kong and Taiwan. *Social Enterprise Journal, 7*(1), 33–49. https://doi.org/10.1108/17508611111130149

Cornforth, C. (2014). Understanding and combating mission drift in social enterprises. *Social Enterprise Journal, 10*(1), 3–20. https://doi.org/10.1108/SEJ-09-2013-0036

Cuddy, A. J., Norton, M. I., & Fiske, S. T. (2005). This old stereotype: The pervasiveness and persistence of the elderly stereotype. *Journal of Social Issues, 61*, 267–285. https://doi.org/10.1111/j.1540-4560.2005.00405.x

Defourny, J., & Kim, S. Y. (2011). Emerging models of social enterprise in Eastern Asia: A cross-country analysis. *Social Enterprise Journal, 7*(1), 86–111. https://doi.org/10.1108/17508611111130176

Defourny, J., & Nyssens, M. (2008). Social enterprise in Europe: Recent trends and developments. *Social Enterprise Journal, 4*(3), 202–228. https://doi.org/10.1108/17508610810922703

Defourny, J., & Nyssens, M. (2010). Conceptions of Social Enterprise and Social Entrepreneurship in Europe and the United States: Convergences and divergences. *Journal of Social Entrepreneurship, 1*, 32–53. https://doi.org/10.1080/19420670903442053

Department for Trade and Industry, United Kingdom. (2003). *Social enterprise: A strategy for success.* Department for Trade and Industry.

Farmer, J., De Cotta, T., McKinnon, K., Barraket, J., Munoz, S.-A., Douglas, H., & Roy, M. J. (2016). Social enterprise and wellbeing in community life. *Social Enterprise Journal, 12*(2), 235–254. https://doi.org/10.1108/SEJ-05-2016-0017

Galera, G., & Borzaga, C. (2009). Social enterprise: An international overview of its conceptual evolution and legal implementation. *Social Enterprise Journal, 5*(3), 210–228. https://doi.org/10.1108/17508610911004313

Gardiner, C., Geldenhuys, G., & Gott, M. (2018). Interventions to reduce social isolation and loneliness among older people: An integrative review. *Health & Social Care in the Community, 26*(2), 147–157. https://doi.org/10.1111/hsc.12367

Garnett, E., Baeza, J., Trenholm, S., Gulliford, M., & Green, J. (2018). Social enterprises and public health improvement in England: A qualitative case study. *Public Health, 161*, 99–105. https://doi.org/10.1016/j.puhe.2018.04.019

Gleibs, I. H., Haslam, C., Jones, J. M., Haslam, S. A., McNeil, J., & Connolly, H. (2011). No country for old men? The role of a Gentlemen's Club in promoting social engagement and psychological well-being in residential care. *Aging & Mental Health, 15*(4), 456–466. https://doi.org/10.1080/13607863.2010.536137

Gordon, K., Wilson, J., Tonner, A., & Shaw, E. (2018). How can social enterprises impact health and well-being? *International Journal of Entrepreneurial Behavior & Research, 24*(3), 697–713. https://doi.org/10.1108/IJEBR-01-2017-0022

Hall, K., Miller, R., & Millar, R. (2015). Public, private or neither? Analysing the publicness of health care social enterprises. *Public Management Review, 18*(4), 539–557. https://doi.org/10.1080/14719037.2015.1014398

Haslam, C., Cruwys, T., & Haslam, S. A. (2014). "The we's have it": Evidence for the distinctive benefits of group engagement in enhancing cognitive health in aging. *Social Science & Medicine, 120*, 57–66. https://doi.org/10.1016/j.socscimed.2014.08.037

Hatzenbuehler, M. L., Phelan, J. C., & Link, B. G. (2013). Stigma as a fundamental cause of population health inequalities. *American Journal of Public Health, 103*(5), 813–821. https://doi.org/10.2105/AJPH.2012.301069

Henderson, F., Hall, K., Mutongi, A., & Whittam, G. (2019). Social enterprise, social innovation and self-directed care: Lessons from Scotland. *Social Enterprise Journal, 15*(4), 438–456. https://doi.org/10.1108/SEJ-12-2018-0080

HM Treasury (2007). *The future role of the third sector in social and economic regeneration* (Final Report). HM Treasury and Cabinet Office. https://assets.publishing.service.gov.uk/government/uploads/system/uploads/attachment_data/file/228900/7189.pdf

Howaldt, J., & Schwarz, M. (2016). *Social innovation and its relationship to social change. Verifying existing social theories in reference to social innovation and its relationship to social change (project: SI-DRIVE).* https://www.si-drive.eu/wp-content/uploads/2016/07/SI-DRIVE-D1-3-Social-Change-final-260416-2.pdf

Jacobson, N. (2007). Dignity and health: A review. *Social Science & Medicine, 64*(2), 292–302. https://doi.org/10.1016/j.socscimed.2006.08.039

Jones, C. (2009). How social enterprises can make a difference in caring for older people. *Working with Older People, 13*(2), 13–16. https://doi.org/10.1108/13663666200900024

Kelly, D., Steiner, A., Mason, H., & Teasdale, S. (2019a). Men's Sheds: A conceptual exploration of the causal pathways for health and well-being. *Health & Social Care in the Community, 27*(5), 1147–1157. https://doi.org/10.1111/hsc.12765

Kelly, D., Steiner, A., Mazzei, M., & Baker, R. (2019b). Filling a void? The role of social enterprise in addressing social isolation and loneliness in rural communities. *Journal of Rural Studies, 70*, 225–236. https://doi.org/10.1016/j.jrurstud.2019.01.024

Kerlin, J. A. (2006). Social Enterprises in the United States and Europe: Understanding and learning from the differences. *Voluntas: International Journal of Voluntary and Nonprofit Organizations, 17*, 247–263. https://doi.org/10.1007/s11266-006-9016-2

Kerlin, J. A. (2013). Defining social enterprise across different contexts: A conceptual framework based on institutional factors. *Nonprofit and Voluntary Sector Quarterly, 42*(1), 84–108. https://doi.org/10.1177/0899764011433040

Kotter-Grühn, D., Kornadt, A. E., & Stephan, Y. (2016). Looking beyond chronological age: Current knowledge and future directions in the study of subjective age. *Gerontology, 62*(1), 86–93. https://doi.org/10.1159/000438671

Leung, S., Mo, P., Ling, H., Chandra, Y., & Ho, S. S. (2019). Enhancing the competitiveness and sustainability of social enterprises in Hong Kong: A three-dimensional analysis. *China Journal of Accounting Research, 12*(2), 157–176. https://doi.org/10.1016/j.cjar.2019.03.002

LifeDB. (2021). *About us* (content in Chinese). https://www.elderlydb.hk/%e9%97%9c%e6%96%bc%e6%a8%82%e6%b4%bb%e6%98%93/

Lisetchi, M., & Brancu, L. (2014). The entrepreneurship concept as a subject of social innovation. *Procedia—Social and Behavioral Sciences, 124*, 87–92. https://doi.org/10.1016/j.sbspro.2014.02.463

Longevity Design House. (2021). *About us.* https://www.longevitygroup.net/about

Luke, B. (2016). Measuring and reporting on social performance: From numbers and narratives to a useful reporting framework for social enterprises. *Social and Environmental Accountability Journal, 36*(2), 103–123. https://doi.org/10.1080/0969160X.2015.1103298

Macaulay, B. (2016). Considering social enterprise involvement in the commissioning of health services in Shetland. *Local Economy, 31*(5), 650–659. https://doi.org/10.1177/0269094216655405

Macaulay, B., Mazzei, M., Roy, M. J., Teasdale, S., & Donaldson, C. (2018a). Differentiating the effect of social enterprise activities on health. *Social Science & Medicine, 200*, 211–217. https://doi.org/10.1016/j.socscimed.2018.01.042

Macaulay, B., Roy, M. J., Donaldson, C., Teasdale, S., & Kay, A. (2018b). Conceptualizing the health and well-being impacts of social enterprise: A UK-based study. *Health Promotion International, 33*(5), 748–759. https://doi.org/10.1093/heapro/dax009

Masi, C. M., Chen, H. Y., Hawkley, L. C., & Cacioppo, J. T. (2011). A meta-analysis of interventions to reduce loneliness. *Personality and Social Psychology Review, 15*(3), 219–266. https://doi.org/10.1177/1088868310377394

McKague, K., & Harrison, S. (2019). Gender and health social enterprises in Africa: A research agenda. *Internal Journal for Equity in Health, 18*, 95. https://doi.org/10.1186/s12939-019-0994-2

Milton, A., Parsons, N., Morant, N., Gilbert, E., Johnson, S., Fisher, A., Singh, S., Cunliffe, D., & Marwaha, S. (2015). The clinical profile of employees with mental health problems working in social firms in the UK. *Journal of Mental Health, 24*(4), 242–248. https://doi.org/10.3109/09638237.2015.1057324

Munoz, S. A., Farmer, J., Winterton, R., & Barraket, J. (2015). The social enterprise as a space of well-being: An exploratory case study. *Social Enterprise Journal, 11*(3), 281–302. https://doi.org/10.1108/SEJ-11-2014-0041

Perissinotto, C. M., & Covinsky, K. E. (2014). Living alone, socially isolated or lonely—What are we measuring? *Journal of General Internal Medicine, 29*(11), 1429–1431. https://doi.org/10.1007/s11606-014-2977-8

Roy, M. J., & Hackett, M. T. (2017). Polanyi's 'substantive approach' to the economy in action? Conceptualising social enterprise as a public health 'intervention.' *Review of Social Economy, 75*(2), 89–111. https://doi.org/10.1080/00346764.2016.1171383

Roy, M. J., Baker, R., & Kerr, S. (2017). Conceptualising the public health role of actors operating outside of formal health systems: The case of social enterprise. *Social Science & Medicine, 172*, 144–152. https://doi.org/10.1016/j.socscimed.2016.11.009

Roy, M. J., Donaldson, C., Baker, R., & Kerr, S. (2014). The potential of social enterprise to enhance health and well-being: A model and systematic review. *Social Science and Medicine, 123*, 182–193. https://doi.org/10.1016/j.socscimed.2014.07.031

Sakulkijkarn, W. (2020). The Role of social enterprise in providing employment for the elderly in Thailand. *Journal of Humanities and Social Science, 13*(25), 2564.

Schaaf, M., Fox, J., Topp, S. M., Warthin, C., Freedman, L. P., Robinson, R. S., Thiagarajan, S., Scott, K., Maboe, T., Zanchetta, M., Ruano, A. L., Kok, M., & Closser, S. (2018). Community health workers and accountability: Reflections from an international "think-in". *International Journal for Equity in Health, 17*(1), 66. https://doi.org/10.1186/s12939-018-0781-5

Schneider, H., Okello, D., & Lehmann, U. (2016). The global pendulum swing towards community health workers in low- and middle-income countries: A scoping review of trends, geographical distribution and programmatic orientations, 2005 to 2014. *Human Resources for Health, 14*, 65. https://doi.org/10.1186/s12960-016-0163-2

Senior Citizen Home Safety Association (SCHSA). (2021). *About us*. https://www.schsa.org.hk/en/introduction/aim/index.html

Shenkin, S. D., Laidlaw, K., Allerhand, M., Mead, G. E., Starr, J. M., & Deary, I. J. (2014). Life course influences of physical and cognitive function and personality on attitudes to aging in the Lothian birth cohort 1936. *International Psychogeriatrics, 26*, 1417–1430. https://doi.org/10.1017/S1041610214000301

Social Enterprise Alliance. (2021). *What is social enterprise?* https://socialenterprise.us/%20about/social-enterprise/

Spear, R., Cornforth, C., & Aiken, M. (2007). *For love and money: Governance and social enterprises*. National Council for Voluntary Organizations, UK. http://oro.open.ac.uk/10328/

Steiner, A., & Teasdale, S. (2017). Unlocking the potential of rural social enterprise. *Journal of Rural Studies, 70*, 144–154. https://doi.org/10.1016/j.jrurstud.2017.12.021

Stevens, R., Moray, N., & Bruneel, J. (2015). The social and economic mission of social enterprises: Dimensions, measurement, validation, and relation. *Entrepreneurship Theory and Practice, 39*(5), 1051–1082. https://doi.org/10.1111/etap.12091

Steves, C. J., Spector, T. D., & Jackson, S. H. (2012). Ageing, genes, environment and epigenetics: What twin studies tell us now, and in the future. *Age and Ageing, 41*(5), 581–586. https://doi.org/10.1093/ageing/afs097

Suchowerska, R., Barraket, J., Qian, J., Mason, C., Farmer, J., Carey, G., Campbell, P., & Joyce, A. (2020). An organizational approach to understanding how social enterprises address health inequities: A scoping review. *Journal of Social Entrepreneurship, 11*(3), 257–281. https://doi.org/10.1080/19420676.2019.1640771

Teasdale, S. (2012). What's in a Name? Making sense of social enterprise discourses. *Public Policy and Administration, 27*(2), 99–119. https://doi.org/10.1177/0952076711401466

Tovel, H., Carmel, S., & Raveis, V. H. (2019). Relationships among self-perception of aging, physical functioning, and self-efficacy in late life. *The Journals of Gerontology: Series B, 74*(2), 212–221. https://doi.org/10.1093/geronb/gbx056

Trombeta, F. M., Ramos, N. P., & Bocchi, S. C. M. (2020). Experience of nurse entrepreneurs in long term institutions for elderly people. *Revista Brasilera Enfermagem, 73*(suppl 3), e20190619. https://doi.org/10.1590/0034-7167-2019-0619

Villotti, P., Corbière, M., Dewa, C. S., Fraccaroli, F., Sultan-Taïeb, H., Zaniboni, S., & Lecomte, T. (2018). A serial mediation model of workplace social support on work productivity: The role of self-stigma and job tenure self-efficacy in people with severe mental disorders. *Disability and Rehabilitation, 40*(26), 3113–3119. https://doi.org/10.1080/09638288.2017.1377294

Wang, K. Y., Lin, Y. L., Han, C. K., & Hung, T. C. (2021). Feasibility study of introducing daily rental suites business model into long-term care institutions. In L. Barolli, A. Poniszewska-Maranda, & H. Park (Eds.), *Innovative Mobile and Internet Services in Ubiquitous Computing. IMIS 2020.* Advances in Intelligent Systems and Computing, vol 1195. Springer, Cham. https://doi.org/10.1007/978-3-030-50399-4_46

Weiss, D., & Freund, A. M. (2012). Still young at heart: Negative age-related information motivates distancing from same-aged people. *Psychology and Aging, 27*(1), 173–180. https://doi.org/10.1037/a0024819

Wong, L., & Tang, J. (2006). Non-state care homes for older people as third sector organisations in China's transitional welfare economy. *Journal of Social Policy, 35*, 229–246. https://doi.org/10.1017/S0047279405009505

Woolhead, G., Calnan, M., Dieppe, P., & Tadd, W. (2004). Dignity in older age: What do older people in the United Kingdom think? *Age and Ageing, 33*(2), 165–170. https://doi.org/10.1093/ageing/afh045

Zasada, M. (2017). Entrepreneurial activity in community health promotion organisations: Findings from an ethnographic study. *Social Enterprise Journal, 13*(02), 144–162. https://doi.org/10.1108/SEJ-07-2016-0030

Ziegler, R. (2017). Social innovation as a collaborative concept. *Innovation: The European Journal of Social Science Research, 30*(4), 388–405. https://doi.org/10.1080/13511610.2017.1348935

Chapter 26
Enhancing Social Capital for Elderly Services with Time Banking

Tommy K. C. Ng, Ben Yuk Fai Fong, and Wilson K. S. Leung

Abstract To relieve the burden of increasing elderly services, enhancing social capital in the community is a practical and feasible strategy. Social capital is about the shared values that a group of individual working together to achieve a positive outcome. It is essential to actively promote social capital in the community because it allows the individuals, particularly volunteers, to link together by sharing their skills, time and even assets. The outcome of enhancing social capital can be tangible or intangible in elderly services. Participation of volunteers is undoubtedly a key element in the services provided for the ageing population. Volunteers, both the young and older adults, can help facilitate the use of social capital in the community. One of the emerging initiatives in social capital is time banking. Time banking is about the exchange of the time of volunteers to provide services for the elderly and earn personal time credit to exchange for services when necessary, usually at a later stage when the individual's need arises. It is a virtuous cycle to sustain the service exchange by enhancing social capital. In achieving a holistic and humanistic care to the elderly, time banking in the community has the potential to alleviate the service demand and burden arising from an increasing ageing population as in the case of Hong Kong. The adoption of time banking in different countries will be analysed for better understanding of the operations and effectiveness of time banking.

Keywords Social capital · Social connection · Time banking · Elderly services

26.1 Introduction

Ageing population is a critical issue worldwide and it leads to a heavy burden to the healthcare system, such as long waiting time of inpatient and outpatient services, insufficient healthcare manpower, etc. Likewise, the demand of social elderly welfare

---

T. K. C. Ng (✉) · B. Y. F. Fong · W. K. S. Leung
School of Professional Education and Executive Development, College of Professional and Continuing Education, The Hong Kong Polytechnic University, Kowloon, Hong Kong, China
e-mail: tommy.ng@cpce-polyu.edu.hk

W. K. S. Leung
e-mail: wilsonks.leung@cpce-polyu.edu.hk

V. T. S. Law and B. Y. F. Fong (eds.), *Ageing with Dignity in Hong Kong and Asia*, Quality of Life in Asia 16, https://doi.org/10.1007/978-981-19-3061-4_26

services, including home cleansing, meal delivery and home visits, shall be increased to meet the needs of the elderly. To relieve the burden of increasing elderly services, enhancing social capital in the community is a practical and feasible strategy. Social capital is about building trust and social network in the community and thus volunteering can enhance the social capital in the community. Since the linkage of different volunteers can share their skills and time, it can provide tangible and intangible positive outcomes to the elderly. Furthermore, the participation of volunteering among older adults is vital for the sustainability of the elderly services. The concept of time banking is to encourage older adults to exchange their time to provide social elderly welfare services for the elderly and earn the personal time credit to exchange for services when necessary, usually at a later stage when an individual's need arises. Time banking can enhance social capital in the community and sustain the elderly services in the long term. First, this chapter aims to review the literature on social capital dimensions and to explain the underlying principle of social capital theory. Second, the influence of social capital combined with the concept of time banking on elderly services will be explored. Third, the results of time banking implementation in different countries will be discussed. Lastly, this chapter offers managerial implications for organisers to promote time banking in the society.

26.2 What is Social Capital

Capital serves a critical role in capitalist societies because it is a distinct commodity (Baker, 1990). In a social system, capital can be presented in various forms. There are three general types of capital in literature, namely, human, physical and social capital, that contribute to business success (Fatoki, 2011; Florin et al., 2003). Past studies mainly focused on the effects of human capital and physical capital on organisational performance from a technical perspective (Lin & Ho, 2011; Wamba et al., 2017). Unlike human and physical capital, social capital inheres within the structure of relations between individuals and among individuals, focusing on the relational aspect (Coleman, 1988). In recent years, the relationship between social capital and public health has dramatically drawn the attention (Gilbert et al., 2013). However, it is still unclear how social capital can play a role in alleviating the stress of public health systems, especially the shortage of community services for the elderly. Hence, there is an urgent need to understand the development of social capital and its application to elderly healthcare services.

Although social capital has been studied in the past 40 years (Coleman, 1988), its definition varies with literature (Wu, 2008). Putnam (1995) referred social capital to "features of social organisation such as networks, norms, and social trust that facilitate coordination and cooperation for mutual benefit" (p. 67). Adler and Kwon (2002) defined social capital as "the resource available to actors as a function of their location in the structure of their social relations" (p. 18). Coleman (1988) defined social capital as a resource deriving from the social structure of individuals that facilitates the achievement of specific goals. In particular, researchers widely agreed the definition of social capital provided by Nahapiet and Ghoshal (1998), which refers to "the sum of the actual and potential resources embedded within, available through, and derived from the network of relationships possessed by an individual or social unit" (Nahapiet and Ghoshal 1998, p. 243). In general, scholars regarded social capital as the goodwill, the structural network of human social interaction and the resources and information that derive from these social structures (Adler & Kwon, 2002). However, researchers conducted their studies on social capital from different dimensions or aspects of social relationships in order to explain the sources and benefits of social capital (Kumi & Sabherwal, 2018).

Drawing on the network concept, Burt (2001) proposed two network structures for social capital creation. From the perspective of network closure, social capital can be established by a network of strongly interconnected components, while the structural hole theory posits that social capital is formulated by a network in which individuals can broker connections between the otherwise disconnected segments (Burt, 2001). In addition to the network concept, Coleman (1988) argued that social capital is created by interpersonal interaction from the social relation perspective, which is intrinsic to social norms and shared values. Nahapiet and Ghoshal (1998) have suggested that social capital can be derived from both social network structures and social relations. They have conceptualised social capital into three dimensions, namely structural, relational, and cognitive capital. The structural dimension refers to the social connections between individuals, that is, who can be reached and how within the personal network (Burt, 1995). In other words, without the network structures, resources, such as information and knowledge, cannot be obtained and interpersonal relationships cannot be established. Researchers often measure this dimension by using network ties, network configurations and appropriable organisations (Nahapiet & Ghoshal, 1998). The relational dimension refers to the level of trust among individuals engendered by interpersonal interactions. Factors in this dimension measure social trust, norms, obligations and identification within a community, which contribute to prosocial behaviours and discourage selfish behaviours (Nahapiet & Ghoshal, 1998). The cognitive dimension refers to the resources offering common understanding and values between individuals, for instance, shared language and vision gather individuals together and achieve common goals within a community (Nahapiet & Ghoshal, 1998). Last but not least, these three dimensions are highly interrelated.

Social capital has enjoyed a rich history of empirical examination across different research areas. In the management discipline, Tsai and Ghoshal (1998) suggested that social capital helped the resource exchange and combination across different business departments of a company and subsequently influences product innovations. Their results confirmed that structural and relational dimensions of social capital positively affected the firm's resource allocation, which in turn influenced the value creation in new product developments. Florin et al. (2003) examined the effect of human, financial and social capital on the performance of 275 ventures in terms of sales growth and return on sales before and after an initial public offering (IPO). Their findings revealed that firm performance is mainly affected by social capital before and after IPO rather than human or financial capital. Moreover, Stam et al. (2014)

conducted a meta-analysis on the effect of social capital on firm performance and found that the structural dimension such as structural holes in entrepreneurs' personal networks was more critical for newly started businesses than old ones, whereas the strong ties (e.g. the relationship between close-knit members) were more favourable for old companies.

In the healthcare context, Lee et al. (2004) investigated social capital of a local community in the United States (US), including individuals' community participation and voting participation. Although their findings reported that the relationship between social capital and hospitals' community accountability was insignificant, they argued that this insignificant result might be caused by these two inapplicable dimensions of social capital. In the context of volunteering behaviour, Wang and Graddy (2008) examined the influence of social capital on individual charitable giving and confirmed the positive relationship between social capital and charitable behaviours. In addition, information systems (IS) researchers moved the concept of social capital from the offline to online environment. Chiu et al. (2006) conducted their study in a professional virtual community and considered the relationship between online members within this community as an online form of social capital. They examined the impact of social capital on prosocial behaviour, that is, knowledge sharing among members and confirmed the positive relationship between social capital and knowledge sharing in the virtual community. In summary, previous empirical studies have confirmed the critical role of social capital in explaining behaviours, no matter commercial or prosocial, across different research areas.

26.3 Relationship Between Social Capital, Volunteering and Elderly Services

Social capital is about social cohesion and social connection to facilitate the accomplishment of broad benefits. The promotion of volunteerism in the community is necessary for the development of social capital so as to maintain sustainability of the community (Miller et al., 2011). To provide elderly services in the community, volunteer work is one of the supportive measures to serve the elderly. The time involvement of the volunteers shall be changed to the helping behaviour in volunteerism and there is often no compensation and reward for the volunteers (Wei et al., 2012). Helping each other, and reduction in loneliness and depression can be the reasons for volunteering. Since there is no relationship or bonding between the volunteer and the service recipients, volunteering behaviour is highly related and can contribute to the social capital. For those who keep volunteering for long period of time, their trust is built and kept in a higher level and they are more likely to sustain their volunteering work (Bekkers, 2012). Besides, the identity of volunteer can promote social trust, which is one of the components of social capital because volunteers need to have trust to provide services to the recipients (Cheung et al., 2016). Thus, volunteers are found to have higher level of generalised trust and involvement in the community

(Stukas et al., 2005). With the development of trust, the cohesion between volunteer and service recipients can be narrowed. Moreover, increase in trust can further motivate and encourage the individual to donate their time and participate in volunteering work (Glanville et al., 2016). Therefore, trust building within the community is associated with volunteering behaviour. Furthermore, social network is also associated with volunteerism.

According to Wilson (2000), individuals who are more likely to be a volunteer due to their social network, such as being active and joining different activities organised by associations. Through the social connection, relatives and friends of the volunteers would be encouraged to join volunteer work and the volunteer community can be extended. In addition, being a volunteer can expand his or her social network by meeting other volunteers for experience sharing (Mannino et al., 2011). On the other side, older adults who are restricted to bond with their relatives have lower likelihood to be invited to participate in volunteering (Dávila, 2018). It indicates that social network of the elderly needs to be expanded to be involving in volunteering behaviour. There are positive impacts of volunteering, from the increase in reputation, recruitment and retention of volunteers, to organisations which provide volunteer services (Rochester et al., 2016). Therefore, volunteering can assist in building social capital in not only the volunteers but also the service recipients, community and organisations.

Volunteerism contributes to elderly services in an indispensable role since the power of volunteers supports part of the elderly services by accompanying the elderly to medical consultations, cleaning the household for the elderly and delivering meals. Providing elderly services by trained older adult volunteers can alleviate the burden on healthcare and domestic services, and help to sustain the development of the community. Since ageing population is emerging, older adults are encouraged to engage in volunteer work. Their participation and support are vital for the development of elderly services in the holistic and humanistic ways. In fact, social connection is not only vital for the volunteers but also the elderly because of the benefits to their physical and psychosocial health (Seppala et al., 2013). Increase in self-rated happiness and life satisfaction as well as decrease in anxiety and depression are proven positive outcomes of being a volunteer. The older volunteers perceive positive personal benefits, such as improved social circle, expanded leadership and productively used time, from the participation in volunteer work (Tang et al., 2010). Moreover, the psychological well-being, including self-acceptance, autonomy and purpose in life, of the elderly participating in volunteering is higher than who do not (Ho, 2017). The reasons of being a volunteer for older adults consist of broadening their horizons and learning new knowledge. Improvement in self-esteem is also found from the older volunteers because volunteering can optimise their sense of belonging and life satisfaction (Russell et al., 2019). Additionally, older volunteers are more satisfied with their health after joining volunteering work because of increased level of physical activity (Sherman et al., 2011). Participation in volunteering has also been found to have less progression of disability in older adults (Carr et al., 2018). There is less loss of physical function of the older adults with higher intensity of volunteer work. It indicates that there are loads of positive outcomes if the older adults participate in volunteering. The elderly services can be improved due to the enhancement of social capital and, conversely, social capital can be enhanced by the engagement of elderly services. Social capital is fundamental and vital to the elderly services as a result of the significant synergy.

The contribution of older adults to volunteering can sustain elderly services in the long term. Since most of the older adults are retired, they can commit more time in volunteering (Morrow-Howell, 2010). Likewise, the motivation of being volunteers in older adults includes staying active and desiring to help others. Obtaining material or non-material rewards, self-fulfilment and enhanced social relationship are also the motives for serving as volunteers (Martinez et al., 2011). On the other hand, health status, limited time and negative experience from past volunteer are barriers that hinder the participation of volunteer work. Transportation is also one of the barriers for elderly volunteering, and so volunteering within the local community can increase the possibility of providing services. To promote older adults volunteering in elderly services, meeting the needs of older adults can help to improve the participation rate. Additionally, volunteering intervention with information regarding the benefits of volunteering as well as setting goals, action plan and outcome, can significantly increase volunteering among older adults (Jiang et al., 2019). Action planning shows an important element of promoting volunteering among the older adults. Furthermore, to increase the commitment of older adult volunteers, adequate training and ongoing support are necessary to strengthen the identity of older volunteers (Tang et al., 2010). Offering high flexibility on choosing volunteer work can overcome barrier for older adults volunteering since they can get involved in other commitments in additional to volunteer work. Moreover, more volunteering should be offered by non-governmental organisation (NGO) at the district level so as to increase opportunities for older adults to volunteer near their residency.

26.4 Relationship Between Social Capital and Time Banking

In recent years, a group of scholars has started to apply the concept of social capital in the context of time banking. Time banking refers to "a unique type of nonprofit peer-to-peer system grounded in a similar logic of service exchange" (Yuan et al., 2018, p. 274). According to Williams (2004), the underlying principle of time banking is paying an hour for each hour of commitment, which can be "cashed in" by requesting an hour's service work in return from a social system at any time in order to promote informal volunteering behaviours within a local community. In other words, the service exchange among individuals is based on the unit of time credit in a community, also known as community currency (Kwon et al., 2019). Researchers have proposed the interrelationship between social capital and time banking. Kwon et al. (2019) claimed that social capital is rooted in the social exchange theory, which posits that individuals justify their decision to stay in a relationship or not by weighing rewards against costs of the exchange relationship, which in turn enables individuals to reduce social insecurity and economic crisis in social exchange. In this regard, Kwon et al. (2019) argued that time credits generated from the time banking system helped promote social capital because it secured social interaction and established trust among members. Their study found that participation in time banking had positively affected social capital in terms of community attachment. Furthermore, Yuan et al. (2018) have integrated the relational dimension of social capital in various virtual communities in an online time banking platform, hOurworld, in the US. They argued that trust and reciprocity (i.e. relational dimension) were relevant to time banking practices and norms. Since time banking practices are regarded as prosocial activities, which require social interactions and commitment between individuals, building trust and reciprocity through the network connection and social interaction among individuals helps to build a sense of online time banking communities (Yuan et al., 2018). Yuan et al. (2018) reported that social trust positively influenced the time banking practices and the sense of community.

In addition, Yuan et al. (2018) contend that the underlying principle of service exchange among individuals is based on generalised reciprocity rather than restricted reciprocity. According to Leung et al. (2019), restricted reciprocity refers to a favour exchange between two exchange parties rather than any third party, whereas generalised reciprocity refers to the exchange of favour and is not limited between two exchange parties but can be reciprocated by anyone in the community. In time banking systems, person A offers one-hour service for person B, and when person A requests to "cash in" this one-hour service, it can be reciprocated by anyone in the system rather than a fixed exchange partner. In this sense, there is a time gap in the service exchange among individuals in time banking systems and it requires a high level of trust between each other because the service is not to be exchanged in real time. Future research on time banking should consider this exchange pattern and further examine how trust can be developed at the initial stage and how it can be sustained in the long run. In summary, recent studies have demonstrated that time banking could be a possible solution to lessen the pressure of a social welfare system such as community elderly care services because the design of time banking system encourages individuals to engage in prosocial and volunteering behaviours (Kakar, 2018; Sasananan et al., 2019). Hence, understanding the development of social capital in the time banking context is critical for promoting community service exchange for the elderly.

26.5 Time Banking in Some Countries or Regions

According to a previous study (Ng, Yim & Fong, 2019), it was noted that the following countries or regions had implemented Time Banking Programmes to alleviate the ageing problems.

26.5.1 The United States

The concept of “time banking” first appeared in the US in the mid-1980s as a form of community currency system (Jacobson & MacMaster, 2000). The initial goal of this “time bank” practice was to encourage people in the community to utilise their time and skills by providing services to others outside the mainstream cash economy. Participants in the “time bank” at that time were not restricted to the elderly population only but to everyone in the community. They earned and spent “time dollars” that were measured by the amount of time required to provide a service instead of the monetary value of the service. These “time bank” programmes were later modified to target the socially and economically marginalised groups of people such as the elderly (Seyfang & Smith, 2002).

The implementation of time banking is comprehensive in the US. There were at least 125 time banks in the US by late 2010 (Collom & Lasker, 2016). The operation expanded to more than 270 time banks and membership reached 27,000 in 2013 (Carroll, 2013). An online platform is available to interested individuals to search for a nearby time bank (TimeBanks USA, n.d.). The contact information and details of hours exchanged are available from the platform, to facilitate individuals to participate. There are two approaches to time banking in the US. One is open to anyone and the other approach is limited to residents within the community, so the number of participants varies among different states. There are operational costs in time banking and the expenditures of coordinators include software support, website maintenance, printing of promotion materials and salary of staff. Overall, time banking gives positive outcomes to the community in the economic, social, health and environmental aspects. Moreover, both the service providers and recipients are satisfied with the operations, particularly in the quality of services (Collom, 2007).

26.5.2 European Countries

26.5.2.1 Switzerland

In Switzerland, the problem of ageing population is expected to become worse (Chastonay, Weber, & Mattig, 2018). The introduction of time banking may ease the challenges arisen from the ageing population. Several cities are initiating time banking. St. Gallen is the first region to introduce the concept of time banking. It was selected as the pilot project because of its previous experience in volunteer programme (Thoele, 2012). The time-saving foundation of St. Gallen operates as a retirement plan with the concept of time banking. The goal of the project is to reduce the cost of social services and to encourage local solidarity in response to a steadily ageing population. During their leisure time, healthy retirees provide care and support to other elderly in need. Every hour of work is recorded as a “deposit” in a special personal account that can later be used to pay for the "time" when the volunteer needs help. However, the technical support of time banking in Switzerland is still at the elementary level (The moneyland.ch, n.d.).

26.5.2.2 United Kingdom

The United Kingdom (UK) had developed time bank and operated over 100 time banks as of 2008 but rapidly expanded the number to about 300 in 2013 (Carroll, 2013; Gregory, 2012b). The number of members grew from 8,000 in 2008 to 20,000 in 2012 (Ryan-Collins et al., 2008). The UK operations of time banking are similar with those in Switzerland and the US but there are three approaches to create co-production, namely person-to-person, person-to-agency and agency-to-agency. Person-to-person is about the exchange of time and service to the individuals in need within the community. Third parties or organisations shall host and coordinate the time bank. Person-to-agency involves contribution to the goals of community and time credits are earned by the hosting organisations. The agency provides choices for members to utilise the credits. The activities are not specific to individuals but the community, including planting trees. Agency-to-agency mainly focuses on the collaboration between agencies to facilitate the exchange of services between organisations and individuals because this approach aims to fully utilise the community assets by sharing of facilities. When an organisation is looking for a room to promote time banking, the other authority can offer underutilised room for this purpose. By sharing resources within the community, it may not only reach the common purposes and goals of improving the services but also share the knowledge and expertise among different discipline of organisations. Ultimately, it creates and establishes a socially inclusive community, maximises the use of community assets, as well as improving the self-esteem, confidence, well-being and social network of the individuals participating in the time banking project (Boyle, Clarke & Burns, 2006; Gregory, 2012a).

26.5.2.3 Finland

In Finland, there are more than 40 time banks countrywide but most of them are inactive (Eskelinen, 2018). "Stadin Aikapankki" is one of the Finnish time banks located in Helsinki and was founded in 2009. The principle of the establishment of "Stadin Aikapankki" is that time, work and needs for help are equally valuable so local assistance between individual strengthens the socially just local economy (Laamanen et al., 2015). Unlike other countries, the unit of exchange is called "Tovi" to exchange services, earning and spending credits. There were around 3,000 members in "Stadin Aikapankki" and a total of 19,000 h exchanged by 2014. The exchangeable services consist of language training, gardening and so on. Nevertheless, the tax authority in Finland has concluded that the transactions of time banks are taxable because the professional activities generate economic benefits to the members (Träskman &

Hyde-Clarke, 2016). Interestingly, the time banks impose 2% of the service credits as an internal tax for supporting the local community organisations, such as food industry and ecological friendly non-governmental organisations, selected by the members of time banking. The internal tax support of the selected local community organisations shall provide goods, such as local organic food, for the time banking members. The selected local community organisations can gain access to the community (Peltokoski et al. 2015). It can create an equal and ecologically sustainable community with justice in the long term.

26.6 Asian Countries or Regions

26.6.1 Japan

Japan is one of the first Asian countries to bring the "time bank" concept to care services for its ageing population. Its time bank currency system is called the "Fureai Kippu" scheme. The development of "Fureai Kippu'" scheme is based on a volunteering system for tackling the limited resources to support the ageing population (Boyle, 2011). Participants can earn credits by providing caring service to the elderly in the community and then use the credits to exchange for similar services they need (Colligan, 2011). The earned credits can be saved and redeemed later in life when necessary. There were more than 660 time banks recorded across Japan and about 250 less known time banks before 2012 (Hayashi, 2012). Two different approaches of time banking are adopted in Japan, consisting of the person-to-person approach and the utilising conventional money approach. In the latter approach, the service recipients may not have enough time credits to exchange for the service and have to pay small amounts of money. The fees are paid to the organisations rather than the service providers. The Japanese time banking system reduces the burden on the service provision and the pressure on community service resources (Ng, 2017).

26.6.2 Taiwan

Taiwan has a similar cultural background to Hong Kong. It started to promote time banks as early as in the 1990s. The Hondao Senior Citizen's Welfare Foundation created the "Volunteer Hours Bank" in 1995 (Hondao Senior Citizen's Welfare Foundation, 2006). Local governments and higher educational institutions also support the advocacy of time banking in Taiwan (Wu & Chou, 2017). Some local governments provide community services for the elderly, including companion for medical consultation, exercise, domestic assistance and meal delivery, to promote charity-related activities. On the other hand, students can learn more about the concept of time banking through service learning in tertiary educational institutions. Both educational and governmental supports have positive impacts on time banking promotion in Taiwan. Instrumental and emotional supports are provided to community services. Instrumental support relates more to actual assistance, such as transportation, and emotional support focuses on caring and understanding to the service recipients. The outcome of time banking has been found positive by both the service providers and recipients. Servers earn a sense of accomplishment after providing services while the receivers in the community feel positive after receiving services (Chou & Lee, 2015). With the platform for reciprocity, it allows community members to help one another in the physical, psychological and social aspects. Furthermore, online platforms, such as social media, are used to invite membership and they can promote time banking in the community (Taiwan Time Bank Association, 2019).

26.6.3 Hong Kong

Compared with other countries, time banking in Hong Kong is grossly underdeveloped because the development and implementation of time banking are still primitive (Hong Kong Sheng Kung Hui, 2018). Only 200 elderly registered in the pilot time banking project launched by the Hong Kong Sheng Kung Hui Welfare Council (TVB News, 2019). The government support on time banking is totally inadequate as the government does not provide any financial support to the non-governmental organisations to launch time banking. Besides, promotion of time banking is rarely found from the Internet in Hong Kong, where the development of time banking falls behind countries of similar economic development and social advancement. Nevertheless, the Research Grants Council had funded a time banking project in 2020 to promote time banking activities in Hong Kong (University Grants Committee, 2020). This is a little big step in the development of time banking in Hong Kong.

26.7 Promoting Time Banking in Community

Governmental support on financial aspect is one of the key elements of promoting and generalising time banking in the community (Seyfang & Smith, 2002). Governments should provide financial subsidisation to NGOs to launch and operate time banking projects in the community. Since the NGOs serve as mediators of time banking, they coordinate and organise service offering and requests. Financial subsidy can facilitate the NGOs to initiate time banking projects, which, similar to volunteering, does not involve any money transition. The organisations operating time banking need to be self-financing but the organisations do not have any profit derived from operating time banking. Hence, financial support from the government can motivate the implementation of time banking in the community. In addition, existing NGOs should be encouraged to engage in the development of time banking because their resources, including manpower and finance, are potentially strong and sufficient to support and sustain the services (Gregory, 2009).

Furthermore, education and promotion of the concept of time banking in the community need to be enhanced because the concept may be new to the community and civilians, particularly young people, who may not be familiar with and have not experienced time banking (Gregory, 2009). Nonetheless, time banking requires a cultural change and paradigm shift, and so education and promotion of time banking would be very challenging. Strong local participation is crucial to the sustainability of time banking because it is very much about neighbours helping neighbours. Without the support of community civilians, it is difficult to develop time banking. The concept of time banking needs to be spread through different channels. The operations and effectiveness of time banking can be promoted by various organisations. Promotional booth, carnival and information leaflet can be targeted to older adults because they are less likely to use the social media. Likewise, social media is useful to promote the concept of time banking to the young adults and adolescents. This can allow them to learn and be familiar with this new social concept. Early community engagement in time banking can help optimising the operations and coordination.

Technical support is fundamental and essential for the implementation and operations of time banking because the offers and requests of services can be enormous. Immediate request may occur and prompt message delivery is paramount. Service providers and recipients can easily and conveniently accept and ask for assistance respectively. Coordination by manual systems cannot effectively or efficiently deliver the messages to service providers and recipients. Although some countries are using web-based applications for users to request the service, the effectiveness of web-based applications cannot support real-time time banking (Han et al., 2014). Moreover, the simplicity and ease of use of online platforms are positively associated with the positive attitude towards time banking (Yuan et al., 2019). Thus, user friendly platform, such as mobile application, can facilitate the implementation of time banking by not only relieving the burden of the organisation but also optimising the users' experience. Peer-to-peer platform can increase the efficiency of services, reduce service costs and enhance service experience. Likewise, the experience and stories of time banking providers should be uploaded to the online platform because such encounters can attract and increase the intention of the potential service provider to participate (Kakar, 2018). On the other side, the experience of service recipients can help promote the usefulness and practicality of time banking. Gamification of online platform can also boost the interest of service providers and recipients to use the platform because they enjoy the mention of badges and levelling up (Hooper et al. 2015). Thus, innovative online platform can help promoting and sustaining time banking.

Youth volunteering is found to have improved psychological well-being and interest in adult volunteering (Kim & Morgül, 2017). Engagement in volunteering early in one's life is beneficial to oneself and also the community. In a study of time banking project involving students, the sense of community and belonging were built because the project provided a platform for students to connect and build relationship with people that they did not know (Matthew, 2020). Participation in time banking can be modified for the youth because their participation can facilitate the continuity of time banking and can practically educate them about the concept and importance of helping others. Likewise, youth participation of providing service in time banking can assist in active participation in services (Marks, 2012). The approach of time banking can allow the youth to provide services to the elderly, such as meal delivery and home visits. Young people can also learn to earn for others by donating the time accumulated to their relatives or the elderly in need as they do not require the services when they are young.

26.8 Conclusion

Social capital is vital for elderly services because social network and trust are fundamental to the sustainability of elderly services. The presence of social network and trust in the community can facilitate the volunteering in elderly services. Besides, well-developed volunteering of elderly services can also expand social capital in the community. The participation of volunteering work by older adults can generate several positive outcomes not only for themselves but also for the entire community. Time banking is an innovative concept to enhance the social capital. It allows older adults to volunteer and provides services to the elderly in the community. The time served by volunteers can be accumulated as time credits for the exchange of services when necessary and getting older. It is definitely a virtuous cycle to enhance social capital and sustain elderly services since trust and social network can be further developed after services provided by time banking. Time banking can also facilitate individuals and communities to take on increased care responsibilities within their communities (Gregory, 2015). However, the adoption of time banking depends on the acceptance of the concept by the community. Hence, promotion of time banking is challenging. Governmental support with financial subsidies to local non-governmental organisations is equally important to operate the scheme. NGOs have strong volunteer networks to initiate time banking in the community. Finally, technical support and youth participation are also crucial to sustain the implementation of time banking within the community, particularly in aged care and elderly services in the pursuit of ageing with dignity for the older adults.

Acknowledgements The work described in this chapter was partially supported by two grants from the Research Grants Council of the Hong Kong Special Administrative Region, China (Project Reference No.: UGC/IDS24/18 and UGC/FDS24/B04/20).

References

Adler, P. S., & Kwon, S. W. (2002). Social capital: Prospects for a new concept. *Academy of Management Review, 27*(1), 17–40. https://doi.org/10.2307/4134367

Baker, W. E. (1990). Market networks and corporate behavior. *American Journal of Sociology, 96*(3), 589–625. http://www.jstor.org/stable/2781065

Bekkers, R. (2012). Trust and volunteering: Selection or causation? Evidence from a 4 year panel study. *Political Behavior, 34*(2), 225–247. https://doi.org/10.1007/s11109-011-9165-x

Boyle, D. (2011). More than money. *NEF, Nesta.* Retrieved from http://www.meansofexchange.com/reportdownloads/LETS-More-Than-Money.pdf

Boyle, D., Clarke, S., & Burns, S. (2006). *Hidden work: Co-production by people outside paid employment*. Joseph Rowntree Foundation.

Burt, R. (2001). Structural holes versus network closure as social capital. In N. Lin, K. Cook, & R. S. Burt (Eds.), *Social Capital: Theory and Research* (pp. 31–56). Routledge. https://doi.org/10.4324/9781315129457-2

Burt, R. S. (1995). *Structural holes: The social structure of competition*. Harvard University Press.

Carr, D. C., Kail, B. L., & Rowe, J. W. (2018). The relation of volunteering and subsequent changes in physical disability in older adults. *The Journals of Gerontology: Series B, 73*(3), 511–521. https://doi.org/10.1093/geronb/gbx102

Carroll, J. M. (2013, June). Co-production scenarios for mobile time banking. In *International Symposium on End User Development* (pp. 137–152). Berlin, Heidelberg: Springer. https://doi.org/10.1007/978-3-642-38706-7_11

Chastonay, P., Weber, D., & Mattig, T. (2018). The health of older people in Switzerland. *Journal of Public Health International, 1*(2), 5–8. https://doi.org/10.14302/issn.2641-4538.jphi-18-2426

Cheung, C. K., Lo, T. W., & Liu, E. S. C. (2016). Sustaining social trust and volunteer role identity reciprocally over time in pre-adult, adult, and older volunteers. *Journal of Social Service Research, 42*(1), 70–83. https://doi.org/10.1080/01488376.2015.1078267

Chiu, C. M., Hsu, M. H., & Wang, E. T. (2006). Understanding knowledge sharing in virtual communities: An integration of social capital and social cognitive theories. *Decision Support Systems, 42*(3), 1872–1888. https://doi.org/10.1016/j.dss.2006.04.001

Chou, W. H., & Lee, L. H. (2015). Investigating the preferences for time banking for senior citizens: Local needs and constraints in the context of Taiwanese culture. *Bulletin of Japanese Society for the Science of Design, 61*(5), 97–106. https://doi.org/10.11247/jssdj.61.5_97

Coleman, J. S. (1988). Social capital in the creation of human capital. *American Journal of Sociology, 94*, S95–S120.

Colligan, P. (2011). *Public services as a platform for giving*. https://assets.publishing.service.gov.uk/government/uploads/system/uploads/attachment_data/file/78914/philip-colligan-essay_0.pdf

Collom, E. (2007). The motivations, engagement, satisfaction, outcomes, and demographics of time bank participants: Survey findings from a US system. *International Journal of Community Currency Research, 11*, 36–83. https://doi.org/10.15133/j.ijccr.2007.004

Collom, E., & Lasker, J. N. (2016). Equal time, equal value: Community currencies and time banking in the US. *Routledge.* https://doi.org/10.4324/9781315580159

Dávila, M. C. (2018). The relationship between social networks and volunteerism among seniors. *Journal of Social Service Research, 44*(1), 38–49. https://doi.org/10.1080/01488376.2017.1395382

Eskelinen, T. (2018). Social space for self-organising: An exploratory study of timebanks in Finland and in the UK. *Nordic Journal of Social Research, 9*, 89–109. https://doi.org/10.7577/njsr.2148

Fatoki, O. O. (2011). The impact of human, social and financial capital on the performance of small and medium-sized enterprises (SMEs) in South Africa. *Journal of Social Sciences, 29*(3), 193–204. https://doi.org/10.1080/09718923.2011.11892970

Florin, J., Lubatkin, M., & Schulze, W. (2003). A social capital model of high-growth ventures. *Academy of Management Journal, 46*(3), 374–384. https://doi.org/10.2307/30040630

Gilbert, K. L., Quinn, S. C., Goodman, R. M., Butler, J., & Wallace, J. (2013). A meta-analysis of social capital and health: A case for needed research. *Journal of Health Psychology, 18*(11), 1385–1399. https://doi.org/10.1177/1359105311435983

Glanville, J. L., Paxton, P., & Wang, Y. (2016). Social capital and generosity: A multilevel analysis. *Nonprofit and Voluntary Sector Quarterly, 45*(3), 526–547. https://doi.org/10.1177/0899764015591366

Gregory, L. (2009). Change takes time: Exploring structural and development issues of time banking. *International Journal of Community Currency Research, 13*, 19–32. https://doi.org/10.15133/j.ijccr.2009.003

Gregory, L. (2012a). Local people rebuilding their communities—An exploration of Welsh time banking. *Contemporary Wales, 25*(1), 40–57.

Gregory, L. (2012b). Time and punishment: A comparison of UK and US time bank use in criminal justice systems. *Journal of Comparative Social Welfare, 28*(3), 195–208. https://doi.org/10.1080/17486831.2012.742452

Gregory, L. (2015). *Trading time: Can exchange lead to social change?*. Policy Press. https://policy.bristoluniversitypress.co.uk/trading-time

Han, K., Shih, P. C., Bellotti, V., & Carroll, J. M. (2014). *Timebanking with a smartphone application.* Collective Intelligence Conference. https://doi.org/10.13140/2.1.1253.3120

Hayashi, M. (2012). Japan's Fureai Kippu time-banking in elderly care: Origins, development, challenges and impact. *International Journal of Community Currency Research, 16*(A), 30–44. https://doi.org/10.15133/j.ijccr.2012.003

Ho, H. C. (2017). Elderly volunteering and psychological well-being. *International Social Work, 60*(4), 1028–1038. https://doi.org/10.1177/0020872815595111

Hooper, C. J., Nind, M., Parsons, S., Power, A., & Collis, A. (2015). Building a social machine: Co-designing a TimeBank for inclusive research. In *Proceedings of the ACM Web Science Conference* (pp. 1–9). https://doi.org/10.1145/2786451.2786472

Hondao Senior Citizen's Welfare Foundation. (2006). *Current services.* http://www.hondao.org.tw/en/index.html

Hong Kong Sheng Kung Hui. (2018, August 12). *Elderly in the Tseung Kwan O Aged Care Complex Serve as Volunteers and Accumulate Credits for the Zhi Fu Scheme (將軍澳安老大樓長者做義工儲分織福).* http://echo.hkskh.org/issue.aspx?lang=2&id=3393&nid=5615

Jacobson, W., & MacMaster, P. (2000). *Family support and time dollars: How to build community using social capital.* Family Support America.

Jiang, D., Warner, L. M., Chong, A. M. L., Li, T., Wolff, J. K., & Chou, K. L. (2019). Promoting volunteering among older adults in Hong Kong: A randomized controlled trial. *The Gerontologist, 60*(5), 968–977. https://doi.org/10.1093/geront/gnz076

Kakar, A. K. (2018). Investigating factors that promote time banking for sustainable community based socio-economic growth and development. *Computers in Human Behaviour*, 105623. https://doi.org/10.1016/j.chb.2018.07.034

Kim, J., & Morgül, K. (2017). Long-term consequences of youth volunteering: Voluntary versus involuntary service. *Social Science Research, 67*, 160–175. https://doi.org/10.1016/j.ssresearch.2017.05.002

Kumi, R., & Sabherwal, R. (2018). Performance consequences of social capital in online communities: The roles of exchange and combination, and absorptive capacity. *Computers in Human Behavior, 86*, 337–349. https://doi.org/10.1016/j.chb.2018.05.008

Kwon, M., Lee, C., Xiao, Y., & McIntosh, W. A. (2019). Community currency activities, community attachment, and quality of life: A case study of the crooked river alliance of TimeBanks. *Time & Society, 28*(3), 1181–1220. https://doi.org/10.1177/0961463X17716737

Laamanen, M., Wahlen, S., & Campana, M. (2015). Mobilising collaborative consumption lifestyles: A comparative frame analysis of time banking. *International Journal of Consumer Studies, 39*(5), 459–467. https://doi.org/10.1111/ijcs.12190

Lee, S. Y. D., Chen, W. L., & Weiner, B. J. (2004). Communities and hospitals: Social capital, community accountability, and service provision in US community hospitals. *Health Services Research, 39*(5), 1487–1508. https://doi.org/10.1111/j.1475-6773.2004.00300.x

Leung, W. K., Shi, S., & Chow, W. S. (2019). Impacts of user interactions on trust development in C2C social commerce. *Internet Research, 30*(1), 335–356. https://doi.org/10.1108/INTR-09-2018-0413

Lin, C.-Y., & Ho, Y.-H. (2011). Determinants of green practice adoption for logistics companies in China. *Journal of Business Ethics, 98*(1), 67–83. https://doi.org/10.1007/s10551-010-0535-9

Mannino, C. A., Snyder, M., & Omoto, A. M. (2011). Why do people get involved? Motivations for volunteerism and other forms of social action. In D. Dunning (Ed.), *Social motivation* (pp. 127–146). Psychology Press.

Marks, M. B. (2012). Time banking service exchange systems: A review of the research and policy and practice implications in support of youth in transition. *Children and Youth Services Review, 34*(7), 1230–1236. https://doi.org/10.1016/j.childyouth.2012.02.017

Martinez, I. L., Crooks, D., Kim, K. S., & Tanner, E. (2011). Invisible civic engagement among older adults: Valuing the contributions of informal volunteering. *Journal of Cross-Cultural Gerontology, 26*(1), 23–37. https://doi.org/10.1007/s10823-011-9137-y

Matthew, R. A. (2020). Banking on community: The use of time banking as an innovative community practice teaching strategy. *Journal of Community Practice, 28*(3), 254–264. https://doi.org/10.1080/10705422.2020.1796877

Miller, A., Simpson, B., Lieben, J., & Simpson, B. J. (2011). Understanding the role of volunteerism in creating social inclusion. *South West Communities Resource Centre.*

Morrow-Howell, N. (2010). Volunteering in later life: Research frontiers. *Journals of Gerontology Series b: Psychological Sciences and Social Sciences, 65*(4), 461–469. https://doi.org/10.1093/geronb/gbq024

Nahapiet, J., & Ghoshal, S. (1998). Social capital, intellectual capital, and the organizational advantage. *Academy of Management Review, 23*(2), 242–266. https://doi.org/10.2307/259373

Ng, D. (2017, April 21). *Time bank lets Japan's seniors swop services for free—from cleaning to companionship.* https://www.channelnewsasia.com/news/asia/time-bank-lets-japan-s-seniors-swop-services-for-free-from-clean-8755056

Ng, T., Yim, N. & Fong, B. (2019). *Time banking for elderly in Hong Kong: current practice and challenges* (CAHMR Working Paper Series No. 2, Issue 1, 2019). The Hong Kong Polytechnic University, College of Professional and Continuing Education, School of Professional Education and Executive Development, Centre for Ageing and Healthcare Management Research, Hong Kong. http://weblib.cpcepolyu.edu.hk/apps/wps/assets/pdf/cw20190102.pdf

Peltokoski, J. Toivakainen, N., Toivanen, T., and van der Wekken, R. (2015). In D. Bollier, & S. Helfrich (Eds.), *Patterns of communing* (pp. 401–409). Commons strategy group and off the Common Press.

Putnam, R. D. (1995). Bowling alone: America's declining social capital. *Journal of Democracy, 6*(1), 65–78. https://doi.org/10.1353/jod.1995.0002

Rochester, C., Paine, A. E., Howlett, S., Zimmeck, M., & Paine, A. E. (2016). Volunteering and Society in the 21st Century. *Springer*. https://doi.org/10.1057/9780230279438

Russell, A. R., Nyame-Mensah, A., de Wit, A., & Handy, F. (2019). Volunteering and wellbeing among ageing adults: A longitudinal analysis. *VOLUNTAS: International Journal of Voluntary and Nonprofit Organizations, 30*(1), 115–128. https://doi.org/10.1007/s11266-018-0041-8

Ryan-Collins, J., Stephens, L., & Coote, A. (2008). *The new wealth of time: How timebanking helps people build better public services.* NEF.

Sasananan, M., Channarong, K., & Kingnakhonthong, S. (2019). Preliminary study of time banking participation. *Quality Production Improvement-QPI, 1*(1), 618–622. https://doi.org/10.2478/cqpi-2019-0083

Seppala, E., Rossomando, T., & Doty, J. R. (2013). Social connection and compassion: Important predictors of health and well-being. *Social Research: An International Quarterly, 80*(2), 411–430.

Seyfang, G., & Smith, K. (2002). *The time of our lives: Using time banking for neighbourhood renewal and community capacity building.* New Economics Foundation.

Sherman, N. E., Michel, R., Rybak, C., Randall, G. K., & Davidson, J. (2011). Meaning in life and volunteerism in older adults. *Adultspan Journal, 10*(2), 78–90. https://doi.org/10.1002/j.2161-0029.2011.tb00127.x

Stam, W., Arzlanian, S., & Elfring, T. (2014). Social capital of entrepreneurs and small firm performance: A meta-analysis of contextual and methodological moderators. *Journal of Business Venturing, 29*(1), 152–173. https://doi.org/10.1016/j.jbusvent.2013.01.002

Stukas, A. A., Daly, M., & Cowling, M. J. (2005). Volunteerism and social capital: A functional approach. *Australian Journal on Volunteering, 10*(2), 35–44.

Taiwan Time Bank Association. (2019). *Home page*. http://www.timebank.org.tw/

Tang, F., Choi, E., & Morrow-Howell, N. (2010). Organizational support and volunteering benefits for older adults. *The Gerontologist, 50*(5), 603–612. https://doi.org/10.1093/geront/gnq020

The moneyland.ch. (n.d.). *Time banking and time-based currency in Switzerland*. https://www.moneyland.ch/en/time-banking-currency-switzerland-guide

Thoele, A. (2012, March 04). Swiss city set to launch elderly care "bank". https://www.swissinfo.ch/eng/swiss-city-set-to-launch-elderly-care--bank-/32209234

TimeBanks USA. (n.d.). *Home page*. https://timebanks.org/

Tsai, W., & Ghoshal, S. (1998). Social capital and value creation: The role of intrafirm networks. *Academy of Management Journal, 41*(4), 464–476. https://doi.org/10.2307/257085

Träskman, T., & Hyde-Clarke, N. (2016). Assessing the potential for "cultural disruption" through sharing economy: A case study of a time bank in Helsinki. *Open Journal of Social Sciences, 4*(6), 111–120. https://doi.org/10.4236/jss.2016.46012

TVB News. (2019, January 6). *Time banking (時間銀行)* [Video file]. http://news.tvb.com/programmes/sundayreport/5c319987e603838f2224e18f/%E6%99%82%E9%96%93%E9%8A%80%E8%A1%8C

University Grants Committee. (2020). *Faculty development scheme (FDS)—project abstract*. https://www.ugc.edu.hk/eng/rgc/funding_opport/fds/funded%20research/fds2021_abstract.html#FDS24/B04

Wamba, S. F., Gunasekaran, A., Akter, S., Ren, S.J.-F., Dubey, R., & Childe, S. J. (2017). Big data analytics and firm performance: Effects of dynamic capabilities. *Journal of Business Research, 70*, 356–365. https://doi.org/10.1016/j.jbusres.2016.08.009

Wang, L., & Graddy, E. (2008). Social capital, volunteering, and charitable giving. *Voluntas: International Journal of Voluntary and Nonprofit Organizations, 19*(1), 23. https://doi.org/10.1007/s11266-008-9055-y

Wei, Y., Donthu, N., & Bernhardt, K. L. (2012). Volunteerism of older adults in the United States. *International Review on Public and Nonprofit Marketing, 9*(1), 1–18. https://doi.org/10.1080/17525098.2010.492653

Williams, C. C. (2004). Informal volunteering: Some lessons from the United Kingdom. *Journal of Policy Analysis and Management, 23*(3), 613–616. https://doi.org/10.1002/pam.20030

Wilson, J. (2000). Volunteering. *Annual Review of Sociology, 26*(1), 215–240. https://doi.org/10.1146/annurev.soc.26.1.215

Wu, M. J., & Chou, Y. H. (2017). Exploratory study on the implementation of time banking in Taiwan: Perspectives from social network analysis. *Journal of Community Work and Community Studies, 7*(2), 45–96. https://doi.org/10.29755/JCWCS

Wu, W. P. (2008). Dimensions of social capital and firm competitiveness improvement: The mediating role of information sharing. *Journal of Management Studies, 45*(1), 122–146. https://doi.org/10.1111/j.1467-6486.2007.00741.x

Yuan, C. W., Hanrahan, B. V., & Carroll, J. M. (2018). Is there social capital in service exchange tools?. Investigating timebanking use and social capital development. *Computers in Human Behavior, 81*, 274–281. https://doi.org/10.1016/j.chb.2017.12.029

Yuan, C. W., Hanrahan, B. V., & Carroll, J. M. (2019). Assessing timebanking use and coordination: Implications for service exchange tools. *Information Technology & People, 32*(2), 344–363. https://doi.org/10.1108/ITP-09-2017-0311

Chapter 27
Redefining Doctor-Patient Relationship and Professional Ethics in Elderly Care

Sukhpreet Kaur and Chor Ming Lum

Abstract The doctor-patient relationship is an essential determinant of quality of healthcare, especially in elderly care as the older adults are more vulnerable in comparison to other age groups. Patients and doctors engage in a consensual relationship in which the patient seeks health-related assistance, and the service provider agrees to provide the highest standard of care, treatment options and to maintain confidentiality. Sometimes information only known by doctors and not disclosed to family members or relatives illustrates the immense trust placed by patients on doctors. This type of care involves four key elements—mutual knowledge, trust, loyalty and regard which will be discussed using the three basic models of the doctor-relationship including Active–Passive Model, Guidance-Cooperation Model and Mutual Participation Model. The American Nurses Association adopts The Code of Ethics to guide professionals towards treatment of their patients to ensure professional ethics in care and to address ethical issues that are likely to arise involving the elderly. Some of the vulnerabilities found in professional ethics in elderly care are incidences of error, neglect and abuse. The aim of this chapter is to discuss doctor-patient relationship and professional ethics in elderly care, and explore what can be done to achieve the highest level of care.

Keywords Doctor-patient relationship · Quality of care · Elderly care · Professional ethics

27.1 Doctor-Patient Relationship

The doctor-patient relationship is a keystone of care. However, it has become challenging with the changing patterns in society, medical advancement and easy access to medical information (Chandra et al., 2018). The medical knowledge of doctors

S. Kaur (✉)
Hong Kong College of Community Health Practitioners, Hong Kong, China
e-mail: izsukhy@gmail.com

C. M. Lum
The Chinese University of Hong Kong, Hong Kong, China

V. T. S. Law and B. Y. F. Fong (eds.), *Ageing with Dignity in Hong Kong and Asia*, Quality of Life in Asia 16, https://doi.org/10.1007/978-981-19-3061-4_27

in particular was previously used for patient management. Today, it is seen as a commodity between the service provider and the patient with treatment being customised to individuals.

The two elements of doctor-patient relationship are instrumental and expressive (Eustice, 2020). The 'instrumental' aspect reviews the ability of the doctor in performing the technical side of care including physical examination, diagnostic tests and treatments. The 'expressive' dimension oversees the affective interaction between the doctor and the patient such as their bonding and showing empathy when appropriate. This chapter discusses doctor-patient relationship, looking into how the vulnerable ageing population faces certain challenges, and how health professionals play a major role to offer assistance to overcome the challenges (Williams et al., 2007).

27.2 Medicine Advancement

The debate over whether medicine is an art or science continues. Many of course think it is science, others believe it is an art or both (Panda, 2006). In the early 1900's, medicine was 'more science than art' (Eustice, 2020). However, cures were often impossible or had limited treatment effects. So the caregivers worked to polish their bedside manners instead. Apparently, words may do as much harm to the patients as does the surgical knife.

Medicine has progressed scientifically while being enriched by integration of cultures (Panda, 2006). It has evolved, based on human values and intuition, and given medicine a strong foundation of practice. Humanistic qualities such as caring and comfort are the cornerstone of medicine without which medicine and healthcare today would be 'suboptimal, useless, even detrimental'. Medical care with humanistic values is of utmost importance for patient welfare, patient autonomy and social justice, the three fundamental principles for physicians and clinical practice. The first principle emphasises the interest, concern and welfare of the patient. Everything else including diagnoses and treatment options are subsidiary to patient welfare. The second principle gives autonomy to the patient of the final decision for treatment options while the doctor gives professional suggestions and/or advice. Lastly, social justice, the third principle, ensures service accessibility to everyone, i.e. universal healthcare strongly advocated by the World Health Organization.

This is why the social skills of health workers are still looked into as an area of further development and training in spite of the emergence of science and technology (Eustice, 2020). However, it is also true that scientific truths are not always true. What is considered right today will probably be invalid or outdated in the next five to ten years. Most surgical procedures used today will be replaced with something better in the future, as in the case of the emerging minimally invasive surgery. Basically, with time, management of diseases including diagnostic methods, will change.

27.3 Quality of Care—Communication and Trust

To manage patients as well as to provide high-quality care, having a healthy doctor-patient relationship is a requisite, and a healthy relationship is dependent on communication and trust. Effective communication is 'one of the ingredients of success in all fields of work' while trust boosts patient care and satisfaction (Chandra et al., 2018). Patients and doctors engage in a consensual relationship in which the patient seeks health-related assistance, and the service provider agrees to the highest standard of care, optimal treatment options and to maintain confidentiality.

Effective communication and trust are extremely important if the doctor is managing patients with two or more chronic conditions (Turabian, 2019). Multimorbidity, mostly found in older patients, is challenging and requires great understanding from the doctor-patient relationship. There can be conflicts on the treatment options and plans arising from managing uncertainty. On the other hand, the doctors in-charge of patients with mental disorders may often seem autocratic (Plesničar, 2016). For patients requiring extra care, the prime rule is to be 'professional, without judgment and be open'. Patients sometimes do not admit their illnesses or do not recognise the symptoms. Therefore, it is important to give them some time to open up, and then communicate and make shared and informed decisions where possible.

27.4 Aspects of Doctor-Patient Relationship

The four key elements that form the doctor-patient relationship are trust, mutual knowledge, regard and loyalty (Chipidza et al., 2015). Often being just seen as a fiduciary relationship, the doctor-patient relationship actually embraces its immense nature. Patients disclose confidential information to their physicians, the act of which the family members or relatives may not be aware of as means to sustain their health by trusting in a doctor and his/her competency. Patients also have the knowledge of the doctor and vice versa, and beliefs to receive the treatment and stay committed until the end. It is basically knowing that the doctor is 'on their side'.

Other than these, there are aspects of the doctor-patient relationship that are subject to parties' needs and preferences. One of them is *informed consent* to medical procedures, giving the patient a choice in the provision of their care (Selinger, 2009). While some rely on the doctor's recommendations, others prefer having a say. *Physician communication style* defines the strength of the doctor-patient relationship. It is found that patient-centred communication has positive outcomes because patients comply better when doctors show interest in them, keep a warm disposition and empathise (Robertson-Jones et al., 2019). Self-disclosure, specifically by patients, is another form of communication that is helpful in building a successful doctor-patient relationship. It encourages the patient to share more information, trust the doctor and continue follow ups or treatments with the doctor. If the doctor responds well, the patient becomes comfortable in sharing more sensitive information. However, some doctors may disregard the needs and information provided by their patients if they think highly of their own skills. It could be even worse if the doctors hold specific biases towards the patient's race, socioeconomic status, culture and gender (Street et al., 2005).

Another aspect is *medical mistrust*. If the patients have little confidence in the doctor or the treatment, they are likely not to follow the doctor's advice and be hesitant in sharing information. This can negatively affect the relationship (Cuevas et al., 2019). Moreover, switching doctors from time to time decreases the quality of care as the doctor-patient relationship is best established by continuity of care. This is rather difficult in integrated care where several care providers and levels of care are involved (Gröne & Garcia-Barbero, 2002).

Since the patient is an equal partner, the bad behaviour of the patient can also have a negative impact on the relationship. For instance, being rude or unnecessarily aggressive can intimidate the doctor, who may likely make mistakes (Riskin et al., 2017). The doctors are normally expected to carry out their job properly but rudeness or bad patient behaviour affect their routines to even perform simple tasks plus impairs the capability to work in critical conditions. Although it is normal for the patients to go through emotions especially during difficult times, under stress or for other reasons, misbehaviour can negatively impact doctor's work and treatment.

27.5 Models of Doctor-Patient Relationship

Years back, Szasz and Hollender (1956) touched on three basic models of the doctor-patient relationship including active–passive model, guidance-cooperation model and mutual participation model. The active–passive model, the oldest of the three, shows power differences between doctors and patients (Chipidza et al., 2015; Eustice, 2020). The patient seeks assistance and information while the doctor makes decisions for the patient. It is most suited during an emergency or when the patient is dazed as it is based on the doctor acting 'upon' the patient (Chipidza et al., 2015). Seeking consent is often forgone in such situations. The guidance-cooperation model, the most prevalent in current medical practice, is when the patient complies with the doctor's advice simply because of the doctor's medical knowledge and the belief that the best interest of the patient prevails (Chipidza et al., 2015; Eustice, 2020). The mutual participation model adopts equal partnership between the patient and the physician. In this model, the patient is perceived as the expert of oneself and therefore, important to be involved in considering treatment options. The doctor pays attention to the needs of the patient and acts accordingly. Both the patient and doctor are respectful of each other's views, expectations and values (Eustice, 2020).

There has been a push for the mutual participation model over the last decades, and understandably so, but application of the models is based on the situations (Chipidza et al., 2015). The effectiveness of the treatment is absolutely dependent on how well the patient is complying with the doctor's plan (Eustice, 2020; Kaba & Sooriakumaran, 2007). Better adherence to treatment is achieved when there is competence and communication in the doctor-patient relationship.

27.6 Doctor-Patient Relationship and Artificial Intelligence

Doctor-patient relationship has evolved to a more patient-centred relationship with technology and automation being increasingly used to improve conventional medicine. However, there is still skepticism about the integration of artificial intelligence (AI) into current medical practice (Aminololama-Shakeri & López, 2019; So et al., 2021). It is believed that AI may provide richer and detailed information about treatment options and intended outcomes but some people worry that the value of human interaction would decline with increased application of technology in achieving diagnostic and treatment accuracy (Aminololama-Shakeri & López, 2019; Nagy & Sisk, 2020).

Doctors have the clinical expertise while the patients have input on matters concerning personal values and preferences. With AI, the doctor-patient relationship will see an upgrade with access to a substantial amount of information, and most importantly, the physicians will be exempted from doing tedious and time-consuming tasks, namely documentation (Aminololama-Shakeri & López, 2019). According to the former chairperson of *Alphabet*, Eric Schmidt, if the AI is implemented, it could allow full concentration on patient engagement as well as assistance with health options for treatment. It could actually allow physicians to be more attentive and listen carefully to their patients instead of being partially occupied with note taking for documentation, thus giving the physicians more time to engage in genuine relationship building (Nagy & Sisk, 2020).

The care of patients is personal. The humanistic approach should remain although it is likely the doctor-patient relationship will be dismissed 'in the name of efficiency, accuracy or cost reduction' (Nagy & Sisk, 2020). This is why when incorporating AI, a step-by-step approach should be followed for the development in the healthcare system to remain consistent with the needs of the patients.

27.7 Elderly Care

Ageing brings physical, psychological, social, economic and lifestyle changes (Williams et al., 2007). There can be drastic changes in social networks and social support with time, specifically from retirement, deaths of friends and family or moving to old age institutions. Moreover, a decline in mobility decreases opportunities for social involvement and puts the elderly at risk of loneliness, stress and depression. Previous studies have found that those with good social support have better health and cognitive functioning, and tend to live longer (Williams et al.,

2007). Psychologically, the older population displays depressive symptoms twice as much as the general population. It is worse when other problems such as limited healthcare coverage, disability, low income and poor health co-exist.

Older people visit their physicians more often than the general population. Hence, they have a higher chance to establish a successful doctor-patient relationship (Williams et al., 2007). The emotional and affective support through effective communication in clinical consultations alongside biomedical information can greatly improve patients' health outcomes. The Accreditation Council for Graduate Medical Education identifies doctor-patient communication and interpersonal skills as one of six areas of medical competence (Al-Temimi et al., 2016). It helps to build a successful relationship between doctors and patients and prevents discrepancy arising from decoding the same information differently. For older patients, effective and empathic communication is an essential part of treatment in addition to having appropriate access to medical services as it serves as a crucial link to health and adaptation to the ageing process (Williams et al., 2007). Many are even interested in discussing end-of-life matters with their doctors (Balaban, 2000). Thus, the quality of doctor-patient relationship is essential for not only people who are dying and their loved ones but also the responsible service providers (Janssen & MacLeod, 2012).

However, effective communication varies across cultures. For instance, in the Chinese culture, consent in medical practice is not only given by the individual patient but also by the family. Many do not even know the final wishes of the family member who is critically ill because communication within one's own family is not very effective (Li, 2013). Furthermore, religious views of the patients or their loved ones on the matter of end-of-life care may differ. Those following Confucian way of life is expected of filial piety. Grown up children should fulfil their duty by bearing the medical expenses and saving the parents. The topic of death is not taken nicely, and this forbids the doctor to discuss the patient's death with the family. In short, it is not easy to establish an effective doctor-patient relationship in terms of communication, but the patients and their loved ones definitely trust the skills of the doctor.

27.8 Professional Ethics in Care

A doctor-patient relationship is deemed the core component in the ethical principles of medicine (Smith, 2019). The doctor tends to a patient's medical needs through check-up, diagnosis and treatment, and therefore, owes a great responsibility towards the management of ailment and successful relationship building. Thus, professional ethics in care is crucial. Ethical values apply to all healthcare workers. The nursing code of ethics by the American Nurses Association (ANA) can be referred to understand what is expected of them. According to the ANA, the code of ethics, believed to have been founded in 1893 and modified several times with the recent change in 2015 (Gaines, 2020), is a guide for carrying out responsibilities in a consistent manner with quality and the ethical obligations of the profession (Epstein & Turner, 2015).

The four main principles of the code of ethics are autonomy, beneficence, justice and non-maleficence (Gaines, 2020). Autonomy is accepting the patient's right to decision-making provided that the patient has received all the information and alternatives to consider, including all potential risks or complications and outcomes. The care plan is then designed based on the medical needs of the patient. It is essential that the needs are supported by care providers for better patient outcomes. Factors that may determine the outcomes include age, gender, cultural, general health, sexual orientation and social support system. Beneficence is having consideration for others and showing kindness in your actions. Justice is about fairness in medical decisions and care regardless of an individual's gender, race, religion, sexual orientation and financial abilities. Lastly, non-maleficence is not to do any harm especially in times of choosing intervention and care for the best possible outcome. This ensures the safety of the patient as well as proper care delivery. When a patient shows suicidal or homicidal signs, it should immediately be reported and the cause be identified.

27.9 Vulnerabilities in Elderly Care

Physicians have been criticised quite often for their insensitive behaviour, for disregarding ethics and for lacking empathy (Panda, 2006). Knowledge is futile if there is no empathy or concern for the patients. Sadly, neglect and abuse of elders is an ongoing issue in many care institutions (Nordström & Wangmo, 2018). Elderly are vulnerable due to their cognitive, physical and verbal limitations, thus are more likely to be mistreated. A study conducted to find out more about the quality of care provided to older patients in nursing homes, geriatrics institutions and ambulant care in Switzerland found that overstraining work demands on the carers often led to incidences of neglect, error and even abuse (Nordström & Wangmo, 2018).

The other areas seen to be affecting the communication between the doctors and elderly patients are stereotypes and prejudices, regression, transference, countertransference and resistance, rapport, empathy and paternalism (Turabian, 2020). Firstly, the physicians may hold unconscious or unintended biases against the term *elderly* which will inevitably lead to discriminatory practices. It is unfortunate that old age is negatively viewed in society which can affect the diagnoses, communication and treatment. Secondly, elderly patients misuse regression by acting immature or seeking continuous attention due to their disease but this can affect the doctor-patient relationship. Thirdly, transference denotes how the older patients feel about the doctor and it can be positive or negative. Countertransference is about the emotional reactions of the doctors towards the patients, and resistance appears when the reactions of the patients go against the doctors and will have a negative impact on the relationship. Fourthly, rapport is being composed during the period of treatment, when the doctor is constantly smiling, being optimistic and patient. If the physician fails to do these, it would be hard to connect with the patient. There is also empathy, which is extremely important when communicating with elderly patients to have a better understanding of the patient's feelings. The lack of empathy takes away opportunities to communicate and recognise their limitations. Lastly, elderly patients are willing to accept the doctor's authority which increases the risk of doctors acting with paternalism. This may lead to making medical decisions without consent, and ignoring the patient's needs and plans. All these should be considered and avoided if communication and relationship building is negatively affected.

In Hong Kong, older adults are encouraged to live independently at home (Lam, 2020). For those who are unable to do so, due to justifiable reasons, are instead put into residential care institutions, namely 'Hostels for the Elderly, Homes for the Aged, Care and Attention and Homes for the Elderly and Nursing Homes'. However, between 2007 and 2018, the demand for these care homes was very high with the average waiting time being about 33 months. Due to the growing number of medical incidents, especially abuses against the elderly, the government has introduced a voluntary certification scheme for elderly care homes to enhance their service standards and establish a practical management system (Zhao, 2018).

The world's population aged 60 and above is expected to reach two billion by 2050. 80 per cent of them will be from low and middle income countries (World Health Organization, 2018). It is essential to align health systems with the needs of older populations and support healthy ageing (Nordström & Wangmo, 2018), and understanding the common health conditions associated with ageing which include diabetes, dementia, depression, hearing loss, chronic diseases and cataracts. To improve monitoring and understanding, and professionalism, early education, continuous training, better management and response are recommended.

27.10 Impact and Suggestions to Foster Doctor-Patient Relationship in Aged Care

Communication between the older patients and their doctors has a positive impact on patient's satisfaction, adherence to clinical management and other health-related outcomes (Williams et al., 2007). The two parties form a relationship which can be remedial for the older patients. They seek emotional support while the physicians engage in open communication and address health-related problems. The doctors can also assist the elderly with daily tasks, for instance, 'simplifying complex treatment regimens', organising medicine and encouraging physical movements.

In China, it has been reported that the doctor-patient relationship has improved significantly during the period of COVID-19 outbreak (Gao & Dong, 2020). With better patient compliance, increased trust and respect, and competent medical staff, China responded quickly to the COVID-19 pandemic. There were no conflicts between the physicians and the patients, and the patients showed great respect indicating that they were able to trust their doctors during major public emergencies. Such doctor-patient relationships in China are usually looked into in three aspects. The first is related to societal reasons, such as the government, investment in healthcare and the health insurance system. The second is the provision of medical care such as clinical management systems, treatment options, physician–patient communication and staff competency. The third is patient satisfaction such as communication and behaviour, and management channels. The pandemic has demonstrated the harmonious relationship between the doctors and patients but it is important to keep the three aspects in mind for further improvement.

27.10.1 Overcoming Vulnerabilities in Ageing

It is always difficult to cater for every need of the elderly patients but there are ways for health professionals to support the older patients to overcome challenges and vulnerabilities related to ageing. Firstly, having guidelines for effective management of care for the older patient so that both parties work together to achieve the health goals and improve quality of life for the elderly (Williams et al., 2007). It is not just about speaking to patients, it is actually paying attention and listening (Cerretani, 2018). The doctor can learn about the patients from their nonverbal cues too. Secondly, the patients should report their health status, previous experiences and current challenges with the aim to reveal more than what is already known to the doctors (Williams et al., 2007). Older patients in particular may forget to share all information and this is why having reminded them from time to time can help the patients to recall details. Moreover, patients are likely to disclose more information if the patient-centred communication style is adopted but the cultural and generational factors may affect the patients' health behaviours (Ashton et al., 2003; Cerretani, 2018). Thirdly, communication competence of the health professionals should be regularly evaluated, either by surveys or interviews (Williams et al., 2007). The evaluation aims to understand and review the gaps and weaknesses in the communication so as to seek ways to improve. Patients are likely to respond positively if the physicians sound optimistic or hopeful of the patient's health outcomes (Cerretani, 2018). Fourthly, as mentioned earlier, older patients are prone to depression. Thus, the physicians should be able to identify signs of depression in their patients and start treatment early. For this reason, training should be provided to physicians working with older patients in order to enhance their familiarity and understanding of the conditions of the elderly (Williams et al., 2007). Lastly, health institutions should provide an in-service training to staff with emphasis on the communication and interpersonal skills to increase their awareness and to serve the patients with better care. At the same time, patients also play a major role in the communication and can be trained to be effective partners. A study has found that trained doctors provide more information, are more compliant in their care and have better outcomes as opposed to those not trained (Adelman et al., 2000).

27.11 Concluding Remarks

Doctor-patient relationship is a keystone of care. Medicine has progressed scientifically but it is mainly evolved based on human values and intuition without which it would be useless or even detrimental. A healthy doctor-patient relationship is dependent on communication and trust. The four key elements of the relationship are trust, mutual knowledge, regard and loyalty. There are other aspects as well, depending on the needs and preferences of both the patients and the physicians. The three models of the doctor-patient relationship include the active–passive model, guidance-cooperation model and mutual participation model. There has been a push for the mutual participation model over the last decades but application of the models is based on the situations. With the doctor-patient relationship being more patient-centred, it is believed that artificial intelligence would provide richer and detailed information on the patient's treatment options and goals. The doctor-patient relationship will see an upgrade with access to a substantial amount of information, and most importantly, the physicians will be exempted from doing tedious and time-consuming tasks namely documentation.

Ageing brings physical, psychological, social, economic and lifestyle changes. Older patients visit their physician more often than the general population, hence having a higher chance to establish a successful doctor-patient relationship. Communication between the older patients and their doctors has a positive impact on patient's satisfaction, adherence to treatment and other health-related outcomes. For older patients, effective and empathic communication is an essential part of treatment in addition to having appropriate access to medical services as it serves as a crucial link to health and adaptation to the ageing process. Older adults are vulnerable due to their cognitive, physical and verbal limitations, thus are more likely to be mistreated. To improve monitoring and understanding, and professionalism in elderly care, early education, continuous training, better management and response are recommended for the achievement of ageing with dignity and humanistic approaches.

References

Adelman, R. D., Greene, M. G., & Ory, M. G. (2000). Communication between older patients and their physicians. *Clinics in Geriatric Medicine, 16*(1), 1–24. https://doi.org/10.1016/S0749-0690(05)70004-5

Al-Temimi, M., Kidon, M., & Johna, S. (2016). Accreditation council for graduate medical education core competencies at a community teaching hospital: Is there a gap in awareness?. *The Permanente Journal, 20*(4). https://doi.org/10.7812/TPP/16-067

Aminololama-Shakeri, S., & López, J. E. (2019). The doctor-patient relationship with artificial intelligence. *American Journal of Roentgenology, 212*(2), 308–310. https://doi.org/10.2214/AJR.18.20509

Ashton, C. M., Haidet, P., Paterniti, D. A., Collins, T. C., Gordon, H. S., O'Malley, K., Peterson, L. A., Sharf, B. F., Suarez-Almazor, M. E., Wray, N. P., & Street, R. L. (2003). Racial and ethnic disparities in the use of health services. *Journal of General Internal Medicine, 18*(2), 146–152. https://doi.org/10.1046/j.1525-1497.2003.20532.x

Balaban, R. B. (2000). A physician's guide to talking about end-of-life care. *Journal of General Internal Medicine, 15*(3), 195–200. https://doi.org/10.1046/j.1525-1497.2000.07228.x

Cerretani, J. (2018, June 5). *How to foster a good doctor-patient relationship.* https://www.volusonclub.net/empowered-womens-health/how-to-foster-a-good-doctor-patient-relationship/

Chandra, S., Mohammadnezhad, M., & Ward, P. (2018). Trust and communication in a doctor-patient relationship: A literature review. *Journal of Healthcare Communications, 3*(3), 36. https://doi.org/10.4172/2472-1654.100146

Chipidza, F. E., Wallwork, R. S., & Stern, T. A. (2015). Impact of the doctor-patient relationship. *The Primary Care Companion for CNS Disorders, 17*(5). https://doi.org/10.4088/PCC.15f01840

Cuevas, A. G., O'Brien, K., & Saha, S. (2019). Can patient-centered communication reduce the effects of medical mistrust on patients' decision making? *Health Psychology, 38*(4), 325. https://doi.org/10.1037/hea0000721

Epstein, B., & Turner, M. (2015). The nursing code of ethics: Its value, its history. *OJIN: The Online Journal of Issues in Nursing, 20*(2), 1–10. https://doi.org/10.3912/OJIN.Vol20No02Man04

Eustice, C. (2020). *The Doctor-patient relationship.* https://www.verywellhealth.com/the-doctor-patient-relationship-188050

Gaines, K. (2020, September 4). *What is the nursing code of ethics?* Nurse.org. https://nurse.org/education/nursing-code-of-ethics/#:~:text=According%20to%20the%20American%20Nurses,how%20a%20person%20will%20conduct.

Gao, B., & Dong, J. (2020). Does the impact of COVID-19 improve the doctor-patient relationship in China? *The American Journal of the Medical Sciences, 360*(3), 305–306. https://doi.org/10.1016/j.amjms.2020.05.039

Gröne, O., & Garcia-Barbero, M. (2002). *Trends in integrated care: Reflections on conceptual issues.* World Health Organization.

Janssen, A., & MacLeod, R. D. (2012). Who cares for whom? Reciprocity of care at the end of life. *Journal of Palliative Care & Medicine, 2*(7). https://doi.org/10.4172/2165-7386.1000129

Kaba, R., & Sooriakumaran, P. (2007). The evolution of the doctor-patient relationship. *International Journal of Surgery, 5*(1), 57–65. https://doi.org/10.1016/j.ijsu.2006.01.005

Lam, G. (2020). Problems encountered by elders in residential care services in Hong Kong. *Asian Education and Development Studies.* https://doi.org/10.1108/AEDS-09-2019-0158

Li, L. B. (2013). Clinical review: Ethics and end-of-life care for critically ill patients in China. *Critical Care, 17*(6), 1–5. https://doi.org/10.1186/cc13140

Nagy, M., & Sisk, B. (2020). How will artificial intelligence affect patient-clinician relationships? *AMA Journal of Ethics, 22*(5), 395–400. https://doi.org/10.1001/amajethics.2020.395

Nordström, K., & Wangmo, T. (2018). Caring for elder patients: Mutual vulnerabilities in professional ethics. *Nursing Ethics, 25*(8), 1004–1016.

Panda, S. C. (2006). Medicine: Science or art? *Mens Sana Monographs, 4*(1), 127. https://doi.org/10.4103/0973-1229.27610

Plesničar, B. K. (2016). Relationship between a doctor and a patient with mental disorder. *Medicine, Law & Society, 9*(1), 11–19. https://doi.org/10.18690/24637955.9.1.11-19

Riskin, A., Erez, A., Foulk, T. A., Riskin-Geuz, K. S., Ziv, A., Sela, R., Pesach-Gelblum, L., & Bamberger, P. A. (2017). Rudeness and medical team performance. *Pediatrics, 139*(2). https://doi.org/10.1542/peds.2016-2305

Robertson-Jones, T. A., Tissue, M. M., Connolly, M., Gallups, S. F., Bender, C. M., & Rosenzweig, M. Q. (2019). Exploring racial differences in patient centeredness of care (PCC) during breast cancer (BC) chemotherapy clinical visits. *Journal of Racial and Ethnic Health Disparities, 6*(1), 94–100. https://doi.org/10.1007/s40615-018-0503-0

Selinger, C. P. (2009). The right to consent: Is it absolute?. *British Journal of Medical Practitioners, 2*(2).

Smith, Y. (2019, June 20). *Doctor–patient relationship.* https://www.news-medical.net/health/DoctorPatient-Relationship.aspx

So, K. H., Ting, C. W., Lee, C. P., Lam, T. T. N., Chiang, S. C., & Cheung, Y. T. (2021). Medication management service for old age homes in Hong Kong using information technology, automation technology, and the Internet of things: Pre-post interventional study. *JMIR Medical Informatics, 9*(2), e24280. https://doi.org/10.2196/24280

Street Jr, R. L., Gordon, H. S., Ward, M. M., Krupat, E., & Kravitz, R. L. (2005). Patient participation in medical consultations: Why some patients are more involved than others. *Medical Care*, 960–969.

Szasz, T. S., & Hollender, M. H. (1956). A contribution to the philosophy of medicine: The basic models of the doctor-patient relationship. *AMA Archives of Internal Medicine, 97*(5), 585–592. https://doi.org/10.1001/archinte.1956.00250230079008

Turabian, J. (2019). Doctor-patient relationship and multimorbidity: The more extraordinary a case seems, the easier it is to solve it. *Archives Family Medicine General Practice, 4*(1), 82–89. https://doi.org/10.36959/577/487

Turabian, J. L. (2020). Psychological phenomena in the doctor-Elderly patient relationship. *Archives of Psychiatry and Mental Health, 4*, 19–23. https://doi.org/10.29328/journal.apmh.1001013

Williams, S. L., Haskard, K. B., & DiMatteo, M. R. (2007). The therapeutic effects of the physician-older patient relationship: effective communication with vulnerable older patients. *Clinical Interventions in Aging, 2*(3), 453–467. https://www.ncbi.nlm.nih.gov/pmc/articles/PMC2685265/

World Health Organization. (2018). *Ageing and health.* https://www.who.int/news-room/fact-sheets/detail/ageing-and-health

Zhao, S. (2018, December 23). Certification system for elderly care homes to launch in next 3 months. *South China Morning Post*. https://www.scmp.com/news/hong-kong/society/article/2179268/certification-system-hong-kongs-elderly-care-homes-launch.

Chapter 28
Quality Assurance in Long-Term and Community Elderly Care Services

Tiffany C. H. Leung and Ray Choy

Abstract The ageing population has increasingly become global social issues to be seriously addressed by healthcare regulators, profit service providers and social service operators in both developed and developing economies. However, there are a number of negative news, such as patient abuse scandals, violation of human rights and data privacy, that pose operational implications in the healthcare sector, and even long-term and community care services for older adults. Contemporary performance measurement systems (CPMS) could be regarded as a management system to record the service quality indicators, thus assisting senior management to control, monitor, and review the organisational performance. Quality assurance (QA) in long-term and community care services for older adults is a series of assessments within an external accreditation scheme to enhance quality service to service users. This chapter is to provide a brief overview of the recent development for QA in long-term and quality indicators for community care services of older adults in the extant literature. There are some practical implications for healthcare regulators, the private sector and non-profit service providers in long-term and community care services for older adults in Hong Kong, to reflect the current services and identify possible improvements in the future.

Keywords Quality assurance · Performance measurement systems · Community care services for older adults

28.1 Introduction

There are four demographic megatrends, including population growth, population ageing, migration, and urbanisation that are critical data to monitor global population progress in order to achieve Sustainable Development Goals (SDGs) by 2030 (United

T. C. H. Leung (✉)
Faculty of Business, City University of Macau, Macau, China
e-mail: tiffanyleung@cityu.mo

R. Choy
Department of Innovative Social Work, City University of Macau, Macau, China
e-mail: raychoy@cityu.mo

V. T. S. Law and B. Y. F. Fong (eds.), *Ageing with Dignity in Hong Kong and Asia*, Quality of Life in Asia 16, https://doi.org/10.1007/978-981-19-3061-4_28

Nations, 2019a). Thus, accurate and timely population data allow governments to forecast demographic trends and develop appropriate government policies, financial planning, and social protection to meet the long-term goals. The global ageing population has increasingly become global social issues to be seriously addressed by healthcare regulators and service providers in both developed and developing economies. One in 11 people in the world was over aged 65 in 2019, while one in six people will be over age 65 by 2050 (United Nations, 2019a). There are three major demographic drivers of the ageing population: declining fertility rates, the technological advancement, and the overall improvement, and increase in longevity of the older adults (United Nations, 2020). In particular, the potential impact of ageing population on labour market and the fiscal pressure of governments reserve pension funds, public healthcare systems, and social security schemes for the older adults will be faced by various countries (United Nations, 2019b). Policymakers, healthcare academics, and care service providers for older adults in different countries should take immediate measures in addressing the increasing demand of the ageing population in the next few decades (Ng et al., 2018a, 2018b).

Policymakers need to address the global ageing population with long-term care and social welfare and consider allocating of long-term healthcare services mainly provided by the local government, the private sector, or mixed models. According to Eurofound's report (2017), nursing and residential care facilities provided by the public sector in European countries have gradually decreased more than that of the private sector in the past decades. To have continuous improvement on the service quality, ensure individual health and safety and cost-effectiveness, policymakers tend to allow the open market competition to enhance the efficiency of operation management and effectiveness of the long-term care service providers. The quasi-markets for the long-term care services might be delivered in more efficient way with a lower operating cost which may imply with a low-quality service (Garavaglia et al., 2011; Zigante & King, 2019). However, the quality of such services was previously difficult to measure and assess without an established framework. Recently, health equity and quality of care have been increasingly regarded as the two important factors for healthcare quality assurance (QA) in European countries (Cookson et al., 2018). Leichsenring et al. (2013) contend that the major concern of policymakers is to control fiscal budget and financial resource rather than improve service quality and promote QA for the public interest.

It is important for long-term care service providers to have accurate, timely, and relevant information about service users' expectations, satisfactions, and identify possible room for improvement. With the independent third-party, accreditation and certification for long-term care service providers could ensure and enhance the service quality for service users and their family members (Lee, 2017). Previous studies have not widely examined the performance management of community care services for older adults in general and in Asia Pacific region in particular (Ng et al., 2018a, 2018b). Thus, this chapter provides a brief overview of the recent development for QA in long term and community care services for older adults in Hong Kong.

This chapter is broadly divided into three main sections. After the introduction, the second section introduces a general understanding of the main concepts of QA in long-term care, quality indicators or instruments to measure service quality in long-term care and provides a brief overview of QA framework for the older adults in Hong Kong. Finally, conclusion will be provided at the last section.

28.2 Main Concepts of Quality Assurance in Long-Term Care

QA is generally defined as the 'activity of third parties to ensure and certify defined quality criteria from an external perspective' (Bauer et al., 2006 cited in Nies et al. 2013). QA is often considered as an important assessment of quality management to deliver good quality of services or products in business operation (Zigante & King, 2019). The commonly used principle in QA is the Plan-Do-Check-Act (PDCA) framework which was proposed by Dr Edward Deminin in 1950s (Jonge et al., 2011). This framework has been widely used in various industries to identify the continuous improvement. However, in the case of long-term care services, the local government will act as the service purchasers or act on behalf of the service users to provide an important governance of QA (Huber et al., 2008). The QA highly depends on how to set the standards, monitor quality performance, and impose punishment when quality standards are failed to meet the minimum requirements (Malley et al., 2015). Thus, the implementation of QA could be considered as a long-term process (Jonge et al., 2011).

Governments or healthcare regulatory bodies tend to be the main regulator of service quality in the long-term care to ensure the safety of service users, maintain quality control, and compliance of public or private healthcare providers (Zigante & King, 2019). The main purpose of QA is to protect the service users and ensure accountability for public financial resources in long-term care (Zigante & King, 2019). The general standards of QA often include staff ratio, living environment, and care provision governance, but the outcome-based standards are widely adopted in the field and tend to focus on quality of life, human rights, and dignity (Zigante & King, 2019).

Registration, licence, and certification are often considered as service accreditation systems which are minimum and optimal standards to operate in the long-term care market (Zigante & King, 2019). This service accreditation is largely based on the evaluation of the service quality offered by service providers, concentrating on capability, competency, and reliability of the regular assessment items (Evans & Lindsay, 2017). The requirements for service accreditation are generally seen as uniform, but such requirements may vary greatly based on different healthcare settings, such as nursing homes, residential home care services, or private nursing homes combined with medical care (Zigante & King, 2019). The service accreditation process is typically divided into two sections: internal and external reviews. The service providers will submit the supporting documents and other supplement information to the review panel, while the external reviewers evaluate the service providers by various assessment criteria and different assessment forms, such as internal reviews, on-site visits, and interviews with staff members, service users, and their family members (Zigante & King, 2019).

28.3 Quality Indicators or Instruments to Measure Service Quality in Long-Term Care

To enhance good quality care, local governments, and healthcare regulatory agencies could choose three general types of policy instruments: regulatory, economic, and information-based instruments (Malley et al., 2015). First, regulatory instruments are often considered as formal rules and regulations in mandatory practices to promote good quality care, while informal rules tend to be found in voluntary practices (i.e. healthcare organisations are free to choose whether to apply accreditation scheme or not) (Malley et al., 2015). However, various types of regulations could lead to unintended consequences or unforeseen outcomes, such as the narrow-mind vision from the senior management (i.e. service providers highly concentrate on what QA matrix is measured rather than providing good quality of service to users), excessive focus on short-term results rather than long-term goals, and choosing less risky clients in order to meet the QA standards (Zigante & King, 2019). Second, economic instruments are often seen as financial incentives, such as government grants, quality-related subsidies, and reimbursement schemes, which appear to reward service providers for spending financial resources to further improve good service quality care in the organisations and meet benefits from the ongoing QA initiatives (Jonge et al., 2011; Zigante & King, 2019). Nevertheless, with such economic incentive schemes, the public service purchasers will impose more quality assessment criteria on their selection process and expect service providers to maintain both service quality at a competitive price in the market (Zigante & King, 2019). Third, information-based instruments are intended to change behaviour of both care users and service providers through different assessment tools, such as quality management systems, knowledge management schemes, and public reporting with the independent third-party assurance (Zigante & King, 2019). This instrument is often seen as education and knowledge management that could highly encourage service providers to adopt the best practice and guideline in the industry to offer good service quality to service users (Malley et al., 2015).

The healthcare service quality indicators vary greatly across jurisdictions and there are no uniform, universal, and comprehensive quality indicators (Jonge et al., 2011). The frequently used measurement items or indicators for service quality have been widely examined in the extant academic literature (Garavaglia et al., 2011; Jonge et al., 2011; Jun et al., 1998; Kalepu, 2014; Lee et al., 2013). Thus, the classic quality indicators could be broadly divided into three types: indicators of structural quality, process indicators, and outcome indicators which is known as the Structure, Process and Outcome (SPO) framework (Donabedian, 1980; Jun et al., 1998). However, quality indicators have evolved over time and have been modified by different scholars in this field (Evans & Lindsay, 2017; Lee et al., 2013). First, indicators of structural quality are widely adopted in long-term care (Donabedian, 1980). These indicators are the major staff and physical characteristics of the service providers, the tangible resources, and the physical settings (including the qualifications of staff members, the employee training levels, and the average number of empty beds) (Garavaglia et al., 2011; Jonge et al., 2011; Zigante & King, 2019). Second, process indicators often refer to the major indicators of the interpersonal interaction between care workers and healthcare users for the service care, such as punctuality, feeding skills, and showering procedure (Jonge et al., 2011; Zigante & King, 2019). Third, outcome indicators are often associated with service users' health status and client satisfaction which have widely received attention in the academic literature (Jonge et al., 2011). Prevalence of injury, falls, and symptoms of depression are included. However, there is a lack of reliable information or richness of data source in the database for efficiency assessment of outcome-related indicators (Garavaglia et al., 2011). In addition, there are three main factors that may affect the outcome indicators: (i) service users may be managed by different healthcare providers, (ii) variance in outcome indicators due to different assessment methods, and (iii) observed differences due to different healthcare providers (Jonge et al., 2011).

The Adult Social Care Outcome Toolkit (ASCOT) measure has made the leading indicator to link the service outcome of the long-term care (Forder et al., 2018). The ASCOT is a set of indicators to measure the impact of service in relation to quality of life of service users, such as personal comfort, food and beverage, health and safety, social participation, accommodation cleanliness, and human dignity, while the indicators of carers include professional qualifications, encouragement, and peer support (Zigante & King, 2019). However, it is difficult to measure and evaluate the outcome in healthcare service quality due to the long assessment period between healthcare service provision and the outcome after the service treatment (Choi et al., 2005). The ASCOT measure has been widely used in the UK and transferred to other European countries, such as Germany, France, Finland, and even in Japan (Zigante & King, 2019).

Other researchers suggest adopting SERVQUAL scale to assess the service quality in healthcare services (Headley & Miller, 1993). The global quality of service could be divided into five SERVQUAL domains: tangible resource (physical facilities, equipment, and appearance of staff members), reliability (delivery of quality service to patients independently and accurately), responsiveness (prompt service to clients), empathy (caring, attention, and consideration), and assurance (competence, courtesy, and credibility) (Parasuraman et al., 1985). Venkatapparao and Gopalakrishna (1995) state that the service outcome is the major concern for clients, while other studies highlight different aspects, such as staff behaviour (Alford, 1998), the perception of nurse caring (Larrabee et al., 2004), and personnel support and accessibility of the healthcare service (Otani et al., 2005). There are different assessment items to evaluate the service quality in healthcare services in the prior studies. Lee (2017) conducts a literature review in measurement items of healthcare service quality and suggests 11 commonly used standardised assessment items, including empathy of clients, responsiveness to users, reliability of service, health and safety, tangible resource, timeliness, accessibility of service, quality assurance, efficiency of operation, cost-effectiveness, and service improvement.

28.4 Quality Assurance Framework for Elderly Services in Hong Kong: An Overview

The Social Welfare Department (SWD) of the Hong Kong SAR Government together with non-governmental organisations (NGOs) provide social welfare services by using the government subventions mode, while the subvented and private sectors, to a lesser extent, offer the social services through service contract. The bulk of services for the older adults are largely rendered by the NGOs and the private sector.

The main purpose of services for the older adults in Hong Kong is to promote the health of the older adults by offering a wide range of social services to enable them to live longer and to offer residential care services that accommodate the different social needs of the ageing population (Social Welfare Department, 2020a, 2020c). The SWD coordinates a number of community care services, such as residential care homes for the elderly (RCHEs) and other supporting healthcare services for the older adults. The main objective of the residential care services is to offer supporting facilities and services for the older adults aged 65 or above and could not fully look after themselves at home, and for those who have any individual issues, health concerns, social needs, and other particular reasons (Social Welfare Department, 2020a).

The 2020–2021 estimated expenditure of the SWD is HK$94,497 million.[1] In Hong Kong, the expenditure for services of the older adults is HK$12,266 million which is the second largest expenditure of social welfare (Social Welfare Department, 2020d). Out of this amount, HK$11,670 million (95%) is for the subvented/private sectors based on the Estimates of Expenditure under the SWD in 2020–21 (Social Welfare Department, 2020d). Due to the large amount of public expenditure and accountability of the use of government funding, it is the responsibility of the SWD to monitor the subvented services and to set up a robust QA mechanism for the industry (Social Welfare Department, 2020d). The SWD assesses service providers based on a set of well-defined QA framework which can be divided into three sections: (i) service performance monitoring system (SPMS), (ii) legislation, licencing and regulation, and (iii) promoting good practice/best practice in service (Social Welfare Department, 2020d).

---

[1] The exchange rate between US dollars and Hong Kong dollars is around 1: 7.8.

28.4.1 Service Performance Monitoring System (SPMS)

For the SPMS, the SWD together with the NGOs operating subvented services offer cost-effective, accountable, and output-driven services for the service users. Service performance within the SPMS is often measured by the Funding and Service Agreements (FSAs) and Service Documents (SDs) prepared between the SWD and NGOs (Social Welfare Department, 2020b).

28.4.1.1 Funding and Service Agreements (FSAs)

NGOs are often required to observe and monitor the respective terms and agreements for various services as written in the FSAs and SDs. These documents generally define the major duties and responsibilities of the service providers. The major role of the SWD is to examine the service performance and standards of the service providers (Social Welfare Department, 2020b). Essential Service Requirements (ESRs) identify some essential features of the service infrastructure and they establish these requirements based on the type of service provided, such as professional qualifications of staff members, availability of suitable physical facilities, and compliance with relevant service manuals (Social Welfare Department, 2020b).

In particular, a number of Output Standards with certain levels of achievement is clearly identified in FSAs and SDs. Output Standards are in the quantitative indicators to measure the major activities in relation to the provision of a specific service, such as enrolment figures, number of registered service users, completion rate of individual healthcare plans, attendance rate, and number of organised events (Social Welfare Department, 2020b).

Regarding the intended outcome, Outcome Standards are expected to assess the efficiency of the service performance. These outcomes are often established based on the type of service provided and the raw data are systematically collected by the particular assessment tools, for example, surveys or identification of the similarity and difference between the results before and after receiving the service. Outcome Standards are normally related to the positive improvement of service users after the service provision, for example, supporting social network, skill and knowledge enhancement, and improved capability in family care management (Social Welfare Department, 2020b).

28.4.1.2 Service Quality Standards (SQSs)

SQSs often define the level of service provision and operation management that service operators are intended to achieve. The SQSs are established based on four major principles which are in line with the essential values of social welfare services. These four principles are: (i) to define the major objectives of the service and design the delivery mode transparent to the general public; (ii) to allocate tangible resources efficiently and continuous quality enhancement; (iii) to recognise and meet particular service users' expectations and needs; and (iv) to respect the rights of service users (Social Welfare Department, 2020b). Each of 16 SQSs is explained by a series of Criteria and Assessment Indicators. A number of handbooks, guidelines, and self-assessment checklist have been developed to assist service operators to adopt approaches for a particular service type in achieving the SQS standards.

28.4.1.3 Service Performance Assessment

Service operators offering subvented services are subject to the three main assessment of SPMS. First, service operators are needed to submit statistical report and self-assessment on ESRs periodically on their service units' achievement with reference to the Output Standards and Outcome Standards. In addition, Self-assessment Report on Service Performance have to be submitted. The SWD would examine all the relevant information against the agreed levels established in the service agreements. Second, a regular review visit or a surprise visit is paid which is the SWD's service performance evaluating activity to be organised at a service unit, with a view of checking the application of SQSs and ESRs. Third, on-site assessment is an intended visit arranged by the SWD, unannounced or at short notice, to analyse and evaluate the quality, and relevant issues to a service operator (Social Welfare Department, 2020b). In particular, on-site assessment is normally conducted to newly established service units and other units with identified service performance issues and problems in service operation. In order to make the assessment transparent and open, the Service Performance Monitoring System Performance Assessment Manual covering all the important features of the SPMS was published (Social Welfare Department, 2020b). As a whole, the current assessment methods highly encourage service providers to take greater responsibility and accountability for their operations, develop a mechanism to have early detection, monitoring, and intervention of poor service performance in order to maintain cost-effectiveness in service quality (Social Welfare Department, 2020b).

28.4.2 Legislation, Licencing, and Regulation

One of the most effective measures to keep, monitor, and enhance the quality of social welfare services is gate-keeping—to control who can provide the services. The SWD develops a licencing system to monitor and regulate RCHEs under the Residential Care Homes (Elderly Persons) Ordinance (Social Welfare Department, 2020a). The SWD through its Licensing and Regulation Branch and Licensing Office of RCHEs is mainly responsible for the registration or licencing schemes in respect of RCHEs to comply with the local regulation (Social Welfare Department, 2020a). The major purposes of licencing and regulation are to make sure that the RCHEs are in accordance with the legislative requirements to offer services at an acceptable standard. Similarly, the Branch implements not only the regulatory mechanism for the service operations of RCHEs, but also applies a number of measures to improve their service quality (Social Welfare Department, 2020a).

For the potential service operators, they are required to demonstrate, among others, the quality of service even before they provide the service. Since 2001, the SWD has introduced a competitive bidding scheme to choose suitable service operators to operate contract with RCHEs at purpose-built premises (Social Welfare Department, 2020a). The bidding exercises are normally opened to private service organisations and NGOs. In particular, the selection criteria place more emphasis on service quality.

28.4.3 Promoting Good Practice/Best Practice in Service Management

There is no doubt that a government department should play a vital role in regulatory and compliance work. However, it is the responsibility of every service provider and practitioner involved to build up and uphold quality of the service. In consultation of the industry operators, the SWD has published a range of good practice/best practice checklists, manuals, and SQS benchmarking reports. The purpose of such endeavours is to promote good practice and best practice in the service for the older adults.

As far as education and training for the practitioners is concerned, the competency standards required for different functional areas of the service of older adults were set up after industry-wide consultation. The competency standards serve as useful reference for design of training programmes and human resources development.

28.5 Concluding Remarks

This chapter introduces a general understanding of the main concepts of QA in long-term care, quality indicators or instruments to measure service quality in the long-term care, and provides a general overview of QA framework for the older adults in Hong Kong. The SWD in Hong Kong assesses service providers according to a set of well-defined QA framework, including (i) SPMS, (ii) legislation, licencing, and regulation, and (iii) promoting good practice/best practice in service.

There are some practical implications for policymakers, healthcare regulators, profit, and non-profit service providers in long-term and community care services for older adults in the Great Bay Area (GBA) of mainland China to reflect the current services and identify possible improvements in the future. The QA framework could help the older adults and their family members gain more confidence when choosing RCHEs and other supporting healthcare services. This study has three limitations and offers some suggestions for future research directions. First, this chapter provides a brief overview of QA in long-term and community care services for older adults in Hong Kong. However, this chapter has been confined to one city. The extent and nature of QA can vary across different provinces in China, institutional settings, and local regulation due to different economic, social, and political factors. Future studies could focus on the QA in long-term and community care services for older adults by comparing differences and similarities among different provinces in China and other Asian countries. Second, this chapter has been limited to the literature review and secondary data available in one city. Further empirical studies, quantitative studies, and longitudinal research could examine whether the QA in long-term and community care services for older adults could change over time. Third, this chapter has been confined to the QA in long-term and community care services for older adults. Future research could focus on the QA as the longitudinal study of the subvented and the non-subvented private sectors which could see the potential challenges or improvement over time.

References

Alford, B. L. (1998). Affect, attribution, and disconfirmation: Their impact on health care service evaluation. *Health Marketing Quarterly, 15*(4), 55–74. https://doi.org/10.1300/J026v15n04_04

Choi, K. S., Lee, H., Kim, C., & Lee, S. (2005). The service quality dimensions and patient satisfaction relationships in South Korea: Comparisons across gender, age and types of services. *Journal of Service Marketing, 19*(3), 140–149. https://doi.org/10.1108/08876040510596812

Cookson, R., Asaria, M., Ali, S., Shaw, R., Doran, T., & Goldblatt, P. (2018). Health equity monitoring for healthcare quality assurance. *Social Science and Medicine, 198*, 148–156. https://doi.org/10.1016/j.socscimed.2018.01.004

Donabedian, A. (1980). *The definition of quality and approaches to its assessment*. Health Administration Press.

Eurofound. (2017). *Care homes for older Europeans: Public, for-profit and non-profit providers*. Publications Office of the European Union. https://www.eurofound.europa.eu/publications/report/2017/care-homes-for-older-europeans-public-for-profit-and-non-profit-providers

Evans, J. R., & Lindsay, W. M. (2017). *Managing for quality and performance excellence*. South-Western Cengage Learning.

Forder, J. F., Vadean, S. R., & Malley, J. (2018). The impact of long-term care on quality of life. *Health Economics, 27*(3), 43–58. https://doi.org/10.1002/hec.3612

Garavaglia, G., Lettieri, E., Agasisti, T., & Lopez, S. (2011). Efficiency and quality of care in nursing homes: An Italian case study. *Health Care Management Science, 14*(1), 22–35. https://doi.org/10.1007/s10729-010-9139-2

Headley, D. E., & Miller, S. J. (1993). Measuring service quality and its relationship to future consumer behaviour. *Journal of Health Care Marketing, 13*(4), 32–41.

Huber, M., Maucher. M., & Sak, B. (2008). *Study on social and health services of general interest in the European Union*. European Centre for Social Welfare Policy and Research.

Jonge, V. D., Nicolaas, J. S., Van Leerdam, M. E., & Kuipers, E. J. (2011). Overview of the quality assurance movement in health care. *Best Practice and Research Clinical Gastroenterology, 25*(3), 337–347. https://doi.org/10.1016/j.bpg.2011.05.001

Jun, M., Peterson, R. T., & Zsidisin, G. A. (1998). The identification and measurement of quality dimensions in healthcare: Focus group interview results. *Healthcare Management Review, 23*(4), 81–96. https://doi.org/10.1097/00004010-199810000-00007

Kalepu, R. N. (2014). Service quality in healthcare sector: An exploratory study on hospitals. *The IUP Journal of Market Management, 13*(1), 7–28. https://ssrn.com/abstract=2494699

Larrabee, J. H., Ostrow, L., Withrow, M. L., Janney, M. A., Hobbs, R. G., Jr., & Burant, C. (2004). Predictors of patient satisfaction with inpatient hospital nursing care. *Research in Nursing and Health, 27*(4), 254–268. https://doi.org/10.1002/nur.20021

Leichsenring, K., Nies, H., & Van der Veen, R. (2013). The quest for quality in long-term care. In K. Leichsenring, J. Billings, & H. Nies (Eds.), *Long-term care in Europe* (pp. 167–190). Palgrave Macmillan.

Lee, S., Lee, D., & Olson, D. (2013). Health-care quality management using the MBHCP excellence model. *Total Quality Management and Business Excellence, 24*(1–2), 119–137. https://doi.org/10.1080/14783363.2012.728853

Lee, D. H. (2017). HEALTHQUAL: A multi-items scale for assessing healthcare service quality. *Service Business, 11*(3), 491–516. https://doi.org/10.1007/s11628-016-0317-2

Malley, J., Trukeschitz, B., & Trigg, L. (2015). Policy instruments to promote good quality long-term care services. In C. Gori, J. L. Fernandez & R. Wittenberg (Eds.), *Long-term care reforms in OECD countries: successes and failures* (pp. 167–194). Policy Press. https://doi.org/10.2307/j.ctt1t88zbz.12

Ng, A. W., Leung, T. C. H., & Ho, J. C. K. (2018a). Development of accreditation approach of elderly care service providers: Experience from East and West. In P. Yuen, A. W. Ng, & B. Fong (Eds.), *Sustainable health and long-term care solutions for an aging population* (pp. 126–144). IGI Global. https://doi.org/10.4018/978-1-5225-2633-9.ch007

Ng, A. W., Leung, T. C. H., & Tsang, K. T. (2018b). Social enterprise for elderly housing: policy for accountability and public-private responsible financing. *Population Ageing, 13,* 365–384. https://doi.org/10.1007/s12062-018-9235-5

Nies, H., R., van der Veen., & Leichsenring, K. (2013). Quality measurement and improvement in long-term care in Europe. In OECD Health Policy Studies (Ed.), *A Good life in old age? Monitoring and improving quality in long-term Care* (pp. 223–246). OECD Publishing.

Otani, K., Kurz, R., Harris, L., & Byrne, F. (2005). Managing primary care using patient satisfaction measures. *Journal of Healthcare Management, 50*(5), 311–325. https://pubmed.ncbi.nlm.nih.gov/16268410/

Parasuraman, A., Zeithaml, V., & Berry, L. (1985). A conceptual model of service quality and its implications for future research. *Journal of Marketing, 49*(4), 41–50. https://doi.org/10.2307/1251430

Social Welfare Department. (2020a). *Hong Kong: The facts—Social welfare.* https://www.swd.gov.hk/en/index/site_pubpress/page_fact/

Social Welfare Department. (2020b). *Service performance monitoring.* https://www.swd.gov.hk/en/index/site_ngo/page_serviceper/

Social Welfare Department. (2020c). *Service for the elderly.* https://www.swd.gov.hk/en/index/site_pubsvc/page_elderly/sub_introducti/

Social Welfare Department. (2020d). *Head 170 — Social Welfare. Department.* https://www.swd.gov.hk/storage/asset/section/4348/en/2021_22_Estimates_of_Expenditure_under_Social_Welfare_Department_(EN).pdf

United Nations. (2019a). *World population prospects 2019a: Highlight.* Department of Economic and Social Affairs – Population Division. https://population.un.org/wpp/Publications/Files/WPP2019a_Highlights.pdf

United Nations. (2019b). *The 2019b revision of world population prospects.* https://www.un.org/development/desa/publications/world-population-prospects-2019b-highlights.html

United Nations. (2020). *Ageing.* https://www.un.org/en/global-issues/ageing

Venkatapparao, M., & Gopalakrishna P. (1995). Mediators vs moderators of patient satisfaction. *Journal of Health Care Marketing, 15*(4), 16–21. https://pubmed.ncbi.nlm.nih.gov/10154639/

Zigante, V., & King, D. (2019). *Quality assurance practices in long-term care in Europe.* European Commission. https://doi.org/10.2767/167648

Chapter 29
Building an Effective Medication Management Service for the Older Adults in Hong Kong

Sau Chu Chiang, Cheuk Wun Ting, Kei Hong So, Yin Ting Cheung, Chui Ping Lee, Daisy Lee, and Gary Chung Hong Chong

Abstract The chapter delineates the practices, significance, and challenges in developing a safe medication management service for institutionalised and community-dwelling older adults. According to the United Nations, one in six people in the world will be aged over 65 by 2050. While a substantial proportion of the older adults live in the community, they are facing many medication-related problems including polypharmacy, non-compliance, failure to understand dosage instructions, and poor general medication knowledge. The traditional and manual medication handling process in Residential Care Homes for the Elderly (RCHEs) is also tedious, labour-intensive, and error-prone. The Hong Kong Pharmaceutical Care Foundation (HKPCF), a charitable organisation, has developed a system for medication management in RCHEs. Through the utilisation of information and communication technologies (ICT), a safer medication management plan can be developed. This chapter introduces two ICT-enabled medication management service models

S. C. Chiang (✉) · K. H. So
Hong Kong Pharmaceutical Care Foundation, Hong Kong, China
e-mail: scchiang@pcfhk.org

K. H. So
e-mail: kennethso@pcfhk.org

C. W. Ting · Y. T. Cheung · C. P. Lee
School of Pharmacy, Faculty of Medicine, The Chinese University of Hong Kong, Hong Kong, China
e-mail: cwfelixting@link.cuhk.edu.hk

Y. T. Cheung
e-mail: yinting.cheung@cuhk.edu.hk

C. P. Lee
e-mail: cplee@cuhk.edu.hk

D. Lee
School of Professional Education and Executive Development, The Hong Kong Polytechnic University, Hong Kong, China
e-mail: daisy.lee@cpce-polyu.edu.hk

G. C. H. Chong
Hospital Pharmacist, Hong Kong, China

V. T. S. Law and B. Y. F. Fong (eds.), *Ageing with Dignity in Hong Kong and Asia*, Quality of Life in Asia 16, https://doi.org/10.1007/978-981-19-3061-4_29

for the older adults living in both elderly homes and in the community, respectively. For elderly homes, the model focuses on the integration of an ICT-enabled drug dispensing process with the Automated Tablet Dispensing & Packaging System (ATDPS) and the Visiting Pharmacist Service (VPS) to achieve a more efficient and accurate workflow. For community-dwelling older adults, the model seeks to enable safe in-home drug administration by patients through the provision of a medication review and reconciliation service by pharmacists, medication repackaging into multi-dose pouches using ATDPS, and technology-assisted drug medication administration and monitoring using mobile apps. The chapter concludes with practical suggestions for the development of a sustainable ICT-enabled medication management service for the older adults to improve medication adherence to better control chronic diseases and related hospitalisations, and reduce the pressure on caretakers.

Keywords Medication management · Automation technology · Detachable tablet adapter · Intelligence-assisted checking · Information and communication technologies

29.1 Introduction

Based on the Hong Kong government's 2016 Population by census, the older adults—people aged 65 or above—made up 15% of the total population in Hong Kong. Of these older adults, 8.1% lived in non-domestic households, which included Residential Care Homes for the Elderly (RCHEs), with the remaining living alone or with family members in the community. As the percentage of the older adult population is expected to increase to 29% by mid-2036, an increase in the need for older adults' care in both RCHEs and the community is foreseeable (Census & Statistics Department, 2018). In this chapter, we will highlight the limitations of the existing medication management practices in Hong Kong's RCHEs. We will then describe the local experience in using information and communication technologies in medication management services at a number of RCHEs (case study I) and among community-dwelling older adults (case study II). Both the preliminary achievements and challenges of this programme will be discussed.

Case Study I: Building a Safe Medication Management Service for Residents in Elderly Homes in Hong Kong

I.1 The Importance in Developing a Safe Medication Management Service in Elderly Homes

I.1.1 The Medication Management Process in RCHEs

In RCHEs, medication management is a critical issue due to the prevalence of polypharmacy in individual older adult residents, as well as the complexity in handling medications for multiple older adult residents. The average number of residents per RCHE in Hong Kong ranges from 49 (25th percentile) to 118 (75th percentile). Statistics from past studies show that up to 92.7% of residents in RCHEs receive chronic medications, with 42.5% taking five or more different types of chronic medications (Census & Statistics Department, 2009). Since older adult residents in RCHEs tend to be more dependent on caregivers to assist in activities of daily living (ADLs), healthcare providers need to take greater responsibility for their medication management (Wilson et al., 2010). Nevertheless, since there is no legal requirement to include pharmacists or dispensing staff in the process, the medication management process becomes the daily responsibility of nursing staff (nurses and health workers) in RCHEs. Though health workers are considered to have a supporting role in the medication management process, they frequently assume primary responsibility when it comes to handling medications (Social Welfare Department, 2020). However, the only requirement to become a health worker in Hong Kong is to pass a training course approved by the Director of Social Welfare (Social Welfare Department, 2020). Approved courses must be at least 296 h in duration (courses are usually between 300–400 h), but only a small portion of the syllabus (12 h) is dedicated to medication management (Social Welfare Department, 2021). Compared with pharmacists, the inadequate training provided to health workers regarding medication poses a safety risk to older adults in RCHEs.

RCHEs collect residents' medications from various sources, such as public hospitals and clinics managed by the Hospital Authority (HA) and the Department of Health (DH), private hospitals, and private clinics operated by general practitioners (GPs) (Wong et al., 2013b). Among these sources, the HA is the major supplier of residents' medications. These are supplied in individual packs. The labelling information includes details such as the name of medication, the dosage, the frequency of administration, and the name of the patient for each medication. After collecting residents' medications, nursing staff in RCHEs register the medications based on the labelled information on in-house paper forms which are used as the medication administration record. Usually, there is no assistance from purpose-made information systems and the staff complete the forms manually or with typing on a spreadsheet. Each day, the nursing staff need to manually prepare the medications for the residents by putting the correct quantity of each medication into small medication cups marked with each resident's name. This is based on information received from various sources and registered in each resident's medication administration record. Another member of the nursing staff then checks the medications that have been prepared. During each medication round, nursing staff administer the medications and record the administration on the in-house paper forms.

The processes look simple but a single error in the medication management process could harm the vulnerable residents in these RCHEs. A local survey revealed that 36.8% of RCHEs administered the wrong drug to a resident at least once between 2005 and 2010 (Leung, 2012). In particular, the inadvertent administration of oral hypoglycaemic agents can have potentially fatal consequences. From June 2005 to March 2006, among the 23 cases of drug-induced hypoglycaemia detected by the Hospital Authority Toxicology Reference Laboratory, 9 of them were related to confirmed or suspected drug administration errors in RCHEs (Ching et al., 2006).

This problem persists even until now, as exemplified by a reported case of coma due to the inadvertent administration of an antidiabetic drug in 2020 (Mingpao, 2020). This worrying situation in RCHEs requires more attention and intervention from healthcare professionals.

I.1.2 The Limitations of the Existing Medication Management Process

The manual medication management process is laborious and time-consuming. Generally speaking, it takes an RCHE nursing staff member around 6 h to prepare medications for 100 residents. The manual handling of large quantities of medications and the use in-house paper forms places a huge burden on nursing staff, who also need to provide other care services to the residents of RCHEs. As a result of long working hours and a heavy workload, the turnover rate of nursing staff is very high with a vacancy rate of 18% (Labour & Welfare Bureau, 2017; Legislative Council, 2013). The shortage of RCHE staff members combined with the time pressures involved pose a threat to the safe administration of medications in RCHEs.

Given the enormous quantity of medications involved, storage and waste are also common problems in RCHEs. Owing to the heavy caseload in the public healthcare system, residents usually have long follow-up periods and receive at least 16 to 52 weeks of medications during each follow-up visit. Storing large quantities of medications is often a challenge within the limited space found in RCHEs. As medication regimens change frequently due to residents' changing medical conditions, it was estimated that more than 10 million units of oral solid medications were discarded annually in all RCHEs, and the total cost of wasted medications annually was over HK$5,800,000 (Wong et al., 2013a).

29.2 Introducing the Use of Information and Communication Technologies for Medication Management Services in Elderly Homes

Given the concerns regarding the existing (and rudimentary) medication management model, the introduction of Information and Communication Technologies (ICT) in the medication process is an obvious and inevitable solution to improve medication safety for older adults.

Residents' medication profiles in RCHEs are complicated and frequently change. To enable the more accurate (and efficient) input and retrieval of related information, an Information Technology (IT) system can be implemented to manage medication records. Unlike paper forms, IT systems allow information to be updated in real time. The use of IT systems is already a common practice in overseas nursing facilities. A study in the United States reported that electronic health records were adopted in 84% of 544 nursing homes surveyed (Vest et al., 2019). It has been demonstrated that IT systems in the healthcare sector help to reduce medication errors, enhance monitoring, and improve patient care (Chaudhry et al., 2006). In Hong Kong, though IT systems like the Clinical Management System (CMS), the Pharmacy Management System (PMS), and the Electronic Patient Record (ePR) are being used in hospital settings, the use of IT in RCHEs lags far behind.

The traditional model of medication management (the manual handling of numerous medications) for RCHE residents is error-prone and time-consuming. To facilitate the medication management process, automation technology (AT) is often adopted to replace manual medication dispensing and packaging to engender higher accuracy and efficiency. The medications for each resident during each medication round are packaged into separate drug pouches, a process which allows for the more accurate and safe administration of drugs. According to a study conducted by Beobide-Tellería et al. (2018), automated packaging reduced dispensing errors by 91% (pre: $n = 1{,}327$; post: $n = 1{,}398$) in seven nursing facilities in Spain. Automated packaging can either be unit-dose (one dose of medications packaged in one drug pouch) or multi-dose (multiple doses of medications for a resident at a particular time packaged in one drug pouch). While unit-dose packaging is commonly adopted in hospital inpatient settings for large-scale drug distribution, multi-dose packaging is usually preferred in RCHEs and community-care settings for individual, patient-based drug administration.

The use of paper forms to check and administer medications is the customary practice in RCHEs, a process that is both tedious and outdated. Instead of in-house paper forms, electronic medication administration records (eMARs) are more convenient for nursing staff. Simply using a mobile app, nursing staff can easily retrieve real-time updates and record drug administration during medication rounds. eMARs are also seen as a way to improve medication safety. For instance, Alenius and Graf reported a statistically significant reduction in the perceived risks of most types of medication errors after using eMARs in two nursing homes in Sweden (Alenius & Graf, 2016).

Different technologies can be interconnected to improve the existing medication management model. With the Internet of Things (IoT), which is defined as 'a network of intelligent objects that is capable of organising and sharing information, data and resources, decision making, and responding to feedback', information from various digital devices can be synchronised to develop a multifaceted network for the entire medication management process (Majumder et al., 2017).

29.3 An ICT-Enabled Medication Management Service Model for Elderly Homes

To achieve a more accurate and efficient workflow, the Hong Kong Pharmaceutical Care Foundation (HKPCF) has developed the Integrated Old Age Home Medication Management Programme with a number of interconnected components, including the SafeMed Medication Management System (SMMS), the Automated Tablet

Dispensing and Packaging System (ATDPS), eMARs, and the Visiting Pharmacist Service (VPS). This dynamic integration of ICT-enabled services provides a more coherent insight into the entire medication management workflow.

29.3.1 Key Features of the Model

Developed by the HKPCF, the SMMS is an IT system designated for RCHEs in Hong Kong to create systematic medical and medication profiles of older adult residents. Residents' personal particulars, medical conditions, current medications, follow-up consultations, and their history of hospital admissions can be maintained and accessed by RCHE nursing staff via the SMMS.

With the SMMS's user-friendly interface for data entry, RCHEs can easily create medication lists for each resident. For example, a comprehensive drug database is embedded in the SMMS which is regularly reviewed and updated by HKPCF pharmacists. The uniqueness of this drug database compared with other existing systems is that it provides a full list of the medications available through the HA, which is the main supplier of medications to older adult residents in Hong Kong. Details of medications, including drug code, generic and trade names, dosage forms, strength, therapeutic class, common dosage regimens, precautions, manufacturer, Hong Kong registration number, and legal classification are included in the database. In addition, photographs of each medication are available for RCHE staff to clearly identify the medications based on their colour, shape, and markings.

Another feature of this model relates to the dispensing and packaging of medications. Tablets and capsules, which are the major dosage forms, are collected by the HKPCF from RCHEs. A centralised dispensing hub was established to provide an automated packaging service for RCHEs. The Automated Tablet Dispensing and Packaging System (ATDPS) in the dispensing hub is a dedicated machine to package medications into drug pouches. Due to limitations in terms of scale, financial resources and physical space, putting an automated packaging machine in each RCHE in Hong Kong is not feasible. To promote economies of scale, a centralised model of packaging was set up and piloted. Replacing the process of manually preparing medications, an off-site automated packaging service improves the efficiency of preparing medications for multiple RCHEs and reduces the workload of RCHE nursing staff. In this centralised model, unused tablets or capsules originally dispensed to a resident can be packaged and supplied to another resident who needs the identical medications, hence potentially reducing medication wastage.

Being closely connected with the IT system, the ATDPS receives the medications and the corresponding dosage instruction information stored in the SMMS for packaging. Multi-dose packaging is adopted so that a resident's medications for a particular administration time are packaged in the same drug pouch. The ATDPS consists of 112 drug canisters, each tailor-made to hold one brand of tablets or capsules. Half-cutters are available in some of the canisters to automatically cut tablets in half if needed. While the 112 canisters cover the most commonly prescribed medications for older adult residents, some less common drugs can also be dispensed, via a detachable tablet adapter (DTA) to be included in the pouch packaging process. Drug pouches generated from an ATDPS are rolled with an automatic winder to allow for easy handling.

Intelligence-assisted checking is performed with the use of a drug verification machine which generates a judgement result list. By getting rid of attention fatigue during manual checking, any incorrect packaging of medications can be easily spotted by the machine. Snapshots of drug pouches are displayed on a screen for re-verification by a pharmacist to further ensure medication safety. The time of manually inspecting medications is also minimised, improving the efficiency of drug verification.

After the packaged medications are delivered to RCHEs by the HKPCF, RCHE nursing staff check and administer the medications based on the eMARs using a convenient tablet computer. The eMARs comply with the Guidelines on Drug Management in Residential Care Homes issued by the Social Welfare Department as well as ensuring the 'five rights' in medication administration: the right patient, the right drug, the right dosage, the right route, and the right time. The real-time updates available via eMARs have replaced the need to manually modify records on printed paper forms. By showing only the medications to be administered at a particular time, the chance of a 'wrong-time' administration is reduced. The time wasted on printing paper forms can also be eliminated, allowing more time to be spent on more useful nursing care tasks.

Along with the implementation of the revamped ICT-based medication management process, the HKPCF also offers the Visiting Pharmacist Service (VPS) for RCHEs. The VPS fills in for the lack of trained personnel in RCHEs when it comes to medication management. Visiting pharmacists are responsible for providing both clinical and practical interventions in order to streamline the medication management system. During each visit, a visiting pharmacist reviews residents' medication profiles to check for any drug-related problems. Medication reconciliation is performed using the SMMS. The visiting pharmacist provides suggestions on the handling and storage of medications and improving the local workflow of medication management in RCHEs. Any enquiries on drug information, disease state management, or the use of the SMMS and eMARs in RCHEs are also addressed by the visiting pharmacist (Figs. 29.1 and 29.2).

In a prospective, pre-post interventional study, after implementing the Integrated Old Age Home Medication Management Programme with the use of IT, AT, and IoT for RCHEs (more details to be discussed in Sect. 29.3), we found that both time efficiency and medication safety were improved. The number of doses prepared and checked in 10-min blocks significantly increased (pre: 41.3, SD 31.8; post: 70.6, SD 22.8; $P < 0.001$), while the number of medication errors were significantly reduced (pre: 10/9504 doses, 0.1%; post: 0/5731 doses; $p = 0.02$) (So et al., 2021).

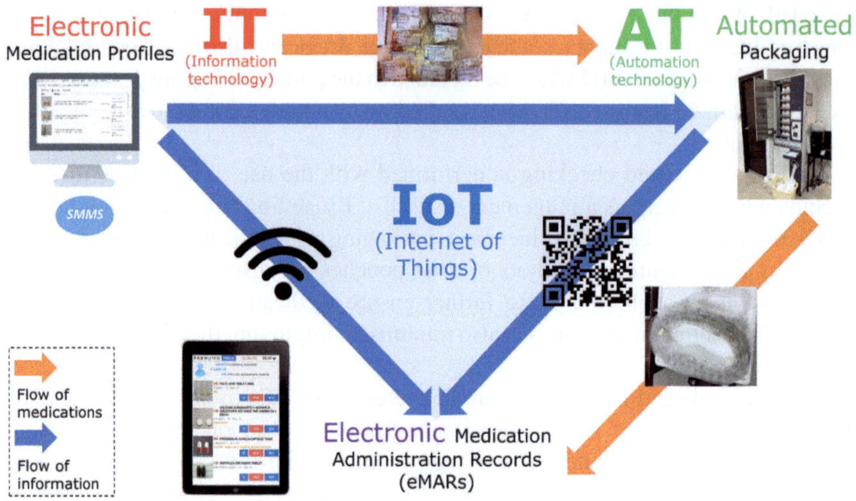

Fig. 29.1 The flow of medications and information with the use of technology (*Source* Adapted from Figure S1 of So et al. [2021]; SMMS: SafeMed Medication Management System)

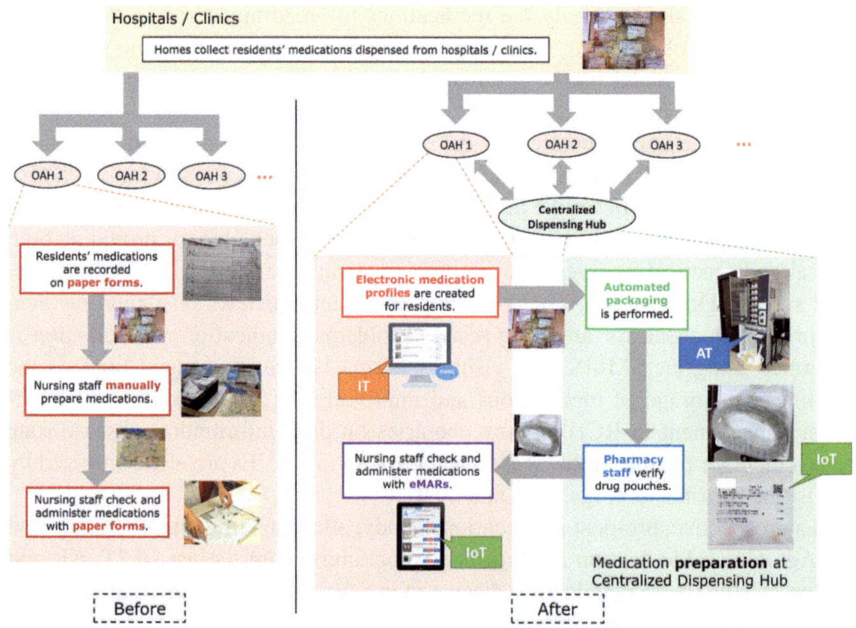

Fig. 29.2 The medication management process before and after implementation of the Integrated Old Age Home Medication Management Programme (*Source* Modified from Fig. 2 of So et al. [2021]; AT: automation technology; eMARs: electronic medication administration records; IoT: Internet of Things; IT: information technology; RCHE: Residential Care Home for the Elderly)

29.3.2 Suggestions for Future Development of ICT-Enabled Medication Management Services for Elderly Homes

The Integrated Old Age Home Medication Management Programme needs to face and tackle various challenges. We would like to share our learnings to facilitate the future implementation of the service model in elderly homes.

First, the service radically changes the usual workflow of nursing staff, and so the attitude and learning capacity of staff in elderly homes could be a major roadblock. As the staff involved are generally older, they may need more time to familiarise themselves with the technologies involved. Sufficient training, full on-site support, adequate run-in times, as well as strong leadership from within the elderly homes are crucial elements to assist staff cope with the changes needed to facilitate the implementation of new service model.

Second, the service model also needs to deal with the prevailing legal and regulatory constraints, which have not been updated despite technological advancements. When the ATDPS was first introduced to an elderly home in Hong Kong, the use of such systems was not specifically supported by the 2008 Guidelines and Code of Practices issued by the Social Welfare Department (SWD) regulating elderly homes. At that time, the HKPCF had to seek assistance from legislators to amend the existing regulations and a new set of Guidelines on Drug Management in Residential Care Homes 2018 was finally released with provisions for the use of ATDPS (Social Welfare Department, 2018).

Finally, financial sustainability is also a major challenge. The cost of the centralised packaging service alone amounts to HK$300 (US$38.5) per resident per month, and it is only made possible through charitable funding. However, the participating beneficiary homes have such tight budget constraints that none are willing to pay for the service out-of-pocket. To solve this problem in the future, we need to identify strategies to fund and optimise the programme by reducing duplication and making better use of the savings incurred from the decreased workload and medication wastage. One example is that medications could be provided by the HA in bulk directly to the dispensing hub instead of being dispensed individually to each patient at each medical follow-up. This eliminates the redundant dispensing of medications in both HA pharmacies and the centralised hub while fully unlocking the potential savings of unused medications.

Case Study II: Building a Safe Medication Management Service for the Older Adults in the Community in Hong Kong

II.1 The Significance in Developing a Safe Medication Management Service for Community-dwelling Older Adults

Outside of RCHEs, the majority of community-dwelling older adults have medication non-compliance problems (Society for Community Organization, 2020), with

68.7% reporting that they did not take their medications at the correct time. Furthermore, 28% also reported self-adjusting dosages or stopping taking their medications completely. Improper storage of medication is also very common among this age demographic, with some older adults storing multiple medications in the same container, and only a small percentage of those surveyed reported discarding expired (34.7%) and obsolete (12%) medications (Communications & Public Relations Office, 2007). Therefore, it is important to assist the older adults who have chronic diseases with their medication management as poor adherence can lead to poor clinical outcomes and increased healthcare costs (Leung et al., 2015).

II.2 Introducing the Use of Information and Communication Technologies (ICT) in Medication Management Services for Community-Dwelling Older Adults

For community patients, it is often a challenge to reconcile multiple medications from multiple prescribing sources, including various specialties in different hospitals and clinics across the public and private sectors. It is therefore important to have an IT platform to allow the recording and sharing of medication information across institutions. In Hong Kong, an electronic platform, namely the eHRSS (electronic Health Record Sharing System), has been developed by the government to create free and lifelong electronic health records for all members of the public (eHealth HK, 2021). In addition, a smart in-home medication dispenser or a medication reminder app can report drug administration patterns of community-dwelling older adults back to a server, which allows caretakers or healthcare professionals to review medication compliance.

29.4 An ICT-Enabled Medication Management Service Model for Community-Dwelling Older Adults

29.4.1 Key Features of the Model

In view of the difficulties in medication management faced by the community-dwelling older adults, the HKPCF started the Community Outreach Programme on Medication Management (COPMM) project. This project aimed to relieve the burden of medication management for the older adults living in the community by providing medication review and reconciliation by pharmacists, an individualised medication packaging service, and assistive reminder technology aids. The details of the operation model are outlined below.

The beneficiary may be referred from various Community Day Care Centres (CDCCs) and non-governmental organisations (NGOs) or directly recruited by the HKPCF. Services from pharmacists are provided either at designated neighbourhood community centres, which the older adults regularly visit and where pharmacists can be stationed to meet them, or at individual patients' homes in selected cases. In view of the COVID-19 pandemic, some sessions have been converted to teleconsultations using communication technologies.

The first step involves pharmacists helping patients to register with the eHRSS (if necessary) and to check the overall medication status of the older adults. This is to make sure the medications that the subject presented are complete and necessary and that the correct administration methods (for example, dosages and frequencies) are in place. During the first session, the pharmacist will interview the patient to fill in the Elderly Participant Assessment Form (EPAF) to assess the patient's medication knowledge, compliance, and handling. The pharmacist will then identify and resolve any problems such as medications with unidentified sources and purposes, as well as medications that are expired or improperly stored. If needed, the pharmacist will fill in an intervention advisory form for appropriate follow-up action to be taken by a doctor or another appropriate caretaker. The pharmacist will determine the exact service that the older adults need and make follow-up plans accordingly. If possible, the EPAF will be filled in again during the second session to assess any change in the patient's self-management of their medications.

A correct medication list is then created for each older adult using the SMMS. The pharmacist will print out a complete list of medications with the names of the medications, drug photos, and the administration instruction for the participant's records. The electronic record in the SMMS allows for the patient's medication regimen to be easily referenced during the next follow-up, and it also facilitates the provision of further services such as medication packaging. The pharmacist will evaluate if the patient has the ability to take care of their own medications and pack their own pillboxes. For those who are not capable of doing this, they are provided with a packaging service using either blister pillboxes or the Semi-Automatic Tablet Dispensing and Packaging System (S-ATDPS). If the patient opts for the S-ATDPS, the machine is connected to the SMMS which generates packaging orders from patients' profiles to enable multi-dose packaging. The S-ATDPS operates similarly to the ATDPS mentioned earlier, except there is no canister and that the medications need to be put manually on the detachable tablet adapter (DTA) tray located at the top of the machine, which allows for a wide variety of medications used by community patients to be packaged. Each pouch is packed with medications for the same administration time slot to enable accurate and convenient administration by the patient.

The patient may opt to use a smart dispenser with the packaged pouches. The dispenser will play music and flashlights at the pre-set time of administration to remind the patient to take the medications. The patient needs to press a button to stop the music and lights and have the relevant pouch dispensed, which will be recorded and available for viewing by the pharmacist on the system's back end. The patient may also opt for a reminder app (for example, MedRemind developed by the HKPCF) which displays a notification on a person's smartphone at the time of administration. The patient acknowledges that they have taken the medication through the notification, which is then recorded on the server to allow pharmacists to review medication compliance and follow up with the patient when necessary (Fig. 29.3).

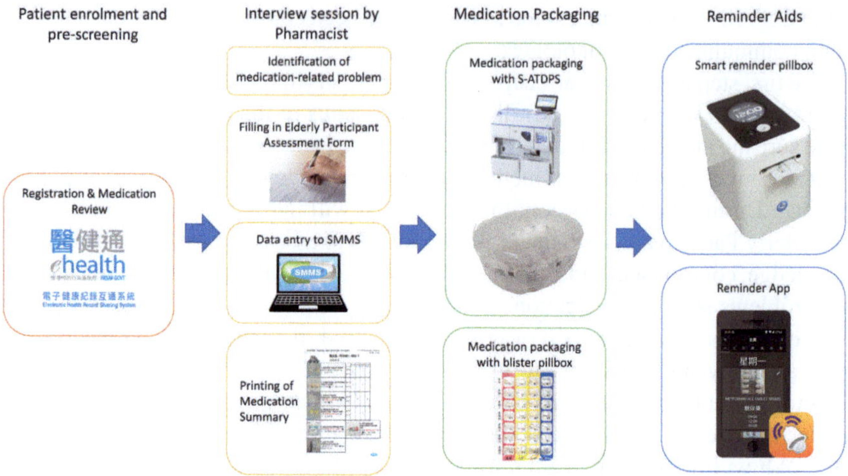

Fig. 29.3 The components and flow of the Community Outreach Programme on Medication Management project (SMMS: SafeMed Medication Management System; S-ATDPS: Semi-Automatic Tablet Dispensing and Packaging System)

A Community Outreach Programme on Medication Management (COPMM) pilot project was conducted in March 2020 with 22 participants. During this pilot phase, the medication self-management ability score of the participants significantly improved by an average of 3.27 points between the two sessions (Wilcoxon signed-rank test (modified by Pratt [1959]): $p < 0.0001$). More participants will need to be observed as the study continues to better determine the effects of a pharmacist's intervention on the participants' medication management (Table 29.1).

Boxplot of the Medication Self-Management Ability Score between two interview sessions from the Community Outreach Programme on Medication Management project pilot study is shown in Fig. 29.4. A higher score is indicative of better ability. This figure shows that the patients have demonstrated significantly better ability in managing their medications after one session of interviews with the pharmacist.

Table 29.1 Descriptive statistics from the Community Outreach Programme on Medication Management project pilot study

No. of participants	22
Gender	Male: 6 (27.3%) Female: 16 (72.7%)
Age (mean)	68.7 (SD: 15.4)
Medication Self-Management Ability Score (1st visit) (mean)	10.6 (SD: 4.0)
Medication Self-Management Ability Score (2nd visit) (mean)	13.9 (SD: 2.8)
Improvement in Medication Self-Management Ability Score (mean)	3.27 (SD: 2.29)

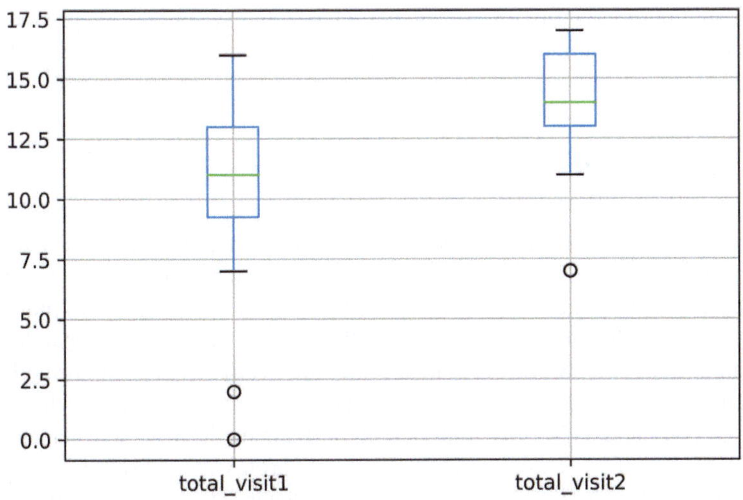

Fig. 29.4 Boxplot of the Medication Self-Management Ability Score between two interview sessions

29.4.2 Suggestions for Future Development of ICT-Enabled Medication Management Services for Community-Dwelling Older Adults

We have faced some challenges during the implementation of this model. First, the service model relies on the use of different platforms and technologies which the service targets may not be the most familiar with. For example, many older adult patients reported difficulty in registering for the eHRSS and providing consent to pharmacists. In this case, the pharmacist had to fall back on the limited information provided by patients and they could not access the complete medication profile of the person in question. The COVID-19 pandemic had made teleconsultation necessary in some cases, but some older adult patients had difficulty in operating the online conferencing software. We suggest that the government should take a proactive role in facilitating the use of technology, such as making the registration process for the eHRSS more user-friendly or sponsoring NGOs to provide technical support to the older adults during the registration process.

Second, the interaction between the model's various components is also a major obstacle. The information from eHRSS was not downloadable, requiring manual data entry from the pharmacist during each visit to build up the medication list. A lot of time had been spent developing and enhancing the reception portal of the S-ATDPS and the relevant testing of communication between S-ATDPS and SMMS. The smart dispenser and reminder app have not been integrated either. We propose the increased adoption of common interoperability standards used worldwide, such as the Fast

Healthcare Interoperability Resources (FHIR), which may ease the integration of the model's different components (Fast Healthcare Interoperability Resources, 2019).

29.5 Conclusion

We have briefly described the processes of adopting technology to address medication safety issues in RCHEs and among community-dwelling older adults. An innovative medication management programme comprising of IT, AT, and IoT components improved the medication safety and time efficiency of medication preparation and medication safety for RCHEs. A unique community outreach programme with pharmacist interviews, IT platforms, packaging services, and reminder aids enhanced the ability of community-dwelling older adults in their medication self-management. Harnessing the expertise of pharmacists and other professional disciplines and more collaborative effort are essential. The adoption of technology to build a safe and efficient medication management service for the older adults would be in keeping with the vision embodied by 'the Smart City Blueprint for Hong Kong' (Innovation & Technology Bureau, 2020), which was introduced by the Government of the Hong Kong SAR to facilitate the use of innovation and technology to improve people's quality of life. The sustainability and expansion of this service to more RCHEs and other targeted populations should remain an important agenda item for future health service planning.

References

Alenius, M., & Graf, P. (2016). Use of electronic medication administration records to reduce perceived stress and risk of medication errors in nursing homes. *CIN: Computers, Informatics, Nursing, 34*(7), 297–302. https://doi.org/10.1097/CIN.0000000000000245

Beobide-Tellería, I., Ferro-Uriguen, Á., Miró-Isasi, B., Martínez-Arrechea, S., & Genua-Goena, M. I. (2018). The impact of automation on the safety of drug dispensing in nursing homes. *Farmacia Hospitalaria, 42*(4), 141–146. https://doi.org/10.7399/fh.10949

Chaudhry, B., Wang, J., Wu, S., Maglione, M., Mojica, W., Roth, E., Morton, S., & Shekelle, P. G. (2006). Systematic review: Impact of health information technology on quality, efficiency, and costs of medical care. *Annals of Internal Medicine, 144*(10), 742–752. https://doi.org/10.7326/0003-4819-144-10-200605160-00125

Ching, C., Lai, C., Poon, W., Lui, M., Lam, Y., Shek, C., Mak, T., & Chan, A. (2006). Drug-induced hypoglycaemia—New insight into an old problem. *Hong Kong Medical Journal, 12*(5), 334–338.

Census and Statistics Department. (2009). *Thematic household survey report no.40—Socio-demographic profile, health status and self-care capability of older persons.* https://www.statistics.gov.hk/pub/B11302402009XXXXB0100.pdf

Census and Statistics Department. (2018). *Thematic report: Older persons.* https://www.statistics.gov.hk/pub/B11201052016XXXXB0100.pdf

Communications and Public Relations Office. (2007). *CUHK discovers poor drug compliance among the Elderly* [Press release]. https://www.cpr.cuhk.edu.hk/en/press/cuhk-discovers-poor-drug-compliance-among-the-elderly/

eHealth HK. (2021). *What's eHealth.* https://www.ehealth.gov.hk/en/whats-ehealth/index.html
Fast Healthcare Interoperability Resources. (2019). *FHIR specification v4.0.1: 2.13 FHIR overview.* https://www.hl7.org/fhir/overview.html
Innovation and Technology Bureau. (2020). *HKSmart city blueprint.* https://www.smartcity.gov.hk/
Labour and Welfare Bureau. (2017). *Replies to LegCo questions—LCQ7: Manpower shortage in elderly service sector.* https://www.info.gov.hk/gia/general/201711/29/P2017112900367.htm
Legislative Council. (2013). *Submission on Manpower situation of residential care homes for the elderly from The Elderly Services Association of Hong Kong.* https://www.legco.gov.hk/yr12-13/chinese/panels/ws/papers/mpws0219cb2-663-1-c.pdf
Leung, D. Y., Bai, X., Leung, A. Y., Liu, B. C., & Chi, I. (2015). Prevalence of medication adherence and its associated factors among community-dwelling Chinese older adults in Hong Kong. *Geriatrics & Gerontology International, 15*(6), 789–796. https://doi.org/10.1111/ggi.12342
Leung, E. (2012). *The project on accreditation system for residential care services for the elders in Hong Kong-Five-year review report (2005–2010).* The Hong Kong Association of Gerontology.
Majumder, S., Aghayi, E., Noferesti, M., Memarzadeh-Tehran, H., Mondal, T., Pang, Z., & Deen, M. J. (2017). Smart homes for elderly healthcare—Recent advances and research challenges. *Sensors, 17*(11), 2496. https://doi.org/10.3390/s17112496
Mingpao. (2020). *Elderly house prescribed wrong medications, elder woman fell in coma for two months, medication for diabetes mellitus was not prescribed, Social Welfare Department issued a warning letter* (Chinese only). https://news.mingpao.com/pns/%E8%A6%81%E8%81%9E/article/20200920/s00001/1600538534594/%E5%AE%89%E8%80%81%E9%99%A2%E6%B4%BE%E9%8C%AF%E8%97%A5-%E8%80%81%E5%A9%A6%E6%98%8F%E8%BF%B7%E5%85%A9%E6%9C%88-%E9%80%81%E9%99%A2%E9%A9%97%E5%87%BA%E6%9C%AA%E7%B6%93%E8%99%95%E6%96%B9%E7%B3%96%E5%B0%BF%E8%97%A5-%E7%A4%BE%E7%BD%B2%E7%99%BC%E8%AD%A6%E5%91%8A%E4%BF%A1
Pratt, J. W. (1959). Remarks on zeros and ties in the Wilcoxon signed rank procedures. *Journal of the American Statistical Association, 54*(287), 655–667.
So, K. H., Ting, C. W., Lee, C. P., Lam, T. T. N., Chiang, S. C., & Cheung, Y. T. (2021). Medication management service for old age homes in Hong Kong using information technology, automation technology, and the internet of things: Pre-post interventional Study. *JMIR Medical Informatics, 9*(2), e24280. https://doi.org/10.2196/24280
Social Welfare Department. (2018). *Guidelines on drug management in residential care homes 2018* (Chinese only). https://www.swd.gov.hk/en/index/site_pubsvc/page_lr/sub_rche/id_introd/
Social Welfare Department. (2020). *Code of practice for residential care homes* (Elderly Persons). https://www.swd.gov.hk/storage/asset/section/2923/en/CoP_RCHE_Eng_20200101.pdf
Social Welfare Department. (2021). *Health workers centralised training courses—Course content and related requirements* (Chinese only). https://www.swd.gov.hk/storage/asset/section/4272/en/Guideline_HWTC_Annex_1_Combined.pdf
Society for Community Organization. (2020). *Press release—Press conference on the investigation of drug needs of grass-root elderly* (Chinese only) [Press release]. https://soco.org.hk/en/pr20200929/
Vest, J. R., Jung, H.-Y., Wiley, K., Jr., Kooreman, H., Pettit, L., & Unruh, M. A. (2019). Adoption of health information technology among US nursing facilities. *Journal of the American Medical Directors Association, 20*(8), 995–1000. e1004. https://doi.org/10.1016/j.jamda.2018.11.002
Wilson, N. M., March, L. M., Sambrook, P. N., & Hilmer, S. N. (2010). Medication safety in residential aged-care facilities: A perspective. *Therapeutic Advances in Drug Safety, 1*(1), 11–20. https://doi.org/10.1177/2042098610381418
Wong, A. Y., Chan, P. W., Chan, E. W., Cheng, M., & Wong, I. C. (2013a). Drug wastage among the elderly living in old-aged homes in Hong Kong. *Hong Kong Pharmaceutical Journal, 20*(1), 16–19.
Wong, A. Y., Chan, P. W., Chan, E. W., Cheng, M., & Wong, I. C. (2013b). The pharmaceutical services to the elderly in the old aged homes in Hong Kong: A scoping exercise. *Hong Kong Pharmaceutical Journal, 20*(1), 11–15.

Chapter 30
The Role of Clinical Pharmacists in the Multidisciplinary Care of Geriatric Patients: Now and the Future

Wilson W. S. Chu and Gary Chung Hong Chong

Abstract There has been an unprecedented growth in population ageing across the world in recent years. In 2017, the Census and Statistics Department of Hong Kong predicted that the number of older adults aged 65 and over will increase from 18% of the whole population in 2020 to 32% in 2050. Medication management in older patients will, therefore, become even more challenging in the years ahead. Nowadays, pharmacists are being integrated into multidisciplinary teams to provide extensive clinical services, including evidence-based medication optimisation, drug therapy-related problem identification, as well as medication adherence and monitoring, in order to provide more holistic and humanistic care to older adults. This chapter first describes the role of a geriatric clinical pharmacist in a multidisciplinary team. Then, the relevance of pharmacists' role in the practice of polypharmacy including de-prescribing is illustrated. Furthermore, the utilisation of innovative technology, or "telepharmacy", to communicate and provide counselling is demonstrated. The appliance of newer technology such as Facial Recognition Technology (FRT) and Artificial Intelligence (AI) to verify medication adherence is introduced, as well as the use of Transdermal Optical Imaging (TOI) to measure vital signs such as blood pressure after taking the medications. Lastly, the use of technology to help in fall detection and prevention, and the adoption of eye movement patterns in face recognition to assess cognitive decline in the older adults is revealed. All these new and innovative initiatives further enhance and demonstrate the important role of clinical pharmacists in the multidisciplinary care for older adults in the pursuit of ageing with dignity.

Keywords Clinical pharmacist · Telepharmacy · Polypharmacy · Artificial intelligence · De-prescribing

---

W. W. S. Chu (✉) · G. C. H. Chong
Hospital Pharmacist, Hong Kong, China
e-mail: ww.chu@yahoo.com

V. T. S. Law and B. Y. F. Fong (eds.), *Ageing with Dignity in Hong Kong and Asia*, Quality of Life in Asia 16, https://doi.org/10.1007/978-981-19-3061-4_30

30.1 Introduction

Population ageing has witnessed unprecedented growth across the world, particularly in growing economies such as the United States, Europe, Japan, and China (National Institutes of Health, 2016). According to the World Health Organization (2011, October), from 2010 to 2050, the percentage of the world's population aged 65 and older will approximately double from about 7.5% to 17% (from 524 million to 1.5 billion). Medication management in older patients has therefore become a more pressing concern than ever. According to Marsh and McLennan Companies' Asia Pacific Research Center (2020), the healthcare costs related to caring for the older adults (those aged 65 and older) across the Asia–Pacific region are expected to increase fivefold from US$0.5 trillion per year to US$2.5 trillion per year by 2030.

The number of older adults in Hong Kong aged 65+ is projected to extend from 18% (1.4 million) of the total population in 2020 to 32% (2.6 million) of the population in 2050 (Census & Statistics Department, 2017). Projections for healthcare expenditure on the older adults have been conducted in various national settings just like the United States, Japan, Singapore, and by international organisations such as the Organisation for Economic Co-operation and Development (OECD) employing a range of various methodologies.

In Hong Kong, the Food and Health Bureau (2008) has commissioned the University of Hong Kong to conduct a study to project the general public and personal health expenditures in Hong Kong up to the year 2033 showing that the Hong Kong's healthcare spending is estimated to double from US$22 billion to US$40 billion. According to the Hong Kong Poverty Situation Report 2015, the estimated expenditure related to the older adults will increase from a total of US$7 billion in 2014–2015 to a total of US$18 billion in 2064–2065.

30.2 Multidisciplinary Medication Management for Geriatric Patients in Hong Kong

As specialty-trained practitioners, clinical pharmacists provide comprehensive medication management and direct care to patients (Patient-Centered Primary Care Collaborative, 2012). They work directly with physicians, other health professionals, and patients to make sure that the medications prescribed for patients contribute to the most effective possible health outcomes (American College of Clinical Pharmacy, 2020).

In 2017, the OECD Health Working Papers stated that medication management and reconciliation is one of the clinical-level interventions and value-based approaches that can reduce patient harm (Slawomirskii et al., 2017). The older adults are at the highest risk due to their high number of comorbidities and drugs usage (Vejar et al., 2015). Within the United States, the American Society of Health-System

Pharmacists (2020) issued Medication Safety Guidelines stating that clinical pharmacists play a crucial role and are equipped with the expertise to prevent Drug-Related Problems (DRPs) that would harm patients. In the United Kingdom, the Royal Pharmaceutical Society (2020) suggests that through regular clinical checks of medical cases and therefore the comprehensive evaluation of all relevant information, including patient characteristics, disease states, laboratory results, and medication regimen, clinical pharmacists could identify pharmacotherapeutic problems.

Geriatric clinical pharmacist service in the hospital with in-patient, day-patient, out-patient, and community care services was started in October 2012. The service was regular and delivered in an in-patient ward setting where patients' charts are reviewed with the geriatrician team of pharmacists who are required to have qualifications and competency as the Board Certified Pharmacotherapy Specialist (The Board of Pharmacy Specialties, 2020) or the Board Certified Geriatric Pharmacist (The Board Certified Geriatric Pharmacist, 2020). British National Formulary, Lexi-comp Drug Information Handbook, the electronic clinical resource tool UpToDate, and an in-house checklist for medication order review are used as the standard to substantiate the correct interventions.

A clinical case example is extracted as follows (Table 30.1). During a consultant ward round, a senior geriatrician inquired if there was any alternative to Quinidine

Table 30.1 Pharmaceutical Care Plan Case 1

Clinical Case Report
Date: 09/1/2020 **Inquiry:** • A senior geriatrician inquired if Quinidine Sulphate Extended Release Tablet 300 mg could be switched to other alternative because of the supply shortage, for a patient with Brugada syndrome **Findings:** • Quinidine Sulphate Extended Release tablet 300 mg was no longer available although several attempts on sourcing this item – Currently, there is one patient on this drug named XX who has Brugada syndrome with implantable cardioverter-defibrillator implanted, using the drug for ventricular fibrillation/ventricular tachycardia control. His current dose is Quinidine Sulphate Extended Release 300 mg three times a day **Recommendations:** • An alternative available would be Quinidine Sulphate plain Tablet 200 mg. Therapy with this Quinidine Sulphate preparation could be begun with 200 mg every six hours, then the dose may be cautiously titrated. According to the product insert, the elimination half-life of this preparation is 6 to 8 h in adults. We understand about the issue of compliance, however, as mentioned the source extended release version could not be identified **References:** • Biquin Durules product monograph (Astra Pharma—Canada), Rev 3/97, Rec 3/97. http://www.rxmed.com/b.main/b2.pharmaceutical/b2.1.monographs/CPS-%20Monographs/CPS-%20(General%20Monographs-%20B)/BIQUIN%20DURULES.html accessed on 09 Jan 2013 • Quinidex package insert (AH Robbins—US), Rec 2/97, Rev 10/87
Number of Hours Involved: 2.5 h

Source The authors

Sulphate Extended Release Tablets 300 mg due to a supply shortage for a patient with Brugada syndrome. The finding was that Quinidine Sulphate Extended Release Tablets 300 mg were no longer available although several attempts were made to source this item. The drug was for ventricular fibrillation and pulseless ventricular tachycardia control. The dose of Quinidine Sulphate Extended Release was 300 mg three times a day in this case. Upon investigation, an alternative medication available in Hong Kong was identified: Quinidine Sulphate Tablet 200 mg. According to the product insert, the elimination half-life of this preparation was six to eight hours in adults. Further literature research was done and it was decided that the Quinidine Sulphate Tablet therapy could be begun with 200 mg every six hours. The dose was then cautiously titrated further.

30.2.1 Documentation

The Pharmaceutical Care Network Europe (PCNE) classifications were adapted to document and record the interventions and findings, with a password-protected Microsoft Access database. The PCNE defines a Drug-Related Problem (DRP) as "*an occasion or circumstance involving drug therapy that actually or potentially interferes with desired health outcomes*". This classification is to be used in analysis into the nature, prevalence, incidence of DRPs, and as an indicator in experimental studies of pharmaceutical care outcomes. It is conjointly meant to assist healthcare professionals to document DRP-information within the pharmaceutical care process (Pharmaceutical Care Network Europe, 2020). All data could be accessed and analysed for reporting purposes (Table 30.2).

30.2.2 De-Prescribing

According to the World Health Organization (2019, June), polypharmacy is that the concurrent use of multiple medications and these include over-the-counter, traditional complementary medicines, and prescription used by a patient. Although there is no standard definition, polypharmacy is usually considered as the routine use of five or more medications (American Society of Health-System Pharmacists, 2020). To combat polypharmacy, the supervised withdrawal of any inappropriate medications could reduce a number of the issues related to polypharmacy (Chui et al., 2017). The method is described as "de-prescribing" and can be used to reduce the overall medication burden. The aim is to reduce both the possible side effects suffered by patients and the complexity of the medication regimen (Garfinkel et al., 2015). De-prescribing can help to scale back polypharmacy in the older adults. Hospitalisation presents a chance to re-evaluate the utilisation of medications (Cheong et al., 2018). Medication review by pharmacists may cause a significantly fewer number of fall-risk medications and therefore the number of falls in the older adults (Marvin

Table 30.2 PCNE classifications

	Code	Primary domains
Problems (also potential)	P1 P2 P3	Treatment effectiveness Treatment safety Other
Causes (including possible causes for potential problems)	C1 C2 C3 C4 C5 C6 C7 C8 C9	Drug selection Drug form Dose selection Treatment duration Dispensing Drug use process Patient related Patient transfer related Other
Planned Interventions	I0 I1 I2 I3 I4	No intervention At prescriber level At patient level At drug level Other
Intervention Acceptance	A1 A2 A3	Intervention accepted Intervention not accepted Other
Status of the DRP	O0 O1 O2 O3	Problem status unknown Problem solved Problem partially solved Problem not solved

Source The Pharmaceutical Care Network Europe (PCNE)

et al., 2017). Moreover, all of these goals are related to better drug compliance and improved overall quality of life (Duncan et al., 2017). The Pharmacy Forum Northern Ireland (2016) supports the de-prescribing process and insists that it could prevent unnecessary drug prescriptions and thus reduce the drug expenditure in healthcare systems.

Two sample cases, 2 and 3, of de-prescribing are described below:

Case 2: Patient MS was an 89-year-old female who was chair-bound. Her past medical history, presenting complaints, and medications are listed in Table 30.3.

Her serum creatinine (SrCr) was 189 umol/L, with calculated Creatinine Clearance (CrCl) using Cockcroft-Gault formula for females being around 20 ml/min (Arora, 2021). Patient MS was on Alendronate, which was a bisphosphonate inhibiting bone resorption, to decrease the rate of bone resorption and increase in bone mineral density indirectly. Use was not recommended when CrCl is less than 35 mL/minute (Lexi-comp, 2020a). The patient was chair-bound and after assessing the risks versus the benefits, the pharmacist recommended that the doctor should discontinue prescribing Alendronate and continue the calcium and vitamin D3 (Miller, 2020).

Case 3: Patient SC is a 96-year-old female. Her past medical history, presenting complaints, and medications are listed in Table 30.4.

Table 30.3 Pharmaceutical Care Plan Case 2

	Admission Date: Feb 2020	Day of Hospitalization: 3 days
Patient	Patient Initial: MS Age: 89	Drug Allergy: Diltiazem, Metoprolol Sex: F
Past Medical History	Renal failure, atrial fibrillation, congestive heart failure, hypertension, iron deficiency anemia, gastrointestinal bleeding	
Presenting Complaints	Pneumonia	
Subjective	Oedema, cough	
Objective	Sodium Na 140 mmol/L (136–145) Potassium K 3.5 mmol/L (3.5–5.1) Creatinine Clearance CrCl (Cockcroft-Gault Equation) was CrCl less than 30 ml/min	
Current Medications	Azithromycin 500 mg daily Ceftriaxone 1 g daily Vitamin D3 1000 units daily Salbutamol 2 puffs every four hours as needed Alendronate 70 mg once per week Calcium Carbonate 1 g daily Enalapril 2.5 mg daily Famotidine 20 mg twice daily Ferrous Sulphate 300 mg twice daily Frusemide 40 mg daily Lactulose 10 ml at night as needed Potassium Chloride Slow Release 600 mg daily Senna 7.5 mg at night as needed	
Assessment/Interventions	Drug-related problem(s): Serum Creatinine = 189 umol/L. CrCl = less than 30 ml/min	

Source The authors

Her blood pressure was 118/78 mm Hg and her target is less than 140/90 mm Hg (James et al., 2014, 2017) or less than 130/80 mm Hg (Arnett et al., 2019). She was on multiple anti-hypertensive drugs: Hydralazine 25 mg twice daily and Amlodipine 10 mg daily. Apart from this, both Frusemide and Isosorbide Mononitrate could lower her blood pressure. She was also on Terazosin which was an alpha one blocker indicated for benign prostatic hyperplasia and hypertension as an alternative agent (Lexicomp, 2020b). Since the blood pressure of SC was controlled and Terazosin might cause dizziness and increased fall risks, the pharmacist recommended to de-prescribe Terazosin 1 mg. Her blood pressure remained stable upon discharge.

Table 30.4 Pharmaceutical Care Plan Case 3

	Admission Date: June 2020	Day of Hospitalization: 5 days
Patient	Patient Initial: SC Age: 96	Drug Allergy: Nil Sex: F
Past Medical History	Anaemia, end-stage renal failure, diabetes mellitus, fracture hip, multiple myeloma	
Presenting Complaints	Fatigue and dizziness	
Blood pressure	BP 118/78 mm Hg	
Objective	Sodium Na 138 mmol/L (136–145) Potassium K 3.2 mmol/L (3.5–5.1) Urea 30.4 mmol/L (2.8–8.1) Serum Creatinine 670 umol/L Creatinine Clearance CrCl less than 10 ml/min Albumin 30 g/L (35–52)	
Current Medications	Aluminum Hydroxide, Magnesium Hydroxide, and Simethicone Liquid 10 ml three times daily Amoxicillin and Clavulanate 375 mg twice daily Frusemide 60 mg daily Hydralazine 25 mg twice daily Isosorbide Mononitrate 20 mg twice daily Allopurinol 100 mg daily Amlodipine 10 mg daily Calcium Carbonate 1 g three times daily Glipizide 2.5 mg daily Terazosin 1 mg at bedtime Paracetamol as needed Senna as needed	
Assessment/Interventions	Drug-related problem(s): SC's BP is well controlled. Terazosin is not a good hypertensive agent and may cause dizziness and increase fall risk	

Source The authors

30.3 The Role of Pharmacists in Preventing Falls in the Older Adults

Falls are the most explanation for morbidity and disability within the older adults. More than one-third of people 65 years of age or older have falls per annum, and in half of the cases, the falls are recurrent (Tinetti & Kumar, 2010). Independent risk factors for falls include, previous falls, balance impairment, decreased muscle strength, visual defect, polypharmacy or psychoactive drugs, walking difficulty, depression, dizziness, functional limitations, age older than 80 years, female sex, incontinence, cognitive impairment, arthritis, diabetes, and pain (Tinetti & Kumar, 2010). Research demonstrates that a collaborative multidisciplinary team can provide individualised patient interventions and reduce both the rate and risk of falls (Gillespie et al., 2012).

Medications are a well-known risk factor for falls. However, it is important to think about the rationale for taking a medicine before deciding to prevent or withdraw it for fall prevention purposes, because the condition the drug is used to treat might itself be a risk factor for falls (Al-Aama, 2011). A complete medication review by the pharmacist includes a review of age-related physical changes that predispose older adults to drug-drug interactions, drug-disease interactions, and medication side effects which will increase a patient's chances of falls (Karani et al., 2016).

As a member of the Fall Assessment Service Team (FAST) within the hospital, the main role of the pharmacist is to screen patients using a standardised protocol to work out falls risk, complete a thorough medication review, and recommend vitamin D supplementation, when appropriate. When conducting a thorough review, the pharmacist works with the patients and caregivers to screen for medications which will increase fall risks using the "Hospital Fall Assessment Service Team Fall Risk Increasing Drug (FRID) List", derived from the American Geriatrics Society Beers Criteria (American Geriatrics Society, 2019), STOPP Screening Tool of Older Persons' Prescriptions (O'Mahony et al., 2015) and START Screening Tool to Alert to Right Treatment (O'Mahony et al., 2015) as the main references.

Case 4: Patient SJ was an 86-year-old female who was chair-bound. Her past medical history, presenting complaints, and medications are listed in Table 30.5.

SJ was on multiple medications and one of her drugs, Amitriptyline 25 mg taken at night time, was prescribed without indication. SJ was not in pain and did not have a sleeping disorder. Given that she was chair-bound and that tricyclic antidepressants should be avoided in the older adults, as it may cause sedation, delirium, urinary retention, constipation, orthostatic hypotension, and increases the risk of falls, the pharmacist recommended discontinuing the Amitriptyline. This recommendation was accepted by her geriatrician.

30.4 Telepharmacy Using Zoom

Video conferencing software Zoom for patient counselling began in August 2020. Patient JC is an 84-year-old female who was admitted to the emergency department ward with exertional chest discomfort and ankle swelling. During her hospital stay, the clinical pharmacist provided counselling on medication adjustment, mainly on reducing the dosage of her Amlodipine prescription from 10 mg to 2.5 mg in the morning, newly prescribed Aspirin 80 mg in the morning (with the recommendation that it should be taken with food), Famotidine 20 mg in the morning (with the recommendation given for gastrointestinal protection), and Nitroglycerin sublingual tablet (with thorough education on proper use). It had been decided to continue with her other current medications including Sertraline 25 mg daily and Zopiclone 3.75 mg at bedtime as required. Upon discharge, a telepharmacy appointment was

Table 30.5 Pharmaceutical Care Plan Case 4

	Admission Date: May 2020	Day of Hospitalization: 3 days
Patient	Patient Initial: SJ Age: 86	Drug Allergy: Nil Sex: F
Past Medical History	Anaemia, atrial fibrillation, osteoporosis, stroke, symptomatic sinus bradycardia, diabetes mellitus	
Presenting Complaints	Admitted for lower respiratory tract infection	
Subjective	General discomfort, fever, respiratory symptoms	
Objective	Sodium Na 141 mmol/L (136–145) Potassium K 3.2 mmol/L (3.5–5.1) Urea 3.6 mmol/L (2.8–8.1) Serum Creatinine 53 umol/L	
Current Medications	Amoxicillin and Clavulanate 1 g twice daily Oseltamivir 75 mg twice daily Calcium Carbonate 1.5 g daily Gliclazide 40 mg in the morning Metformin 500 mg twice daily Metoclopramide 10 mg three times daily Lansoprazole 30 mg daily Simvastatin 20 mg at night Vitamin D3 1000unit daily Rivaroxaban 15 mg daily Digoxin 62.5mcg daily Amitriptyline 25 mg at night	
Assessment / Interventions	Drug-related problem(s): Amitriptyline is a tricyclic antidepressants in Beers Criteria. The drug has no indication for SJ and the pharmacist recommended discontinuing the drug	

Source The authors

arranged with JC to possess follow-up discussions regarding her medications, especially regarding reducing her dosage of Amlodipine. Telepharmacy provides pharmacists real-time and direct communications with patients unbound by geographic or time constraints. This humanistic approach enables the pharmacists to contribute efficiently to improving medication use of patients especially the aged population, who are physically unable or should not travel to a pharmacy or meet face to face with a pharmacist. Telepharmacy can provide pharmaceutical education and look after selected older patients. It also reduces travelling time and provides cost-effective engagement with patients. Telepharmacy helps pharmacists to deliver appropriate treatments, at the appropriate time, in the appropriate place, and for the appropriate patient. In addition, pharmacists could save and record counselling videos such as inhaler technique, eye drops application for unlimited review. Telepharmacy, at the same time, safeguards patient privacy as the patient could be at home and maintain the dignity of older people.

30.5 The Future—Using Artificial Intelligence in Older Adults' Care

Artificial Intelligence (AI) was initially conceptualised within the 1950s with the goal of enabling a machine or computer to think and learn like humans. The SKYNET computering system was described as "self-aware" in the movie Terminator 2 in 1991 (Cameron, 1991). Nowadays, AI is employed used by companies like Facebook (facial recognition) and Google (search suggestions).

AI has played a critical role in manufacturing industries for many years, but it has only recently begun to take a leading role in healthcare. According to Rai (2018), AI systems were projected to be a US$6 billion industry by 2021. A recent McKinsey review predicted that healthcare would be one of the top 5 industries to use AI, citing more than 50 user cases and over US$1 billion were already raised in start-up equity (Batra et al., 2018). From patient self-service to chatbots, computer-aided detection systems for diagnosis, and image data analysis to spot candidate molecules in drug discovery, AI is already at work, increasing convenience and efficiency, reducing costs and errors, and usually making it easier for more patients to receive the healthcare they need. Craft (2017) has classified the AI applications into three categories as follows:

1. Patient-oriented AI
2. Clinician/Pharmacist-oriented AI
3. Administrative- and operational-oriented AI

Examples of applications of AI in older adults' care are described in six case studies:

Case Study 1: Patient-Oriented AI—Face-Recognition Technology (FRT)
Older adults are at greater risk of adverse drug reactions due to the metabolic changes and reduced drug clearance related to ageing (Brahma et al., 2013). For instance, older adult patients are at increased risk of haemorrhage with oral anticoagulants.

In 2017, a study proved the effectiveness of AiCure's medication adherence solution, which used a form of facial recognition AI to verify that patient had taken the right medication (Labovitz et al., 2017). Facial Recognition Technology (FRT) is a method used to identify any individual based on their specific facial features like bone structure and skin texture. Its functional algorithm relies on existing databases that compare these features in order to produce a result. Using the front-facing camera of a phone, AiCure (https://aicure.com/) visually confirms when each dose is taken or missed. In the study, the findings were based on a 12-week randomised, controlled trial that measured the tool's effect on adherence rates for Dabigatran, Rivaroxaban, Apixaban, and Warfarin compared with a control group. Patients were randomised to receive daily monitoring by the AI platform (intervention) or to receive no-daily monitoring (control). The AI application visually identified the patient, the medication, and the confirmed ingestion. Adherence was measured by pill counts and plasma sampling in both groups. Plasma drug concentration levels indicated that adherence was 100% (15 of 15) and 50% (6 of 12) in the intervention and control groups, respectively.

Case Study 2: Patient-oriented AI—Smart Mirrors and Transdermal Optical Imaging

Accurate vital signs such as blood pressure measurement in the older adults is a very important and widely applicable subject (Reddy et al., 2014). It is done by combining FRT into a simple mirror with built-in skin analysis and Transdermal Optical Imaging (TOI) to measure blood pressure and stress level. Optical sensors on smartphones can capture red light reflected from patients' haemoglobin under the skin, which allows TOI to visualise and measure blood flow changes. TOI technology uses several state-of-the-art techniques in photoplethysmography with respect to the extraction of a raw signal (e.g., the region of interest tracking, multiple raw signals, three coloured channels) and the estimation of a plethysmographic signal (e.g., bandpass filtering). However, unlike other video-based technology, TOI separates each video image into several layers called "bitplanes" in each of the three coloured channels. Then, employing a machine learning-based algorithm developed to gather blood flow data (Luo et al., 2019), such "mirror" technology could monitor and track patients' blood pressure before and after they take their anti-hypertensive medications, and thus aid medication adherence. It could also go a step further by referring patients to their doctor if there are any abnormal fluctuations in blood pressure, especially for those older adults who live alone. A new "cuffless" approach involves capturing a short video of a patient's face and hands lasting for a few seconds combined with analysis beneath the skin to estimate the heart rate and blood pressure (Kloberdanz, 2018).

Case Study 3: Patient-Oriented AI—Smartwatches Revolutionising the Delivery of Care

With the launch of latest electrodes found within the devices, it is now possible for patients to perform electrocardiography directly from their wrist. The built-in mobile application (app) also can monitor rapid and skipped heartbeats. Patients could receive a notification if an irregular cardiac rhythm such as atrial fibrillation is detected. These applications also allow vital data, that may otherwise be missed, to be provided to the physicians.

Case Study 4: Patient-Oriented AI—digitalAngel, ANGEL4, and Fall Detection in the Older Adults

Devices like digitalAngel (https://www.digitalangel.eu) and ANGEL4 (https://www.sense4care.com/tienda/angel4-fall-detection/) have begun to use machine learning models to make informed decisions around incidents that have occurred within a particular setting. Hospitals and aged care facilities might apply this technology to observe falls and incidents, contributing to workforce optimisation to make sure care is provided where and when it is needed most. Through proactive observance and alert functions that are based on machine decision-making capabilities, residents and patients can be monitored within personalised settings for a range of frequently occurring incidents that may have tangible negative effects on the well-being, recovery, and overall care of older adults. Monitoring functions can include fall alerts, wandering, circadian rhythm deviation, etc. Moreover, predictive analysis AI can even analyse sounds to make decisions around potential incidents occurring within rooms. This technology contributes to elderly care without the necessity need for intrusive devices and wearables (Syno Global, 2018).

Case Study 5: Patient-Oriented AI—Eye Movement Patterns to Assess Cognitive Decline in the Older Adults

In 2008, an investigation looked into the link between eye movement patterns and cognitive performance during natural ageing through modelling and comparing the movement of young (18–24 years) and older (65–81 years) adults using a new approach (Chan et al., 2018). The research noted associations among cognitive status, recognition performance, and eye movement patterns. The more holistic strategy an adult used, the more likely he or she encountered a false alarm situation. This suggested an association between the holistic eye and movement strategy and false alarms in facial recognition.

In another research published in July 2020, Nie et al. (2020) found that patients with mild cognitive impairment had lower novelty preference scores on the visual paired comparison than healthy controls. They concluded that eye movement parameters related to cognitive functions could be helpful in the early identification of dementia and in the development and evaluation of preventive and therapeutic strategies.

These studies have demonstrated that wearable technologies are slowly being repurposed or augmented to improve medical outcomes, which historically could only be done in a hospital. AI is leveraged to gather, analyse, and interpret massive amounts of data which may improve the quality of life of patients everywhere, without geographical limitations and ensuring that older adult patients continue to age healthily and are treated with dignity.

Case Study 6: Pharmacist-Oriented AI—A Pharmacist Chatbot

It is suggested that using online chatbots enables the pharmacies to have a knowledgeable, virtual assistant available round the clock to answer health-related queries, give directions on using specialised healthcare devices and information on advanced drug administration, and send treatment reminders (Forbes, 2020).

A chatbot is a computer programme that permits humans to interact with technology using a variety of input methods such as voice, text, gesture, and touch at all times in the year. If speech is used, the chatbot first turns the voice data input into text using the automated speech recognition technology. Text only chatbots such as text-based messaging services skip this step. AI chatbots are powered by AI code that are more complex than the rule-based chatbots, which tend to be more conversational, data-driven, and predictive. AI chatbots are generally more sophisticated, interactive, and personalised than task-oriented chatbots. Over time and through machine learning with data, they become more contextually aware and leverage linguistic communication, and apply predictive intelligence to personalise the user's experience (Artificial Solutions, 2020).

The latest chatbot technology like Kore.ai is used by pharmacies to answer common medication queries on matters such as composition, drug interactions, recommended dosages, side effects, differences between generics and name-brands. These bots can remind patients once they got to take their medication or perform exercises, as in the case of physical therapy. It can also send patients reminders that their prescription has to be refilled, that they are due for a routine check-up, and for other health-related issues (Kore.ai, Inc, 2020).

30.6 Conclusion

Pharmacists are equipped with professional knowledge to handle drug-related problems which may be explicit risks for older adult patients. The worth of geriatric clinical pharmacists in improving the general quality of prescribing and consequently minimising drug-related problems has been illustrated. As an essential member of the multidisciplinary team, interventions by pharmacists have a positive effect on prescribing in older adults, making certain that they receive effective, safe, and efficient drug therapy. Pharmacist-initiated de-prescribing can facilitate cut back polypharmacy and hospitalisation in the older adults and it presents a chance to re-evaluate the use of "high-risk" medications. Additionally, the pharmacist in the Fall Assessment Service Team (FAST) is one of the strategies to reinforce the safety and quality of pharmaceutical care among older adult patients in the hospital, and in turn improves patients' quality of life. Telepharmacy is also provided to older adult patients, particularly those with travel difficulties. Recorded video could also be used to provide counselling such as inhaler techniques rather than using traditional patient information leaflets. Furthermore, the appliance of newer technology, such as using Facial Recognition Technology (FRT) and Artificial Intelligence (AI) could assist pharmacists to verify medication adherence. Soon, the utilisation of Transdermal Optical Imaging (TOI) could routinely help geriatric patients to measure their blood pressure after taking medications. Most significantly, equipped with good communication skills, pharmacists perceive how patient's feel could help the older adult patients age with dignity.

References

Al-Aama, T. (2011). Falls in the elderly spectrum and prevention. *Canadian Family Physician, 57*(7), 771–776. https://pubmed.ncbi.nlm.nih.gov/21753098/

American College of Clinical Pharmacy. (2020). *About clinical pharmacists.* https://www.accp.com/about/clinicalpharmacists.aspx

American Geriatrics Society. (2019). *American geriatrics society 2019 updated AGS beers criteria®for potentially inappropriate medication use in older adults.* https://agsjournals.onlinelibrary.wiley.com/doi/epdf/10.1111/jgs.15767

American Society of Health-System Pharmacists. (2020). *ASHP guidelines on preventing medication errors in hospitals.* https://www.ashp.org/-/media/assets/policy-guidelines/docs/guidelines/preventing-medication-errors-hospitals.ashx

Arnett, D. K., Blumenthal, R. S., Albert, M. A., Buroker, A. B., Goldberger, Z. D., Hahn, E. J., ... & Ziaeian, B. (2019). 2019 ACC/AHA guideline on the primary prevention of cardiovascular disease: A report of the American College of Cardiology/American Heart Association task force on clinical practice guidelines. *Circulation, 140*(11), e563–e595. https://doi.org/10.1161/CIR.0000000000000677

Arora, P. (2021). *What is the cockcroft-gault formula for estimating creatinine clearance (CrCl) and how is it used in patients with chronic kidney disease (CKD)?* https://www.medscape.com/answers/238798-105315/what-is-the-cockcroft-gault-formula-for-estimating-creatinine-clearance-crcl-and-how-is-it-used-in-patients-with-chronic-kidney-disease-ckd8

Artificial Solutions. (2020). *What is a chatbot?* https://www.artificial-solutions.com/chatbots

Batra, G., Queirolo, A., & Santhanam, N. (2018, January 8). *Artificial intelligence: The time to act is now.* https://www.mckinsey.com/industries/advanced-electronics/our-insights/artificial-intelligence-the-time-to-act-is-now

Brahma, D., Wahlang, J., Marak, M., & Sangma, M. (2013). Adverse drug reactions in the elderly. *Journal of Pharmacology and Pharmacotherapeutics, 4*(2), 91. https://doi.org/10.4103/0976-500x.110872

Cameron, J. (Director) (1991). *Terminator 2: Judgment Day* [Film]. Carolco Pictures.

Census and Statistics Department. (2017). *Hong Kong population projections 2017–2066.* https://www.statistics.gov.hk/pub/B1120015072017XXXXB0100.pdf

Chan, C., Chan, A., Lee, T., & Hsiao, J. (2018). Eye-movement patterns in face recognition are associated with cognitive decline in older adults. *Psychonomic Bulletin & Review, 25*, 2200–2207. https://doi.org/10.3758/s13423-017-1419-

Cheong, S. T., Ng, T. M., & Tan, K. T. (2018). Pharmacist-initiated deprescribing in hospitalised elderly: Prevalence and acceptance by physicians. *European Journal of Hospital Pharmacy, 25*, 35–39. https://doi.org/10.1136/ejhpharm-2017-001251

Chui, K., Chong, G., & Chu, W. (2017, December 5). *Effectiveness of identifying drug-related problems (DRPs) at an outpatient hospital pharmacy in Hong Kong* [Poster presentation]. Midyear Clinical Meeting and Exhibition 2017, Orlando, USA. https://www.eventscribe.com/2017/ASHP-Meeting/ajaxcalls/PosterInfo.asp?efp=WUFORk1KUU8yMDk5&PosterID=117676&rnd=0.2697316

Craft, L. (2017, June 30). *Emerging applications of AI for healthcare providers.* https://www.gartner.com/en/documents/3753763/emerging-applications-of-ai-for-healthcare-providers

Duncan, P., Duerden, M., & Payne, R. (2017). Deprescribing: A primary care perspective. *European Journal of Hospital Pharmacy, 24*(1), 37–42. https://doi.org/10.1136/ejhpharm-2016-000967

Food and Health Bureau. (2008). *Projection of Hong Kong's healthcare expenditure.* https://www.fhb.gov.hk/beStrong/files/consultation/projecthealthexp_eng.pdf

Forbes, E. (2020, May 24). *Artificial intelligence—A potential game-changer for the pharmacy sector!.* http://thetechnews.com/2020/05/24/artificial-intelligence-a-potential-game-changer-for-the-pharmacy-sector/

Garfinkel, D., Ilhan, B., & Bahat, G. (2015). Routine deprescribing of chronic medications to combat polypharmacy. *Therapeutic Advances in Drug Safety, 6*(6), 212–233. https://doi.org/10.1177/2042098615613984

Gillespie, L., Robertson, M., Gillespie, W., Sherrington, C., Gates, S., Clemson, L., & Lamb, S. (2012). Interventions for preventing falls in older people living in the community. *Cochrane Database Systematic Reviews, 12*(9), 1–3. https://doi.org/10.1002/14651858.CD007146.pub3

James, P. A., Oparil, S., Carter, B. L., Cushman, W. C., Dennison-Himmelfarb, C., Handler, J., ... & Ortiz, E. (2014). 2014 evidence-based guideline for the management of high blood pressure in adults: report from the panel members appointed to the Eighth Joint National Committee (JNC 8). *The Journal of the American Medical Association, 311*(5), 507–520. https://doi.org/10.1001/jama.2013.284427

Karani, M., Haddad, Y., & Lee, R. (2016). The role of pharmacists in preventing falls among America's older adults. *Frontiers in Public Health, 4*(250), 1–4. https://doi.org/10.3389/fpubh.2016.00250

Kloberdanz, K. (2018). *Selfies against hypertension? This smartphone app could measure blood pressure just by scanning your face and hand.* https://www.ge.com/news/reports/ai-hypertension-smartphone-app-measure-blood-pressure-just-scanning-skin

Kore.ai, Inc. (2020). *Personalized care: Virtual assistants trigger innovation in healthcare.* https://kore.ai/solutions/industries/healthcare/

Labovitz, D., Shafner, L., Gil, M., Virmani, D., & Hanina, A. (2017). Using artificial intelligence to reduce the risk of nonadherence in patients on anticoagulation therapy. *Stroke, 48*(5), 1416–1419. https://doi.org/10.1161/STROKEAHA.116.016281

Lexicomp. (2020a). *Alendronate: Drug information.* https://www.uptodate.com/contents/alendronate-drug-information?search=bisphosphonates&selectedTitle=1~133&usage_type=panel&display_rank=1&kp_tab=drug_general&source=panel_search_result

Lexicomp. (2020b). *Terazosin: Drug information.* https://www.uptodate.com/contents/terazosin-drug-information?search=terazosin&source=panel_search_result&selectedTitle=1~27&usage_type=panel&kp_tab=drug_general&display_rank=1

Luo, H., Yang, D., Barszczyk, A., Vempala, N., Wei, J., Wu, S., Zheng, P., Fu, G., Lee, K., & Feng, Z. (2019). Smartphone-based blood pressure measurement using transdermal optical imaging technology. *Circulation: Cardiovascular Imaging, 12*(8), e008857. https://doi.org/10.1161/CIRCIMAGING.119.008857

Marsh and McLennan Companies' Asia Pacific Research Center. (2020). *Advancing into the golden years: Cost of healthcare for Asia Pacific's elderly.* Marsh and McLennan Companies. https://www.mmc.com/content/dam/mmc-web/Files/APRC/APRC%20Ageing%20report%20EXEC%20SUMM.pdf

Marvin, V., Ward, E., Poots, A., Heard, K., Rajagopalan, A., & Jubraj, B. (2017). Deprescribing medicines in the acute setting to reduce the risk of falls. *European Journal of Hospital Pharmacy, 224*(1), 10–15. https://doi.org/10.1136/ejhpharm-2016-001003

Miller, P. (2020). *Osteoporosis in patients with chronic kidney disease: Management.* https://www.uptodate.com/contents/osteoporosis-in-patients-with-chronic-kidney-disease-management

National Institutes of Health. (2016). *World's older population grows dramatically—NIH-funded Census Bureau report.* https://www.nih.gov/news-events/news-releases/worlds-older-population-grows-dramatically

Nie, J., Qiu, Q., Phillips, M., Sun, L., Yan, F., Lin, X., … Li, X. (2020). Early diagnosis of mild cognitive impairment based on eye movement parameters in an aging Chinese population. *Frontiers in Aging Neuroscience, 12*, 221. https://doi.org/10.3389/fnagi.2020.00221

O'Mahony, D., O'Sullivan, D., Byrne, S., O'Connor, M., Ryan, C., & Gallagher, P. (2015). STOPP/START criteria for potentially inappropriate prescribing in older people: Version 2. *Age and Ageing, 44*(2), 213–218. https://doi.org/10.1093/ageing/afu145

Patient-Centered Primary Care Collaborative. (2012). *The patient-centered medical home: Integrating comprehensive medication management to optimize patient outcomes resource guide.* http://www.pcpcc.org/sites/default/files/media/medmanagement.pdf

Pharmaceutical Care Network Europe. (2020). *New version (9) PCNE DRP-Classification.* https://www.pcne.org/news/87/new-version-9-pcne-drp-classification

Rai, S. (2018). *Cognitive computing and artificial intelligence systems market in healthcare.* BCC Publishing. https://www.bccresearch.com/market-research/healthcare/cognitive-computing-artificial-intelligence-systems-market-healthcare.html

Reddy, A., Jogendra, M., & Rosendorff, C. (2014). Blood pressure measurement in the geriatric population. *Blood Pressure Monitoring, 19*(2), 59–63. https://doi.org/10.1097/MBP.0000000000000021

Slawomirskii, L., Auraaeni, A., & Klazingai, N. (2017). *The economics of patient safety* (OECD Health Working Papers, No. 96). OECD Publishing. https://www.oecd-ilibrary.org/social-issues-migration-health/the-economics-of-patient-safety_5a9858cd-en

Syno Global. (2018). *Artificial intelligence for fall detection and proactive care.* https://syno.global/artificial-intelligence-for-fall-detection-and-proactive-care/

The Board Certified Geriatric Pharmacist. (2020). *Geriatric pharmacy.* https://www.bpsweb.org/bps-specialties/geriatric-pharmacy/#1517761118361-6c02bae3-f5a01517848269340

The Board of Pharmacy Specialties. (2020). *Pharmacotherapy.* https://www.bpsweb.org/bps-specialties/pharmacotherapy/#1517746856979-c1fe2e04-8ffb15177800157771517854077689151785833382515178634536801517864316733

The Pharmacy Forum Northern Ireland. (2016). *Clinical check guidance.* Pharmaceutical Society of Northern Ireland. https://www.pfni.org.uk/wp-content/uploads/2017/05/Pharmacy-Forum-Clincial-Guidance.pdf

The Royal Pharmaceutical Society. (2020). *Clinical checks—Quick reference guide.* https://www.rpharms.com/resources/quick-reference-guides/clinical-checks

Tinetti, M., & Kumar, C. (2010). The patient who falls "it's always a trade-off." *The Journal of the American Medical Association, 303*(3), 258–266. https://doi.org/10.1001/jama.2009.2024

Vejar, M., Makic, M., & Kotthoff-Burrell, E. (2015). Medication management for elderly patients in an academic primary care setting: A quality improvement project. *Journal of the American Association of Nurse Practitioners, 27*(2), 72–78. https://doi.org/10.1002/2327-6924.12121

World Health Organization. (2011, October). *Global health and aging.* National Institutes of Health Publication. https://www.who.int/ageing/publications/global_health.pdf

World Health Organization. (2019, June). *Medication safety in polypharmacy.* The WHO Document Production Services. https://apps.who.int/iris/bitstream/handle/10665/325454/WHO-UHC-SDS-2019.11-eng.pdf?ua=1

Index

V. T. S. Law and B. Y. F. Fong (eds.), *Ageing with Dignity in Hong Kong and Asia*, Quality of Life in Asia 16, https://doi.org/10.1007/978-981-19-3061-4

MIX
Papier aus verantwortungsvollen Quellen
Paper from responsible sources
FSC® C105338

If you have any concerns about our products,
you can contact us on
ProductSafety@springernature.com

In case Publisher is established outside the EU,
the EU authorized representative is:
Springer Nature Customer Service Center GmbH
Europaplatz 3, 69115 Heidelberg, Germany

Printed by Libri Plureos GmbH
in Hamburg, Germany